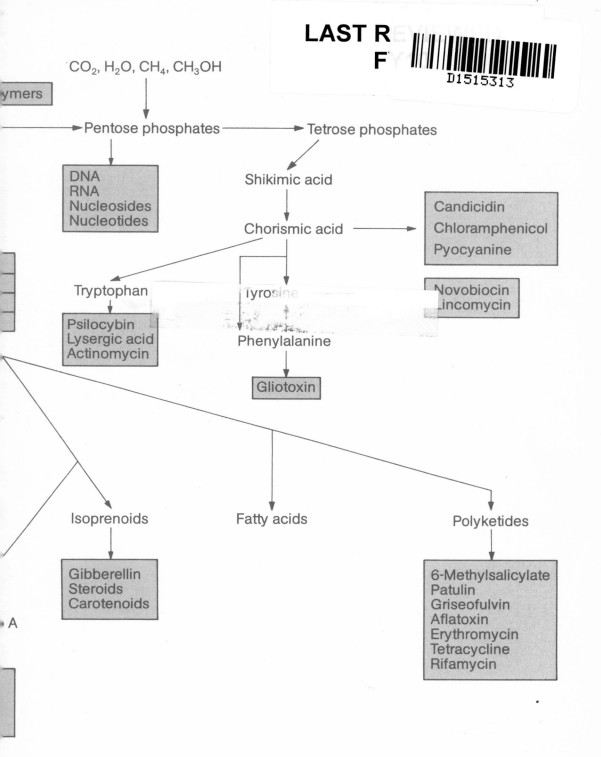

CO_2, H_2O, CH_4, CH_3OH

ymers

Pentose phosphates → Tetrose phosphates

DNA
RNA
Nucleosides
Nucleotides

Shikimic acid

Chorismic acid → Candicidin
Chloramphenicol
Pyocyanine

Novobiocin
Lincomycin

Tryptophan   Tyrosine

Psilocybin
Lysergic acid
Actinomycin

Phenylalanine

Gliotoxin

Isoprenoids   Fatty acids   Polyketides

Gibberellin
Steroids
Carotenoids

6-Methylsalicylate
Patulin
Griseofulvin
Aflatoxin
Erythromycin
Tetracycline
Rifamycin

A

Fundamentals of Biotechnology

Edited by
Präve/Faust/Sittig/Sukatsch

S

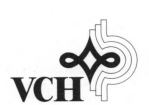

© VCH Verlagsgesellschaft mbH, D-6940 Weinheim (Federal Republic of Germany), 1987

Distribution:
VCH Verlagsgesellschaft, P.O. Box 1260/1280, D-6940 Weinheim (Federal Republic of Germany)
USA and Canada: VCH Publishers, Suite 909, 220 East 23rd Street, New York NY 10010-4606 (USA)

ISBN 3-527-26144-3 (VCH Verlagsgesellschaft) ISBN 0-89573-224-6 (VCH Publishers)

Fundamentals of Biotechnology

Edited by
Paul Präve, Uwe Faust, Wolfgang Sittig
and Dieter A. Sukatsch

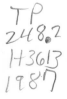
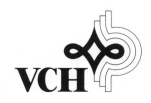

Original Title: Handbuch der Biotechnologie
Copyright 1982 by Akademische Verlagsgesellschaft, D-6200 Wiesbaden

Translated by B. J. Hazzard

Editorial Director: Dr. Hans-F. Ebel
Production Manager: Heidi Lenz

Library of Congress Card No. 87-10604

Deutsche Bibliothek, Cataloguing-in-Publication Data
Fundamentals of biotechnology / ed. by P. Präve ... [Transl. by B. J. Hazzard]. –
Weinheim; Deerfield Beach, FL: VCH, 1987.
  Einheitssacht.: Handbuch der Biotechnologie ⟨engl.⟩
  ISBN 3-527-26144-3 (Weinheim);
  ISBN 0-89573-224-6 (Deerfield Beach, FL)
NE: Präve, Paul [Hrsg.]; EST

Composition and printing:
Zechnersche Buchdruckerei, D-6720 Speyer
Bookbinding: J. Schäffer OHG, D-6718 Grünstadt
Printed in the Federal Republic of Germany

Preface

Biotechnology covers a wealth of specialized disciplines which includes not only the new genetic engineering techniques but also old fermentation processes which our ancestors practised thousands of years ago. In recent years many exciting developments have taken place, and – especially in the eyes of the public – the field has gained greatly in importance. It took some time for the literature to catch up with the rapid progress being made both in university and industrial laboratories. One of the first books to give a comprehensive description of the entire field was a predecessor of the present book (published in Germany in 1982). The success of this book and the considerable interest shown by English-speaking colleagues have prompted us to prepare an English version. *Fundamentals of Biotechnology* is based on the second edition of the German book; the entire contents have been brought up to date and in part revised.

Fundamentals of Biotechnology is not only an advanced textbook but is intended for everyone who is interested in biotechnological questions. In a field involving people with widely different backgrounds – microbiologists, engineers, chemists and many others – it was our idea to provide colleagues with a ready source of information. The different faces of biotechnology are presented by various authors. We have not attempted to suppress the individuality of the authors completely. Experience has shown us that this yields a coverage which is more vivid and provides a better view of specific subjects than if the editors had taken excessive pains to unify contributions. Chapters 1 to 8, which present the basic concepts of biotechnology, are followed by chapters dealing with special processes and products. Each chapter includes a detailed list of references. In the Appendix useful information on sources, products and biotechnological processes is collected. The extensive index will be especially appreciated by those wishing to use the book as a reference work.

We are indebted to Frau A. Christ for her invaluable assistance in the preparation of this book. To the translator, Mr B. J. Hazzard, we offer our special thanks for his careful translation of the German book and for his helpful comments. Finally, we wish to thank Dr I. Umminger for her painstaking editorial management and for compiling the index.

January 1987   The Editors

Contents

Part III
Processes and Products

Appendix

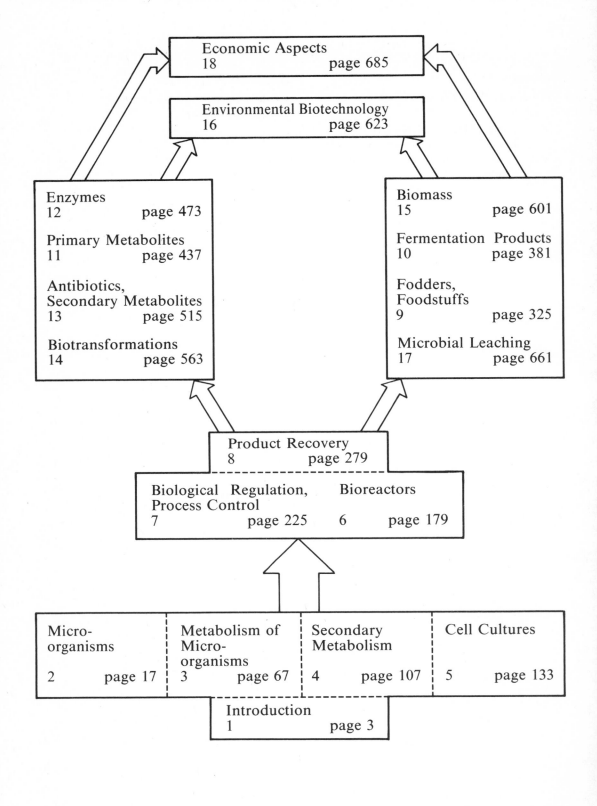

Economic Aspects
18   page 685

Environmental Biotechnology
16   page 623

Enzymes
12   page 473

Primary Metabolites
11   page 437

Antibiotics,
Secondary Metabolites
13   page 515

Biotransformations
14   page 563

Biomass
15   page 601

Fermentation Products
10   page 381

Fodders,
Foodstuffs
9   page 325

Microbial Leaching
17   page 661

Product Recovery
8   page 279

Biological Regulation,   Bioreactors
Process Control
7   page 225   6   page 179

Micro-
organisms

2   page 17

Metabolism of
Micro-
organisms
3   page 67

Secondary
Metabolism

4   page 107

Cell Cultures

5   page 133

Introduction
1   page 3

Part I: Introduction

Chapter 1

Biotechnology – History, Processes, and Products

Hans-Jürgen Rehm and Paul Präve

1.1 Definition

At the present time, by biotechnology is understood the use of biological processes within the framework of technical operations and industrial production.

It is therefore an application-oriented science of microbiology and biochemistry that is very closely connected with technical chemistry and chemical engineering. Biotechnology always deals with reactions which, in principle, are of biological nature. These reactions are performed either by living microbial cells or plant and animal cells and their tissues, or by enzymes from cells or parts of cells. The production of biomass from the organisms or parts of organisms mentioned is also an area of biotechnology [DECHEMA (German Society for Chemical Apparatus), 1976].

This definition does not include the field of agriculture, which could undoubtedly be regarded as a part of biotechnology. The field of medical technology, which deals with the manufacture of apparatuses for biological purposes, such as heart-lung machines, is not included in this definition, either. This medical technique is often called **biotechnique.**

1.2 Development of Biotechnology

On the basis of this definition it can be seen that biotechnology is a very old field. In prehistoric times, ethanol was probably the first organic substance prepared deliberately, and this by a biotechnological process: alcoholic fermentation. Several stages of development can be recognised in the history of biotechnology, and these are shown in Table 1-1.

1.2.1 Unconscious Use of Biotechnology: Processes in the Manufacture of Foodstuffs

Almost all primitive peoples became acquainted with **alcoholic fermentation** through the fact that sugar-containing fruits underwent spontaneous fermentation on storage. Later, as is still customary today with many peoples, these fermentations were carried out deliberately in earthenware vessels, hollowed-out tree-trunks, nutshells, leather bags, or other vessels. Such was the practical development of the first technological process based on microbiological phenomena.

The production of **wine** from grapes depends on the cultivation of the vine. Evidence for the existence of the vine before 2000 BC in Assyria has been found. As a rule, wine fermentation is left to the yeasts that occur on the grapes. An advanced wine culture developed particularly in the Greek and Roman areas and to some extent this has lasted to the present. The Roman emperor Marcus Aurelius Probus promoted wine growing in Germany on the Moselle and on the Rhine (276 to 282 AD). Wine growing was brought from Europe to South America, especially Chile, Argentina, and Brazil, and also to North America, especially California. For a good 100 years, there have also been significant wine-growing areas in South Africa and Australia.

Beer was mentioned by the Sumerians on a famous clay tablet, the "Monument Bleu," which is kept in the Louvre. There is also a number of documents on the manufacture of beer in the prehistoric era both from Babylonia and from Egypt.

The preparation of beer does not presuppose the cultivation of cereals, since beer can also be made from grass seeds. Greater technical knowledge is necessary for the manufacture of beer than for the simple fermentation of fruits to give wine. This led to the situation that beer was frequently brewed in relatively

Table 1-1. Information on the Historical Development of Biotechnology (Recent period not Included).

Proving bread with leaven	prehistoric period (before 3000 BC)
Fermentation of juices to alcoholic beverages in almost all natural populations	prehistoric period (before 3000 BC)
Knowledge of vinegar formation from fermented juices	prehistoric period (before 3000 BC)
Cultivation of the vine in Assyria	before 2000 BC
Manufacture of beer in Sumer and Babylonia and in Egypt	3rd century BC or even earlier
Wine growing promoted by Marcus Aurelius Probus in Germany	3rd century AD
Manufacture of beer by Celts and Germans	BC and AD
Production of spirits of wine (ethanol)	from 1150 AD, possible indications even earlier
Vinegar manufacturing industry near Orléans	14th century
Artificial growing of mushrooms in France	after about 1650
Visualization of yeast cells by Leeuwenhoek	about 1680
Discovery of the fermentation properties of yeasts by Erxleben	1818
Description of lactic acid fermentation by Pasteur	1857
Assumption of the dependence of fermentation on enzymes by M. Traube	1858
Discovery of Acetobacter by Hansen	1879
Microbiological production of lactic acid	1881
Artificial growth of mushrooms in the USA	after about 1885
Detection of fermentation enzymes in yeast by Buchner	1897
First communal sewage plants in Berlin, Hamburg, Munich, Paris, and other cities	from the end of the 19th century
German process for the manufacture of bakers' yeast	1915
Process for the large-scale production of food and fodder yeast by Delbrück, Hayduck, and Henneberg	1914–1916
Weizmann process for the manufacture of butanol and acetone	1915/1916
Sulfite process for the manufacture of glycerol by Connstein and Lüdecke	1915/16
Manufacture of citric acid in a surface process	from about 1920
Discovery of penicillin by Fleming	1928/29
Microbiological transformations discovered by Mamoli and Vercellone	1937

Beginning of penicillin manufacture	1941/44
Discovery of streptomycin by Schatz and Waksman	1944
Discovery of chlortetracycline by Duggar	1948
Submerged process for the production of acetic acid	1949
Manufacture of vitamin B_{12}	from about 1949
Technical microbiological transformations	after about 1949
Discovery of many other antibiotics	from 1950
Discovery of the structure of deoxyribonucleic acid by Watson and Crick thus providing the foundation for genetic engineering	1953
Manufacture of glutanic acid by Kinoshita et al.	after 1957
Manufacture of citric acid in the submerged process	about 1955/60

large operations. It is known that as early as in the third millenium BC there were commercial breweries in Babylonia with expert brewers who could prepare malt from barley or emmer. Even at that time it was known that germinated grain dissolves more readily therefore can be fermented to beer better than ungerminated cereals.

The manufacture of beer was carried out somewhat as follows: barley or glume-containing emmer was moistened and allowed to germinate. So-called "beer loaves" were made from this "green malt." Part of the germinated cereal was dried in the hot sun – this corresponds to some extent to our present kiln-drying process – and was stored as stock materials for periods in which no cereal was available. Malt and beer bread were stirred with water and the residue was separated from the clear liquid with the aid of a wickerwork basket. This corresponds roughly to our clarification process. Fermentation was carried out in earthenware vessels provided with lids.

The **Babylonian beers** had slightly acidic taste which arose from an accompanying lactic acid fermentation (caused in part by the lactic acid bacteria adhering to the cereal). The lactic acid substantially increased the keepability of the beer. However, the amount of acid was not controlled, so that beers with very different acidities were produced. In Bab-

ylonia there were about twenty different types of beer, and even the Egyptians prized the "Babylonian export beer." There were precise brewing instructions and laws for the manufacture of beer for inns and innkeepers in the Hammurabi Codex.

The **Egyptian beers** were manufactured mainly from roasted beer loaves, so that they were dark-colored beers. Here the beer was spiced with safflower plants and the fruit of various other plants. Many beers had an alcohol content of 12 to 15% which could only be achieved by sugar replenishment during fermentation, since otherwise a repression of fermentation by the sugar would have been unavoidable. With sugar replenishment during the consumption of the sugars by alcoholic fermentation further sugars had to be formed continuously from the starch and the dextrin of the thick mash by the action of the malt enzymes so that the yeasts always found favorable sugar concentration. Such replenishment required a good knowledge of the fermentation process. At this time, so far as concerns yeasts, it was known that the fermentation process started up more rapidly when the deposit from old fermentation batches was used again for a new fermentation.

The Romans, with their refined culture, enjoyed wine more, as the Greeks had done before them. The Celts and Germans, on the other hand, apparently preferred beer. They brewed mainly top-fermented beers with an acidic taste which were stored in vessels with capacities of up to 500 L at about 10 °C in the ground. The Arabs also drank a large amount of beer. They introduced the manufacture of beer into Spain in about the eighth century AD.

Since the sixteenth century, brewery techniques have been introduced into the American continent. Today, the manufacture of beer from cereals, particularly from barley, is known throughout the world. It has even been introduced into the East Asian area although a beer-like drink, so-called rice wine, has been brewed there for centuries.

Ethanol is believed to have been recognized for the first time about 1150. It was obtained by distillation from alcoholic beverages. Since it was very frequently manufactured from wine, it was also called spirits of wine. The name is derived from the Latin spiritus vini. Paracelsus then gave spirits of wine the Arabic name "al ko'hol" (the finest, the noblest). However, steppe people had probably obtained spirits from fermented milk even earlier.

Metal, clay, or earthenware boilers were used for distillation. They were fitted with lids containing one or more openings. Hollow wooden pipes, hollowed-out bamboo tubes, etc., were inserted in these openings and were sealed to the lid by luting with loam, clay, cow dung or similar substances. For cooling, the receiver was usually placed in a trough filled with water, which had to be replaced from time to time. "Technologically" better equipped distilleries made use of a stream, i.e., flowing water, as cooling liquid.

The manufacture of ethanol has spread throughout the world. Thin sugarcane juice has been fermented to ethanol for more than 50 years in Brazil and is used on the large scale as a fuel for automobiles.

Very many foodstuffs have been prepared with the aid of microorganisms for several hundred or sometimes several thousand years. Examples are all **curdled milk products,** most types of **cheese,** and, not least, very many **East Asian** and **oriental foodstuffs.** In the fermenting of bread dough with the aid of **leaven** an inoculation of mixed cultures of microorganisms from one starter to another has been practised for many thousand years. It is interesting that even today, in spite of our great microbiological knowledge, we have not succeeded in composing a mixture from pure cultures leading to a good enough leavening of the dough to be comparable with a natural starter.

In addition to ethanol, another primary metabolite, **acetic acid,** was manufactured with the aid of microorganisms. The formation of vinegar from fermented alcoholic beverages was already known to the cultures of the Babylonians, Assyrians, and Egyptians. Later, the Greeks and Romans enjoyed certain good wine vinegars diluted with water as refreshing drinks. Until the early Middle Ages, vinegar was prepared exclusively in the home, and only towards the end of the fourteenth century did an independent vinegar-manufacturing industry develop in France, particularly in the Orléans area. Here vinegar was first manufactured from beer and wine mash by a slow surface process, the so-called Orléans process.

A new method for the manufacture of vinegar was described by Boerhaave (1668 to 1738). This process is performed with a flowing liquid and no longer with a stationary liquid as in the Orléans process. The Boerhaave process is a forerunner of the quick vinegar process which was substantially developed by Schützenbach, in particular. In 1824, J. Hamm developed the generator process. In the last two processes, the acetic acid is formed in a vinegar generator filled with beechwood shavings bearing colonies of Acetobacter sp., by the trickling of ethanol over the carrier-bound bacterial colonies. The bacteria oxidize the ethanol to acetic acid. The necessary air passes from below upwards over the bacterial cultures due to the density difference caused by the heat of oxidation. Thus, even at that time an extraordinarily interesting three-phase system was developed, working with the solid bacterial phase, the liquid substrate phase, and the countercurrent gas phase.

Only since 1949 has this process been superseded by a submerged process for the manufacture of acetic acid developed by Hromatka and Ebner.

This first period of the historical development of biotechnology continues to influence present trends and is currently still being extended in parallel to other, more modern, areas of biotechnology.

1.2.2 Biotechnological Processes without Absolute Prohibition of Foreign Infections

In the second half of the nineteenth century, the pioneering work of Pasteur and a number of other microbiologists and chemists showed that in microorganisms many important physiological metabolic reactions take place which could be considered for technical utilization. Following this realization, manufacturing processes for a whole series of primary metabolic products were rapidly developed.

Although Robert Koch had already developed the technique for the preparation of pure cultures of microorganisms, these processes always took place with the risk of infections by species of microorganisms that were not directly involved in the process. Merely by the choice of the ecological conditions for the species of microorganisms with which the process was performed were foreign microorganisms to be excluded. Products such as lactic acid, citric acid, ethanol, butanol/acetone, etc., were obtained with the aid of microorganisms in this way.

The production of **butanol/acetone** played an important role particularly in the First, and

then also in the Second, World War (see Chapters 11 and 18). It was brought to a state of technical maturity in the First World War by Weizmann, who later became the first President of the state of Israel.

The manufacture of **glycerol** has also been of great importance in both World Wars.

The beginning of the microbial production of **citric acid** at the beginning of the twenties has made the cultivation of lemon trees unnecessary, particularly in Italy. This led to a loss of jobs in these areas until the plantations were turned over to other citrus fruits.

The first **biological sewage clarification plants** had been developed by the end of the 19th century. These involved continuous biotechnological processing. In addition, the mass production of **bakers' yeast,** i.e., a biomass process, and also the manufacture of **fodder yeast** from the wastes of, for example, pulp mills, were developed. In all these processes, small amounts of foreign microbes occurring have no disturbing effects.

1.2.3 Biotechnological Manufacture of Products with the Exclusion of Foreign Microbes

The discovery of the antimicrobial effect of penicillin by Alexander Fleming (1928/29) made it desirable to obtain this material in large amounts. Since, however, penicillin is cleaved by the enzymes of various foreign microbes and so made ineffective, the development of biotechnological processes which could be carried out with the **absolute exclusion of foreign microbes** was necessary. The "Oxford group" introduced such a development of chemical engineering from 1940 onwards. Since then it has been possible to allow the producing microorganism to grow and produce to its absolute optimum degree without worrying about foreign organisms. These were prevented from developing during the process by means of a complicated operating technique and no longer, as in the older technique, solely by suitable ecological conditions. In this way it also became possible to obtain substances which are normally formed in only small amounts and to carry out microbiological transformations and many similar processes.

The development of penicillin led to the discovery of many other antibiotics (see Chapter 13). The names of Waksman, Schatz, Abraham, Chain, Umezawa, and many others are associated with these discoveries and developments. Other known secondary metabolic products are also being manufactured by these processes, such as vitamin B_{12}, gibberellins, and alkaloids. The manufacture of cortisone/cortisol and of estrogenic ovulation inhibitors (the "pill"), in particular, has become economically possible by means of microbial transformations. This phase of development is still continuing. The chemical engineering involved is complicated and expensive. The products are not cheap; in most cases they are not mass products.

1.2.4 Application of Important Results of Basic Research to Biotechnology

While the search for other secondary metabolic products and their manufacture is being carried on intensively, further developments can be recognized in the field of biotechnology.

Basic research has produced a large number of results in the fields of microbiology, biochemistry, enzyme research, molecular biology, and genetic engineering, and, not least, also chemical engineering which are being made practical use of today in biotechnology.

The results in the field of enzyme research have led to the development of processes with **immobilized enzymes** and also with **immobilized cells** (see Chapter 12). The results of microbiology and biochemistry – particularly our knowledge of the biosynthesis of a number of important substances and of the regulation of these biosyntheses – have led to the **directed manufacture** of a whole number of **secondary metabolic products** (see Chapter 13). Many results in the field of molecular biology have already been applied to biotechnology (e.g., "genetic engineering") as well. Investigations in chemical engineering have led to the production of new reactors, optimized processes in new and old reactors, and the improvement of measuring and controlling technique, and, finally, to the computer-controlled performance of some processes.

1.3 General Observations on Biotechnological Processes

Basically, most biotechnological processes can be reduced to a simple equation:

$$\text{Substrate} + \begin{matrix}\text{microbial}\\\text{cells}\end{matrix} \xrightarrow{\overset{\text{process}}{\text{engineering}}} \text{product}$$

Process engineering consists of the **manufacturing process (fermentation)** proper and the subsequent **recovery procedure** (isolation of the product or of the cells). The product may be cell biomass, a metabolic product of the cells, or a transformation product of a given starting material. The living microorganisms may be replaced by parts of them, e.g., by components of microorganisms or by enzymes. Furthermore, an initially complex substrate can be replaced by a definite chemical compound which is converted into a product in one or a few steps. Then the equation runs, for example:

Substance + enzyme $\xrightarrow{\text{process engineering}}$ product

These reactions are already very simplified biotechnicological processes. In general, however, biotechnological processes are altogether more complex. They can be formulated by a scheme (Fig. 1-1) which is based essentially on the working equation of biotechnology given above.

Microorganisms – **the deciding factor of a biotechnological process** – occur ubiquitously and can be found all over the Earth. To isolate them, generally, samples of soil, water, or air are collected and suitable species are isolated from them and are bred pure **(screening).** For this purpose, the samples are diluted with sterile nutrient medium or isotonic solutions to such an extent that on the subsequent plating onto solid agar nutrient media individual microorganisms, after incubation, give single colonies which can easily be isolated with inoculation needles. The choice of the samples for the medium, the incubation temperature, the pH, and many other factors depend on which organisms are to be isolated (identification manuals: Bergey (1974); Lodder (1971)).

Of the multitude of known genera and species of microorganisms, only a small proportion is utilized biotechnologically (see Chapter 2). Most of the strains described are kept in a large number of **collections** (see Appendix) and can be obtained from these collections.

Protracted development work must often be performed before a process can come into use. First there is the **detection** of the desired product. Since wild strains usually form only very minute amounts of the product, the methods of detection must be very sensitive. As a rule, the methods used are physicochemical (e.g., chromatography) or microbiological (e.g., inhibition plate test). In the **development** of a process, a variety of methods is often used, but in **production** a reduction of this multiplicity again to one or a few methods, is aimed at.

Rapid, certain, and sensitive methods of detection for desired products are also necessary in the course of process development in order to improve the strains. The yield of the product is raised by **selection** and **mutation.** In parallel to this, the substrate is optimized, since the isolation medium is not usually identical with the production medium. If possible the **production medium** (Table 1-2) must contain cheap raw materials, but at the same time special requirements for improved biosynthesis of the product must be borne in mind. The substrate costs frequently amount to as much as 50% of the total manufacturing costs (see Chapter 15 and 18).

The actual manufacture of the product in the reactor is, in ordinary usage, the **fermentation** proper (Dellweg, 1979). A reactor must be constructed in such a way that, in aerobic processes, the cells are well supplied with air, the carbon dioxide produced can be led off, and each cell be kept in contact with all parts of the substrate. For many fermentations the **sterility** of the reactor and of the medium is a prerequisite, since only then can an optimum productivity of the strain used be ensured. Table 1-3 shows the time required for the destruction of various commonly occurring bacterial spores (see Appendix). **Anaerobic fermentation processes** frequently run for relatively long times and therefore generally require simpler plants (barrels, vats, fermentation tanks) (Rehm, 1980). In **aerobic processes,** on the other hand, the standard reactor is the aerated stirring vessel of which, again, there is a wealth of designs (see Chapter 6). In order to be able to compare developments and results better, DECHEMA (Deutsche Gesellschaft für chemisches Apparatewesen e.V., Frankfurt, FR Germany) has developed the "standard reactor" (reactor for comparative studies) in which the multifold experience of university and industry has been incorporated. Recently, new developments of a technical nature have been introduced which are

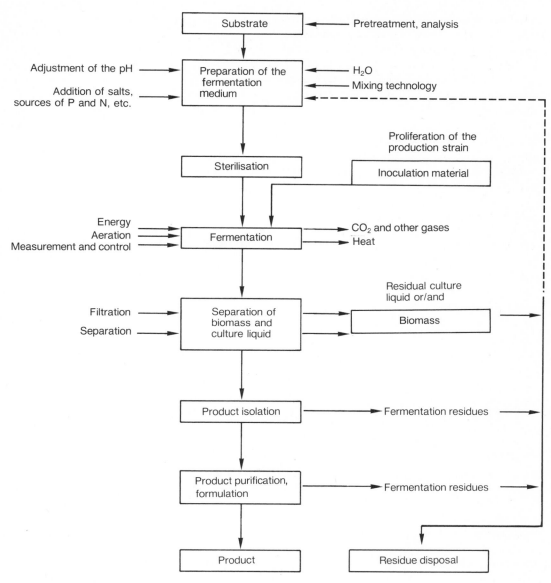

Fig. 1-1. Flow sheet of biotechnical processes.

more adapted to special requirements (high levels of oxygen supply, continuous operation, etc.) (see Chapter 6).

The **recovery of the product** often takes place at the end of the fermentation, at the moment of highest yield. In the production of cell mass, the recovery is carried out continuously, since these processes can usually be operated continuously. Downstream processing may range from a simple drying of the solution up to complicated multistage processes including extraction or ion-exchange steps (see Chapter 8).

The last step of a biotechnological process is the **product formulation,** for which a large amount of "know-how" from other manufactures, is available.

1.4 Importance of Biotechnology

Biological processes have had central importance in the foodstuffs industry, in particular, for thousands of years, but it is only in the last hundred years that they have been applied more intensively in chemical technology.

Table 1-2. Raw Materials for Fermentation.

Pure C-containing substrates	Mono-, di-, and polysaccharides Hydrocarbons Alcohols CO_2
Complex substrates	Molasses Cellulose waste liquors Saccharified wood solution Spent wash Corn steep liquor Pharmaceutical media Whey
Sources of N	NH_3, NO_3, urea Amino acids Soybeans
Inorganic salts	Phosphates, sulfates, chlorides
Trace elements	K, Na, Mg, Ca, Fe, Co, Zn

Table 1-3. Times Necessary to kill Bacterial Spores when Exposed to Dry Heat.

Spores of	Killing times in minutes at temperatures of						
	120°C	130°C	140°C	150°C	160°C	170°C	180°C
Bacillus anthracis	—	—		60–120	9–90		3
Clostridium botulinum	120	60	15–60	25		10–15	5–10
Clostridium tetani		20–40	5–15	30	12	5	1
Soil bacteria				180	30–90	15–60	15

H. G. Schlegel, *Allgemeine Mikrobiologie,* p. 166. G. Thieme Verlag, Stuttgart 1969.

At the present time, modern biotechnology is capable of becoming a part of industry of increasing economic importance.

The field of operation of biotechnology consists of three large areas:

1. **Microbiology,** including microbial genetics;
2. **Biochemistry,** physical chemistry, and technical chemistry; and
3. **Process engineering** and apparatus constructions.

Biotechnology is developing by close interweaving between these areas and can develop further only by means of an interdisciplinary cooperation between them.

Many products can be manufactured only biotechnologically. This applies particularly to most of the secondary metabolic products such as, for example, antibiotics, vitamin B_{12}, and many others, but it also applies to many products that are manufactured by a microbial transformation and which cannot be produced profitably in any other way, such as, for example, steroids and many estrogenic ovulation inhibitors that are used as "antibaby pills". At the present time about 90 **antibiotics** for medical use are manufactured industrially. The production of antibiotics is in the order of more than 30000 tons per year. Even special antibiotics, such as monensin, a coccidiostat and animal feed supplement, and validamycin, which is used in Japan for the control of phytopathogenic bacteria, are already being manufactured on the ton scale.

More than 20 amino acids are offered by various industries as biotechnologically prepared products. Of these glutamic acid is particularly important with a current production of about nearly 300000 tons per year.

More than 25 **enzymes** are produced technically. It is impossible nowadays to imagine the economy without their use, for example, as rennet in the USA, for the manufacture of cheese, and as proteases and amylases in many branches of industry. The situation is similar with citric acid, the manufacture of which has assumed an important place in foodstuffs chemistry.

Millions of people in the world owe their lives to the use of **antibiotics.** The same applies to other therapeutic agents, including vaccines, which are likewise largely produced biotechnologically. Many people do not realize that for us the antibiotics practically represent the "philosophers' stone" of the Middle Ages which was sought and pursued with such great labor.

Together with many different chemical and physical purification processes, the **biotechnological purification of sewage** is the most important means of rendering sewage harmless and clarifying it so that it can be returned to the natural water cycle (see Chapter 16).

Recent developments of biotechnology in close connection with its neighboring areas make up an increasing proportion of **environmental protection.** Recycling processes with biomass are currently being intensively studied and tested in order to achieve processes for the degradation of environmentally harmful substances with the aid of microorganisms.

Biotechnological industries often use ecologically beneficial processes. They frequently require less energy, since many reactions are performed at low temperatures and without substantial overpressure.

In the technical field, it has been possible in the last few years, particularly through investigations in the field of the **production of biomass,** to apply measuring and controlling technology, including the use of computers, to the vital processes of cells taking place in reactors. The importance of this application of modern technologies for living systems will certainly increase in the future.

Another highly interesting field is the use of **fixed systems.** By being fixed to matrices, both living cells and also their enzymes can be used repeatedly, and at the same time the advantages of smaller dimensions of plants are obtained, since biotechnology is usually carried out in highly diluted aqueous solutions.

Molecular biology, with its first attempts at application as **genetic engineering,** is certainly capable of opening up completely new possibilities for biotechnology. It has become likely that by manipulating cells, in combination with measuring and controlling techniques and the technical developments of the last few years, complicated natural substances normally very difficult to obtain can be manufactured in controlled fashion. If basic science is to understand Nature and technology is to apply what is understood, a broad field is opened up here to biotechnology which could possibly be a decisive factor in human society during the next few decades.

1.5   Literature

[1] *Biotechnologie. Eine Studie über Forschung und Entwicklung*. DECHEMA, Frankfurt/M. 1982.
[2] Maurizio, A.: *Geschichte der gegorenen Getränke*. Paul Parey, Berlin 1933.

Textbooks and Reviews

Blakebrough, N. (ed.): *Biochemical and Biological Engineering Science,* Vol. 1 and 2. Academic Press, London, New York 1967/68.
Bruchmann, E. E.: *Angewandte Biochemie*. Eugen Ulmer, Stuttgart 1976.
Dellweg, H. (ed.): *4. Symposium Technische Mikrobiologie Berlin 1979*. Versuchs- und Lehranstalt für Spiritusfabrikation und Fermentationstechnologie, Berlin 1979.
Esser, K.: *Kryptogamen*. Springer-Verlag, Berlin, Heidelberg, New York 1976.
Fritsche, W.: *Biochemische Grundlagen der Industriellen Mikrobiologie*. VEB Gustav Fischer, Jena 1978.
Gerstenberg, H., Sittig, W. and Zepf, K.: *Chem. Ing. Techn.* **52,** 19 (1980).
Gottschalk, G.: *Bacterial Metabolism*. Springer-Verlag, Berlin, Heidelberg, New York 1979.
Karlson, P.: *Kurzes Lehrbuch der Biochemie für Mediziner und Naturwissenschaftler*. 9th Ed. Georg Thieme-Verlag, Stuttgart 1974.
Lehninger, A. L.: *Biochemistry*. Worth Publishers, New York 1970.
Metz, H.: *GIT Fachz. Lab.* **23** (6), 602 (1979).
Perlman, D. and Tsao, G. T. (eds.): *Annual Reports on Fermentation Processes*. Vol. 1 and 2. Academic Press, New York, San Francisco, London 1977/78.
Präve, P., Sukatsch, D. A. and Faust, U.: „Biotechnology: The Industrial Production of Natural Substances", *Interdiszip. Sci. Rev.* **1** (1), 85 (1976).
Rehm, H. J.: *Industrielle Mikrobiologie*. 2nd Ed. Springer-Verlag, Berlin, Heidelberg, New York 1980.
Rehm, H. J. and Reed, G. (ed.): *Biotechnology*. Vol. 1–8. Verlag Chemie, Weinheim 1981 ff.
Schlegel, H. G.: *Allgemeine Mikrobiologie*. Georg Thieme-Verlag, Stuttgart 1972.
Smith, G.: *An Introduction to Industrial Mycology*. 6th Ed. Edward Arnold, London 1969.
Weide, H. and Aurich, H.: *Allgemeine Mikrobiologie*. Gustav Fischer-Verlag, Stuttgart, New York 1979.
Yamada, K.: *Japan's most advanced industrial fermentation technology and industry*. The International Technical Information Institute, Tokyo 1977.

Part II: Fundamentals of Biotechnology

Chapter 2

Microorganisms – Biology and Genetic Procedures for Strain Improvement

Karl Esser and Friedhelm Meinhardt

2.1   Introduction

The idea of this chapter is to give a summarizing account of the most important microorganisms that are used for biotechnological processes. After a definition of terms in tabular form for organization, the biotechnically relevant bacteria and fungi are described in separate sections corresponding to their taxonomic classification. Here, value is placed on **morphogenesis** and also, and particularly, on ontogenesis since it is just a knowledge of life cycles that is of decisive importance for the handling of the corresponding microorganisms, particularly in relation to their cultivation. Consequently, at the corresponding points the genetic methods are also described. This contribution is not intended to replace any textbook of microbiology; it is specially intended as an introduction for persons working in biotechnology, whether as biologists as biochemists, or as process engineers. We have therefore placed value on a point-by-point description of individual organisms important for practice.

2.2   Bacteria (Schizomycetes)

The bacteria are **prokaryotes.** Their genetic information is not localized in chromosomes but lies freely in the protoplasm, usually as circular double-stranded DNA. Bacteria lack the cell organelles that are typical for the eukaryotes, such as mitochondria and plastids. There is in addition no compartmentation of the protoplasts by an endoplasmic reticulum. They are mainly **heterotrophic** and live ubiquitously as **saprophytes** or **parasites.** There are mobile and immobile unicellular and multicellular representatives. In the typical case, their cell wall is a murein sacculus.

Summarizing literature

General bacteriology: Clifton, 1958; Thimann, 1967.
Physiology: Clifton, 1957; Doelle, 1969; Gottschalk, 1979.
Genetics: Bresch and Hausmann, 1970; Hayes, 1968; Knippers, 1971; Watson, 1976.
Taxonomy: Bergey, 1975; Kandler and Schleifer, 1980; Sherman, 1967.
Practical introduction: Clowes and Hayes, 1968; Winkler, Rüger and Wackernagel, 1972.
Special groups of bacteria: Clarke and Richmond, 1975; Young and Wilson, 1972.

2.2.1   Definition of Terms

Bacterial Cells

Typical prokaryote organization, i.e., only nuclear equivalent; no plastids and mitochondria; other cell organelles typical for eukaryotes such as, for example, endoplasmic reticulum are also absent; cell wall usually with a murein skeleton, frequently surrounded by a slime layer (= capsule).

Types of Cells

The great morphological variety can be brought down to a few basic types.

Cocci: Spherical, diameter usually 0.5 to 1 µm; classified according to direction of division and arrangement into

 Diplococci: one direction of division, two cells adhere to one another;

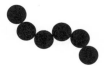 Streptococci: one direction of division; several cells adhere to one another in the form of chains;

Tetracocci: two directions of division; four cells remain attached to one another;

Staphylococci: three directions of division, irregular arrangement of the cells;

Sarcinas: three directions of division, cubic arrangement of the cells.

The terms given still find use as trivial names but to some extent they are also used in the binary nomenclature.

Rods: Elongated. Widths usually 0.2 to 2.2 μm, length usually 1.2 to 7.0 μm.

Bacteria: cylindrical, rounded at the ends;

Vibrios: bent in the form of commas;

Spirilla: with many bends, frequently tapering to a point at the end, length up to 50 μm;

Spirochaetes; with several bends, bent, flexible, length up to 60 μm;

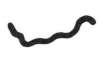

Flaviform (Corynebacterium), thread-like outgrowths (Caulobacter), and mucus stalks (e.g., Gallionella) are other variants of this basic type.

However, not all bacteria can be unambiguously assigned to these two basic types, e.g., **mycoplasmae**

have no cell wall and therefore vary in shape and size and the same applies to rickettsiae (cell parasites). In addition, many bacteria can change their form with a change in the external conditions (L forms, transition from rods to coccoid cells). Such changes in form are known as **pleomorphism.**

Motion

Either by "gliding" or with the aid of flagella, which can be arranged in different ways:

monopolar, monotrichous: a single flagellum inserted at a pole (Vibrio);

monopolar, polytrichous = lophotrichous: bundle of flagella inserted at a pole (Thiospirillum);

bipolar, polytrichous = amphitrichous: bundle of flagella inserted at the poles at both ends (Spirillum);

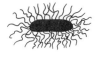

peritrichous: flagella inserted in the longitudinal sides or over the entire surface (Bacillus).

Vegetative Bodies

Unicellular organisms: Cocci, rods, pleomorphs (see above).
Cell associations (coenobia): Agglomeration of physiologically independent individual cells to form ordered or unordered groups after one or more cell divisions (see also under Types of cells).

a) Spherical forms: various types and cocci (see above).
b) Filamentous forms: branched or unbranched threads.

Following Bergey's Manual, to denote these types of coenobia we use only the expression "filament" and include among them those forms that are given by other authors under the term "trichomes."

freely mobile (Beggiatoa)

sessile (Thiotrix, Leucothrix)

Fig. as ——— individual threads (Beggiatoa)

bundles (Thioploca, Peloploca)

Fig. as ——— uniform (Beggiatoa)

polar (Thiotrix)

straight (Leucothrix)

spirally coiled (Thio-spirilopsis)

here we must also include the "giant forms": Caryophanon, and Oscillospira.

Multicellular Organisms: The cells are no longer physiologically independent. In the case of prokaryotes, these include only the mycelium-producing forms.

The term mycelium (see p. 28) has been taken over from the eukaryotic fungi, since the mycelium-forming bacteria were previously included among these. Of course, in the case of prokaryotes we are not dealing with mycelia in the true sense. This also follows from the fact that within the actinomycetes there are all possible transitional forms between cell aggregates and multicellular mycelium-forming organisms.

In the Actinomycetales a progression is found from the predominantly unicellular Mycobacterium species through occasionally filamentous cell associates in the genus Nocardia to the coenocytic mycelial Streptomyces, and with this a progression of propagation is associated.

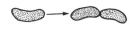

Mycobacterium: binary fission

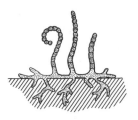

Nocardia: }
Actinomyces: }   fragmentation of the mycelium

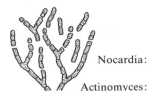

Streptomyces: conidia

Propagation

Transmission of genetic information, usually associated with cell multiplication;

asexual: no recombination of the genetic material.

a) Binary fission: schizotony or fission (an old term was schizomycetes or fission fungi); in the case of rods always perpendicular to the longitudinal axis;

b) spore formation;

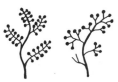

Conidiospores: conidia, vegetative propagation units usually formed exogenously on specific sporophores;

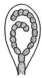

sporangiospores: flagellate or nonflagellate spores formed endogenously in specific spore containers (sporangia);

endospores: highly heat-resistant resting forms with multilayer spores sheaths formed endogenously;

parasexual: recombination of genetic material: replaces sexual propagation, which does not take place;

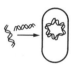

conjugation: association of cells; the unilateral transfer of genetic material takes place through protein tubuli (pili) (e.g., *Escherichia coli,* F factor);

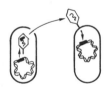

transformation: uptake of free DNA by the bacterial cell usually possible only in vitro (e.g., pneumococci, rough and smooth cells);

transduction: transfer of genetic material from bacterium to bacterium with the aid of a bacteriophage as vector.

Organization of the Genetic Material

Bacterial chromosome: double-stranded DNA circular, so far known (length about 1 mm in the case of *Escherichia coli*).

The expression chromosome is not correct in the strict sense since it is reserved for the differently organized chromosomes of eukaryotes; also customary are the terms: nucleus equivalent, nucleoid.

Plasmid: additional circular DNA molecule (length range 1 to 150 μm).

The term episome which was formerly customary is no longer used.

Types of Nutrition

autotrophic: acquisition of energy from light (photoautotrophic) or inorganic compounds (chemoautotrophic);

heterotrophic: acquisition of energy from organic compounds.

Mode of acquiring energy

aerobic: requires oxygen (respiration) as an electron acceptor, high acquisition of energy;

anaerobic: does not use oxygen as electron acceptor or for fermentation, small acquisition of energy.

Mode of Life

saprophytes: feed on dead organic material;

parasites: feed on living material of a host organism;

commensals: organisms of different species that live together without either being detectably harmed;

symbionts: organisms of different species both of which obtain advantages by living together. The transitions between all four types are fluid.

2.2.2 Classification

In contrast to the taxonomy of plants and animals, which takes into account so far as possible the natural evolutionary relationship, a bacterial system is governed by **artificial criteria** such as, for example, shape, motility, nutrition, propagation.

One of the oldest classification criterion of bacteria that is still used today is **Gram staining**; this is based on differences in cell wall structure.

Gram-positive bacteria after being stained with Crystal Violet/iodine followed by treatment with ethanol, retain the blue-black dye complex. **Gram-negative** bacteria on the other hand, are decolorized.

The standard work on bacterial taxonomy since 1923 has been Bergey's Manual which, in the eighth edition (1975) differentiates the bacteria into the following 19 "parts" each of which is subdivided on the usual principles into orders, families, genera, and species:
With the exception of the actinomycetes, all biotechnically relevant bacteria (in list marked) belong to the group of Eubacteria.

2.2.3 Bacteria of Biotechnological Importance

Rehm (1979) has recently summarized the most important bacterial species that are involved in biotechnological processes on the basis of the classification from Bergey's manual (Table 2-1). The Table can be used as a reference basis for the processes described in this and the other chapters of the book.

2.2.4 General Remarks on Cultivation, Maintenance, and Storage

Nutrient Media

The cultivation of microorganisms in the laboratory, as also on the technical scale, presupposes a knowledge of their nutritional demands. The common environmental factors such as temperature, oxygen demand, light,

Part	Title
1	**Phototrophic bacteria**
2	**The gliding bacteria**
3	**The sheathed bacteria**
4	**Budding and/or appendaged bacteria**
5	**The spirochaetes**
6	**Spiral and curved bacteria**
7	**Gram-negative aerobic rods and cocci**
8	**Gram-negative facultative anaerobic rods**
9	**Gram-negative anaerobic rods**
10	**Gram-negative cocci and coccobacilli**
11	**Gram-negative anaerobic cocci**
12	**Gram-negative chemolithotrophic bacteria**
13	**Methane-producing bacteria**
14	**Gram-positive cocci**
15	**Endospore-forming rods and cocci**
16	**Gram-positive asporogenous rod-shaped bacteria**
17	**Actinomycetes and related organisms**
18	**The rickettsiae**
19	**The mycoplasmae**

group of Eubacteria

Table 2-1. Summary of Bacteria of Biotechnological Importance (based on Rehm, 1980).

Group and family of bacteria	Important genera involved in technical processes	Group and family of bacteria	Important genera involved in technical processes
Gram-negative, aerobic rods and cocci		**Endospore-forming rods and cocci**	
Pseudomonadaceae	Pseudomonas: assimilation of hydrocarbons, SCP, oxidation of steroids, oxidation of hydrogen including: Acetobacter: oxidation of alcohols, e.g., ethanol → acetic acid, sorbitol → sorbose	Bacillaceae	Bacillus: formation of antibiotics (especially polypeptide antibiotics), enzymes. Clostridium: formation of butanol, acetone, butyric acid, botulins
Methylomonadaceae	Methylomonas, Methylococcus: oxidation of methane and methanol	**Gram-positive, non-spore-forming bacteria**	
Azotobacteriaceae	Azotobacter: nonsymbiotic binding of nitrogen	Lactobacillaceae	Lactobacillus: formation of lactic acid and milk products, silage, many lactic acid foodstuffs, spoilage of foodstuffs
Gram-negative facultative anaerobic rods		**Actinomycetes and related organisms**	
Enterobacteriaceae	Escherichia and Aerobacter: many different processes, e.g., formation of nucleotides and of 2-ketoglutaric acid	Coryneform group of bacteria	Corynebacterium and Arthrobacter: oxidation of hydrocarbons, formation of amino acids. Cellulomonas: degradation of cellulose
Gram-negative chemolithotrophic bacteria		Propionibacteriaceae	Propionibacterium: formation of vitamin B_{12} and propionic acid; also in cheese
	Thiobacillus: leaching of copper, zinc, iron, manganese, and other sulfides	Mycobacteriaceae	Mycobacterium: oxidation of hydrocarbons and other substrates, such as steroids

Table 2-1. Summary of Bacteria of Biotechnological Importance (based on Rehm, 1980).

Group and family of bacteria	Important genera involved in technical processes
Methane-forming bacteria	
Methanobacteriaceae	Methanobacterium, Methanosarcina, Methanococcus: formation of methane, especially in digestion towers (2nd stage) in sewage treatment
Nocardiaceae	Nocardia: oxidation of hydrocarbons and other substrates such as steroids
Gram-positive cocci	
Micrococcaceae	Micrococcus: oxidation, e.g., of hydrocarbons and steroids
Streptococcaceae	Streptococcus: formation of lactic acid and biacetyl; Leuconostoc: formation of dextran
Streptomycetaceae	Streptomyces: formation of very many antibiotics, enzymes, and vitamin B_{12}

etc., are usually species-specific and cannot be summarized briefly.

Bacteria require a **source of carbon** and a **source of nitrogen,** and, in addition **minerals, trace elements,** and frequently, also **vitamins** or other growth factors. While autotrophic forms assimilate carbon dioxide as the source of carbon, the heterotrophic forms require an organic source of carbon.

All these demands are satisfied by the traditional standard medium of bacteriology, the **nutrient broth,** which is made up as follows: 1000 mL of meat extract, 10 g of peptone, and 5 g of sodium chloride.

Preparation of meat extract: grind meat without sinews and fat and add the double amount of water, leave overnight at 4°C, boil for 30 min and then, after cooling, filter. In peptone, soluble amino acids are present as the result of tryptic or peptic digestion of the proteins. The sodium chloride acts as osmostabilizer.

This medium is adequate for the cultivation of most bacteria. Corresponding to the specific nutritional requirements of some species, other substances are added to the standard medium such as, for example, grape sugar, serum, blood, or liver.

Standardized preprepared media are offered in dried form by various manufacturers, and information about them can be found in the literature, e.g.: Difco manual, 9th edition, 1953, or E. Merck AG, Mikrobiologisches Handbuch (no date).

Pure Cultures

For any laboratory work and for technical purposes it is necessary to prepare pure cultures from natural isolates, i.e., individual bacterial cells must be separated from the others and the colonies arising from them, in this case called **clones,** be isolated. The most certain way of achieving this is a **manual singling out** of the bacterial cells under the preparation microscope or with the aid of a micromanipulator, as is possible in the case of fungal spores or yeast cells. However, because of the smallness of bacterial cells it is often impossible to apply these techniques to them.

There are two other methods, both of which offer the highest possible degree of probability of obtaining pure bacterial clones. Both are based on the principle of a dilution series and finally lead to individual cultures, one being carried out on a solid medium and the other in a liquid medium.

a) **Dilution streak.** If from a bacterial culture applied in the form of a streak subsidiary streaks are made with an inoculating loop as shown in Fig. 2-1 (the inoculating loop is flamed between sucessive streaks), individual colonies are finally obtained. These are treated by the same method again until the colonies are uniform at least in morphological and physiological aspects.

To single out obligate anaerobes, the individual dilutions are suspended in an agar medium in test-tubes and are incubated under an atmosphere of nitrogen.

The disadvantage of the dilution streak method is due to the fact that the possibility cannot be excluded that two bacteria may adhere to one another, for example, a bacterium without a slime layer in the slime layer (capsule) of another bacterium so that in this way a "permanent" mixed culture arises.

b) **Dilution series.** The bacterial culture is suspended in a liquid nutrient medium and its concentration (titer) is determined with the aid of a hematocytometer. After appropriate dilution, 1 mL of the suspension is then pipetted on to a Petri dish and streaked out on it. Depending on the capacity for multiplication, any desired number of individual cells (in the case of Petri dishes with a diameter of 9 cm, not more than 50) can be allowed to grow into clones.

A detergent can be added to the nutrient solution in order to limit to a minimum the adhesion of the cells to one another described above for the streaking-out method.

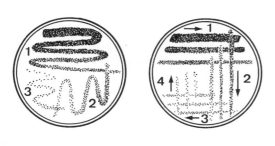

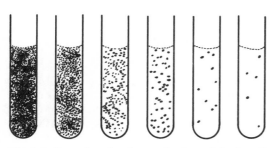

Fig. 2-1. Procedure for the production of single-cell bacterial cultures: a) streaking process; b) dilution series.

Cultivation of Bacteria with Different Oxygen Demands

The oxygen demand of bacteria can easily be determined with the aid of an **agar shake culture**: in test-tubes, an agar medium (about 10 mL in each) is allowed to cool to 45°C and is inoculated with a strain. After vigorous shaking and the setting of the agar, each tube is incubated at the temperature specific for the organism concerned. After about one day the following pattern is obtained:

The **obligate aerobes** are capable of growing only in the presence of atmospheric oxygen and their cultivation presents no difficulties if sufficient oxygen is supplied

The **facultative aerobes** grow best under anaerobic conditions but they can tolerate oxygen

The **facultative anaerobes** multiply in the optimum manner under aerobic conditions but oxygen is not essential for their growth

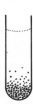

The **obligate anaerobes** can be cultivated only if oxygen is excluded

During the cultivation of aerobic and facultative anaerobic bacteria no problems arise, but in the case of obligate anaerobes special precautionary measures must be taken in order to exclude the atmospheric oxygen that is "poisonous" for them. This can be achieved in various ways:

Physical: hermetically sealed vessels are evacuated and if necessary an oxygen-free gas mixture is admitted (Knorr's anaerostat) (Zeissler, 1969; Knorr, 1930).

Chemical: absorption of the oxygen by pyrogallol soaked in potassium hydroxide solution (pyrogallol process); other absorbing reagents such as dithionite may also be used.

Biological: by the simultaneous cultivation of oxygen-consuming organisms.

All these methods for cultivating obligate anaerobes have, naturally, been developed for laboratory use and usually can be applied to fermenter cultures only with difficulty. In those cases, one must have recourse to special aeration systems which prevent the access of oxygen by the introduction of nitrogen or carbon dioxide.

Maintenance and Storage

Both in the laboratory and in industry it is necessary to have available for relatively long periods important strains such as, for example, type strains or good producing agents. It is in fact a question of having available "fresh" material exhibiting the original characteristics when after fairly long vegetative multiplication **degenerative phenomena** (senescence, etc.) appear.

Previously it was customary to maintain strains on slope agar at low temperatures in the refrigerator. In this way, the metabolic activity as a whole and, consequently, the whole rate of multiplication as well were greatly reduced. This method requires that the cultures are transferred at relatively long intervals, but regularly to fresh nutrient medium. In this way, degenerative phenomena are highly reduced but cannot be avoided entirely.

Today, to achieve **better preservation,** the following techniques are used:

a) Storage under **chemically inert liquids:** for example, agar cultures are covered with a layer of paraffin oil and stored under cool conditions. In this way, on the one hand, the metabolism is reduced further and, on the other hand, drying out is prevented. This method is used more in the case of filamentous fungi than in the case of yeasts and bacteria. In this way, cultures can be kept for several years.

b) **Freezing:** this is usually carried out in liquid nitrogen ($-196\,°C$). Freezing must take place rapidly, since otherwise the cells are damaged or destroyed by the formation of ice crystals. Subsequently, the cultures are stored either in liquid nitrogen or at least at $-80\,°C$. On reuse, thawing out must also be carried out very rapidly, if possible at $37\,°C$. This method is suitable for unicellular organisms and for relatively small amounts of filamentous fungi that have to be bred in liquid cultures.

c) **Drying:** the drying of suspensions (bacteria, yeasts, conidiospores) in vacuum is carried out by adding these to a carrier (such as, for example, silica gel or sand) and an emulsifying agent (such as, for example, skim milk or serum); storage is preferably carried out in closed ampuls or in a desiccator at low temperatures.

d) **Freeze-drying** (lyophilization): this is carried out after the previous rapid freezing of concentrated cell suspensions with liquid nitrogen followed by drying in vacuum in the presence of a protective liquid (e.g., serum, glycerol). Storage is carried out in closed ampuls under inert gases, if possible in the refrigerator.

When this method is used, it is true that the mutability and therefore the regeneration of the cultures is greatly reduced, so to a certain extent is their **viability.** The "rate of regeneration" differs from organism to organism, so that it may be recommended to store several preparations of each strain. In addition, it has proved to be desirable before practical application first to evaluate a sample on an agar or liquid medium of each culture stored for a relatively long time.

2.3 Fungi (Mycophyta)

The fungi are **eukaryotes** which may be derived from the colorless representatives of the unicellular algae. Since they are not capable of forming plastids, they are **heterotrophic.** They live as **saprophytes** or **parasites** in fresh water (rarely in salt water) and on land. The saprophytes, and also many of the parasites, can be cultivated in the laboratory. Within the fungi are found all transitions from motile unicellular organisms up to multicellular but usually coenocytic thalli of complicated structure. True tissues are not formed, but only

plectenchyma. Apart from a few forms having no cell walls, their cell walls contain chitin and only in some taxa do they contain cellulose.

Summarizing literature

General mycology: Ainsworth and Sussman, 1965 to 1968; Burnett, 1968; Gäumann, 1964; Ingold, 1973; Müller and Löffler, 1971; Webster, 1980; Esser, 1982.
Physiology: Cochrane, 1963; Lilly and Barnett, 1951; Smith and Berry, 1971; Turner, 1971.
Genetics: Burnett, 1975; Esser and Kuenen, 1967; Fincham, 1983; Raper, 1966.
Taxonomy: Kreisel, 1969; Bessey, 1968.
Practical instructions: Alexopoulos and Beneke, 1964; Bothe, 1971; Dade and Gunnel, 1969; Esser, 1982; Koch, 1972; Stevens, 1974.
Special groups of fungi: Chang and Hayes, 1978; Gray, 1970, 1973; Lincoff and Mitchell, 1970.

The treatment of individual groups of interesting fungi, particularly from methodological aspects such as, for example, composition of nutrient media and laboratory techniques is described in King, 1974.

2.3.1 Definitions of Terms

The following definitions have been taken from Esser, 1982.

Cell

Typical eukaryote organization (with the exception of the fact there are no plastids). Cells generally contain several nuclei; they are polyenergid.

Vegetative Body

Plasmodium: amoeboid thallus of the Myxomycetes, without cell walls.

Hyphae: filamentous branched vegetative structures which are either nonseptate (Phycomycetes) or are partitioned by septa (Ascomycetes, Basidiomycetes). The septa are generally perforated.

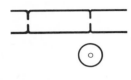

Simple septum: annular perforation permits the passage of cell nuclei and other cell organelles.

Doliporic septum: annular perforation constricted to such an extent by its barrel-shaped structure that, while there is in fact a cytoplasmic continuity between neighboring cells which even permits a passage of smaller cell organelles, it permits the passage of cell nuclei only after the breakdown of the doliporus (occurs only in Holobasidiomycetes).

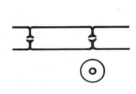

Mycelium: the hyphae as a whole.

Even when the hyphae of a mycelium are septate, this can be regarded as a coenocyte if an exchange of cytoplasm and cell organelles between the individual cells is possible.

When below in the case of fungi we call the individual compartments of a mycelium cells, this is done only for reasons of simplicity and analogy in relation to the other eukaryotes with unperforated cell walls.

Heterokaryon: mycelium containing genetically different nuclei.

Homokaryons: mycelium containing genetically identical nuclei.

Dikaryon: a special form of heterokaryon containing only two genetically different nuclei per cell that divide in conjugated fashion by certain mechanisms.

Monokaryon: special form of homokaryon in which each cell contains only one nucleus.

Sprout cells: spherical or ellipsoidal cells that in vegetative multiplication

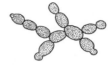

"sprout" out from the mother cell like bubbles. As sprout mycelia, sprout cells form looser cell associations.

Plectenchyma: felted or plaited tissues are not true tissues; the tissue-like cohesion is achieved by the swelling of the cell walls to form water-insoluble gels that ensheathe the complete hyphal system. Prosoplectenchyma: the individual hyphae are still recognizable. Paraplectenchyma: hardly to be distinguished from true tissues, since pronounced thickening of the cell walls and also pit-like structures may occur.

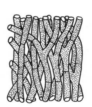

Sclerotia: resting multicellular plectenchymatic organs.

Paraphyses: sterile upward-growing hyphae which start from the hyphae of a hymenium and are to be found in branched or unbranched form between asci or basidia.

Propagation Cells and Propagation Organs

Holocarpy: the whole vegetation body is transformed into a propagation cell container.

Eucarpy: only a part of the thallus forms a propagation cell container, while the remainder continues its vegetative activity.

Auxiliary fruiting forms: serve for vegetative propagation; no alternation of nuclear phases.

a) Planospores = zoospores: 1 to 2 flagella arise in planosporangia (zoosporangia). Occur in aquatic fungi and some parasites.

b) Aplanospores: in terrestrial forms,

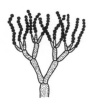

endogenous in multiplicity in sporangia

exogenous, conidiospores (known for short as conidia) are usually formed on typical conidiophores.

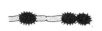

oidiospores (called oidia for short) arise as spherical or extended cells after the breakdown of septate hyphae.

chlamydospores (also called gemmae) are thick-walled resting spores. They arise terminally or within the hyphae from one or more septa after local contraction of the plasma. Thus, between individual chlamydospores there may be plasma-free spaces in the hyphae.

Main fruiting forms: serve for sexual propagation; alternation of nuclear phases.

In the **lower fungi** a resting organ, (e.g., a spore) arises from the zygote, which usually germinates after meiosis to form a sporangium.

In the **higher fungi** frequently there is no formation of a resting organ. The nucleus of the zygote divides meiotically, and typical meiosporangia arise.

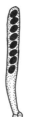

Ascus: sheath-like sporangium in which the meiospores (usually eight) arise by free cell formation.
Characteristic feature of the class of ascomycetes.

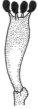

Basidium: club-shaped sporangium on which exogenous meiospores (usually four) are segmented off.
Characteristic feature of the class of basidiomycetes.

Hymenium: sporangia-bearing layer which may be permeated by sterile hyphae (paraphyses).

The sporangia may be formed in unordered fashion or in hymenia in plectenchymatic fruit bodies (ascocarps or basidiocarps).

Modes of Fertilization

Fertilization sensu stricto is **karyogamy.** It takes place after the fusion (plasmogamy) of propagation elements the morphological state of which may differ very considerably. The great variety of the modes of fertilization due to this can be seen from the following review:

Gametogamy: fusion of individual gametes, which are formed in gametangia. Corresponding to the habitus of the gametes, distinctions are made between:

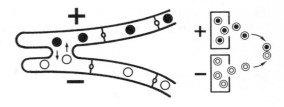

    isogamy: fusion of gametes of the same shape and size.

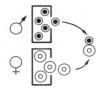   anisogamy: fusion of gametes of the same shape but of different size.

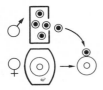   oogamy: fusion of gametes of different shape and different size.

Gametangiogamy: fusion of gametangia, with no (free) gamete formation.

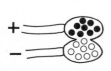   In analogy with gametogamy, a distinction can be made here also on the basis of the same criteria between isogametangiogamy, anisogametangiogamy and oogametangiogamy.

Gameto-gametangiogamy: fusion of a gamete with a gametangium.

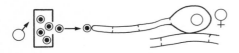

Somatogamy: fusion of vegetative cells that exhibit no kind of specific differentiation.

Obstacles to Fertilization

In many organisms, the individual modes of fertilization are subject to limitations. Such an obstacle to fertilization leads to the situation that, for example, in oogamy not every male cell can fuse with every female cell. Corresponding to the genetic control of this **incompatibility** there are certain groups within the male and within the female gametes which fuse with one another only in certain combinations. The term mating type has been used for this phenomenon and it is frequently denoted by the symbols + and − (or a and α). Similarly, when isogamy or somatogamy exists there are often genetically different mating types.

Life Cycles

a) **Sexual Cycles.** In accordance with sexual propagation, the life cycle of a species begins with the zygote arising by plasmogamy (P) and karyogamy (K) and ends with the formation of gametes, which can take place immediately after meiosis (M) or some time later. These types of nuclear phase alternation are not directly linked with one another but are separated from one another by a series of mitotic nuclear divisions which mostly lead to the formation of a vegetative body. The various life cycles are classified according to whether these mitoses take place in the haploid phase, the diploid phase, or in both phases.

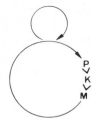

Haplont: the vegetative body is haploid, since meiosis takes place immediately after karyogamy. The diploid phase is restricted to the zygote. Vegetative multiplication is possible by means of haplomitospores.

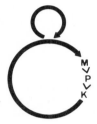

Diplont: the vegetative body is diploid, since a series of mitotic divisions occurs between karyogamy and meiosis. The haploid phase is limited to the gametes. Asexual reproduction is possible by means of diplomitospores.

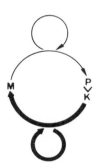

Haplodiplont: since numerous mitotic divisions take place both between meiosis and karyogamy (as in haplonts) and between karyogamy and meiosis (as in diplonts), in this type the nuclear phase alternation is linked with an alternation of generations.

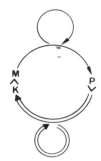

Haplodikaryont: the vegetative body is haploid. The dikaryophase is restricted to some early stages of fruit body formation. The sheaths of the fruit bodies are haploid. The diploid phase is confined to the nucleus of the zygote. Asexual multiplication by haplomitospores is possible.

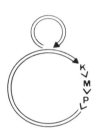

Dikaryont: the vegetative body (including sheaths of the fruit bodies) is dikaryotic, since immediately after the formation of the haplomeiospores these themselves or the cells arising from them undergo fusion (somatogamy). The diploid phase is limited to the zygote, and the haploid phase, in general, to the meiospores. Asexual multiplication by dikaryotic mitospores is possible.

In this connection, two other specific life cycles must be mentioned which, however, occur only in fungi. They are characterized by the fact that after the fusion of the gametes (plasmogamy) karyogamy does not follow immediately, i.e., between the haploid and diploid phases a further, so-called dikaryotic, phase is inserted in which the haploid nuclei multiply by mitotic divisions. Since these nuclear divisions generally take place in conjugated fashion, this ensures that at the end of the dikaryotic phase in the formation of zygotes the descendents of the two gamete nuclei are present in approximately equal numbers. Two cycles are distinguished:

b) **Parasexual Cycle.** For the sake of completeness within the framework of these considerations one more phenomenon must be mentioned which cannot be classified unambiguously either in the life cycles or in the propagation systems to be described in the next section. This is the so-called parasexual cycle which has so far been detected only in fungi. As the name itself indicates, in this cycle there is an occurrence of sexuality-like processes, particularly in relation to the recombination of the genetic material which has already been described as the essence of sexual propagation. In the parasexual cycle, however, recombination does not take place during a meiosis but in the course of mitotic divisions, which is expressed in the prefix "para-".

While the first step of the parasexual cycle usually takes place regularly when haploid cells come into contact with one another (for exceptions, see p. 48), the frequency of the last steps is very low: nuclear fusion 10^{-6} to 10^{-7}; crossingover $5 \cdot 10^{-2}$ per nuclear fission; haploidization 10^{-3} per nuclear fission.

It can be seen from this that the parasexual cycle plays practically no role in the fungi that are capable of a sexual multiplication. Its significance and its necessity first become clear in the case of the **Fungi imperfecti,** which have lost the capacity for sexual propagation (p. 42). Here the parasexual cycle provides the only possibility for the exchange of genetic material and therefore takes the place of the nonexistent sexual propagation at least to some extent. Thus, in the organisms otherwise referred only to asexual propagation, "survival in the sense of a continuous evolution is ensured" (see also the discussion of propagation systems on p. 28).

Organization of the Genetic Material

Chromosomal DNA: The chromosomes contain as their main constituents, in addition to double-stranded linear DNA, approximately equal amounts of basic histones and also small amounts of other proteins and chromosomal RNA. Their number is species-specific. They are delimited from cytoplasm by a nuclear membrane.

Extrachromosomal DNA: mitochondrial DNA is found in the mitochondria and in its organization corresponds substantially to the bacterial chromosome (see above, p. 21). **Plasmids** (for definition, see bacteria, p. 21) were first discovered in yeast and in the ascomycete *Podospora anserina* (Guerineau, 1979; Stahl et al., 1978) but quite recently they have also been found in many other fungi (for reference, see Esser et al., 1983).

Nutrition, Mode of Life, Supply of Energy

All fungi are heterotrophic (saprophytes or parasites) and predominantly aerobic.

2.3.2   Classification

The taxonomic classification of the fungi substantially reflect the subjective opinions of the systematician (Müller, 1974). The classification into four classes used here, must therefore be regarded purely pragmatically as a classification principle. In the following review, only those orders are given to which representatives with biotechnological relevance belong.

Parents

Recombination

no mitotic crossing-over   mitotic crossing-over

Recombinants

The individual steps of the parasexual cycle, which were first discovered in Aspergillus, are: The formation of heterokaryons: the fusion of haploid cells with genetically different nuclei. The appearance of diploid nuclei after the fusion of the haploid nuclei of the heterokaryon. Mitotic crossing-over: processes of chromosomal exchange in the course of the mitoses of the diploid nuclei in the heterokaryon. Haploidization: reduction of the diploid nuclei to haploid in the course of numerous mitoses (e.g. by loss of chromosomes).

1st Class: Myxomycetes

Slime molds, saprophytes or parasites, yellow, reddish, or lilac to brown slimy coatings on rotting parts of plants. Vegetative body = plasmodium, no cell wall, react to external stimuli with amoeboid motility, phagotrophic nutrition. Cell walls (chitin, cellulose) only during the formation of spores, and therefore intermediate in position between animals and plants.

2nd Class: Phycomycetes

Lower fungi, earlier incorrectly called algaelike fungi. Vegetation body of microscopically small unicellular to macroscopically recognizable mycelia without transverse walls, transverse walls only during the segmentation of propagation cell containers. Asexual propagation by planospores (aquatic forms) or aplanospores (terrestrial forms). Sexual propagation shows great variety in the mode of fertilization. Life cycle: mainly haplonts, but also diplonts and even haplodiplonts.

Orders:

1. Chytridales
2. Blastocladiales
3. Monoblepharidales
4. Hyphochytriales
5. Oomycetales

6. Zygomycetales
Terrestrial forms: Asexual propagation by spores (formed endogenously in sporangia, or conidia (segregated off exogenously on carriers).

Sexual propagation by fusion of gametangia (formation of juga).

Among the total of three families, only the Mucoraceae with 30 genera are important biotechnologically; the remainder are mold fungi, usually saprophytes on plant or animal substrates and more rarely parasitic on plants. All are haplonts, and the index form is generally regarded as *Phycomyces blakesleeanus,* which prefers fatty acids and fat-containing substrates ("oil fungus") (Fig. 2-2).

The genus Rhizopus which, with the species *nigricans* is probably the oldest fungus used biotechnologically (production of citric acid, see Table 2-2, p. 43) differs from the scheme shown in Fig. 2-2 by the following characteristics: the sporangia do not arise individually but in bundles of two or three and at their starting position from the mycelium form small root-like (which explains "Rhizopus") processes into the substrate. On copulation, the gametangia do not raise themselves above the substrate but pair in a plane. The antler-like processes are not present either. The representatives of the genus Mucor correspond substantially to the morphology of Rhizopus with the exception that the sporangiophores are not branched, and no rhizoid-like processes are formed.

3rd Class: Ascomycetes

Asci-bearing fungi, with the exception of a few unicellular species, highly branched mycelia with perforated transverse walls which enable cell nuclei and other cell organelles to pass through (and they are therefore coenocytes). Mode of life: saprophytes, including many coprophilic species that live on animal feces, or parasites, including many causative agents of plant diseases. Asexual propagation through exogenously formed conidiospores or by oidiospores. Sexual propagation by ascospores: greater uniformity than in the case of the Phycomycetes. Mode of fertilization: gametogamy or gametogametangiogamy. Life cycle: a so-called dikaryotic phase frequently occurs between haploid phase and karyogamy (see also p. 31).

Division into subclasses according to the way in which the fruit body is formed:

Subclass Protoascomycetidae:
no fruit bodies

a) 1st Order: Endomycetales (Saccharomycetales)

All yeasts belong to this taxon. Although the yeasts are mostly unicellular organisms, their

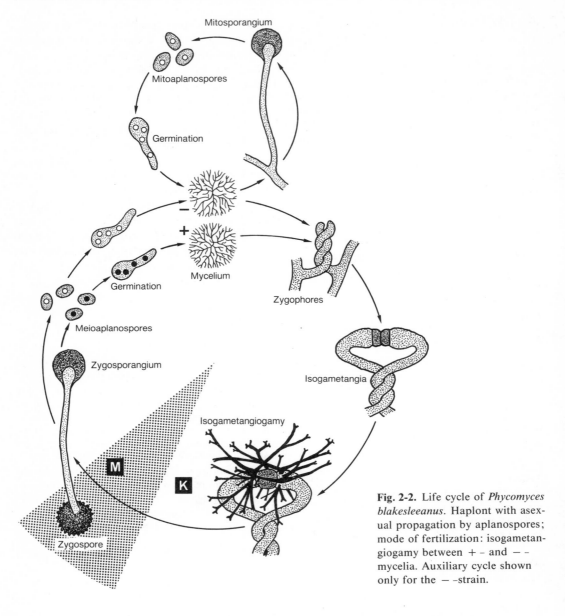

Fig. 2-2. Life cycle of *Phycomyces blakesleeanus*. Haplont with asexual propagation by aplanospores; mode of fertilization: isogametangiogamy between + – and – – mycelia. Auxiliary cycle shown only for the – –strain.

spherical to elongated cells can aggregate to form cell associates, and there are also hyphae-producing forms. The property of forming hyphae may be a species characteristic but in many species it may occur only transiently, depending on the external conditions. The further systematic subdivision of the yeasts into genera is governed by morphological characteristics, and the classification of species within the genera according to physiological characteristics, such as, for example, the assimilability of certain sources of carbohydrate. The standard work on their taxonomy is Lodder's book (1974).

In this connection it appears necessary to point out that, because of mutability, erroneous determinations can very easily be made if only physiological criteria are used. Details are given by Stahl and Esser (1979).

With regard to their life cycle, the yeasts include not only haplonts but also diplonts and haplodiplonts.

Of great importance, for basic research as well as for other purposes, is the bakers' or brewers' yeast *Saccharomyces cerevisiae* (Fig. 2-3). It can be taken as an example of a diplont. A typical representative of the haploid yeasts is the fission yeast *Schizosaccharomyces pombe* (pombe beer, production of arrack), in which the diploid phase is restricted to the zygote. A special illustration can therefore be renounced. An example of a haplodiplont is the alkane yeast *Saccharomycopsis lipolytica*. As can be seen from Fig. 2-4, haploid and diploid vegetative cells of the same shape

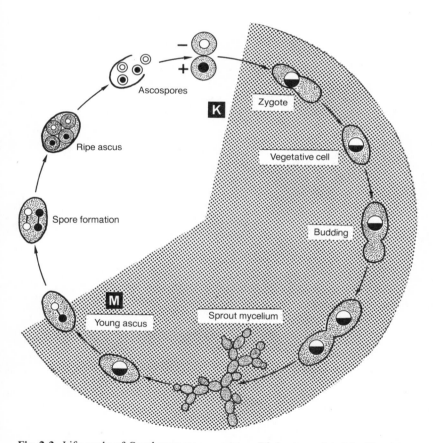

Fig. 2-3. Life cycle of *Saccharomyces cerevisiae*. Diplont; mode of fertilization: somatogamy between + – and – –mating types.

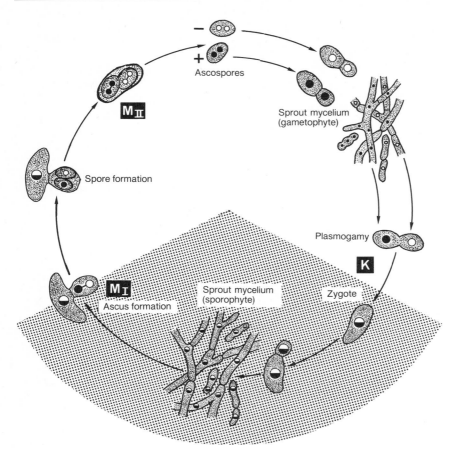

Fig. 2-4. Life cycle of *Saccharomycopsis lipolytica*. Diplont; mode of fertilization: somatogamy between + – and − –cells.

are present. Yeasts of this type are used in many countries for the production of single-cell protein from paraffins.

On a consideration of Figs. 2-3 and 2-4, it is clear that in both species of yeasts there are two different mating types because of an obstacle to fertilization. This is the case with by no means all yeasts. Other biotechnologically relevant forms such as, for example, Pichia and Hansenula, are self-fertile.

On the basis of their morphological and physiological characteristics, a number of imperfect forms, which also play a part in the

fermentation industry, are also reckoned among the yeasts.

b) 2nd Order: Taphrinales (Exoascales)

Subclass *Plectomycetidae*:

Cleistothecium: closed spherical fruit body; the spores of the asci are liberated only after the breakdown or tearing of the wall of the fruit body (peridium).

a) 1st Order: Plectascales (Eurotiales)

To this taxon belong the classical objects of the fermentation industry, namely the repre-sentatives of the genera Penicillium and Aspergillus and also the genus Cephalosporium, which has only recently come into

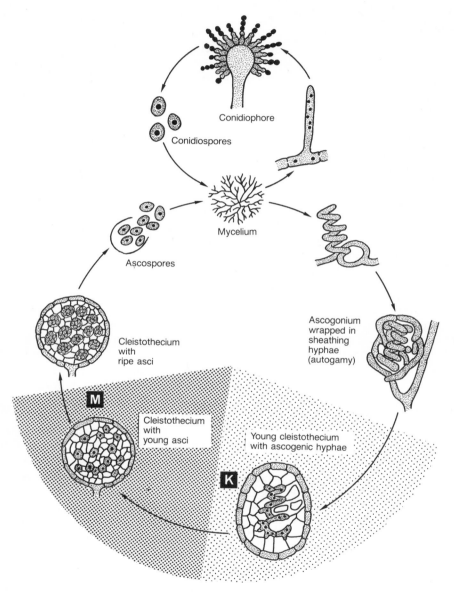

Conidiophore

Conidiospores

Mycelium

Ascospores

Cleistothecium with ripe asci

Ascogonium wrapped in sheathing hyphae (autogamy)

M

Cleistothecium with young asci

Young cleistothecium with ascogenic hyphae

K

Fig. 2-5. Life cycle of *Aspergillus repens*. Haplodikaryont with asexual propagation by conidiospores; mode of fertilization: autogamy.

prominence. Most species of these three genera are imperfect and are placed in this order of perfect fungi only because of their typical conidiophores. One of the less perfect representatives, namely *Aspergillus repens* serves as the index form. As can be seen from Fig. 2-5, this, like all higher ascomycetes, is a haplodikaryont which, however, can propagate asexually by conidiospores.

b) 2nd Order: Erysiphales (true powdery mildew)

Subclass *Loculomycetidae:*

Pseudothecium: only after the formation of the spherical primordia of the fruit bodies are the gametangia formed in cavities (loculi); the spores of the asci are thrown out through openings which arise locally through the gelatinization of the peridium.
Five Orders, no biotechnological relevance, mainly plant parasites.

Subclass *Pyrenomycetidae:*

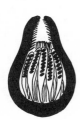

Perithecium: closed, bottle-shaped fruit body; asci arise as a closed layer (hymenium) frequently together with sterile hyphae (paraphyses); expulsion usually takes place successively through a preformed opening (ostiolum) of the "bottle neck", which is lined with sterile hyphae (periphyses). Several to many of the perithecia can be embedded in plectenchymatic stroma of special structure.

a) 1st Order: Sphaeriales

Although some of the most important fungi for **basic research** such as Neurospora, Podospora, and Sordaria belong to the Sphaeriales, this group is of subordinate importance in biotechnology. In this connection only the genus Gibberella needs to be mentioned; this is a fungus that has become known by the production of the growth agent gibberellin, and a number of imperfect species of this genus which were earlier included under the name Fusarium. Exhaustive information on the "genus Fusarium" is given by Booth (1971).

Large numbers of the perithecia of Gibberella are embedded in plectenchymatic structures. Since the life cycle of this haplodikaryont has not yet been elucidated in all its details, we shall not give an account of it here. However, it corresponds in principle to that of *Claviceps purpurea* (see Fig. 2-6).

b) 2nd Order: Clavicipitales

In the only family of this order, the Clavicipitaceae, there are two genera, namely Claviceps and Epichloe, which are both plant parasites. *Claviceps purpurea,* which, mainly on rye, but also on other graminaceous plants, evokes the formation of the so-called **ergot,** even though it has already been known for centuries, is still of biotechnological interest today. In fact, it is possible to produce the alkaloids that it forms in fermenter cultures, as well. These substances are the starting materials for a large number of drugs. Its life cycle, which has only recently been elucidated, is shown in Fig. 2-6. Typical for this haplodikaryote are the eight rod-shaped ascospores. Although the formation of the perithecia on germinating sclerotia, the germination of the ascospores, and the cultivation of the mycelium can be carried out under laboratory conditions, passage through a host is necessary for the performance of crossings. References are given by Esser and Tudzynski, 1978.

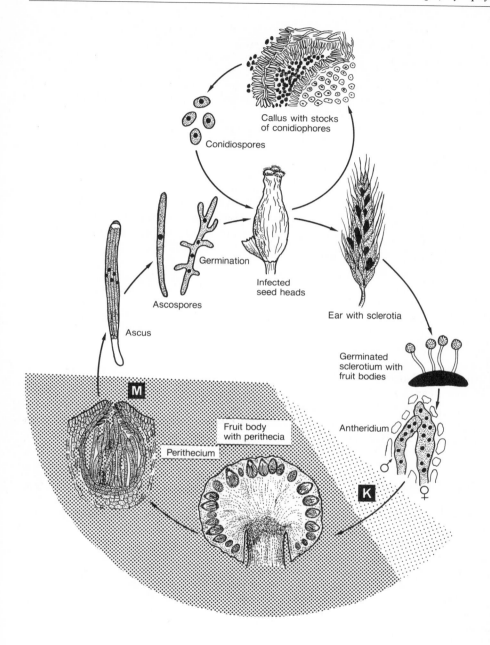

Fig. 2-6. Life cycle of *Claviceps purpurea*. Haplodikaryont with asexual propagation by aplanospores; mode of fertilization: anisogametangiogamy.

c) 3rd Order: Laboulbeniales

Subclass Discomycetidiae:

 Apothecium: disk- or cup-shaped fruit body which, in the mature state, bears a hymenium on its surface.

a) 1st Order: Pezizales

b) 2nd Order: Helotiales

c) 3rd Order: Phacidiales

d) 4th Order: Tuberales

This taxon includes, in particular the various Tuber species that have long been of great interest as edible truffles. Since it has not so far been possible to keep truffle mycelium in laboratory cultures to a worthwhile extent (rate of growth 1 to 2 mm per month), with these mycorrhizal fungi (e.g., oak, hazel) one must, as before, have recourse to outdoor production. Apart from natural occurrence, recently experiments have been carried out on the large scale on the growing of these fungi in culture gardens in the Mediterranean area (literature in Grente (1974) and Delmas (1976)).

4th Class: Basidiomycetes

Basidial fungi, richly branched mycelia with perforated transverse walls which, however, are closed by a barrel-like structure (doliporus). Cell nuclei and other cell organelles can pass through the septa only after the breakdown of the doliporus. Mode of life: saprophytes and parasites almost exclusively terrestrial. In the case of the saprophytes, the best known are the edible fungi, and in the case of the parasites the rust fungi and smuts (Uredinales, Ustilaginales) as the causative agents of plant diseases. The so-called wood-destroying fungi (mostly saprophytes) are of practical importance for the degradation of lignin and cellulose, and their fruit bodies can also be used as edible fungi. Many basidiomycetes live

as symbionts in the roots of bushes and trees (Mycorrhiza). Asexual propagation by conidio-, oidio-, or chlamydospores. Specific conidiophores such as occur in the ascomycetes, are rarely formed. Sexual propagation by basidiospores; mode of fertilization: mainly somatogamy. Life cycle: the dikaryotic phase predominates.

Division into subclasses according to the structure of the basidium. In the subclass Phragmobasidiomycetidae (Heterobasidiomycetidae, Hemibasidiomycetidae) the basidium is subdivided by transverse walls. Since **no biotechnologically relevant forms** are found in this group, no further breaking down into orders is given.

Subclass: Holobasidiomycetidae

(Homobasidiomycetidae, Autobasidiomycetidae). The basidium is not subdivided.

a) 1st Order: Exobasidiales:

Endoparasites, hymenium on the upper side of the fallen parts of plants; no fruiting bodies.

b) 2nd Order: Poriales (Aphyllophorales, Boletaceae, Polyporaceae):

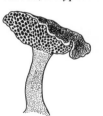 Hymenium in tubes, on crests and only rarely on gills: fruit bodies crust-like, console-shaped, more rarely pileus-like.

Representatives of this order are predominantly **wood-rotting fungi,** the so-called brown rot fungi (degradation of cellulose) and white rot fungi (degradation of cellulose and lignin). Both the fungi as such and also the enzymes obtained from them are used for **processes of recycling** wood, straw, and other cellulose and lignin-containing wastes. No special index form will be described since their development cycles, where known, agree with those of the Agaricales (see also Fig. 2-7).

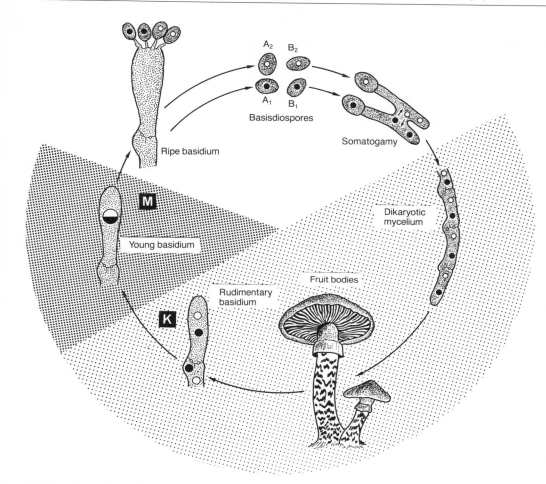

Fig. 2-7. Life cycle of *Agrocybe aegerita*. Dikaryont; mode of fertilization: somatogamy between genetically different mating types.

c) 3rd Order: Agricales (Phyllophorales, agarics, gill-fungi):

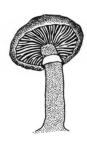

Hymenium predominantly on gills, more rarely in tubes; fruiting bodies generally with pileus having a central stalk.

In this order, in addition to the best-known **edible fungi (mushroom, shii-take fungus) there is also a large number of wood-degrading fungi** and **antibiotics-producers** (Anke, 1978). As the index form we may give *Agrocybe aegerita,* which has not only been investigated accurately from the genetic aspect but is also used as an edible fungus (poplar mushroom), as well as for the degradation of wood and straw and as a producer of antibiotics (Meinhardt, 1980). As follows from Fig. 2-7, this is a typical dikaryont, the mating behavior of which is determined by complex genetic factors (A, B). A definite gene sequence is also responsible for the formation of the fruit body which follows the dikaryotic mycelium.

d) 4th Order: Gasteromycetales:

 Hymenium in a chambered inner cavity of the usually stalked or unstalked bulb-like fruiting body.

Some producers of antibiotics have also recently been found in this group (Anke et al., 1977).

Fungi Imperfecti (Deuteromycetes)

In contrast to all other plant divisions, within the fungi there is a large number of organisms that have lost the **capacity for sexual** reproduction. Since the taxonomy of the fungi is based predominantly on the form of the organs of propagation, these fungi cannot be assigned to the existing classes of fungi with a "perfect" life cycle. They are therefore collected together as "Fungi imperfecti" or Deuteromycetes in a special taxon which is added on as a so-called form class to the four classes of perfect fungi.

In this taxon there is a wealth of biotechnologically relevant fungi which, as already described above for Aspergillus, Penicillium, and Cephalosporium, are, so far as possible, placed in the orders of the perfect fungi on the basis of certain morphological characteristics.

2.3.3 Biotechnologically Important Fungi

The fungi of biotechnological relevance are listed in Table 2-2 on the basis of the taxonomic classification given above. This compilation obviously makes no claim to completeness.

2.3.4 General Remarks on Cultivation, Maintenance, and Storage

In the following sections, reference can be made to a large extent to an earlier publication (Esser, 1982).

Nutrient Media

Apart from the obligate parasites, the cultivation of which in the laboratory is impossible, and the few saprophytes, which grow only on their natural substrates, the fungi can, in general, be grown on **natural media** for our purposes. Here the following natural products are used alone or in various combinations.

Corn meal extract*, malt extract*, yeast extract*, peptone*, sucrose (commercial product), glucose, and, especially for the coprophilic fungi, feces from plant-eating animals, especially horse droppings. These natural media, which can be prepared without a great expenditure of time, also contain the necessary minerals, trace elements, and vitamins, so that these need not be added.

Universal media:

– **Corn meal medium:** Standard medium for most fungi. 1000 mL of maize meal extract, 5 g of malt extract, 2 mL of a 10% solution of potassium hydroxide. Maize meal extract: suspend 250 g of maize meal in 10 L of tap water and incubate overnight at 60°C. Decant off the supernatant and discard the deposit. The maize meal should be derived from the ordinary commercial variety of "yellow corn" and not be ground too finely so that husks and aleurone are not lost.

* Corn meal can be obtained from the Getreidemühle H. Niewind, 4364 Datteln-Klostern, Federal Republic of Germany; malt extract from Diamalt AG, 8000 München [Munich] 40, Friedrichstr. 18; Federal Republic of Germany; yeast extract (Merck 3751), peptone (Merck 7216).

Table 2-2. Summary of Fungi of Biotechnological Importance (using information from Rehm, 1980).

Order	Genera	Products
Zygomycetales	Phycomyces Mucor Rhizopus	Organic acids, enzymes
	Blakeslea Choanephora	*β*-Carotene
Endomycetales	Ashbya Candida Cryptococcus Eremothecium Rhodotorula Saccharomyces Saccharomycopsis Torulopsis	Riboflavine Citric acid Protein Riboflavine Lipids Ethanol Proteins Citric acid
Plectascales	Aspergillus Cephalosporium Penicillium	Antibiotics, organic acids, enzymes Antibiotics Antibiotics, organic acids, enzymes Enzymes, mycotoxins
Sphaeriales	Fusarium Gibberella	Gibberellins, protein, fats Substances with hormone-like action
Clavicipitales	Claviceps	Alkaloids
Tuberales	Tuber	Biomass
Poriales	Polyporus Trametes	Conversion of lignin Enzymes
Agaricales	Agaricus Agrocybe Lentinus Pleurotus Oudemansiella Volvariella	Biomass Biomass Biomass, pharmaceuticals Antibiotics, biomass Antibiotics Biomass
Gasteromycetales	Cyathus	Antibiotics

– **Corn meal-malt medium:** Modification of the maize medium, particularly for holobasidiomycetes, using 30 g instead of 5 g of malt extract. Media ready for the laboratory of similar compositions are supplied by Difco and Merck (Bacto Corn Meal Agar B 386, Bacto Corn Meal with dextran B 114; prepared medium: Merck 13840).

- **Corn meal-acetate medium:** Standard medium for the germination of ascospores of coprophilic fungi. In addition to corn meal medium: 2.3 mL of a 10% solution of potassium hydroxide, 4.4 g of ammonium acetate (for Podospora) or 5 g of sodium acetate (for Sordaria).

- **Malt medium** for liquid cultures of asco- and basidiomycetes: 15 g of malt extract, 4 mL of a 10% solution of potassium hydroxide, 1000 mL of tap water.

- **Horse manure.** Universal medium for all coprophilic fungi, which, in particular promotes the germination of spores because of its high acetate content. Fresh horse dung, which should be derived from animals that have been fed with oats and must not be soaked with horse urine (uric acid!) is well moistened with tap water and pressed into the desired culture vessels and sterilized.

- **Horse manure medium** can be used in place of horse dung. After the addition of agar, it has a smooth surface and does not dry out as rapidly as horse dung. 100 mL of horse dung extract, 5 g of maltose, 0.5 g of magnesium sulfate heptahydrate ($MgSO_4 \cdot 7 H_2O$), 0.5 g of calcium nitrate ($Ca(NO_3)_2$), 0.25 g of dipotassium hydrogen phosphate (K_2HPO_4), 0.19 g of peptone, and 100 mL of distilled water.

- **Horse manure extract:** boil one "horse dropping" per 150 mL of tap water in an Erlenmeyer flask with an absorbent cotton plug in the water bath for 1 to 2 hours, and after decantation and filtration use the supernatant. Prepare this extract afresh each time, since it easily decomposes and does not withstand repeated sterilization.

Presporulation medium for *Saccharomyces cerevisiae:*

20 g of glucose, 2 g of ammonium sulfate (($NH_4)_2SO_4$), 2 g of potassium dihydrogen phosphate (KH_2PO_4), 5 g of yeast extract, and 1000 mL of distilled water. Before use, this medium should be kept in the sterile state for at least 7 days.

Sporulation medium for *Saccharomyces cerevisiae:*

1 g of glucose, 8.2 g of potassium acetate, 2.5 g of yeast extract, 1.86 g of potassium chloride (KCl), 0.35 g of magnesium sulfate heptahydrate ($MgSO_4 \cdot 7H_2O$), 1000 mL of distilled water. In contrast to the presporulation medium, this medium must be used immediately after sterilization.

Pure Cultures

a) **Single-Spore or Single-Cell Cultures: Manual isolation** under the **preparation microscope** is the simplest method. However, it requires cells with a size of at least 10 µm.

For this purpose, so-called hard agar is used, i.e., a 5% sterile aqueous agar filled into Petri dishes in such a way that the upper edge of the agar is just below the rim of the dish (this facilitates manipulation with the preparation needle since it is possible to work in the regions near the edge, as well). Since under certain circumstances it is necessary to work with the bottom light of the preparation microscope, only highly purified agar (e.g., Difco Bacto-agar) should be used so that the gel is clear and transparent.

This technique is suitable, in particular, for fungi that throw off active spores. The Petri dish filled with aqueous agar is placed upside down on a fungal culture that has been grown in a Petri dish of equal size, and the edges are sealed with transparent adhesive tape. After sufficient spores have been thrown off, under the preparation microscope with the aid of the preparation needle by gently moving the spores over the agar it is possible to isolate individual spores and, after cutting them out with a small piece of agar, to transfer them to the appropriate nutrient medium. Petri dishes marked on the bottom are best used for this purpose. After the incubation of the culture, the formation of mycelium can also be followed under the preparation microscope, and stock cultures can be set up by reinoculation in slope agar tubes.

This method can also be applied when it is desired to isolate vegetative cells, which are previously transferred from suitable cultures to the hard agar. Manual isolation has the advantage that even mixed cultures can be used, since with larger objects under the preparation microscope the spores or cells of different plants can be distinguished. However, limits are set to this method by the size of the cells to be manipulated. Thus, the ascospores of yeasts (diameter about 3 μm) cannot be isolated under the preparation microscope. The same also applies to many conidiospores. In these cases, the very accurate but also laborious method of **micromanipulation** must be used. This involves performing the appropriate manipulations under a special microscope by means of minute glass tools manufactured under the microscope which are included in a hydraulic system capable of moving in three dimensions (de Fonbrune, 1949).

The **plating method** is used particularly in the case of smaller objects. Here the process starts from suspensions of cells or spores; the medium used is either sterile nutrient medium or 1/4 strength Ringer solution.* After the titer of the suspension has been determined with the aid of a counting chamber**, such as is used in the determination of the erythrocyte number in the clinic, and appropriate dilution, about 2 mL of the suspension is pipetted into a Petri dish containing nutrient agar and is uniformly distributed in it by tipping the dish back and forth. The number of cells transferred is governed by the rate of growth, e.g., in the case of unicellular algae or yeasts that form only colonies, up to 100 cells per dish are plated out, while, on the other hand, in the case of mycelium-forming fungi which, like, for example, Neurospora, have a growth rate of several cm/day, only about ten. With this method, as well, it is unconditionally necessary to check under the microscope after not more than 24 h whether and which cells are growing.

However, the plating method is associated with a certain safety risk. Since in no case is it possible with 100% certainty to exclude the possibility that two or even more cells have remained attached to one another, the possibility exists that colonies or mycelia from several cells have developed.

b) **Selective Methods of Cultivation:** Bacterial infections in fungal cultures can be relatively easily eliminated by the **addition of antibiotics** to the agar nutrient medium.

The antibiotic must in no case be autoclaved with the nutrient medium. Dissolved in or diluted with sterile water, it is added to Petri dishes filled with agar media after the contaminated cultures have grown. Then after only a short time it is usually possible to cut out bacteria-free cells or pieces of mycelium from the edge zones of the culture with the preparation needle and the preparation microscope.

With rapidly growing hyphal fungi that are infected with bacteria, as a rule the use of antibiotics can be renounced and bacteria-free hyphal tips be cut out from the edge zones after one or two passages of the culture.

---

* Preparation: 0.9 g of sodium chloride, 0.042 g of potassium chloride, 0.048 g of calcium chloride (CaCl$_2$·6H$_2$O), 0.02 g of sodium carbonate, and 400 mL of distilled water autoclaved at 120°C for 20 min. The salts can be obtained in tablet form from Merck (10113).

** E.g., counting chamber according to Neubauer: instructions for use can be obtained from Hallman, L: *Klinische Chemie und Mikroskopie,* 9th Ed. Thieme-Verlag, Stuttgart 1960.

Maintenance and Storage

In principle, the procedure here may be the same as has been described for bacteria (see p. 26). However, it must be pointed out that freezing and freeze-drying are preferably applied only to those fungi that sporulate copiously. Nonsporulating hyphal fungi do not withstand this treatment. In this connection, it must necessarily be mentioned that there are also a number of thermosensitive fungi which do not survive storage even at temperatures below 10°C, e.g., numerous aquatic phycomycetes and also the straw-degrading basidiomycete Volvariella (further information in Esser, 1976).

2.4 Strain Improvement

In biotechnology, as soon as one has a microorganism available that forms a certain useful product, the aim exists to **increase its yield.** This can be done, on the one hand, by changing or **improving the external conditions** (process optimization) or, on the other hand, by genetic manipulation (see section 2.4.4).

The genetic methods that have been used so far are directed, on the one hand, to the organism and its characteristics (e.g., eukaryote/prokaryote, sexual cycle/no sexual cycle), but on the other hand they may be historically determined and be directed according to the current state of basic research.

2.4.1 Selection

This is the oldest and simplest method and has been used since the beginning of human technology – more or less unconsciously – particularly in the breeding of plants and animals when from among the production strains the best-producing are continuously selected out. This method by the **"seek and discard principle"** is frequently called **screening** and even today represents the beginning of any process of strain improvement.

2.4.2 Selection with Subsequent Mutation

When the artificial initiation of mutations (constant hereditary changes in the genome) by means of energy-rich radiation became known, this process was used relatively early in the plant-breeding field (Knapp, 1938).

It found entry into microbial genetics only with the further development of mutational genetics and, namely, with the knowledge that mutations can also be induced by chemical agents. It is just by this process that considerable improvement in production has been achieved in the last few years.

Initiation of Mutation

a) **Chemical Mutagenesis.** Chemical mutagens are usually classified in textbooks according to their action mechanism, i.e., whether they change, replace, or eliminate bases. Without going into details that are not necessary for practical application, the following classification can be undertaken:

Base analogs cause a transition, i.e., an interchange, of a purine or a pyrimidine base; e.g., 5-bromouracil leads to the replacement of cytosine by thymidine (C-T).

2-Aminopurine leads to the replacement of adenine by guanine (A-G).

Deaminating and alkylating substances can also cause transitions, e.g., nitrite ($NaNO_2$) deaminates A and C, and on replication AT pairs are replaced by GC pairs, and conversely.

$CH_3SO_3CH_2CH_3$

Ethyl methanesulfonate (EMS) and methylnitro-nitrosoguanidine (MNNG) also mainly cause transitions through the alkylation of bases. MNNG is probably the most promising mutagen since it causes only a relatively low lethality – as compared with its mutation-inducing effect.

Intercalating substances, such as acridine dyes (e.g., proflavine), by becoming inserted between the base pair, cause a so-called frame shift, i.e., the genetic information is read incorrectly because of a displacement.

b) **Physical Mutagenesis.** Energy-rich rays of various origins are used as physical mutagens.

- **X-Rays.** Since Müller (1927) discovered that these ionizing rays caused mutations in the fruit fly Drosophila, up to about the middle of the forties X-rays were used almost exclusively for the production of artificial mutants. In general, however, particularly in the case of mi-

croorganisms, these have the disadvantage that **chromosomal mutations** such as breaks, deletions, etc., are initiated to a large, and point mutations to only a small, extent.

- **Ultraviolet rays.** After the discovery by Knapp (1938) that DNA absorbs UV at 260 nm and on the basis of his subsequent first mutation experiment with UV, this agent was widely used in the subsequent period. Since after UV treatment it is mainly **point mutations** that occur, even today it is impossible to consider practical operations without it. In contrast to X-rays, in the case of UV something about the molecular action mechanism is known, namely that far-reaching thymine dimerizations are initiated. Also connected with this is the so-called **photorepair;** i.e., if, after UV irradiation, the organism is kept in the light a reversion of the effect takes place. It is therefore customary after UV mutagenesis to keep the objects treated in the dark for a relatively long period. Details in Esser and Kuenen (1967).
- **Radioisotopes.** Only recently in the course of improvements in labeling techniques with radioactive material have isotopes also been used for the initiation of mutations.

In practice, with no object is it possible to predict what type of mutagenesis offers the greatest prospects for a given purpose. It is therefore indispensable first to test various mutagens in a kind of screening operation.

Isolation of mutants

Here, the terms **variants** and **mutants** must first be clearly defined. Unfortunately, in the last three years the custom has arisen that many authors, when they obtain functionally changed organisms by treatment with mutagens, call these organisms mutants. Originally, however, **mutants** was the term given only to those organisms in which the spontaneous or induced change reappeared constantly even after a passage through a sexual cycle. This was natural at a time when work was being carried out exclusively with eukaryotes.

It is difficult to apply this definition to prokaryotes and Fungi imperfecti. Here, nevertheless, one should only speak of mutants when after relatively long vegetative multiplication the changed characteristic is retained. In other cases it is better to speak of **variants.**

For the isolation of any type of mutants from a population of irradiated genetic material a **selection system** is required. This is governed by the type of the desired mutation. Selection mechanisms for nutritionally defective mutants, resistance mutants, and temperature-sensitive and similar types of mutations that are used in basic research predominantly as **genetic labels** are relatively simple. The establishment of a selection system for mutations which aim at **improving the yield** in the production of given primary and secondary metabolites or of certain enzymes is more complicated.

Procedures for the isolation of mutants are given in a short review (Table 2-3). This compilation makes no claim whatever to completeness. For this purpose the relevant textbooks should be used such as, for example, for bacteria Hayes (1974), for fungi Esser and Kuenen (1967), for general microbiology Schlegel (1976), and for applied microbiology Crueger and Crueger (1982).

2.4.3 Selection and Mutation with Subsequent Recombination

Obviously, even at an early period use was made, if always unconsciously, of a **new combination of the genetic material** particularly in animal and plant breeding. However, in the past this was used deliberately in the improvement of microorganisms by breeding only to a relatively small extent, and this mostly because with these organisms the technical prerequisites for performing recombination such as,

for example, an accurate knowledge of the life cycle and the system of propagation, were not available.

An important prerequisite for the use of this method is the possibility of determining the results of recombinations with certainty and rapidity. In the first cases, naturally, so far as the eukaryotes are concerned, the haplonts offered an advantage, since in them the phenotype is identical with the genotype, and, of course, this also applies to all prokaryotes in which likewise there is only one genome per cell.

The fastest possibility of determining recombinants is provided by the so-called **tetrad analysis,** a method that can be applied to eukaryotes (as, for example, in the case of the yeast *Saccharomyces cerevisiae,* see Fig. 2-3). It consists in the possibility of isolating the four products of a meiotic division (in this fungus, four spores) and cultivating them separately (details in Esser and Kuenen, 1967).

With many other eukaryotes, the performance of tetrad analysis is not possible for various reasons: either because the spores are too small or because the four products of meiosis do not remain together in the course of development. Here one must have recourse to **random analysis,** which already requires a selection to a certain degree, which, particularly for the prokaryotes, is an invariable procedure for the determination of recombinants.

When a sexual cycle is either unknown or, because of deficient knowledge of culture conditions, cannot be performed in the laboratory, for the preparation of recombinants recourse must be made to the various **mechanisms of the parasexual cycle.** In the case of fungi, this means in the first place mitotic recombination; in the case of bacteria use can be made of conjugation, transformation, or transduction, depending on the object. In each case, both with eukaryotes and also with prokaryotes, of course, the rate of recombination is far lower and the experimental effort is higher than when the sexual cycle is used. A review of the practical use of the sexual cycle

Table 2-3. Procedure for the Isolation of Mutants.

Type of mutant		Enrichment	Recognition test
Auxotrophic	bacteria	Cultivation in minimal medium with the addition of an antibiotic which acts only on growing cells (e.g., penicillin)	Plating out on complete medium and replica plating (Lederberg technique) on to minimal medium with various supplements
	fungi	a) See Bacteria b) Cultivation in minimal medium and filtration off of the germinated mycelia	Plating out on complete medium and replating on minimal medium with the filter paper replica technique. Testing of suspects on minimal medium with various supplements
Resistant	bacteria and fungi	Plating out a large number of cells on solid nutrient media with the addition of the inhibiting substance	Direct, since only the resistant cells grow in colonies
Temperature-sensitive	bacteria and fungi	a) At higher temperatures, see resistant b) At lower temperature; "penicillin technique", see auxotrophic	a) Direct, since only temperature-sensitive mutants grow b) Incubation at normal temperature leads to the dying off of the wild-type cells and then cultivation at a low temperature shows up the temperature-sensitive mutants
Constitutive, catabolic, enzymes		a) Simulation of catabolite repression by an antiinductor b) Cultivation with substrate as limiting factor c) Alternating cultivation on two substrates	a) Direct, since only those colonies grow that possess the enzyme constitutively b) Direct c) Constitutive organisms become established faster
Constitutive, anabolic, enzymes		Cultivation with the addition of a antimetabolite that possesses end-product repression	Direct, since only those cells grow that do so in spite of the antimetabolites

in fungi has been published elsewhere (Esser and Stahl, 1981). A corresponding summary for bacteria is unnecessary, since with these prokaryotes, by definition, only parasexual mechanisms can lead to a recombination.

In this connection, it is unconditionally necessary to go into another problem, namely the **combination of genetic material from different organisms.** In the perfect eukaryotes, in general, there are no difficulties, since the sexual process is induced by the **fusion of sex cells** or sex organs. Here, as well, the obstacles to fertilization that frequently occur (see p. 30) can be circumvented by certain techniques and methods. The combination of genetic material in the case of organisms that exhibit no sexual cycle is more difficult. As already mentioned, in the case of fungi it is possible to induce mitotic recombination by the **formation of heterokaryons.** As a rule, however, this process requires that the genetic material should be forced together, which takes place if the two partners are brought together by a **complementation of auxotrophic characteristics** (forced heterokaryons). In a number of other cases, however, the **formation of heterokaryons** fails because of the inability of the two partners to break down their cell walls and fuse. This difficulty can be bridged over by the **artificial production of protoplasts,** in which the cell walls of fungi, and also of bacteria, are degraded enzymatically, this being carried out in a medium isotonic for the cell. Experience has shown that the protoplasts prepared in this way fuse relatively easily under suitable conditions but after fusion they divide only a few times and then regenerate their cell walls. The principle of the protoplast method is shown in Fig. 2-8 using as example the alkane yeast *Saccharomycopsis lipolytica.* In many cases it is not necessary to degrade the cell wall completely. Such cells in which cell wall residues still adhere to the plasmalemma are called **sphaeroplasts.**

A practical introduction to the production of protoplasts has been published by Peberdy (1979). As an example of the application of these techniques through the improvement of strains, the investigations of Hamlyn and Ball (1979) may be given.

2.4.4   Gene Manipulation

The techniques for the exchange of genetic material that have been described so far, whether within a sexual or a parasexual system, find their limitation – quite apart from methodological difficulties – where it is required to go beyond the boundaries of a genus and in many cases even that of a species, since it has been possible to do this with the aid of the technique described above in only a few cases – e.g., in the case of antibiotics producing Aspergillaceae.

Starting from the fact that it is possible to cleave DNA at quite definite points by specific enzymes (endonucleases, restriction enzymes) and then to link it up again subsequently by means of another type of enzyme (ligases), in the last few years the **method of genetic engineering** (gene manipulation) has been developed. A very clear and simple summary of the method and results of this technique is given by Old and Primrose (1980).

The principle of this technique is that genetic information is isolated from a donor organism and is cleaved by restriction enzymes into individual pieces. These pieces are incorporated in a carrier DNA and transferred with this vector into another cell.

Practical experience with this technique has been obtained essentially for the transfer of genetic information within bacteria (Maniatis et al., 1982).

An essential prerequisite for a successful application of gene manipulation in practice is the availability of a suitable vector which ensures both replication and maintenance not only of the vector DNA but also of integrated foreign genetic material.

For any vector system and especially for plasmids the following features are considered to be of particular importance:

1. **Selectable markers:** Apart from the "classical" antibiotic resistance genes of *E. coli* plasmids, auxotrophic markers or other genes phenotypically easy to recognize are required.

2. **Restriction sites:** These sites represent the loci at which foreign DNA is integrated. The insertion of foreign DNA into the

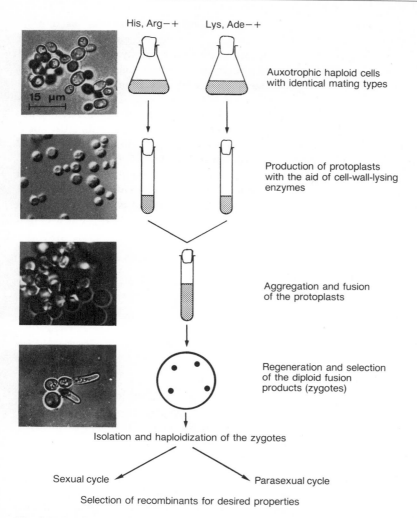

His, Arg—+   Lys, Ade—+

Auxotrophic haploid cells
with identical mating types

Production of protoplasts
with the aid of cell-wall-lysing
enzymes

Aggregation and fusion
of the protoplasts

Regeneration and selection
of the diploid fusion
products (zygotes)

Isolation and haploidization of the zygotes

Sexual cycle   Parasexual cycle

Selection of recombinants for desired properties

Fig. 2-8. Production, fusion, and regeneration of protoplasts as prerequisite for the recombination of genetic material shown for the case of the alkane yeast *Saccharomycopsis lipolytica*. Details in Stahl (1978, 1980).

sequence coding for an antibiotic resistance leads to the inactivation of the gene concerned. Cells lacking growth in the presence of the antibiotic may easily be detected. Thus it is desirable to have marker genes with unique restriction sites.

3. **Molecular weight:** In order to avoid damages by shearing forces during the process of preparation, vectors should have a molecular weight as low as possible. In addition, low molecular weight is normally accompanied by a high copy number.

The most effective and widely used vector systems will be presented below. Additionally, examples showing their biotechnological relevance will be given.

Cloning with Plasmids

The best known cloning vehicle is probably the bacterial plasmid pBR 322. This vector was created artificially by using different parts of certain naturally occuring plasmids; for details see Bolivar et al. (1977a, b). In *E.coli* the pBR 322 confers resistance against the antibiotic ampicillin (ApR) as well as tetracycline (TcR). Within the regions coding for the antibiotic resistances many unique restriction sites for different endonucleases exist. Taken together with its low molecular weight (4.3 kbp; 2.8 MD; 1.39 μm), it becomes obvious why this plasmid has been used for gene cloning throughout the world since its creation.

The principle of gene cloning with pBR 322 is outlined in Fig. 2-9.

In the last few years it has been shown repeatedly that even the **eukaryote/prokaryote boundary** can be crossed with the aid of this technique (Struhl et al., 1976; Ratzkin and

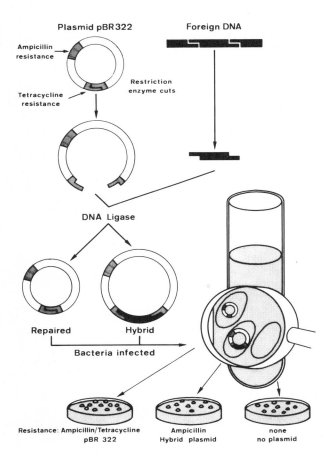

Fig. 2-9. Principle of gene cloning using the *E.coli* plasmid pBR 322. The vector and the foreign DNA are cleaved with the same restriction enzyme; the restriction site is located within the TcR resistance gene of pBR 322. After mixing and ligation two types of plasmids are recovered: the original vector (religated) and a hybrid molecule consisting of the vector and a piece of foreign DNA. After infection of the bacteria with the ligation mixture 3 types of cells can be differentiated on the appropiate media: 1) Cells carrying the (religated) vector exhibit tetracycline resistance as well as ampicillin resistance. 2) Cells carrying the hybrid plasmid exhibit only ampicillin resistance because the tetracycline resistance is inactivated by the integration of the foreign DNA. 3) Cells carrying no plasmids are sensitive to both antibiotics.

Carbon, 1977). These experiments have found a great response in the mass media, particularly since they relate to such sensational transmission of information as, for example, the transfer of genetic information for the production of insulin or interferon from animal cells into bacterial cells (Gilbert and Villa-Komaroff, 1980; Goedell et al., 1979). The expectations that were roused particularly by the popularization of this technique have, however, frequently not been confirmed in practice when the necessary criterion of an **economic production** has been made the basis of industrial application. The problems arising in the transfer and realization of genetic information from eukaryotes into prokaryotes have recently been pointed out by McLeod (1980).

Bacteriophages and Cosmids

One of the most thoroughly studied *E. coli* viruses is the bacteriophage lambda. The DNA of this virus is about 47 kbp in size and linear when isolated directly from phage particles. The 5′ ends of the double-stranded (ds) lambda-genome exhibit short single-stranded (ss) regions which are 12 nucleotides in size. By the association of these cohesive termini upon injection into the host cell the **cos site** is formed and the lambda-DNA adopts a circular structure.

It is not very convenient to use wild-type lambda for gene cloning because – among many other reasons – there are too many sites on the lambda-genome for the restriction enzymes normally used.

Derivatives carrying only one site for a special restriction endonuclease have been constructed. Foreign DNA (insertion vectors) can be integrated into this target site. The removal of phage DNA which is not essential and which is replaced by foreign DNA is another way to use lambda for gene cloning (replacement vectors), (Thomas et al., 1974; Murray and Murray, 1975; Leder et al., 1977).

The in vitro packaging of the recombined DNA molecules into phage particles markedly enhances transformation frequency: normally 10^4 to 10^6 plaques/µg DNA in transfection experiments using recombinant DNA; up to 10^7 plaques/µg using in vitro packaged DNA (Sternberg et al., 1977).

The DNA of phage lambda is replicated via a special mechanism (rolling circle) which leads to the formation of concatemers. This concatemeric form of phage DNA is the substrate for the packaging reaction. (Details in Hohn and Murray, 1977).

During packaging, at each **cos site** nicks are introduced 12 bp apart on opposite strands of the DNA generating the cohesive termini that are found in λ DNA in phage particles. Packaging takes place only if the DNA to be packaged fulfills two criteria: (1) a small recognition region near the **cos site** must be present and (2) the distance between **cos sites** in the concatemeric DNA must be about 47 kbp, thus resembling the size of wild-type lambda DNA (Hohn, 1975).

A recombinant phage constructed in vitro that carries the *E. coli* DNA ligase gene induces after infection of the host a five-hundredfold overproduction of the enzyme which then represents 5% of total protein. (Panasenko et al., 1977). More detailed information about expression of genes cloned in lambda will be found in Hopkins et al. (1976), Moir and Brammar (1976).

Plasmids which contain a fragment of DNA including the above mentioned **cos site** are called **cosmids** (Collins and Brüning, 1978; Collins and Hohn, 1978). These plasmids are used as vectors in connection with the in vitro packaging of DNA. This cloning system (cosmid together with in vitro packaging) permits selection for fragments of the desired size (see also Fig. 2-10), because the DNA to be packaged must be in the range of total natural lambda DNA.

After infection of the recombinant DNA into a susceptible *E. coli* strain the molecule

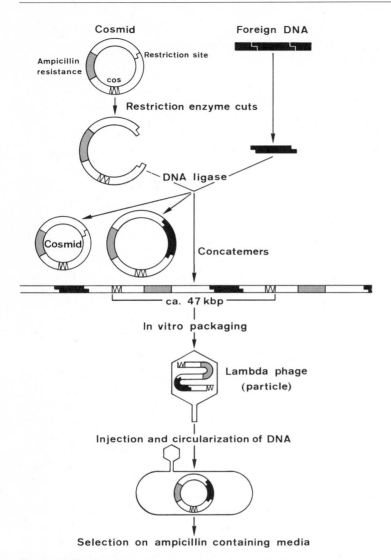

Fig. 2-10. Cloning using cosmids and in vitro packaging. For details see text.

circularizes and is replicated as a normal plasmid without the expression of any phage function. Transformants can be selected through antibiotic resistances as described above. Cosmids are therefore an excellent tool for cloning large DNA fragments, as is normally required for the establishment of so called genomic libraries.

Another Coli phage – M 13 –, which has a completely different genome organization and life cycle, has recently been developed as cloning vehicle (Messing et al., 1977; Barnes,

1979). M 13 is a filamentous *E. coli* phage containing ss DNA and may vary in size, so that it can easily harbor additional DNA. Within the infected cell the ss DNA is converted to a ds replicative form which amplifies up to 300 copies per cell. The phage does not lyse its host but growth is retarded. This causes the formation of turbid plaques when the material is plated on suitable bacteria. The properties of M 13 have been exploited in establishing a cloning system specially used for DNA sequencing, where large amounts of ss DNA are required. A **multiple cloning site** containing 10 or more unique restriction sites and, in addition, an effective selection system for the detection of recombinant phages were integrated into an inessential region of the M 13 genome. This system comprises the promotor/operator of the lac-operon plus the DNA sequence coding for 145 N-terminal amino acids of β-galactosidase. After the infection of certain *E. coli* strains carrying deletions into appropriate regions of the β-gal gene complementation results in an active enzyme.

Enzyme synthesis is experimentally stimulated by the inducer IPTG (isopropyl β-D-thiogalactopyranoside). Positive clones are easily detected on agar plates containing x-gal (5-bromo-4-chloro-3-indolyl β-D-galactopyranoside). The β-galactosidase converts this substrate into a blue dye (bromochloroindole).

A recombinant phage which contains a piece of foreign DNA in the multiple cloning site located within the β-galactosidase gene is not capable of complementing the deletion in the gene of the bacterial host. Recombinant phages will therefore cause white plaques on x-gal plates. The color reaction thus allows the direct detection of recombinant clones. For details see: Messing et al. (1981), Messing and Vieira (1982). The β-gal complementation system has also been used to construct other cloning vehicles such as plasmids (Rüther et al., 1981). Because of its general and still increasing importance this system is outlined

in Fig. 2-11. For reasons of clarity it is represented as being integrated into a plasmid.

Cloning in several organisms

Prokaryotes

The preceding paragraphs clearly show that the production of recombinant DNA is usually performed with *E. coli*. For practical applications cloning in other organisms will be of special interest: the Gram-positive, non-pathogenic bacteria of the genus Bacillus produce large amounts of extracellular enzymes (Henner and Hoch, 1980) and that is why gene cloning using this organism plays an important role for many biotechnological processes.

Molecular cloning systems in Bacillus have been developed following two different lines of research:

1. **Endogenous plasmids and phages:** Extrachromosomal DNA in bacilli was first described for *B. megaterium* and there have now been many reports of plasmids in this species (Carlton and Smith, 1974; Carlton and Brown, 1979; Rostas et al., 1980; Stahl and Esser, 1983). Consequently efforts have been made to develop a plasmid-mediated cloning system for *B. megaterium* (Brown and Carlton, 1980).

   The majority of the plasmids described for *B. megaterium,* as well as those for *B. subtilis* (Lovett and Bramucci, 1975; Tanaka and Koshikawa, 1977; Bernhard et al., 1978; Uozumi et al., 1980), lack identifiable markers and thus do not seem to be capable of use as cloning vehicles at this time.

   However, Bernhard et al. (1978) have isolated a tetracycline resistance (TcR) plasmid from a strain of *B. cereus* and Bingham et al. (1979) have found two TcR plasmids in thermophilic Bacillus species.

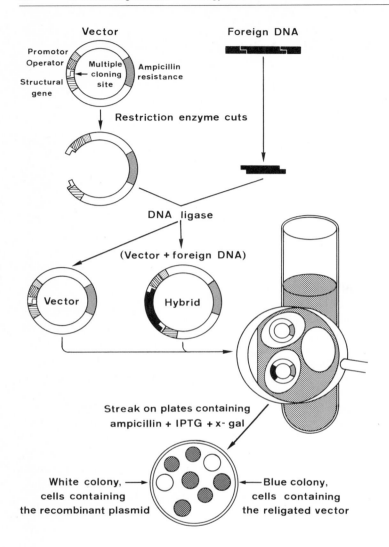

Fig. 2-11. Selection of recombinant DNA-molecules using the β-gal complementation system. The vector and the foreign DNA to be cloned are cleaved with the same restriction enzyme producing cuts in the multiple cloning site and in the foreign DNA. After infection of the appropiate *E.coli* strain with the ligation mixture and subsequent plating on medium containing the antibiotic ampicillin, IPTG as an inducer for enzyme synthesis, and x-gal as the substrate two types of colonies are recovered: 1) Blue colonies carrying the religated vector which complements the defect of the host strain resulting in an active β-galactosidase. 2) White colonies carrying hybrid plasmids. Insertion of foreign DNA has led to noncomplementation and therefore no active β-galactosidase is formed.

The TcR plasmid of *B. cereus* can also be used to transform *B. subtilis* (Bernhard et al., 1978). The plasmid is stable for more than 100 generations without selection pressure. Digestion with restriction enzymes and religation yielded small TcR plasmids with high copy numbers and single sites for some restriction enzymes (Kreft et al., 1978).

A fragment of the TcR resistance plasmid isolated from the above-mentioned *B. thermophilus* is also capable of autonomous replication in *B. subtilis*. A recombinant plasmid consisting of DNA from *E. coli* and *B. subtilis* has been successfully used to transform *B. subtilis* (Tanaka and Kawano, 1980).

Most of the plasmids described above are of limited value as cloning vehicles, because they carry only one marker and hence do not allow the identification of recombinants by insertional inactivation. Colony hybridization and immunologic methods may help to solve this problem.

Transducing phages have been used for cloning of heterologous DNA (Kawamura et al., 1980; Nomura et al., 1979), but these systems are far from being as effective as those described for *E. coli*. The development of comparable highly sophisticated techniques for gene cloning as available in *E. coli*, e.g., in vitro packaging, appears to be a prerequisite for successful and effective gene cloning in bacilli.

2. **Foreign plasmids:** As pointed out above, plasmids of various bacilli can be used for cloning in *B. subtilis* (for review see Kreft and Hughes, 1982). The search for vectors originating from distantly related organisms has also led to the development of potential cloning vehicles (for review see Ehrlich et al., 1982). A number of small, high-copy-number, antibiotic resistance plasmids originating from *Staphylococcus aureus* have been transferred into *B. subtilis*

(Ehrlich, 1977). Some of these plasmids were used for cloning without any modification. Foreign DNA was integrated into unique restriction sites located outside the only antibiotic resistance gene (Ehrlich, 1978; Gryczan and Dubnau, 1978; Keggins et al., 1978). An insertional inactivation vector (comparable to pBR 322 in *E. coli*) carrying two antibiotic resistance genes and having unique restriction sites within one of these loci was also used for cloning (Löfdahl et al., 1978; Gryczan et al., 1980).

Combining different plasmids of *S. aureus* with one other, with *E. coli* plasmids, or with Bacillus DNA has led to the construction of the so called **bridge plasmids** (= shuttle vectors) which are capable of replication in *B. subtilis* as well as in *E. coli* (Ehrlich, 1978; Michel et al., 1980; Gray and Chang, 1981). These vectors have the advantage that any method developed for *E. coli* can be used to construct hybrids and these may subsequently be tested in *B. subtilis*. For practical applications it is of special importance that *S. aureus* plasmids may be used as vectors in a palette of other organisms, since they are able to replicate not only in *B. subtilis* but also in *E. coli* (Goze and Ehrlich, 1980) and even yeast (Goursot et al., 1982).

The outstanding problem in the successful use of cloning in *B. subtilis* is the high degree of instability of the hybrid plasmids, observed either as the loss of plasmids or as rearrangements (Gryczan et al., 1980; Grandi et al., 1981; Gray and Chang, 1981). Studies concerning recombination in *B. subtilis* should help to overcome these difficulties.

Cloning systems have also been developed for other bacteria, e.g., Pseudomonas. For reviews see Sakaguchi (1982), Bagdasarian and Timmis (1982) and Streptomyces (Chater et al., 1982). The use of these systems for industrial purposes is still in its initial stages for reasons comparable in most cases to those outlined for *B. subtilis*.

Eukaryotes

Cloning in higher eukaryotes such as mammals and higher plants is beyond the scope of this contribution, but for those who are especially interested in this field we refer to the following reviews and monographs:

Mammalian cells:
Grass and Khoury (1982), Colbere-Garapin et al. (1982), Howard (1983).

Higher plants:
Hohn et al. (1982), van Montagu and Schell (1982), von Wettstein (1983) and a booklet edited by Pühler (1983).

The **vectors** currently in use **for transformation of eukaryotic microorganisms** (yeasts and filamentous fungi) are predominantly hybrids consisting of DNAs from *E. coli* plasmids and from the respective eukaryote.

The first transformation experiments with **yeast** were performed with strains carrying a nonrevertible mutation at the leu-2 gene locus. Transformation was achieved with hybrid plasmids consisting of the sequence of the wild-type leu-2 yeast gene integrated into a bacterial plasmid (Hinnen et al., 1978). Similar experiments were performed with plasmids carrying other yeast genes (Hicks et al., 1979). In almost every case the involvement of chromosomal DNA sequences resulted in a stable integration of the vector DNA into the yeast nuclear genome and, thus, no extrachromosomally replicating vectors were detected. In addition, the transformation frequency was quite low, i.e., in the range of about 10 transformants/μg DNA.

Plasmids replicating extrachromosomally and giving high transformation frequencies in yeast were obtained in two different ways:

1. Since most strains of *Saccharomyces cerevisiae* contain a small plasmid – ca. 2 μm in length – (Hollenberg et al., 1970; Royer and Hollenberg, 1977; Kielland-Brandt et al., 1980), it was tempting to combine its origin of replication with a selective marker (Beggs, 1978; Hicks et al., 1979; Struhl et al., 1979). Vectors based on 2-μm DNA are relatively unstable (structurally and segregationally), but the use of the recipient strains free of 2-μm plasmids created by Hollenberg and coworkers has enhanced stability markedly. For details concerning cloning with 2-μm DNA-vectors and the expression of foreign genes in *Saccharomyces cerevisiae*, see Hollenberg (1982).

2. Other vectors transforming yeast with a high frequency have been described by Struhl et al. (1979) and Kingsman et al. (1979). These vectors consist of a bacterial plasmid and yeast DNA carrying a chromosomal origin of replication (Stinchcomb et al., 1979, 1980; Tschumper and Carbon, 1980; Beach et al., 1980). Following this line of research even DNA sequences of other eukaryotes capable of acting as origins of replication in yeast have been detected, e.g. *Neurospora crassa, Dictyostelium discoideum, Drosophila melanogaster, Zea mays* (Stinchcomb et al., 1980).

The construction of an additonal **artificial circular minichromosome** containing a chromosomal origin of replication and the centromer of a yeast chromosome has been reported by Clarke and Carbon (1980). This minichromosome is stably inherited and behaves in crosses like an additional linkage group. Minichromosomes like this have interesting properties since they ensure a certain degree of stability and can be manipulated with classic formal genetic procedures.

Cloning in filamentous fungi received a strong impetus after the discovery of a plasmid in the ascomycetous fungus *Podospora anserina* (Stahl et al., 1978). Comparable elements were subsequently found in other fungi and also in higher plants. These genetic traits often show homology with the mt DNA and in some cases they are correlated with certain phenotypes which exhibit typical extrachromosomal inheritance, e.g. senescence in *Podospora anserina.*

Since it was found that the plasmids of *Podospora anserina* and other fungi represent amplified parts of mt DNA which presumably carry a replicon, two alternative approaches to the construction of vectors from mt DNA were followed:

1. The use of mt plasmids.

2. The use of sequences of mt DNA that carry replicons. Following this approach, mt DNA from any organism carries at least one replicon and thus makes any organism available for genetic engineering irrespective whether there are plasmids or not.

Details of this concept for genetic engineering in eukaryotes are given in Esser et al. (1983). The principle is outlined in Fig. 2-12. For general information see: Esser et al., 1985.

Last but not least one should mention that efforts are being undertaken to develop a **recombinant RNA technology.** The first promising steps towards such a system have been made (Miele et al., 1983, and for review see Lewin, 1983). Perhaps in future this will represent another efficient tool for microbiology with relevance to biotechnology, in addition to the procedures that already exist.

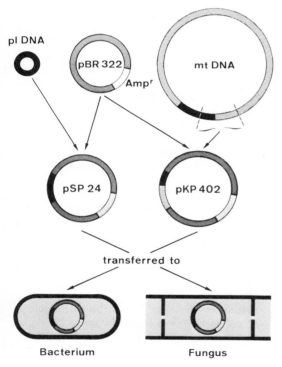

Fig. 2-12. Construction of shuttle vectors with the integration of mitochondrial DNA from *Podospora anserina* into a bacterial plasmid, pBR 322. In using either the Podospora mitochondrial plasmid (top left) or a part of mitochondrial DNA containing an autonomously-replicating sequence (top right), both hybrid vectors replicate and also express equally in *E. coli* and in Podospora (adopted from Esser, 1983).

2.5 Literature

Ainsworth, G. C. and Sussman, A. S. (eds.): *The Fungi.* Vol. I–III. Academic Press, New York, London 1965–1968.

Alexopoulos, C. J. and Beneke, E. S.: *Laboratory Manual for Introductory Mycology.* Burgess, Minneapolis 1964.

Anke, T., Oberwinkler, F., Steglich, W. and Höfle, G., "The striatins – new antibiotics from the basidiomycete *Cyathus striatus*", *J. Antibiot.* **30,** 221–225 (1977).

Anke, T., "Antibiotika aus Basisdiomyceten", *Z. Mykol.* **44,** 131–141 (1978).

Bagdaserian, M. and Timmis, K. N., "Host: vector systems for gene cloning in Pseudomonas", *Curr. Top. Microbiol. Immunol.* **96,** 47–67 (1982).

Barnes, W. M., "Construction of an M13 histidine-transducing phage: a single-stranded cloning vehicle with one Eco R1 site", *Gene* **5**, 127–139 (1979).

Beach, D., Piper, M. and Shall, S., "Isolation of Chromosomal origins of replication in yeast", *Nature* **284**, 185–187 (1980).

Beggs, J. D., "Transformation of yeast by a replicating hybrid plasmid", *Nature* **275**, 104–109 (1978).

Bergey's Manual of Determinative Bacteriology. 8th Ed., Buchanan, Z. E., Gibbons, N. E. (eds.). Williams + Wilkins Co., Baltimore 1975.

Bernhard, K., Schrempf, H. and Goebel, W., "Bacteriocin and antibiotic resistance plasmids in *Bacillus cereus* and *Bacillus subtilis*", *J. Bacteriol.* **133**, 897–903 (1978).

Bessey, E. A., *Morphology and taxonomy of fungi.* Hafner, New York, London 1968.

Bingham, A. H. A., Bruton, C. J. and Atkinson, T., "Isolation and partial characterization of four plasmids from antibiotic-resistant thermopilic bacilli", *J. Gen. Microbiol.* **114**, 401–408 (1979).

Bolivar, F., Rodriguez, R. L., Betlach, M. C. and Boyer, H. W., "Construction and characterization of new cloning vehicles. I. Ampicillin-resistant derivatives of the plasmid pMB9", *Gene* **2**, 75–93 (1977a).

Bolivar, F., Rodriguez, R. O., Geene, P. J., Betlach, M. V., Heynecker, H. L., Boyer, H. W., Crosa, J. H. and Falkow, S., "Construction and characterization of new cloning vehicles. II. A multipurpose cloning system", *Gene* **2**, 95–113 (1977b).

Booth, C., *The Genus Fusarium.* Commonwealth Mycol. Inst., Kew 1971.

Both, C. (ed.), *Methods in Microbiology.* Vol. 4. Academic Press, London 1971.

Bresch, C. and Hausmann, R.: *Klassische und molekulare Genetik,* 3rd Ed. Springer-Verlag, Berlin, Heidelberg, New York 1972.

Brown, B. J. and Carlton, B. C., "Plasmid-mediated transformation in *Bacillus megaterium*", *J. Bacteriol.* **142**, 508–512 (1980).

Burnett, J. H., *Fundamentals of Mycology.* Arnold, London 1968.

Burnett, J. H., *Mycogenetics.* John Wiley, London 1975.

Carlton, B. C. and Smith, M. P. W., "Size distribution of the closed circular deoxyribonucleic acid molecules of *Bacillus megaterium*. Sedimentation velocity and electron microscope measurements". *J. Bacteriol.* **117**, 1201–1209 (1974).

Carlton, B. C. and Brown, B. J., "Physical mapping of a plasmid from *Bacillus megaterium* by restriction endonuclease cleavage", *Plasmid* **2**, 59–68 (1979).

Chang, S. T. and Hayes, W. A. (eds.), *The Biology and Cultivation of Edible Mushrooms.* Academic Press, New York, San Francisco, London 1978.

Chater, K. F., Hopwood, D. A., Kieser, T. and Thompson, C. J., "Gene Cloning in Streptomyces", *Curr. Top. Microbiol. Immunol.* **96**, 69–95 (1982).

Clarke, L. and Carbon, L., "Isolation of a yeast centromere and construction of a functional small circular chromosome", *Nature* **287**, 504–509 (1980).

Clarke, P. H. and Richmond, M. H. (eds.), *Genetics and Biochemistry of Pseudomonas.* John Wiley, London, New York, Sydney, Toronto 1975.

Clowes, R. C. and Hayes, W., *Experiments in Microbial Genetics.* Blackwell, Oxford, Edinburgh 1968.

Clifton, C. E., *Introduction to Bacterial Physiology.* McGraw-Hill, New York, Toronto, London 1957.

Clifton, C. E., *Introduction to Bacteria.* McGraw-Hill, New York, Toronto, London 1958.

Cochrane, V. W., *Physiology of Fungi.* Wiley and Sons, New York 1963.

Colbere-Garapin, F., Garapin, A. and Kourilsky, P., "Selectable markers for the transfer of genes into mammalian cells", *Curr. Top. Microbiol. Immunol.* **96**, 145–157 (1982).

Collins, J. and Brüning, H. J., "Plasmids usable as gene-cloning vectors in an in vitro packaging by coliphage λ: 'cosmids'", *Gene* **4**, 85–107 (1978).

Collins, J. and Hohn, B., "Cosmids: a type of plasmid gene-cloning vector that is packageable in vitro in bacteriophage λ heads", *Proc. Natl. Acad Sci. USA* **75**, 4242–4246 (1978).

Crueger, W. and Crueger, A., *Lehrbuch der Angewandten Mikrobiologie.* Akademische Verlagsgesellschaft, Wiesbaden 1982.

Dade, H. A. and Gunnel, J., *Class Work with Fungi,* 2nd ed. Commonwealth Mycological Institute, Kew 1969.

De Fonbrune, P., *Technique de micromanipulation.* Masson et Cie., Paris 1949.

Delmas, J., *La truffe et sa culture.* INRA, SEI, Etude No. 60, Versailles 1976.

Difco Manual of Dehydrated Culture Media and Reagents for Microbiological and Clinical Laboratory Procedures. 9th Ed.: Difco Laboratories, Detroit/Mich. 1953.

Doelle, H. W., *Bacterial Metabolism.* Academic Press, New York, London 1969.

Ehrlich, S. D., Niaudet, B. and Michel, B., "Use of plasmids from *Staphylococcus aureus* for cloning of DNA in *Bacillus subtilis*", *Curr. Top. Microbiol. Immunol.* **96,** 19–29 (1982).

Ehrlich, S. D., "Replication and expression of plasmids from *Staphylococcus aureus* in *Bacillus subtilis*", *Proc. Natl. Acad. Sci. USA* **74,** 1680–1682 (1977).

Esser, K., *Cryptogams – Cyanobacteria, Algae, Fungi, Lichens.* Cambridge University Press, 1982.

Esser, K., Kück, U., Lamy-Hinrichs, C., Lemke, P., Osiewacz, H. D., Stahl, U. and Tudzynski, P., *Plasmids of Eukaryotes, Fundamentals and Applications.* Springer-Verlag, Berlin, Heidelberg, New York 1985.

Esser, K., Kück, U., Stahl, U. and Tudzynski, P., "Cloning vectors of mitochondrial origin for eukaryotes, a new concept in genetic engineering", *Curr. Genet.* **7,** 239–243 (1983).

Esser, K. and Kuenen, R., *Genetik der Pilze,* expanded new impression. Springer-Verlag, Berlin, Heidelberg, New York 1967.

Esser, K. and Stahl, U., "Hybridization". In: H. J. Rehm and G. Reed (eds.), *Handbook of Biotechnology,* Vol. 1. Verlag Chemie, Weinheim, New York 1981.

Esser, K. and Tudzynski, P., "Genetics of the ergot fungus *Claviceps purpurea*. I. Proof of a monoecious life cycle and segregation patterns for mycelial morphology and alkaloid production", *Theor. Appl. Genet.* **53,** 145–149 (1978).

Esser, K. and Tudzynski, P., "Genetic control and expression of senescence in *Podospora anserina*". In: P. A. Lemke (ed.), *Viruses and Plasmids in Fungi.* Marcel Dekker Inc., New York 1979, pp. 595–615.

Esser, K., Tudzynski, P., Stahl, U. and Kück, U., "A model to explain senescence in the filamentous fungus *Podospora anserina* by the action of plasmid like DNA", *Mol. Gen. Genet.* **178,** 213–216 (1980).

Fincham, J. R. S., *Genetics.* Wright, Bristol 1983.

Gäumann, E., *Die Pilze,* 2nd Ed. Birkhäuser, Basel, Stuttgart 1964.

Gilbert, W. and Villa-Komaroff, L., "Fremde Proteine aus Bakterien", *Spektrum der Wissenschaft* **6,** 99–108 (1980).

Goedell, D. V., Heynecker, H. R., Aozumi, T., Arentzen, R., Itakura, K., Yansura, D. W., Ross, M. H., Miozzari, G., Crea, R. and Seeburg, P. H., "Direct expression in *Escherichia coli* of a DNA sequence coding for human growth hormon", *Nature* **281,** 544–548 (1979).

Goursot, R., Goze, A., Niaudet, B. and Ehrlich, S. D., "Plasmids from *Staphylococcus aureus* replicate in yeast *Saccharomyces cerevisiae*", *Nature* **298,** 488–490 (1982).

Goze, A. and Ehrlich, S. D., "Replication of plasmids from *Staphylococcus aureus* in *Escherichia coli*", *Proc. Natl. Acad. Sci. USA* **77,** 7333–7337 (1980).

Grandi, G., Mottes, M. and Sgaramella, V., "Instability of *Escherichia coli* HisG gene cloned in *Bacillus subtilis:* an example of convergent macro and micro evolution in plasmids", *Plasmid* **6,** 99–111 (1981).

Gray, O. and Chang, S., "Molecular cloning and expression of *Bacillus licheniformis* β-lactamase gene in *Escherichia coli* and *Bacillus subtilis, J. Bacteriol.* **145,** 422–428 (1981).

Gray, W. D., *The Use of Fungi as Food and in Food Processing,* Part II. Butterworth, London 1970.

Grente, J., *Perspectives pour une trufficulture moderne.* 4th edition revized and supplemented by the author.

Gruss, P. and Khoury, G., "Gene transfer into mammalian cells: use of viral vectors to investigate regulatory signals for the expression of eukaryotic genes", *Curr. Top. Microbiol. Immunol.* **96,** 159–170 (1982).

Gryczan, T. J. and Dubnau, D., "Construction and properties of chimeric plasmids in *Bacillus subtilis*", *Proc. Natl. Acad. Sci. USA* **75,** 1428–1432 (1978).

Gryczan, T. J., Contente, S. and Dubnau, D., "Molecular cloning of heterologous chromosomal DNA by recombination between a plasmid vector and a homologous resident plasmid in *Bacillus subtilis*", *Mol. Gen. Genet.* **177**, 459–467 (1980a).

Gryczan, T. J., Shivakumar, A. G. and Dubnau, D., "Characterization of chimeric plasmid cloning vehicles in *Bacillus subtilis*", *J. Bacteriol.* **141**, 246–253 (1980b).

Guerineau, M., "Plasmid DNA in Yeast". In: P. A. Lemke (ed.), *Viruses and Plasmids in Fungi*. Marcel Dekker, New York, Basel 1979.

Hamlyn, P. F. and Ball, C., "Recombination Studies with *Cephalosporium acremonium*", *Am. Soc. Microbiol.* **1979**, 185–191.

Hayes, W., *The Genetics of Bacteria and their Viruses*, 2nd Ed. Blackwell, Oxford, Edinburgh 1974.

Henner, D. J. and Hoch, J. A., "The *Bacillus subtilis* Chromosome", *Microbiol. Rev.* **44**, 57–82 (1980).

Hernalsteens, J. P., "The *Agrobacterium tumefaciens* Ti plasmid as a host vector system for introducing foreign DNA in plant cells", *Nature* **287**, 654–656 (1980).

Hicks, J. B., Hinnen, A. and Fink, G. R., "Properties of Yeast Transformation", *Symp. Quant. Biol.* **43**, 1305–1313 (1979).

Hinnen, A., Hicks, J. B. and Fink, G. R., "Transformation of Yeast", *Proc. Natl. Acad. Sci. USA* **75**, 1929–1933 (1978).

Hohn, B., "DNA as substrate for packaging into bacteriophage lambda in vitro", *J. Molec. Biol.* **98**, 93–106 (1975).

Hohn, B. and Murray, K., "Packaging recombinant DNA molecules into bacteriophage particles in vitro", *Proc. Natl. Acad. Sci. USA* **74**, 3259–3263 (1977).

Hohn, T., Richards, K. and Lebeurier, G., "Cauliflower mosaic virus on its way to recoming a useful plant vector", *Curr. Top. Microbiol. Immunol.* **96**, 193–220 (1982).

Hollenberg, C. P., Borst, P. and van Bruggen, E. F. J., "Mitochondrial DNA. V. A 25 μ closed circular duplex DNA molecule in wild-type yeast mitochondria. Structure and genetic complexity", *Biochim. Biophys. Acta* **209**, 1–15 (1970).

Hollenberg, C. P., "Cloning with 2-μm DNA vectors and the expression of foreign genes in *Saccharomyces cerevisiae*", *Curr. Top. Microbiol. Immunol.* **96**, 119–144 (1982).

Hopkins, A. S., Murray, N. E. and Brammar, W. J., "Characterization of top-transducing bacteriophages made in vitro", *J. Molec. Biol.* **107**, 549–569 (1976).

Howard, B. H., "Vectors for introducing genes into cells of higher eukaryotes", *Trends Biochem. Sci.* **8**, 209–212 (1983).

Ingold, C. T., *The Biology of Fungi*, 3rd Ed. Hutchison Educational, London 1973.

Itakura, K., Hirose, T., Crea, R., Riggs, A. D., Heynecker, H. R., Bolivar, F. and Boyer, H. W., "Expression in *Escherichia coli* of a chemically synthesized gene for the hormone somatostatin", *Science* **198**, 1056–1063 (1977).

Kandler, O. and Schleifer, K. H., "Systematics of Bacteria", *Prog. Bot.* **42**, 234–246 (1980).

Kawamura, F., Saito, H. and Ikeda, Y., "Bacteriophage Φ 1 as a gene cloning vector in *Bacillus subtilis*", *Mol. Gen. Genet.* **180**, 259–266 (1980).

Keggins, K. M., Lovett, P. S. and Duvall, E. J., "Molecular cloning of genetically active fragments in *Bacillus subtilis* and properties of the vector plasmid pUB110", *Proc. Natl. Acad. Sci. USA* **75**, 1423–1427 (1978).

Kielland-Brandt, M. C., Wilken, B., Holmberg, S., Petersen, L. J. G. and Nilsson-Tillgren, T., "Genetic evidence for nuclear location of 2-micron DNA in yeast", *Carlsberg. Res. Commun.* **45**, 119–124 (1980).

King, R. C. (ed.), *Handbook of Genetics*, Vol. I, Bacteria, Bacteriophages and Fungi. Plenum Press, New York, London 1974.

Kingsman, A. J., Clarke, L., Mortimer, R. K. and Carbon, J., "Replication in *Saccharomyces cerevisiae* of plasmid pBR313 carrying DNA from the yeast trpl region", *Gene* **7**, 141–152 (1979).

Klingmüller, W., *Genmanipulation und Gentherapie*. Springer-Verlag, Berlin, Heidelberg, New York 1976.

Klingmüller, W., "Genetic engineering for practical application", *Naturwissenschaften* **66**, 182–189 (1979).

Klingmüller, W., "Möglichkeiten und Grenzen der genetischen Manipulation", *Naturwissenschaften* **68**, 120–127 (1981).

Knapp, E., "Die Mutation". In: *Handbuch der Pflanzenzüchtung*, Vol. 1. 1938, pp. 178–199.

Knippers, R., *Molekulare Genetik*. Thieme-Verlag, Stuttgart 1971.

Knorr, M., *Zentralbl. Bakteriol. Parasitenk. Infektionskr. Hyg. Abt. 1 Orig.* **117**, 154 (1930).

Koch, W. J., *Fungi in the Laboratory, a Manual and Text,* 2nd Ed. Carolina Student Stores 1972.

Kreft, J., Bernhard, K. and Goebel, W., "Recombinant plasmids capable of replication in *B. subtilis* and *E. coli*", *Mol. Gen. Genet.* **162,** 59–67 (1978).

Kreft, J. and Hughes, C., "Cloning vectors derived from plasmids and phage of Bacillus", *Curr. Top. Microbiol. Immunol.* **96,** 1–17 (1982).

Kreisel, H., *Grundzüge eines natürlichen Systems der Pilze.* Cramer, Lehre 1969.

Kück, U., Stahl, U. and Esser, K., "Plasmid-like DNA is part of mitochondrial DNA in *Podospora anserina*", *Curr. Genet.* **3,** 151–156 (1981).

Leder, P., Tiemeier, D. and Enquist, L., "EK2 derivatives of bacteriophage lambda useful in the cloning of DNA from higher organisms: the λ gt WES system", *Science* **196,** 175–177 (1977).

Lewin, R., "The birth of recombinant RNA technology", *Science* **222,** 1313–1315 (1983).

Lilly, V. G. and Barnett, H. L., *Physiology of the Fungi.* McGraw Hill, New York 1951.

Lincoff, G. and Mitchell, D. H., *Toxic and Hallucinogenic Mushroom Poisoning.* van Nostrand Reinhold Comp., New York 1970.

Lodder, J. (ed.): *The Yeasts,* 2nd Ed. North Holland, Amsterdam, Oxford – American Elsevier, New York 1974.

Löfdahl, S., Sjöström, J. E. and Philipson, L., "A vector for recombinant DNA in *Staphylococcus aureus*", *Gene* **3,** 161–172 (1978).

Lovett, P. S. and Bramucci, M. G., "Plasmid deoxyribonucleic acid in *Bacillus subtilis* and *Bacillus pumilus*", *J. Bacteriol.* **124,** 484–490 (1975).

Maniatis, T., Fritsch, E. F. and Sambrook, J., *Molecular Cloning: A Laboratory Manual.* Cold Spring Harbor Laboratory, 1982.

Martin, S. M., Quadling, C., Jones, M. L. and Skerman, V. B. D., *World Directory of Collections of Cultures of Microorganisms.* Wiley Interscience, New York, London, Sydney, Toronto 1972.

McLeod, A. J., "Biotechnology and the production of proteins", *Nature* **285,** 136 (1980).

Meinhardt, F., "Untersuchungen zur Genetik des Fortpflanzungsverhaltens und der Fruchtkörper- und Antibiotikabildung des Basidiomyceten *Agrocybe aegerita*", *Bibliotheca Mycologica* **75** (1980).

Merck, A. G., *Mikrobiologisches Handbuch.*

Messing, J., Gronenborn, B., Müller-Hill, B. and Hofschneider, P. H., "Filamentous coliphage M13 as a cloning vehicle: insertion of a Hind II fragment of the lac regulatory region in M13 replicative form in vitro", *Proc. Natl. Acad. Sci. USA* **74,** 3642–3646 (1977).

Messing, J., Crea, R. and Seeburg, P. H., "A system for shotgun DNA sequencing", *Nucl. Acid. Res.* **9,** 309–321 (1981).

Messing, J. and Vieira, J., "A new pair of M13 vectors for selecting either DNA strand of double-digest restriction", *Gene* **19,** 269–276 (1982).

Michel, B., Palla, E., Niaudet, B. and Ehrlich, S. D., "DNA cloning in *B. subtilis.* III. Efficiency of random-segment cloning and insertional inactivation vectors", *Gene* **12,** 147–154 (1980).

Miele, E. A., Mills, D. R. and Kramer, F. R., "Autocatalytic replication of a recombinant RNA", *J. Mol. Biol.* **171,** 281–295 (1983).

Moir, A. and Brammar, W. J., "Use of specialized transducing phages in amplification of enzyme production", *Mol. Gen. Genet.* **149,** 87–99 (1976).

Montagu, M. van and Schell, J., "The Ti plasmids of Agrobacterium", *Curr. Top. Microbiol. Immunol.* **96,** 237–254 (1982).

Müller, E., "Taxonomy and phylogeny of fungi", *Fortschr. Bot.* **36,** 247–262 (1974).

Müller, E. and Löffler, W., *Mykologie,* 2nd Ed. Thieme-Verlag, Stuttgart 1971.

Müller, H. J., "Artificial transmutation of the gene", *Science* **66,** 84–87 (1927).

Murray, K. and Murray, N. E., "Phage lambda receptor chromosomes for DNA fragments made with restriction endonuclease III of *Haemophilus influenzae* and restriction endonuclease I of *Escherichia coli*", *J. Molec. Biol.* **98,** 551–564 (1975).

Nomura, S., Yamame, K., Masuda, T., Kawamura, F., Mizukami, T., Saito, H., Tatuki, M., Tamura, G. and Maruo, B., "Construction of transducing phage p11 containing α-amylase structural gene of *Bacillus subtilis*", *Agric. Biol. Chem.* **43,** 2637–2638 (1979).

Old, R. W. and Primrose, S. B., "Principles of Gene Manipulation". In: *Studies in Microbiology,* Vol. 2. Blackwell, Oxford, London, Edinburgh 1980.

Panasenko, S. M., Cameron, J. R., Davis, R. W. and Lehmann, I. R., "Five hundredfold overproduction of DNA ligase after induction of a hybrid lambda lysogen constructed in vitro", *Science* **196,** 188–189 (1977).

Peberdy, J. F. (ed.), *Protoplasts – Application in Microbial Genetics.* University of Nottingham, 1979.

Pühler, A., *Molecular Genetics of the Bacteria-plant Interaction.* Springer-Verlag, Berlin, Heidelberg, New York, Tokyo 1983.

Raper, J. R., *Genetics of Sexuality in Higher Fungi.* Ronald Press, New York 1966.

Ratzkin, B. and Carbon, J., "Functional expression of cloned yeast DNA in *Escherichia coli*", *Proc. Natl. Acad. Sci. USA* **74,** 487–491 (1977).

Rehm, H. J., *Industrielle Mikrobiologie,* 2nd Ed. Springer-Verlag, Berlin, Heidelberg, New York 1980.

Rostas, K., Dobritsa, S. V., Dobritsa, A. P., Koncz, C. and Alföldi, L., "Megacinogenic plasmid from *Bacillus megaterium* 216", *Mol. Gen. Genet.* **180,** 323–329 (1980).

Royer, H. D. and Hollenberg, C. P., "Saccharomyces 2 μm DNA. An analysis of the monomer and its multimers by electron microscopy", *Mol. Gen. Genet.* **150,** 271–284 (1977).

Rüther, U., Koenen, M., Otto, K. and Müller-Hill, B., "pUR 222, a vector for cloning and rapid chemical sequencing of DNA", *Nucl. Acid Res.* **9,** 4087–4098 (1981).

Sakaguchi, K., "Vectors for gene cloning in Pseudomonas and their applications", *Curr. Top. Microbiol. Immunol.* **96,** 31–45 (1982).

Schlegel, H. G., *Allgemeine Mikrobiologie,* 4th Ed. Thieme-Verlag, Stuttgart 1976.

Skerman, V. B. D., *A Guide to the Identification of Genera of Bacteria,* 2nd Ed. Williams + Wilkins, Baltimore 1967.

Smith, H. E. and Berry, D. R., *An Introduction to Biochemistry of Fungal Development.* Academic Press, London, New York 1971.

Stahl, U. and Esser, K., "Inconsistency in the species concept for yeasts due to mutations during vegetative growth", *Eur. J. Appl. Biotechnol.* **8,** 271–278 (1979a).

Stahl, U. and Esser, K., "Subsequent transfers of yeast may lead via single gene mutations to alterations of the species", *Biotechnol. Lett.* **1,** 383–385 (1979b).

Stahl, U. and Esser, K., "Plasmid heterogeneity in various strains of *Bacillus megaterium*", *Eur. J. Appl. Microbiol. Biotechnol.* **17,** 248–251 (1983).

Stahl, U., Lemke, P. A., Tudzynski, P., Kück, U. and Esser, K., "Evidence for plasmid-like DNA in a filamentous fungus, the ascomycete *Podospora anserina*", *Mol. Gen. Genet.* **162,** 341–343 (1978).

Stahl, U., Kück, U., Tudzynski, P. and Esser, K., "Characterization and cloning of plasmid-like DNA of the ascomycete *Podospora anserina*", *Mol. Gen. Genet.* **178,** 639–646 (1980).

Stahl, U., Tudzynski, P., Kück, U., and Esser, K., "Replication and expression of a bacterial-mitochondrial hybrid plasmid in the fungus *Podospora anserina*", *Proc. Natl. Acad. Sci. USA* **29,** 3641 (1982).

Sternberg, N., Tiemeier, D. and Enquist, L., "In vitro packaging of a λ Dam vector containing EcoRI DNA fragments of *Escherichia coli* and phage P1", *Gene* **1,** 255 (1977).

Stevens, R. B., *Mycology Guidebook.* University of Washington Press, Seattle, London 1974.

Stinchcomb, D. T., Struhl, K., Davis, R. W., "Isolation and characterisation of a yeast chromosomal replicator", *Nature* **282,** 39–43 (1979).

Stinchcomb, D. T., Thomas, J., Kelly, J., Selker, E. and Davis, R. W., "Eukaryotic DNA segments capable of autonomous replication in yeast", *Proc. Natl. Acad. Sci. USA* **77,** 4459–4563 (1980).

Struhl, K., Cameron, J. R. and Davis, R. W., "Functional expression of eukaryotic DNA in *Escherichia coli*", *Proc. Natl. Acad. Sci. USA* **73,** 1471–1475 (1976).

Struhl, K., Stinchcomb, D. T., Scherer, S. and Davis, R. W., "High-frequency transformation of yeast: autonomous replication of hybrid DNA molecules", *Proc. Natl. Acad. Sci. USA* **76,** 1035–1039 (1979).

Tanaka, T. and Koshikawa, T., Isolation and characterization of four types of plasmids from *Bacillus subtilis* (natto), *J. Bacteriol.* **131,** 775–782 (1977).

Tanaka, T. and Kawano, N., "Cloning vehicles for the homologous Bacillus subtilis host-vector system", *Gene* **10,** 131–136 (1980).

Thimann, K. V. (ed.): *The Life of Bacteria,* 2nd Ed. Macmillan Co., New York 1967.

Thomas, M., Cameron, J. R. and Davis, R. W., "Viable molecular hybrids of bacteriophage lambda and eukaryotic DNA", *Proc. Natl. Acad. Sci. USA* **71**, 4579–4583 (1974).

Tschumper, G. and Carbon, J., "Sequence of a yeast DNA fragment containing a chromosomal replicator and the TRP1 gene", *Gene* **10**, 157–166 (1980).

Tudzynski, P., Stahl, U. and Esser, K., "Transformation to senescence with plasmid-like DNA in the ascomycete *Podospora anserina*", *Curr. Genet.* **2**, 181–184 (1980).

Turner, W. B., *Fungal Metabolites.* Academic Press, London, New York 1971.

Uozomi, T., Ozaki, A., Beppu, T. and Arima, K., "New cryptic plasmids of *Bacillus subtilis* and restriction analysis of other plasmids found by general screening", *J. Bacteriol.* **142**, 315–318 (1980).

Watson, J. D., *Molecular Biology of the Gene,* 3rd Ed. Benjamin Inc. London, Amsterdam, Sydney 1976.

Webster, J., *Introduction to Fungi,* 2nd Ed. University Press, Cambridge 1980.

Wettstein, D. von, "Genetic engineering in the adaptation of plants to evolving human needs", *Experientia* **39**, 687–713 (1983).

Winkler, U., Rüger, W. and Wackernagel, W., *Bakterien-, Phagen- und Molekulargenetik.* Springer-Verlag, Berlin, Heidelberg, New York 1972.

Young, E. E. and Wilson, G. A., "Genetics of *Bacillus subtilis* and other sporulating gram-positive bacilli". In: H. O. Halvorson, R. Hanson and L. L. Campbell (eds.): *Spores* V. Am. Soc. Microbiol., Washington/D.C. 1972, pp. 77–106.

Zeissler, J., *Handbuch der pathogenen Mikroorganismen,* 3rd Ed. Jena 1929.

Chapter 3

The Metabolism of Microorganisms

Hans Günter Schlegel

3.1 Introduction

The **biotechnologist** will, as a rule, deal with the microbial transformation of simple raw materials into biomass or products of primary or secondary metabolism and also with biotransformations. He has to deal do with living cells, extraordinarily complex formations the investigation of which has advanced far but is by no means yet concluded. Each species of bacteria and yeasts has its peculiarities and requires individual treatment. Dealing with microorganisms, studying their metabolism and its regulation, investigating their individual requirements and tolerances, and defining the conditions under which a certain organism can be used for technical purposes are the tasks of the **microbiologist.** The task of the **biotechnologist** is, then, the conversion of microbiological knowledge into practice. A number of textbooks give an idea of the basic principles of the metabolic physiology and biochemistry of pro- and eucaryotes (Brock, 1979; Schlegel, 1981; Stanier et al., 1978). They also cite other textbooks, monographs, and the latest review papers. We cannot go into details here; on the contrary, an attempt will be made to describe the basic metabolism of microorganisms in a simplified manner and to show its importance for biotechnology.

In his youth, Feodor Lynen characterized the cell (yeast) as "a sack full of enzymes." This statement has rightly been contradicted. It is, however, possible in order to simplify the complicated situation to regard the cell of a microorganism as a **reactor** and, in the first instance, to disregard the fact that a reactor model lacks, at least, the capacity for self-reduplication. All questions connected with the genetic constitution and replication of the genetic material, and also multiplication and growth cannot be considered here. Furthermore, it is quite unnecessary to deal with all enzyme reactions. It is sufficient to present the precursors and products of metabolic pathways, the control steps and switching points in the metabolism and their basic interrelationship.

3.2 Basic Metabolism

The metabolism of the cell aims at **maintaining and multiplying the cell substance,** i.e., the synthesis of the cell components. Cell synthesis requires not only structural components but also energy. Both are obtained by a controlled transformation of substrates in the cell. The sources of energy are, as a rule, nutrients (substrates) taken up from the environment, e.g., glucose. Other nutrients are required for the synthesis of the cell constituents, such as mineral salts, trace elements, and vitamins. The nutrients are transformed in the cell by a multiplicity of successive enzyme reactions via specific metabolic pathways. These fulfil two main functions: they provide precursors for the **synthesis of the cell constituents** that must be available and they supply **energy for synthetic processes** (Fig. 3-1).

Metabolism can be divided into three main sections: (a) the nutrients are first decomposed into small fragments. We speak of degradation or **catabolism.** The degradation pathways may be short (e.g., in the case of acetate) or long (e.g., benzoic acid). The special degradation pathways serve for the production of small molecules (metabolites). These are channeled into the (b) intermediate metabolism or **amphibolism.** The central metabolic pathways serve for the generation of energy or its preparation and also for the synthesis of a large variety of low-molecular-weight compounds from which the building blocks of the cell are synthesized. Building blocks of the cell are the amino acids, purines, pyrimidines, sugar phosphates and other sugar derivatives, organic acids, and other metabolites. In the next step (c), the cell poly-

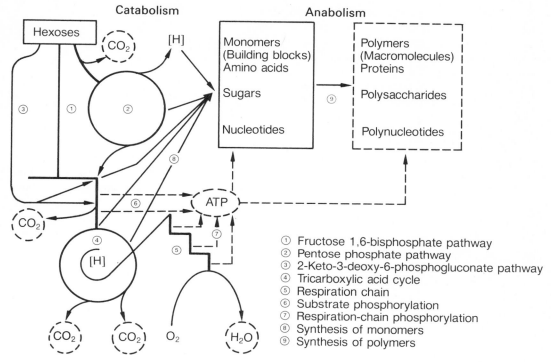

Fig. 3-1. The main divisions of the metabolic pathways in respiring cells. – This and the majority of the following Figures have been taken with the kind permission of the Georg-Thieme-Verlag, Stuttgart, from H. G. Schlegel's textbook: "Allgemeine Mikrobiologie", 5th edition, 1981.

mers such as proteins, nucleic acids, cell wall constituents, and reserve substances are synthesized from these building blocks. The synthesis of the building blocks and that of the cell polymers are comprised under the terms biosynthetic metabolism or **anabolism.**

These basic metabolic pathways which, for example, already make the fermentation metabolism possible are supplemented by special mechanisms for the generation of energy. Complex enzyme systems localized in a cytoplasmic membrane are responsible for the generation of energy by respiration or by photosynthesis. In respiration, the hydrogen [H] split off in the central metabolic pathways is fed into an electron transport chain in such a way that protons (H^+) are transported to the cell exterior and electrons (e^-) are finally transferred to oxygen.

The proton potential at the cell boundary, the cytoplasmic membrane, so arising, is then the driving force for the regeneration of ATP. In photosynthetic microorganisms, light yields energy which leads to the formation of a proton potential.

3.2.1 Function of the Enzymes

The metabolic reactions are catalyzed by enzymes. In practice, all the protein of unicellular organisms is present in the form of enzyme proteins. In many bacteria, almost no structural proteins are present. Regulatory mechanisms ensure that only those enzymes are formed in the cell that are necessary for the assimilation of a given substrate for the synthesis of the cell constituents. A special enzyme is responsible for the conversion of each metabolite into another one. The essential functional properties of an enzyme are the **recognition** of the corresponding metabolite, **catalysis,** and the **controllability** of the catalytic activity. The enzyme-catalyzed transformation begins with the binding of the metabolite, i.e., the enzyme substrate, to the enzyme protein. Binding occurs at the catalytic site. Many enzymes are converted into the active state (the active conformation) only by the binding of the substrate. As a rule, each enzyme deals with only one metabolite, its substrate; it possesses **substrate specificity.** It also catalyzes only one out of many possible transformation processes that the metabolite can undergo; it possesses **action specificity.** Enzymatic catalysis results in the formation of one or several products. However, the transformation continues only until the equilibrium between substrate and product has been reached. A distinction is made between simple and regulatory enzymes, and this will be discussed in section 3.2.9.

3.2.2   Coenzymes and Prosthetic Groups

For the uptake and passing on of fragments of the substrate, the enzyme proteins have available low-molecular-weight compounds which are known as coenzymes and prosthetic groups (Table 3-1). To some extent, they serve the enzyme proteins as tweezers for handling amino groups, methyl groups, hydrogen, electrons, or other small fragments. The coenzymes are of special importance because they cannot be synthesized by many organisms and must be taken in with the food as **vitamins.**

Table 3-1. Coenzymes and Prosthetic Groups, their Functions as Hydrogen-, Group-, or Electron-Carriers, and their Relationships to the Vitamins.

Coenzyme or prosthetic group	Function: transfer of	Vitamin
NAD(P)	Hydrogen, e^-	Nicotinic acid
FMN	Hydrogen, e^-	Riboflavin
FAD	Hydrogen, e^-	Riboflavin
Quinones	Hydrogen, e^-	
Cytochromes	e^-	Heme derivatives
Biotin	Carboxy group	Biotin
Pyridoxal phosphate	Amino group	Pyridoxine
Tetrahydrofolate	Formyl group	Folate, 4-hydroxybenzoate
Coenzyme A	Acyl group	Pantothenate
Lipoate	Acyl group and hydrogen	Lipoate
Thiamine diphosphate[a]	Aldehyde group	Thiamine
B_{12}-Coenzyme	Carboxy group, Methyl group	Cobalamine

[a] Thiamine pyrophosphate

3.2.3 Hydrogen Transfer Reactions

All nonphotosynthetic organisms rely on oxidation processes for the production of energy. The oxidation of organic compounds takes place through the **release of electrons.** The electrons are transferred from the electron donor to the electron acceptor. As a rule, two electrons are transferred simultaneously, two protons being split off from the substrate. We speak of the oxidation or the dehydrogenation of a substrate (hydrogen donor) and the reduction or hydrogenation of a hydrogen acceptor. The catalyzing enzymes here are the **dehydrogenases.** They transfer the hydrogen split off from the substrate to one of the two coenzymes nicotinamide adenine dinucleotide (NAD) and nicotinamide adenine dinucleotide phosphate (NADP). These coenzymes can diffuse freely in the cell and with the aid of other dehydrogenases are capable of transporting the hydrogen to hydrogen acceptors.

3.2.4 Mechanisms of ATP Regeneration

The chemical form in which the energy obtained by fermentation, respiration, or photosynthesis is made available to and is utilized by the cell metabolism is **adenosine triphosphate** (ATP). ATP transfers chemical energy between energy-producing and energy-consuming reactions. It enables the energy-consuming syntheses of metabolites and polymeric macromolecules and also processes involved in movement and osmotic regulation to take place. Many metabolites must be activated by ATP before transformation. ATP is therefore the coenzyme of the activation of metabolites. This activation takes place through **group transfer,** in which either ADP or AMP arises from ATP.

There are three processes through which ATP is regenerated; namely: photosynthetic phosphorylation, oxidative or respiratory-chain phosphorylation, and substrate-level phosphorylation. The first two processes have in common with one another the fact that they are localized in membranes and that ATP is formed by ATP synthase.

Substrate-Level Phosphorylation

Substrate-level phosphorylation can take place in several transformations in the central metabolic pathways. The most important reactions for the regeneration of ATP in the carbohydrate metabolism are catalyzed by phosphoglycerate kinase [1], pyruvate kinase [2], and acetate kinase [3]. In these processes, adenosine diphosphate (ADP) is used as acceptor.

$$\text{Glycerate-1,3-bisphosphate} \underset{\underset{\text{ADP}+P_i \quad \text{ATP}}{}}{\overset{1}{\rightleftharpoons}} \text{3-Phospho-glycerate [1]}$$

$$\text{Phosphoenolpyruvate} \underset{\underset{\text{ADP}+P_i \quad \text{ATP}}{}}{\overset{2}{\longrightarrow}} \text{Pyruvate [2]}$$

$$\text{Acetyl phosphate} \underset{\underset{\text{ADP}+P_i \quad \text{ATP}}{}}{\overset{3}{\longrightarrow}} \text{Acetate [3]}$$

The first two reactions are used by almost all organisms, but the third only by those bacteria which produce acetate, butyrate, butanol, acetone, and isopropanol.

Respiratory-Chain Phosphorylation

Respiratory metabolism is characterized by the capacity for producing energy by **respiratory-chain phosphorylation** or electron-transport phosphorylation (Fig. 3-2). In it, the reducing equivalents

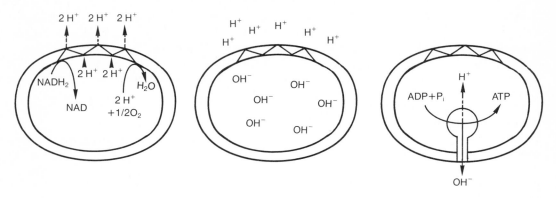

Fig. 3-2. Respiration-chain phosphorylation. The cells of bacteria and mitochondria resemble vesicles enclosed on all sides by the cytoplasmic membrane. The hydrogen transported by the coenzymes to the inner side of the membrane is passed to the outer side of the membrane where protons are released the electrons return to the inside and take up protons. The hydrogen is again passed to the outside of the membrane. Electron transport pumps protons outwards (a). This has the consequence of the formation of an electrochemical gradient with a positive potential outside and a negative potential inside (b). This potential is the driving force that keeps the regeneration of ATP going (c).

(hydrogen or protons and electrons) given up by the substrate are transported to the cytoplasmic membrane or the inner mitochondrial membrane and are then passed through the membrane in such a way that an electrochemical gradient is formed between the inner and outer sides of the membrane, with a positive potential on the outside and a negative potential on the inside. This charge gradient (proton potential) comes about by the arrangement of the components of the electron-transport chain in the membrane. Some of these components transfer electrons, and others hydrogen. The arrangement of the carriers in the membrane means that during the transport of the electrons from the supplying coenzyme to oxygen, protons are taken up on the inner side of the membrane and released on the outer side of the membrane. It is considered that in the membranes the electrons pass around loops. In view of its function, the respiratory chain is also referred to as a "proton pump". A special enzyme, ATP synthase, which synthesizes ATP from ADP and orthophosphate (P_i), is localized in the membrane. In the synthesis of ATP, protons flow back from the outside to the inside of the cell.

Photosynthetic Phosphorylation

Photosynthetic phosphorylation is based on the fact that photochemical reaction centers localized in the membrane transfer electrons from a **donor** to an **acceptor** against the thermodynamic gradient. At least part of these electrons returns via an electron-transport chain to the reaction centers. Through a suitable arrangement of the components in the membrane, as in respiration, there is an ejection of protons from the cell with the formation of a proton potential. The photosynthetic apparatus is a light-driven proton pump. The regeneration of the ATP occurs via a mechanism similar to that in the membrane of the respiring bacteria or mitochondria. In the case of the anaerobic phototrophic bacteria to be discussed later, photosynthesis serves exclusively for the generation of energy. In the case of green plants and cyanobacteria, there are two reaction centers and two successive photoreactions which make it possible to raise the energy level of the electrons to such an extent that water can be utilized as a source of electrons. This combination leads not only to the production of energy but also to the production of reducing power at the level of $NADPH_2$ and the liberation of oxygen.

3.2.5 Uptake of Substrates into the Cell

The nutrients must penetrate through the cell envelope before they can be transformed within the cell. The essential barrier is the cytoplasmic membrane (Fig. 3-3). Only a few substances are taken up by **simple diffusion,** but for most substances spezific enzymes, the so-called **permeases,** are responsible. In practice, a specific permease is necessary for the transport of each individual sugar. The formation of this enzyme is induced by the sugar. Several mechanisms of substrate transport are distinguished. Apart from the simple diffusion assumed for some poisons, inhibitors, and other substances foreign to the cell, a specific permease is responsible for the subsequent three transport processes for each substance.

In the case of **facilitated diffusion,** the substrate is in fact transported specifically but it cannot be accumulated against a concentration gradient in the cell. The other processes, active transport and group translocation, are energy-dependent. If metabolic energy is available, the substance can be accumulated in the cell against a concentration gradient. The two processes mentioned differ only in the nature of the product that is liberated in the interior of the cell. In **active transport,** the same molecule is released into the cytoplasm as was taken up from the nutrient solution. In **group translocation,** the molecule is changed – for example, phosphorylated – during transport.

Special transport mechanisms and iron-complexing compounds, the so-called **sidero-phores,** are responsible for the **transport of iron,** which, as a trace element, plays an important role in nutrition. In an aerated nutrient solution, iron is present as iron(III) compounds; their solubility is very low

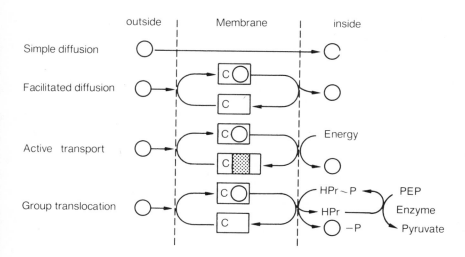

Fig. 3-3. The four mechanisms of the transport of substances into the cell. – Symbols: circle = substrate to be transported; C = carrier or permease; C with gray hatching = energetic carrier; PEP = phosphoenol pyruvate; HPr = the substrate-phosphorylating enzyme.

$(10^{-18}$ M). The siderophores are excreted by the microorganisms, and they bring the iron into solution and transport it into the cell.

3.2.6 Degradation of Carbon and Energy Sources

The two most important metabolic pathways for the degradation of sources of carbon and energy are shown for the case of **glucose degradation,** as an example. Glucose is not only the quantitatively predominating product of photosynthesis but also the most important substrate for the growth of microorganisms. In addition to this, several important cell substances, such as the peptidoglycan cell wall, glycogen, and starch, contain or consist of glucose. When the cells grow on a substrate other than glucose (for example, acetate), the glucose degradation pathway is again used as a synthetic pathway. The degradation of glucose to pyruvate is the backbone of cell metabolism. It begins with two phosphorylation reactions and the cleavage of fructose bisphosphate, then runs through an oxidation and two phosphorylation reactions, and ends with pyruvate. The pathway is well known as **glycolysis** or the **Embden-Meyerhof pathway** (Figs. 3-4a and 3-5).

Many procaryotes use hexoses by a different pathway which is known for its characteristic intermediate as the **2-keto-3-deoxy-6-phosphogluconate pathway** or the **Entner-Doudoroff pathway** (Figs. 3-4b and 3-6). Here, the glucose is first oxidized and is then cleaved to pyruvate and glyceraldehyde 3-phosphate. The latter product is also oxidized to pyruvate via reactions of the glycolysis pathway. Gluconate is also degraded by this pathway, and in many bacteria which degrade glucose by the Embden-Meyerhof pathway gluconate is degraded by the last-mentioned pathway.

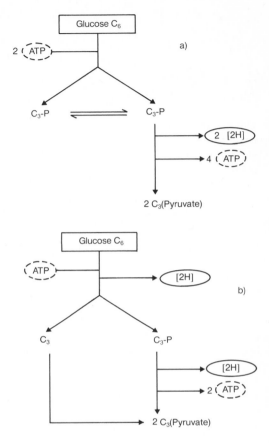

Fig. 3-4. Simplified representation of the metabolic pathways for the degradation of glucose to pyruvate. a) Glycolysis or the Embden-Meyerhof pathway; b) Entner-Doudoroff pathway. In each case, glucose is phosphorylated and is oxidized by several steps to C_3 (pyruvate). The hydrogen split off is transferred to a coenzyme [NAD(P)]. During the oxidation, ATP is regenerated. Pyruvate can be used for various purposes in various ways.

In addition to these two pathways the cell has available the possibility of degrading glucose via the **pentose phosphate pathway.** This is a cyclic process in which the hexose phosphate (C_6) is shortened by only one C atom (CO_2) with the splitting off of hydrogen, and

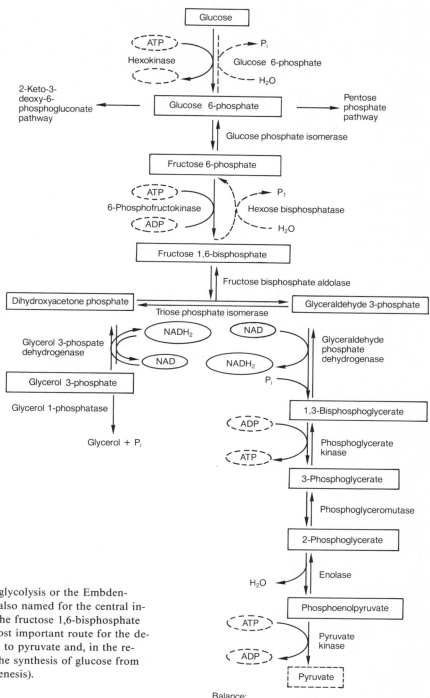

Fig. 3-5. Scheme of glycolysis or the Embden-Meyerhof pathway, also named for the central intermediate product the fructose 1,6-bisphosphate pathway. It is the most important route for the degradation of hexoses to pyruvate and, in the reverse direction, for the synthesis of glucose from pyruvate (gluconeogenesis).

Balance:
Glucose → 2 Pyruvate + 2 ATP + 2 NADH₂

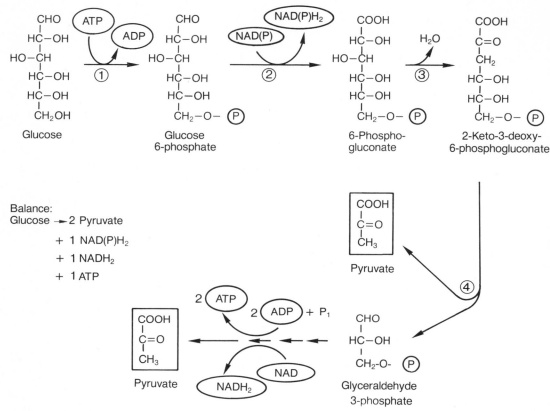

Balance:
Glucose ⟶ 2 Pyruvate

    + 1 NAD(P)H₂

    + 1 NADH₂

    + 1 ATP

Fig. 3-6. The Entner-Doudoroff pathway of glucose degradation, also named for the characteristic intermediate product as the 2-keto-3-deoxy-6-phosphogluconate pathway, is the route for the degradation of hexoses and gluconate used most frequently in bacteria.

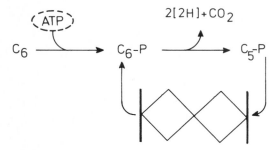

Fig. 3-7. Simplified representation of the pentose phosphate pathway for the oxidation of glucose. The lower part of the scheme symbolizes the fully reversible transformation of 3 C_5-P to 2 C_6-P + C_3-P.

the resulting pentose phosphate (C_5) is reconverted into hexose phosphate and glyceraldehyde phosphate via several rearrangement reactions. The pathway is represented schematically in Fig. 3-7 and is shown in detail in Fig. 3-8.

Pyruvate, which is located in the center of the intermediate metabolism and is necessary for the synthesis of many metabolites, can be oxidized further. Different organisms make use of different enzymes for this purpose (Fig. 3-9). Common to oxidation processes catalyzed by a pyruvate dehydrogenase or an oxi-

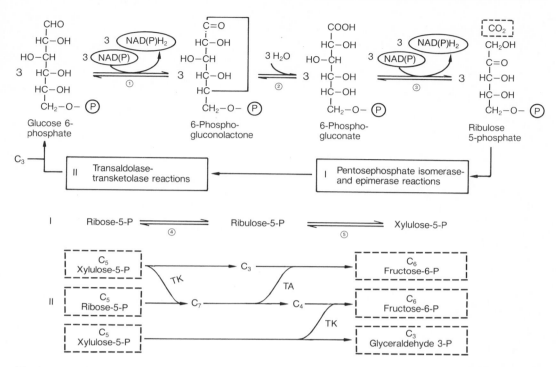

Glucose 6-phosphate

6-Phospho-gluconolactone

6-Phospho-gluconate

Ribulose 5-phosphate

C_3 — II Transaldolase-transketolase reactions ← I Pentosephosphate isomerase-and epimerase reactions

I   Ribose-5-P ⇌ ④ Ribulose-5-P ⇌ ⑤ Xylulose-5-P

II

C_5 Xylulose-5-P		
C_5 Ribose-5-P		
C_5 Xylulose-5-P		

TK C_3 TA C_6 Fructose-6-P

C_7 C_4 C_6 Fructose-6-P

TK C_3 Glyceraldehyde 3-P

Fig. 3-8. Reactions of the pentose phosphate pathway. The cycle shown at the top indicates the oxidation of three hexoses (C_6) to three pentoses (C_5), three molecules carbon dioxide and six 2[H]. The various pentose phosphates can be converted into one another (I). Three C_5 can be converted into two C_6 and one C_3 via the reaction sequence II. Reaction sequence II is completely reversible and, in the reverse direction is used for the production of pentose phosphates for the synthesis of nucleic acids and for fixing carbon dioxide or formaldehyde. – TK = transketolase; TA = transaldolase.

doreductase is the formation of acetyl-CoA (Figs. 3-9a and 3-10); only yeast decarboxylates pyruvate to acetaldehyde (Fig. 3-9b). The hydrogen split off in the oxidation to acetyl-CoA is transferred either to NAD or to ferredoxin, and carbon dioxide is liberated. In one case, formate is liberated.

The **acetyl-CoA** formed is the precursor for numerous biosynthetic pathways. However, it can be also included in a cyclic process, the tricarboxylic acid cycle, which, on the one hand, provides precursors for biosynthetic processes and, on the other hand, serves for

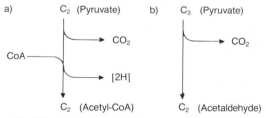

Fig. 3-9. Oxidation of pyruvate to acetyl-CoA (a) or acetaldehyde (b). In different organisms, different enzymes are involved in oxidation to CoA, either formate or carbon dioxide and 2[H] being formed. In the latter case, 2[H] can be transferred to NAD or ferredoxin.

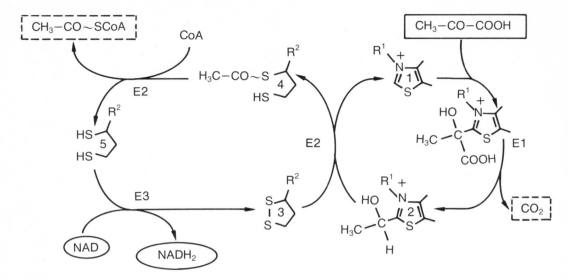

Fig. 3-10. The commonest reaction by far for the oxidation of pyruvate to acetyl-coenzyme A. The transformation takes place on a multienzyme complex including three enzymes (E 1, E 2, and E 3), thiamine pyrophosphate (1) and lipoate (3).

the oxidation of acetate to coenzyme-bound hydrogen ($NADH_2$) and carbon dioxide (Figs. 3-11 and 3-12).

3.2.7 Synthesis of the Low-Molecular-Weight Constituents of the Cell

Numerous biosynthetic pathways leading to the building blocks of the macromolecules start from the intermediate products of the central metabolic pathways. It is astonishing with how few intermediate products (a total of six) the 20 amino acids necessary for the formation of proteins can be synthesized (Fig. 3-13). Other pathways lead to the purines, pyrimidines, lipids, phospholipids, and numerous other metabolites. Individual pathways of biosynthesis include from two to twelve successive enzyme reactions.

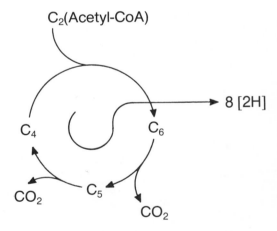

Fig. 3-11. Simplified scheme of the tricarboxylic acid cycle. It is used, on the one hand, for the oxidation of acetate to 2 carbon dioxide and coenzyme-bound hydrogen and, on the other hand, for the preparation of metabolites that are necessary for biosynthetic processes, such as 2-oxoglutarate, succinyl-CoA, and oxaloacetate.

The nitrogen required for the biosynthesis of N-containing substances is available in the cell as ammonium. If the nutrient solution contains nitrate, this must be reduced to ammonium in the course of the assimilatory nitrate reduction process (see 3.2.10). The mercapto sulfur required for the synthesis of sulfur-containing amino acids is made available by assimilatory sulfate reduction.

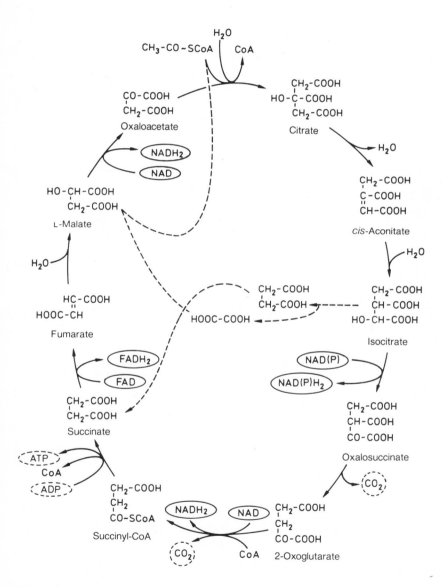

Fig. 3-12. Tricarboxylic acid cycle for the oxidation of acetyl-CoA.

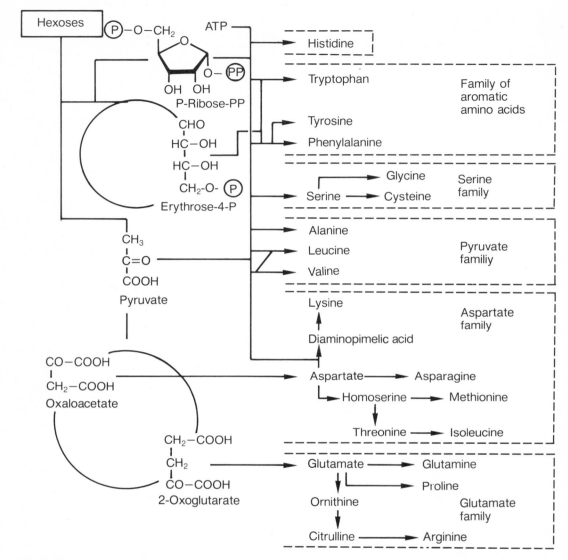

Fig. 3-13. Metabolic pathways for the synthesis of the 20 amino acids that are required for the synthesis of proteins.

3.2.8 Synthesis of Macromolecular Constituents of the Cell

During the growth of the cell, numerous macromolecules are formed from the low-molecular-weight building blocks. The **essential macromolecules** include **deoxyribonucleic acid** (DNA), **ribonucleic acid** (RNA), **proteins**, and **peptidoglycans**. In addition, nonessential macromolecules can be synthesized and accumulated which act as **reserve substances** and are not formed by all microorganisms. This relates to polysaccharides and **poly-β-hydroxybutyric acid.** The macromolecules are also synthesized from activated metabolites which are present in the form either of phosphate esters, adenylate derivatives, or derivatives of coenzyme A.

Deoxyribonucleic acid, which makes up about 3 to 5% of the dry matter of the cell, is synthesized from deoxyribonucleotides by DNA polymerase in the course of DNA replication. The various forms of **ribonucleic acid,** which make up a total of about 5 to 20% of the dry mass, are synthesized from ribonucleotides in the course of transcription by RNA polymerase. The amount of RNA, especially ribosomal RNA, in the cells depends on the rate of growth of the cells; it is high (20%) in fast-growing and low (5%) in slow-growing cells.

Proteins are synthesized from amino acids or activated amino acids present in the form of aminoacyl-transfer RNAs (-tRNAs) in the process of translation on the ribosomes by peptide-bond-linking enzymes. Messenger RNA (mRNA) which contains information on the amino acid sequence, is involved in the process. The cells consist largely of proteins (50 to 70% of the dry matter).

Peptidoglycan, which is the basic skeleton of the bacterial cell, is synthesized from glucose derivatives bearing amino acid side chains; during the synthesis of the macromolecule, glucose derivatives that have first been activated by nucleotides, are transferred to a lipid, transported to the cell wall, and assembled outside the protoplasts. The relative amounts of the macromolecules mentioned in the cells can be influenced to only a very limited extent by changing the conditions of growth.

On the other hand, the **nonessential** macromolecular compounds, such as **polysaccharides** and **poly-β-hydroxybutyric acid (PHB)** can be formed only under certain conditions of growth. Their accumulation can be provoked experimentally. **Polysaccharides** (glycogen and starch) are synthesized by synthetases from nucleotide-activated glucose molecules. PHB is a polymer of β-hydroxybutyric acid and is synthesized from hydroxybutyryl-CoA by means of an appropriate synthase. Both reserve substances are accumulated up to high percentage levels in the cell if carbohydrates or other carbon-containing nutrients are available in excess, but growth is affected by lack of nitrogen or sulfur or because of inadequate aeration. While glycogen and starch are common as reserve materials in both pro- and eucaryotes, whether aerobic or anaerobic, the occurrence of PHB is limited to aerobic procaryotes.

3.2.9 Regulation

The processes of the **uptake** and **degradation of the substrates,** the **generation of energy,** and the **synthesis of metabolites and polymers** in the growing cell are, as a rule, highly coordinated. The coordination of the individual metabolic reactions, which constitutes the harmony of cell metabolism, can be ascribed to the properties of the enzyme proteins, their synthesis, and their function. Regulation of cell metabolism takes place on two levels: on the one hand, by controlling the formation of enzymes and, on the other hand, by modifying their activities.

Regulation by Induction and Repression

The concentration of an enzyme in the cell is a function of the rate at which it is formed. Putting it more accurately, the concentration of the enzyme depends on the frequency of transcription of mRNA. Many enzymes are formed always, regardless of the conditions of the medium; they are **constitutive enzymes.** In contrast to these are the **inducible** and **repressible enzymes.**

The enzymes involved in **substrate degradation** are, as a rule, inducible. They are formed only when the corresponding substrate (the external inducer) is present in the nutrient solution.

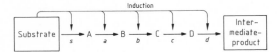

The formation of anabolic enzymes is regulated by enzyme repression.

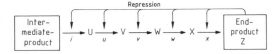

The enzymes involved in the synthesis of amino acids are always formed, for example, when the cells grow in a simple mineral solution containing only energy and nitrogen sources but no amino acids. If an amino acid is added to the nutrient solution, the formation of the enzyme involved in the corresponding synthetic pathway is suppressed or repressed. One speaks of an end-product repression. If two different substrates are available to the cells, then, as a rule, that substrate is preferred which permits faster growth. The enzyme necessary for the degradation of this substrate is formed, and the enzyme necessary for the degradation of the other substrate is repressed, as long as the first substrate is still present.

As a rule, induction and repression relate to all enzymes involved in a pathway of degradation or biosynthesis. Usually, the enzymes belonging to a specific synthetic pathway are formed in a coordinated fashion. In the case of degradation pathways, there may be a coordinated or a sequential induction of the formation of enzymes.

The enzymes of the central metabolic pathways may also undergo regulation at the level of enzyme formation. For example, in aerobically growing cells of *Escherichia coli,* the enzymes of the tricarboxylic acid cycle are present in high concentration. In cells growing anaerobically, the specific activity of these enzymes is only 5 to 10% of the level under aerobic conditions. The formation of 2-oxoglutarate dehydrogenase is actually suppressed completely.

Induction and repression act slowly and can be regarded as a coarse form of regulation.

Regulation by Changing the Catalytic Activities of the Enzymes

As a rule, the **key enzymes** in cell metabolism are subject to regulation at the level of their catalytic activity. The catalytical activities of each enzyme included in a specific degradation or synthetic pathway can be changed in a controllable manner. Because of the controllability of its activity, catalysis can be adapted very rapidly to abruptly changed metabolic situations. The regulation of enzymatic activity can be regarded as fine regulation.

In the case of the majority of enzymes with given properties, the enzymatic activity depends only on the concentration of the substrate and the product and rises hyperbolically with an increase in the substrate concentration (Fig. 3-14). Such enzymes obeying the Michaelis-Menten relation are also called **simple** or **hyperbolic enzymes.** Their activity can be changed only by competing isosteric substrates or by inhibitors. They possess only a few types of centers, namely, the catalytic centers with substrate-binding sites.

In contrast to the simple enzymes are the **regulatory enzymes.** These have considerably more complicated properties (Fig. 3-15b). Most are characterized by substrate saturation the course of which deviates from a paraboloid curve and is frequently sigmoid. The sigmoid curve shows that the enzyme is composed of subunits between which **cooperative interactions** exist. The saturation curve has a very steep section in which the enzyme is highly sensitive, i.e., it reacts to a small change in the substrate concentrations with a large change in enzymatic activity, which almost corresponds to a switching-on or switching-off of the process.

In addition to this, the regulatory enzymes possess, as well as the catalytic centers that recognize and bind the substrates, other, allosteric, centers, likewise stereospecific, which are also known as regulatory centers (Fig. 3-15a). To these are bound **effectors** which modify the activity of the enzyme. There are binding sites for positive effectors (activators) and binding sites for negative effectors (inhibitors). The regulatory enzymes, frequently also called **allosteric** or **sigmoid enzymes,** have a key position in metabolism.

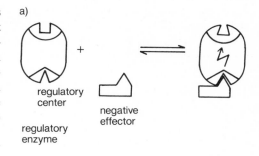

a)

regulatory center

negative effector

regulatory enzyme

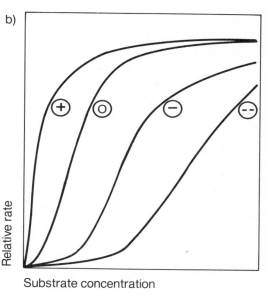

b)

Relative rate

Substrate concentration

Fig. 3-15. A regulatory enzyme binds effectors (a) at the regulatory center that can bring about a lowering (indicated symbolically in the drawing) or a raising of the enzymatic activity. The regulatory enzymes are characterized by a sigmoid substrate saturation curve. The sigmoidity is enhanced by negative effectors and weakened by positive ones (b).

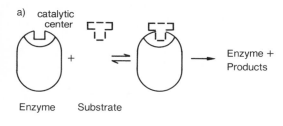

a) catalytic center

Enzyme   Substrate

Enzyme + Products

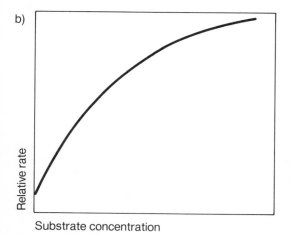

b)

Relative rate

Substrate concentration

Fig. 3-14. A simple enzyme recognizes and binds the substrate at the catalytic center and catalyzes the transformation of the substrate (a). The enzyme activity increases hyperbolically with the substrate concentration (b).

Allosteric effectors are always compounds of low molecular weight, either end-products of biosynthetic pathways or substances the concentration of which can reflect the metabolic situation in the cell, such as adenylates (ATP, ADP, AMP, cAMP, NADH$_2$), or phosphoenol pyruvate. Of the enzymes of a biosynthetic chain, it is usually only the first for the biosynthetic pathway that can be regulated; it is inhibited by the end product.

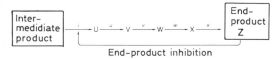

End-product inhibition

Some enzymes are controlled by covalent chemical modification. Here, enzymatic activity is modified by phosphorylation, adenylation, or acetylation. These include glutamine synthetase, citrate lyase, and glycogen synthetase.

As an example of the interlinked nature of regulation, we may show here the essentially allosteric regulation of the central metabolic pathways (Fig. 3-16).

The regulation has the consequence that the microorganisms utilize their nutrients efficiently and that, normally, no building blocks that are to be used for the synthesis of the cell substances are secreted. The overproduction of enzymes and intermediate products is also avoided. From this point of view, the secretion of numerous metabolites and secondary metabolites can be regarded as consequences of a faulty control of the metabolism. Biotechnology makes use of this idea and produces "faultily" regulated mutants which overproduce, accumulate, and secrete a particular metabolite. A knowledge of the metabolic plans of organisms and of the regulation of the pathways of degradation and synthesis can be utilized for a **selection of high-output mutants** for the production of all substances that can be obtained by means of microorganisms. Many methods for the adaptation or programming of microorganisms for the production of antibiotics and other metabolites are based on the selection and combination of faultily regulated mutants.

3.2.10 Substrates of Microorganisms and Degradation Pathways

All substances produced biosynthetically are degradable by microorganisms. For every compound, however complicated, a microorganism exists which is capable of degrading it partially or completely. In their totality, microorganisms appear to be **biochemically omnipotent.** The individual genera or species of bacteria and fungi are, however, characterized by a **limited substrate spectrum** and **specialization to certain groups of substrates.** The commonest substrates are carbohydrates, organic acids, and amino acids. Many bacteria are so highly specialized that they grow very rapidly on aliphatic hydrocarbons but not at all or only very slowly on carbohydrates. While carbohydrates can be channeled into the central metabolic pathways through a few transformation steps, long (peripheral) degradation pathways exist for aromatic and aliphatic hydrocarbons. In many cases, the genetic information for the corresponding enzymes is localized on **plasmids.**

Carbohydrates

Hexoses such as glucose, galactose, fructose, and mannose are taken up into the cell by means of specific permeases and are phosphorylated directly in the cell during transport with conversion into fructose 6-phosphate or glucose 6-phosphate. The hexose phosphate is degraded via the fructose bisphosphate pathway and included in the central pathways. Many bacteria transform hexoses by means of the Entner-Doudoroff pathway. In many microorganisms, the enzymes necessary for the degradation of hexoses are present constitutively; in the overwhelming majority of bacteria these enzymes are inducible.

Disaccharides, such as saccharose, lactose,

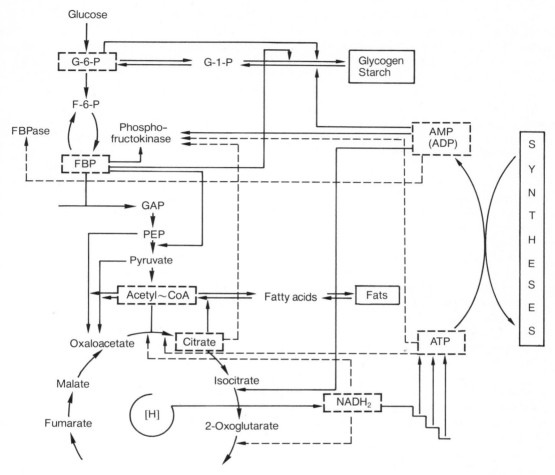

Fig. 3-16. Control of the activity of some of the enzymes involved in the degradation of glucose and the synthesis of storage materials by some metabolites that have a signal function. The thin black arrows proceeding from these metabolites indicate positive, and the red arrows negative, effector functions. If, for example, $NADH_2$ accumulates in the cell (high $NADH_2/NAD$ ratio), the 2-oxoglutarate dehydrogenase is inhibited and 2-oxoglutarate is secreted. An inhibition of the citrate synthase and a blockage of acetyl-CoA may also take place, which leads to the formation of fats. A particularly important control-member of glucose degradation is phosphofructokinase. It is inhibited by ATP and other metabolites; these signal the fact that sufficient ATP (energy) and metabolites are present. Phosphofructokinase therefore acts as a regulatory valve controlling the flux of material. – FBP = Fructose bisphosphate; FBPase = fructose bisphosphatase; GAP = glyceraldehyde 3-phosphate; PEP = Phosphoenolpyruvate.

maltose, and cellobiose are, as a rule, likewise taken up into the cell and processed as entities. The assimilation of disaccharides presupposes the presence of disaccharide-splitting enzymes (invertase, β-galactosidase, maltase, cellobiase). The cleavage products, i.e., the monosaccharides (hexoses) are included in the metabolism on one of the hexose degradation pathways mentioned.

Pentoses are, as a rule, assimilated by only a small number of microorganisms. The wood sugar xylose and many other pentoses are common in plants and pass with plant extracts into the nutrient solution. Part of them is converted into hexoses and glyceraldehyde 3-phosphate through cleavage by phosphoketolase and part of them by transformation via the transketolase-transaldolase system and are then degraded by the known pathways.

Polysaccharides such as starch, glycogen, cellulose, inulin, and other glycans are not taken up as such by the cell but are cleaved outside the cells by secreted **exoenzymes.** Although these polysaccharides are quantitatively some of the predominating products of the formation of biomass on the earth, the number of microorganisms capable of degrading the polymers is not very large. The spore-forming bacteria and many fungi, in particular, are capable of forming starch-degrading enzymes, amylases. The capacity for forming cellulose-degrading enzymes, cellulases, is restricted to a still smaller number of bacteria and fungi. As a rule, the polysaccharides are degraded outside the cell to disaccharides and monosaccharides; both these products can be taken up and subjected to further transformation by the cells. The fact that some polysaccharides can be degraded by microorganisms only with difficulty is of biological importance, since the extracellularly accumulated polysaccharides produced by bacteria and fungi (glucans, fructans, curdlan, xanthan, pullulan, and others) are finding use in the household and in industry.

Organic Acids

The **sugar acids** such as gluconic acid and 2-keto- and 2,5-diketogluconic acids are, in general, good substrates for microorganisms. They are frequently suitable for those bacteria which are incapable of assimilating individual sugars and possess a permease only for fructose but not for glucose, for example. They are introduced into the central pathways via special reactions and the Entner-Doudoroff (ED) pathway. The controlling element of the Entner-Doudoroff pathway is glucose 6-phosphate dehydrogenase; this enzyme regulates the material flow in the ED pathway in a similar manner as phosphofructokinase in the Embden-Meyerhof pathway (see Fig. 3-16). Circumventing this enzyme, gluconate is included in the ED pathway via gluconokinase; the degradation of gluconate is therefore poorly regulated and is suitable for the production of metabolites the formation of which requires a high metabolite pressure (high metabolite concentration) in the cell. Many bacteria grow on organic acids at a high rate and with a good yield. Many organic acids arising in industry as waste products and hitherto unused are suitable for the production of biomass.

C₂ Compounds

Acetate, as a substrate for microorganisms, plays an important role because in activated form (acetyl-CoA) it is a central intermediate of metabolism and takes part in numerous syntheses. When it is supplied as the only substrate, however, additional enzymes of the intermediate metabolism (malate synthase and isocitrate lyase; Fig. 3-17) that are not formed for growth on glucose as substrate (see Fig. 3-16) must be synthesized. For many bacteria, acetate is a readily assimilable growth substrate. Acetate promotes the formation of fatty acids and PHB and is suitable as a substrate in

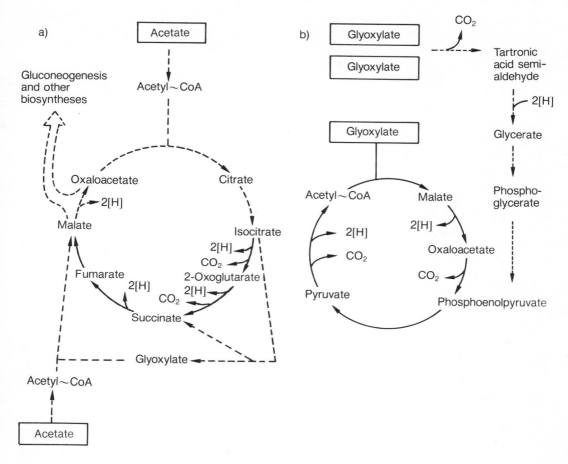

Fig. 3-17. Pathways for the assimilation of acetate (a) and of glyoxylate (b) in metabolism.

those cases where emphasis is placed not on the production of protein-containing biomass but on secretion products.

Glyoxylate is present to only a slight extent in the free form. However, it is the only constituent appearing in the degradation of purines that can be utilized for the production of energy and the synthesis of building blocks. Glyoxylate can be converted with acetyl-CoA into malate or, more frequently, via tartronic semialdehyde into glycerate and 3-phosphoglycerate (see Fig. 3-17).

C_1 Compounds

The C_1 compounds methane, methanol, carbon dioxide, and carbon monoxide have attracted the interest of modern microbiologists since they are available cheaply and in very large amounts. Only special types of microorganisms are capable of assimilating them. **Methane** is assimilated by only a small group of procaryotes, the methane-oxidizing (methylotrophic) bacteria. **Methanol** can be assimilated by bacteria and yeasts. Likewise, only a small group of bacteria (carboxydobacteria) grow on **carbon monoxide**. **Carbon dioxide** can serve as a source of carbon for large groups of bacteria, the **chemolithoautotrophic bacteria** and **photosynthetic organisms**, including anaerobically phototrophic bacteria, aerobic phototrophic bacteria (cyanobacteria), the blue-green algae, and green plants.

Under the action of methane-oxidizing bacteria **methane** is first oxidized to methanol by methane-oxygenase in a reaction consuming one reduction equivalent, and this is then dehydrogenated. The hydrogen liberated in the oxidation of methanol to carbon dioxide is used as a source of energy for methane- and methanol-oxidizing organisms.

$$CH_4 \xrightarrow[H_2O]{O_2+[2H]} CH_3OH \xrightarrow{} HCHO \xrightarrow[\quad]{H_2O} HCOOH \xrightarrow{} CO_2$$
$$\qquad\qquad\quad [2H] \qquad [2H] \qquad [2H]$$

The synthesis of the cell substance starts from the intermediate product formaldehyde and can take place via various routes:

a) Through the **ribulose monophosphate cycle** for fixing formaldehyde (Fig. 3-18). Here ribulose

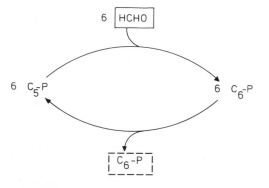

Fig. 3-18. Ribulose monophosphate cycle for the fixation of formaldehyde.

5-phosphate acts as an acceptor of the formaldehyde molecule and hexulose 6-phosphate is formed by hexulose phosphate synthase and is converted by hexulose phosphate isomerase into fructose 6-phosphate. Ribulose 5-phosphate is regenerated via the transaldolase-transketolase reactions.

b) Through the **serine pathway.** Here the formaldehyde group is transferred to glycine, and serine is formed which is included in the central metabolic pathway.

c) Via the **triokinase pathway.** Here formaldehyde and xylulose 5-phosphate are converted by means of transketolase into glyceraldehyde phosphate and dihydroxyacetone. The latter is phosphorylated by triokinase to dihydroxyacetone phosphate. The products are included in the Embden-Meyerhof pathway.

Carbon monoxide, which is available in large amounts in synthesis gas and blast-furnace waste gas, is used by bacteria (carboxydobacteria) for growth. The carbon monoxide (CO) is oxidized by carbon monoxide oxidase to carbon dioxide, and the reducing equivalents arising are used for the aerobic generation of energy. The synthesis of building blocks takes place via the ribulose bisphosphate cycle of carbon dioxide (CO_2) fixation (Fig. 3-19).

All organisms that are capable of obtaining the necessary metabolic energy by the oxidation of inorganic compounds or of hydrogen or by photosynthesis can assimilate **carbon dioxide** via the Calvin cycle or the ribulose bisphosphate cycle. Ribulose bisphosphate acts as the primary carbon dioxide acceptor being cleaved with the fixation of carbon dioxide into two 3-phosphoglycerate molecules. These are included in the sugar metabolism and are partially reconverted into the acceptor via the transaldolase-transketolase reactions.

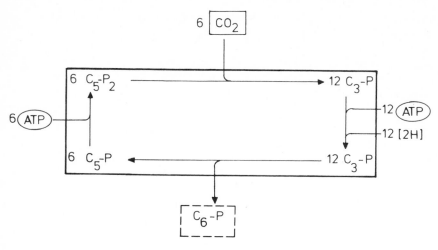

Fig. 3-19. Ribulose bisphosphate cycle for the fixation of carbon dioxide.

Hydrocarbons

Since many bacteria and some yeasts grow very well on **aliphatic hydrocarbons** (alkanes), great hopes have been placed on these raw materials as substrates for the production of biomass and organic acids. There are several bacteria and yeasts which grow faster on hydrocarbons (hexadecane, tetradecane) than on sugars. The degradation of hexadecane takes place only in the presence of oxygen and is initiated by oxygenase reactions (Fig. 3-20). The acetyl-CoA derivatives obtained by β-oxidation are included directly into the central metabolic pathways.

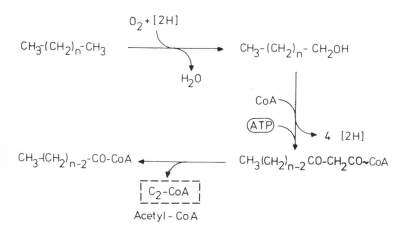

Fig. 3-20. Oxidation of an aliphatic hydrocarbon in the presence of oxygen by a monooxygenase followed by β-oxidation of the fatty acid.

Aromatic compounds, including organic acids (benzoic acid, mandelic acid), amino acids (phenylalanine, tyrosine), and benzene and phenol are also accessible to microorganisms. They likewise undergo conversion only in the presence of oxygen. The initiating oxidation of benzene takes place via a dioxygenase.

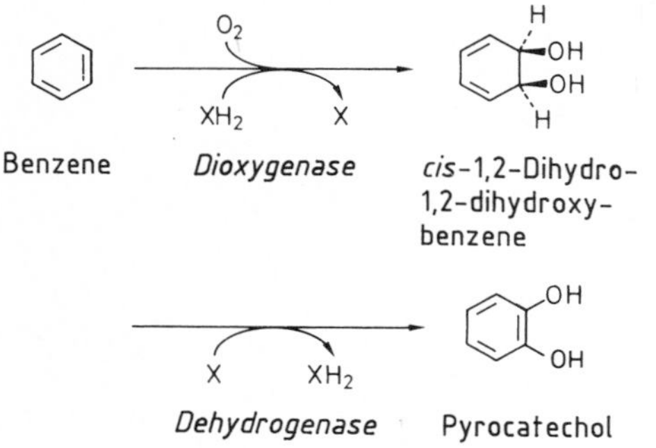

Phenol is oxidized by a monooxygenase to pyrocatechol.

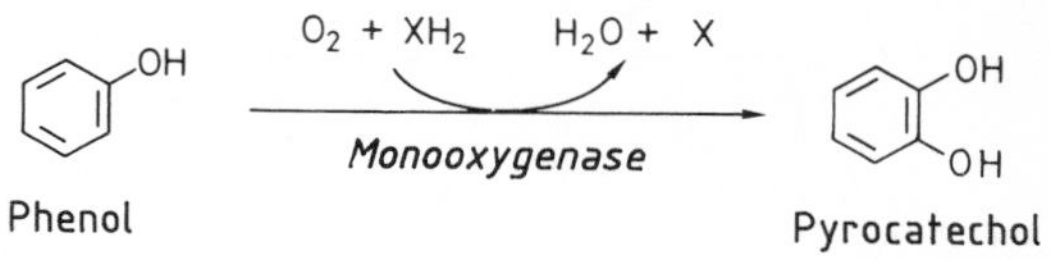

Phenol   Monooxygenase   Pyrocatechol

Benzene   *Dioxygenase*   *cis*-1,2-Dihydro-1,2-dihydroxy-benzene

Dehydrogenase   Pyrocatechol

Only this is cleaved by a dioxygenase to an aliphatic dicarboxylic acid (cis,cis-muconic acid) which is finally converted into known metabolites (acetyl-CoA and succinate) and is included in this way in the intermediate metabolism (Fig. 3-21).

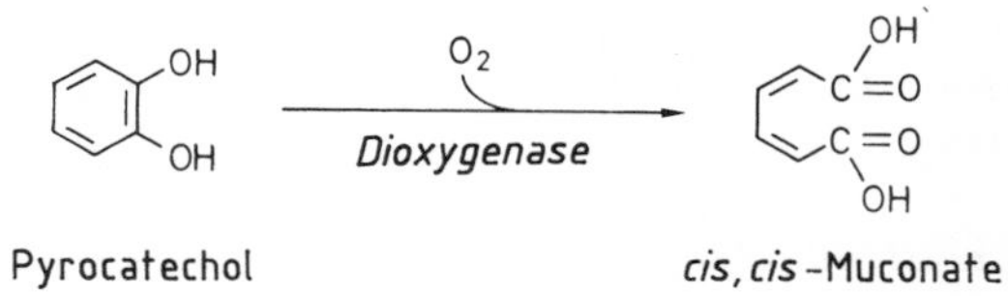

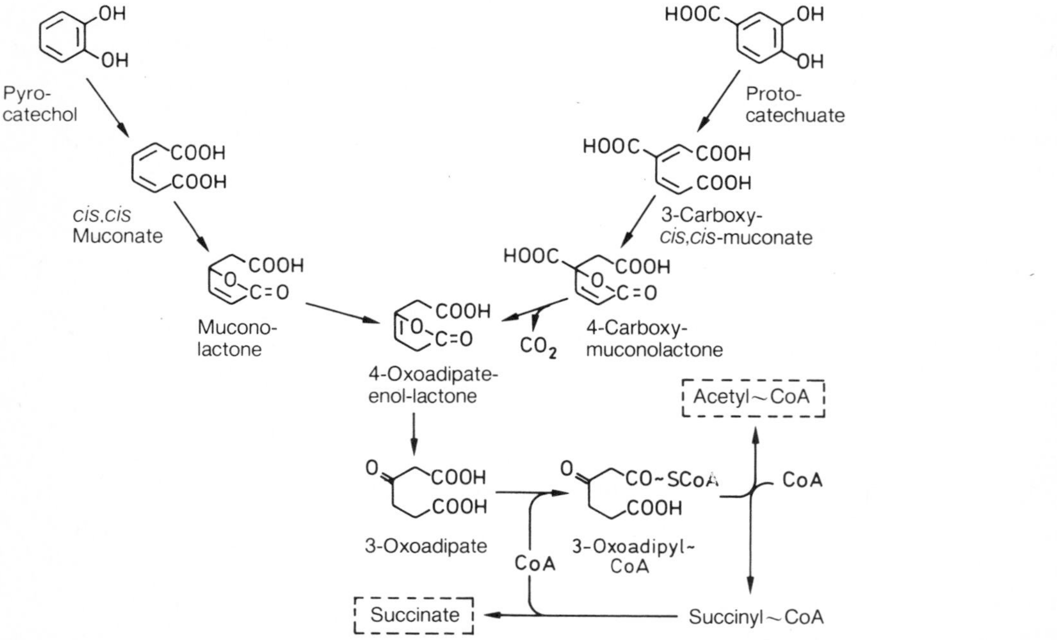

Pyrocatechol   *Dioxygenase*   *cis, cis* -Muconate

Fig. 3-21. Cleavage of the aromatic ring and inclusion of the dicarboxylic acid via the 3-oxoadipate pathway in the central metabolic pathways.

The raw material **lignin,** produced in large amounts in nature, consists largely of aromatic rings and is degraded by fungi and bacteria, but only very slowly and with the partial formation of humic acids.

Sources of Nitrogen

The commonest source of nitrogen for the growth of microorganisms is **ammonium** (Fig. 3-22). Numerous microorganisms are also capable of assimilating **nitrate** or, in low concentrations, **nitrite** and reducing it to ammonia via assimilatory nitrate or nitrite reduction. The capacity for utilizing **urea** is also widespread; it is cleaved by urease. The enzyme is regulated by derepression. As a rule, microorganisms form so much urease that the urea added to the nutrient solution is cleaved completely and ammonium appears. For many production processes, it is necessary to cover the nitrogen demand by the addition of amino acids – either glutamate, aspartate, or alanine – or by the supply of hydrolyzed protein (casamino acids, peptone). If regulatory processes and the avoidance of free ammonia are important, complex sources of nitrogen are indicated.

Only a small number of microorganisms is capable of assimilating **molecular nitrogen** (dinitrogen N_2). However, there is probably a large number of bacteria in which the capacity for nitrogen fixation has not yet been discovered, since the enzyme nitrogenase is extraordinarily oxygen-sensitive.

Oxygen

All strictly aerobic organisms require oxygen (O_2) for growth. They use oxygen as the electron acceptor of the aerobic electron transport process. In this, the oxygen is reduced to water. The microbial assimilation of alkanes and aranes is possible only in the presence of oxygen; in this process, oxygen is incorporated into the carbon skeleton of the organic molecules. Oxygen is soluble in aqueous media in only low concentrations, and the affinity of microorganisms for oxygen is, in general, very high. Oxygen permits a very efficient production of energy and the complete oxidation of the substrates to carbon dioxide and water. However, oxygen can also exhibit harmful effects, particularly when it is supplied at excessively high partial pressures.

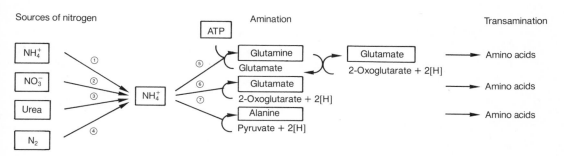

Fig. 3-22. Inclusion of the most important sources of nitrogen in amino acids. – (1) Uptake of ammonium (NH_4^+); (2) assimilatory reduction of nitrate (NO_3^-); (3) cleavage of urea by means of urease; (4) dinitrogen fixation; (5) assimilation of ammonium with the aid of glutamine synthetase having a high affinity for NH_4^+ (small K_m value); (6) assimilation of ammonium with the aid of glutamate dehydrogenase having a low affinity for NH_4^+ (large K_m value); (7) alanine dehydrogenase.

Nitrogen-fixing and autotrophic bacteria are the most sensitive to an excess of oxygen.

The toxicity of oxygen is due primarily to the fact that oxygen can be activated in three different ways.

1. $O_2 + 4e^- \rightarrow 2O^{2-}$
2. $O_2 + 2e^- \rightarrow O_2^{2-}$
3. $O_2 + 1e^- \rightarrow O_2^-$

The tetravalent transfer of electrons to oxygen (1.) is catalyzed by cytochrome oxidase, the terminal enzyme of the electron transport chain. Two oxide ions (O^{2-}) arise which, with two protons each, together lead to the formation of water. The bivalent transfer of electrons to oxygen (2.) leads to the formation of the peroxide anion (O_2^{2-}), i.e., the formation of hydrogen peroxide. This reaction is characteristic for some flavin-containing enzymes. Hydrogen peroxide is toxic for the cell and oxidizes mercapto (SH) groups, for example. Catalase and peroxidase exert protective functions. The monovalent transfer of one electron to oxygen (3.) leads to the formation of the superoxide anion (O_2^-). The reaction is catalyzed by a large number of oxidases, including xanthine oxidase, aldehyde oxidase, and NADPH oxidase, and also by iron-sulfur proteins. As a radical, the superoxide ion is very reactive and leads to the formation of very reactive compounds in the cell. A protective action is shown by superoxide dismutase. This enzyme is apparently present in all strictly aerobic organisms. Due attention must always be paid to the undesirable side-reactions of these enzymes when the organisms are aerated or when hyperbaric oxygen or air under pressure is used.

3.3 Assignment of the Most Important Secretion Products to the Metabolic Types of Microorganisms

The use of microorganisms in industry generally aims at the production of **biomass** or the formation of **primary or secondary metabolites.** Among the primary metabolites, two large groups must be distinguished:

a) Those of anaerobic fermentation (in Pasteur's sense) in which reduced metabolic products are secreted that play a role in the energy metabolism of the fermenting microorganisms.

b) In contrast to these products there is a series of similar compounds which are secreted by strictly aerobic or facultative aerobic microorganisms in the course of an overflow metabolism.

The products of anaerobic fermentations include a series of alcohols, organic acids, and gases: ethanol, propan-2-ol, butanol, butanediol, acetone, formate, acetate, lactate, propionate, butyrate, succinate, caproate, molecular hydrogen, and carbon dioxide.

The products of incomplete oxidations include citrate, glutamate, malate, fumarate, lactate, succinate, 2-oxoglutarate, gluconate, acetate, and many others.

3.4 Metabolic Types

For scientists interested in physiology, biochemistry, and biotechnology, the diversity of microorganisms is visible at a glance when they are included in groups with respect to their metabolic type. The distinguishing characteristics at the basis of this grouping are as follows:

a) Capacity for growth without oxygen (anaerobically) or without alternative inorganic hydrogen acceptors, or incapacity for this (key words: fermentative metabolism – respiratory metabolism).

b) Generation of energy by the utilization of chemical energy (reduction and oxidation reactions) or of light energy (key words: chemotrophic – phototrophic).

c) Generation of energy only by substrate-level phosphorylation or additionally by electron-transport phosphorylation (key words: fermentative production of energy – respiratory production of energy).

d) Generation of the reducing equivalents (hydrogen, electrons) necessary for energy transformation by utilizing inorganic compounds or organic compounds (key words: lithotrophic – organotrophic).

e) Capacity for assimilating carbon dioxide (CO_2) as the sole source of carbon (C) (autotrophic) or otherwise (heterotrophic).

When these different specific features are taken into account (Table 3-2), the microorganisms are divided into the groups mentioned under 3.4.1 to 3.4.5. Overlappings and exceptions are not considered here.

3.4.1 Basic Properties of Fermentative Organisms

Almost only **bacteria** are capable of growth with the **generation of energy by fermentation.** Fermentation takes place in the absence of oxygen, under anaerobic conditions. It is an ATP-regenerating metabolic process in which the cleavage products of the organic substrate (hexose) act simultaneously as hydrogen donors and hydrogen acceptors. In this process, part of the substrate is oxidized and the energy so liberated is utilized for the regeneration of ATP. The cell gets rid of the oxidized carbon in the form of carbon dioxide. The reduction equivalents formed during oxidation are transferred to the residue of the substrate and secreted with these residues (Fig. 3-23).

Most fermentative organisms are **strict anaerobes;** they are capable of growing only under absolutely anaerobic conditions, and oxygen is a poison for them. These include the strictly anaerobic spore-forming bacteria

Table 3-2. Key-Word Description of the Modes of Nutrition of Microorganisms in Relation to their Source of Energy, their Hydrogen Donor, and their Source of Carbon.

Source of energy, hydrogen donor or source of carbon	Type of nutrition
1. Source of energy	
a) Radiation (light)	Phototrophic
b) Oxidation of inorganic or organic compounds	Chemotrophic
2. Hydrogen donor	
a) Reduced inorganic compounds	Lithotrophic
(NH_4^+, NO_2^-, S^{2-}, S, $S_2O_3^{2-}$, Fe^{2+}, CO, H_2)	
b) Organic compounds	Organotrophic
3. Source of carbon	
a) Carbon dioxide as the main source of carbon	Autotrophic
b) Organic compounds	Heterotrophic

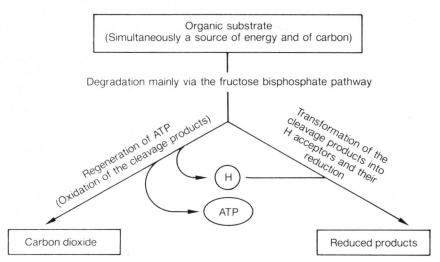

Fig. 3-23. The principle of fermentative metabolism such as is realized for example, in alcoholic fermentation by yeast and bacteria, heteroenzymatic lactic fermentation, propionic acid fermentation, formic acid fermentation, and butyric acid-butanol fermentation.

(clostridia). Many fermentative organisms are **aerotolerant** and microaerophilic; they are capable of tolerating oxygen at relatively low partial pressures or even of assimilating it. These include the lactic acid bacteria, propionic acid bacteria, and others. The Enterobacteriaceae are **facultative anaerobes,** i.e., they are capable of generating energy and growing by respiration and also of performing anaerobic fermentation.

On the basis of the particularly characteristic or quantitatively predominating secretion products (Fig. 3-24), a distinction is made between alcoholic fermentation, lactic acid fermentation, propionic acid fermentation, formic acid fermentation, butyric acid fermentation, and homoacetic acid fermentation.

Alcoholic fermentation by yeasts and bacteria

Ethanol appears as a fermentation product with many fermenting organisms (see Chapter

10). As the quantitatively predominating product it is formed by yeasts and a few bacteria.

The ethanol-forming bacteria and yeasts are used in biotechnology mainly for the production of ethanol and glycerol and for microbial transformation.

Lactic Acid Fermentation

The lactic-acid-forming bacteria do in fact obtain their metabolic energy solely through fermentation, but they behave as aerotolerant, i.e., they grow even in the presence of air. The lactic acid bacteria in the narrower sense have very complex requirements for growth factors. They grow very well on milk, whey, and plant juices where many growth factors and intermediate products are available. They are capable of cleaving milk sugar (lactose) by phosphorylation with the aid of β-galactosidase into glucose and galactose and of assimilating both constituents. For the manufacture of lactic acid, use is made of homofermentative lac-

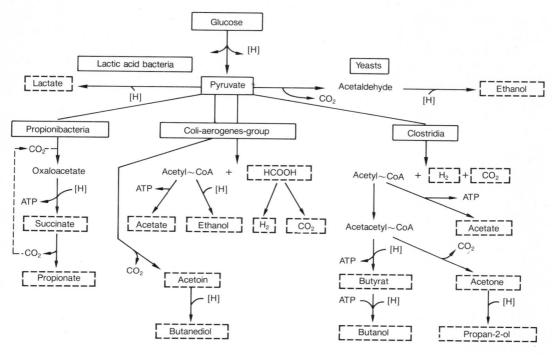

Fig. 3-24. The products of the fermentation of glucose by the most important groups of fermenting organisms.

tic acid bacteria which convert the sugar into lactate with a yield of more than 90%. In the case of the heterofermentative lactic acid fermentation, acetate and/or ethanol also appear in addition to lactate.

The **fields of application of lactic acid bacteria** are extraordinarily manifold. They are used for the souring of milk and milk products, for the manufacture of cheese, bread, and sourdough, for the preparation of sauerkraut and silage and of raw sausage and fermented meat products, and also for the manufacture of technical lactic acid (see Chapter 9). Reference may be made to the fact that pure lactic acid can also be obtained by the fermentation of hexoses by fungi, and the lactic acid prepared in this way is easier to purify than

that obtained with the aid of lactic acid bacteria.

Propionic Acid Fermentation

Propionic acid is the product of the fermentation of lactic acid or carbohydrates by propionibacteria, and also by numerous other bacteria and also by worms. The propionibacteria are microaerotolerant bacteria, which, under strictly anaerobic conditions, ferment lactic acid to propionic acid and succinic acid, but with access of oxygen they carry out limited respiration and, under these conditions, secrete acetic acid as well as propionic acid.

Biotechnologically, the propionibacteria probably have their main field of application in the manufacture of Emmentaler cheese (p. 363) and vitamin B_{12} (p. 456).

Formic Acid Fermentation

Formic acid appears as a fermentation product mostly together with other organic acids such as acetoacetate, succinate, and lactate and the alcohols butanediol, ethanol, and glycerol. Consequently, a "mixed acid fermentation" is also referred to. This type of fermentation is characteristic for the Enterobacteriaceae and for the luminescent bacteria, some bacilli, and a few other forms. The Enterobacteriaceae are facultative anaerobic bacteria; they are capable of carrying out a respiratory metabolism in the presence of oxygen and of fermentation when oxygen is excluded.

Of biotechnical importance are, in the first place, the bacilli belonging physiologically to this group, such as *Bacillus macerans* and *Bacillus polymyxa,* which are used not only because of their fermentation products (butanediol) but also because of the secretion of amylases and proteases.

Butyric Acid – Butanol Fermentation

Butyrate, butanol, acetone, propan-2-ol, and other organic acids and alcohols are typical products of the fermentation of carbohydrates by anaerobic spore-forming organisms (clostridia). The clostridia have available a pronounced fermentative metabolism and grow only under anaerobic conditions. However, there are transitions from strictly anaerobic to almost aerotolerant species. Among the clostridia there are several extremely thermophilic species the temperature optimum of which lies between 60 and 75°C. Taken all together, the clostridia ferment a wide range of natural materials; e.g., polysaccharides such as starch, glycogen, cellulose, hemicellulose, and pectins, and also nucleic acids, proteins, amino acids, purines, and pyrimidines. Many clostridia are strictly specialized for the degradation of only individual natural products out of those mentioned.

From the point of view of biotechnology, the bacteria are of great interest for the manufacture of the products mentioned, and it also appears possible to isolate new fermentation types. Since most of the fermentative organisms belonging here also produce carbon dioxide and molecular hydrogen, they play an eminent role in the anaerobic food chain and in the production of methane.

Homoacetate Fermentation

The homoacetate fermenters (*Clostridium formicoaceticum, C. thermoaceticum*) are characterized by the fact that they form acetate from hexose and, indeed, more than 2 (almost 3) moles of acetate per mole. The reason for this is that these bacteria are capable of using carbon dioxide as hydrogen acceptor and of transferring the fermentation hydrogen to carbon dioxide with the formation of acetate. It appears possible that these bacteria may acquire biotechnological importance for the manufacture of acetate from carbohydrates. They are present in sewage, where they convert hexoses into acetate, which is utilized by methane-forming bacteria to generate methane (see Chapter 16).

3.4.2 Basic Properties of the Organotrophic Aerobically Respiring Microorganisms

The respiratory metabolism with oxygen as hydrogen acceptor is by far the commonest type of metabolism among organisms. It is found in the **strictly aerobic bacteria** as well as in all **nonphotosynthetic eucaryotes,** i.e., fungi, including yeasts, protozoa and metazoa. As a rule, the organic substances are finally oxidized to water and carbon dioxide and are partially incorporated in the cell substance. For most organisms, oxygen is the obligatory terminal hydrogen acceptor but some bacteria are capable, when oxygen is absent and nitrate is present, of obtaining energy by "anaerobic respiration." Taken all together, the aerobically respiring microorganisms have all natural materials available as substrates; however, for individual species of bacteria there are more or less pronounced substrate specificities.

The aerobically respiring microorganisms are of biotechnological importance particularly for the production of biomass, single-cell protein, poly-β-hydroxybutyric acid, endotoxins, and other cell substances. Since respiration is a very efficient process of ATP regeneration, a large part of the substrate is converted into biomass. As a rule, the ratio of biomass production and respiration depends on the energy content (state of reduction) of the substrate; for example, only 50% (w/w) of biomass can be formed from glucose, but 100% (w/w) from hexadecane.

However, the aerobically respiring microorganisms have their outstanding importance for technical microbiology as a result of their capacity not only for completely oxidizing the substrate but also for oxidizing it only **partially** and secreting it again in partly oxidized form. These processes are called "**incomplete oxidation,**" or, because of the similarity of the products secreted to those of anaerobic fermentation, they are also called "oxidative fermentations."

Finally, the aerobically respiring microorganisms also play a role as producing agents of so-called secondary metabolites, i.e., antibiotics, alkaloids, pigments, etc. (see Chapters 4 and 13).

Aerobic Acetic Acid Formation

The acetic-acid-forming bacteria (Acetobacter, Gluconobacter) are characterized by the fact that they oxidize their substrates (alcohols, sugars) only incompletely even when oxygen is supplied in excess. For growth, they use the hydrogen derived from the substrate as a source of energy and transfer it via the electron-transport chain to oxygen with the formation of water; the cell substance is built up from a small part of the substrate with the involvement of vitamins and some building blocks, the presence of which in the nutrient solution is required by many of these bacteria.

$$CH_3-CH_2OH \xrightarrow{\quad} CH_3-CHO \xrightarrow{\ H_2O\ } CH_3COOH$$

Ethanol $\quad$ [2H] Acetaldehyde [2H] $\quad$ Acetic acid

Well-known examples are the oxidation of ethanol to acetate, of propanol to propionic acid, of propan-2-ol to acetone, of glycerol to dihydroxyacetone, of sorbitol to sorbose, of xylose to xylonate, and of glucose to gluconate, 2-keto-gluconate, and 2,5-diketogluconate.

Aerobic Formation of Acid by Fungi

Almost all fungi, including the yeasts, are strictly aerobic. They have a respiratory metabolism available and are capable of oxidizing substrates to water and carbon dioxide. Depending on the conditions of the medium and the availability of oxygen, through certain additives these organisms can, however, give rise to the **secretion of metabolites.** When brought under anaerobic conditions or incubated with a deficiency of oxygen, they secrete ethanol or lactic acid or other acids. This is utilized in the formation of ethanol by yeast. Among the lower fungi (phycomycetes) there are many species that, under anaerobic conditions, produce lactic acid, which, as the fungi are capable of growth in quite simple synthetic nutrient solutions, can be isolated in very pure form. With the aid of fungi, by means of the glucose oxidase secreted into the medium, gluconic acid can also be obtained from glucose. With suitable aeration and at a low pH, *Aspergillus niger* forms citric acid; some yeasts have also proved to be capable of this which can actually utilize aliphatic hydrocarbons as substrates. Fungi can also be used for the production of oxalate, malate, fumarate, succinate, lactate, 2-oxoglutamate, and itaconate.

Production of Amino Acids by Bacteria

Several bacteria of the coryneform, Gram-positive group (Corynebacterium, Brevibacterium, Arthrobacter) can be used for the **production of amino acids.** Hexoses or acetate serve as substrates. Secretion takes place on aeration or suboptimal aeration. As a rule, the secretion of amino acids is greatest when the rate of aeration of the bacteria does not permit the maximum rate of respiration, i.e., when the actual rate of respiration is smaller than the maximum (Hirose et al., 1978; Schlegel and Vollbrecht, 1980) (see Chapters 11 and 15).

Chemical Transformation by Bacteria

Microorganisms are used on a large scale for modifying organic compounds (Kieslich, 1978). The microbial transformations may involve oxidations, hydrogenations, hydrolyses, esterifications, methylations, decarboxylations, dehydrations, deaminations, and aminations. Most of the microorganisms used for these purposes have a strictly aerobic respiratory metabolism (see Chapter 14).

Production of Antibiotics

Antibiotics are secondary metabolites which are mainly secreted by strictly aerobic fungi and by actinomycetes and other bacteria (see Chapters 4 and 13).

Production of Polysaccharides and Waxes

Strictly aerobic bacteria are used primarily for the production of exopolysaccharides such as dextran, xanthan, fructan, curdlan, and alginates (Sutherland and Ellwood, 1979) (see Chapter 11). Waxes and hydrocarbons can also be manufactured with the aid of bacteria (Tornabene, 1977).

Production of Enzymes

Many bacteria and fungi secrete enzymes such as invertase, proteases, pectinase and pectinolytic enzymes, lipase, glucose oxidase, hexose isomerase, amylases, and cellulases and are used for the technical production of these enzymes (see Chapter 12).

3.4.3   Basic Properties of the Lithotrophic Aerobically Respiring Bacteria

Included in the group of aerobic chemolithotrophic bacteria are several groups of soil and water bacteria which are capable of obtaining their metabolic energy by the **oxidation of inorganic compounds or ions** (ammonium, nitrite, sulfide, thiosulfate, sulfite, and iron(II) ions) as well as elemental sulfur or hydrogen as electron donors (Fig 3-25). In this way they obtain reducing equivalents and energy for synthetic processes. The production of energy

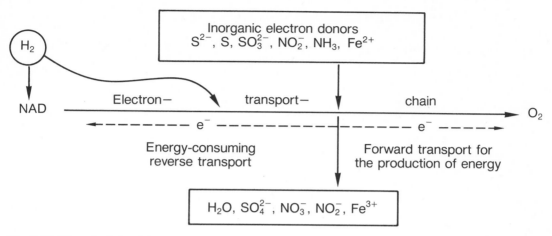

Fig. 3-25. The principle of the energy metabolism of lithotrophic aerobically respiring bacteria. Inorganic electron donors are oxidized. The electrons appearing in this process are included in the electron-transport chain and used partly for the production of energy and partly for the reduction of NAD.

takes place through electron-transport phosphorylation, and oxygen is the terminal hydrogen acceptor. They obtain the carbon for the synthesis of the cell substances through the fixation of carbon dioxide via the ribulose bisphosphate cycle. Some chemolithoautotrophic bacteria are obligately bound to the above-mentioned mode of life; others are also capable, alternatively, of growing chemoorganoheterotrophically, and are therefore facultative chemotrophs. Many have a monopolistic position; the oxidation of ammonium, nitrite, and inorganic sulfur compounds is linked to the activity of the nitrifying and sulfur-oxidizing bacteria.

Nitrification

The only organisms that are capable of converting ammonium into nitrate, i.e., of nitrification, are the nitrifying bacteria or nitrifiers. No bacterium is known that converts ammonium directly into nitrate; on the contrary, two groups of bacteria are involved in this oxida-

tion; the ammonium oxidizers (e.g., *Nitrosomonas europaea*) form nitrite and the nitrite oxidizers (e.g., *Nitrobacter winogradskyi*) form nitrates. Since in the mineralization of organic matter the nitrogen becomes available in the form of ammonium and the liberation of nitrogen in the form of dinitrogen can start only from nitrate, the nitrifiers play a large part in the nitrogen cycle and in **sewage plants** (see Chapter 16).

The Oxidation of Sulfur and of Iron(II)

Only a group of strictly aerobic bacteria is capable of oxidizing reduced sulfur compounds under aerobic conditions and several species of them are combined to form the genus Thiobacillus. They also include one type of spirillum and the genus Sulfolobus. They oxidize the sulfur compounds (sulfides, sulfur, and thiosulfate) to sulfuric acid; the oxidation process and acidification due to *Thiobacillus ferrooxidans* is utilized for the

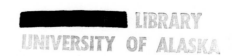

production of heavy metals (copper, zinc, uranium) from poor ores in the presence of pyrite-containing ores (iron sulfide) (see Chapter 17).

Oxidation of Molecular Hydrogen

Molecular hydrogen (H_2) is assimilated by many aerobic and anaerobic bacteria. The aerobic hydrogen-oxidizing bacteria include numerous genera and species *(Alcaligenes eutrophus [= Hydrogenomonas], Pseudomonas facilis, Paracoccus denitrificans)*. They can all grow with hydrogen as the source of energy, carbon dioxide as the source of carbon, and oxygen as the terminal electron acceptor. A small group of bacteria, carboxydobacteria, are capable of oxidizing carbon monoxide under aerobic conditions. Most of them are also capable of growing with hydrogen and carbon dioxide. The biotechnological role of these bacteria resides primarily in the **production of biomass** from hydrogen, carbon monoxide and carbon dioxide if hydrogen can be made available cheaply in the future.

3.4.4 Basic Properties of the "Anaerobically Respiring" Bacteria

A few groups of bacteria are also capable, even when atmospheric oxygen is excluded, of utilizing electron-transport phosphorylation for the production of energy if nitrate, sulfate, sulfur, carbonates, or other compounds are available as hydrogen acceptors. In this process, the compounds are converted into nitrite, dinitrogen, hydrogen sulfide, methane, acetic acid, or other highly reduced compounds (Fig. 3-26). The organisms and processes mentioned are of great practical importance.

Although the term "respiration" should be restricted to processes taking place with the uptake of atmospheric oxygen, when the above-mentioned highly oxidized compounds are used as electron acceptors one also refers colloquially to "anaerobic respiration." The choice of this term is justified by the fact that in both groups, the aerobically and the anaerobically respiring bacteria, there is a respiratory generation of energy by electron-transport phosphorylation.

Denitrification and Nitrate Reduction

Denitrification is the name given to the process of nitrate reduction in which dinitrogen oxide (N_2O) and nitrogen (N_2) are formed. Under anaerobic conditions, the electrons are transferred to nitrate.

$$NO_3^- \rightarrow NO_2^- \rightarrow NO \rightarrow N_2O \rightarrow N_2$$

Numerous bacteria are capable of producing energy with denitrification; they are all aerobic bacteria which are incapable of growing in the absence of oxygen or nitrate. They therefore perform a respiratory metabolism with oxygen or nitrate as electron acceptors. No obligate anaerobes are known among the denitrifiers. The denitrifiers are the only organisms that can reconvert bound nitrogen into molecular nitrogen. They are responsible for the loss of nitrogen by the soil during the occasional anaerobiosis of the soil; the process can also be utilized in sewage plants if nitrified water with organic substrates is kept under anaerobic conditions and the bound nitrogen is converted into free nitrogen (N_2).

The bacteria belonging to a second group, mainly Enterobacteriaceae, likewise reduce nitrate under anaerobic conditions, but only the reduction of nitrate to nitrite is to be regarded as an electron-transport process; the reduction of nitrite to ammonium is linked to fermentation, and nitrite acts as an external

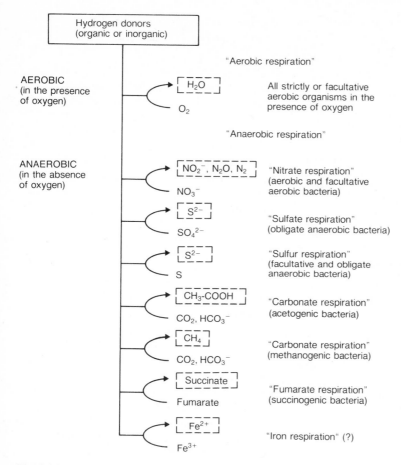

Fig. 3-26. Review of the groups of bacteria with respiratory energy generation, arranged according to their electron acceptors.

electron acceptor. The total process is also known as nitrate ammonification.

$$NO_3^- \rightarrow NO_2^- \rightarrow HNO \rightarrow NH_2OH \rightarrow NH_3$$

Formation of Hydrogen Sulfide by the Reduction of Sulfate

A small group of bacteria is capable of obtaining energy by electron-transport phosphoryla-tion under anaerobic conditions with sulfate as the terminal electron acceptor; the product of the reduction of the sulfate is **hydrogen sulfide**. The major amount of the hydrogen sulfide arising in nature results from this metabolic process. The biogenic sulfur deposited in sediments also owes its origin to these bacteria.

The sulfate-reducing bacteria, of which only the genera Desulfovibrio, Desulfotomaculum, Desulfobacter, and Desulfosarcina may be mentioned here, are of enormous biotechnical importance (see Chapters 16 and 17).

a) Under anaerobic conditions, in the presence of sulfates they form hydrogen sulfide and hydrogen; both products lead to the anaerobic corrosion of iron and other heavy metals.

b) In the digesters of sewage plants, sulfate is preferred to carbonate as electron acceptor; in the presence of sulfate, therefore, the formation of hydrogen sulfide predominates over the formation of methane. When there is a shortage of sulfur for industrial processes, hydrogen sulfide or elemental sulfur could be obtained very easily from seawater sulfate and organic wastes.

Formation of Methane by the Reduction of Carbonate

The main sources for the methane occurring in nature or obtainable by microbial transformation are acetate, on the one hand, and carbon dioxide and molecular hydrogen, on the other. While only a few methane-forming (methanogenic) bacteria are capable of using acetate as a source of methane, all methanogenic bacteria are capable of utilizing hydrogen and carbon dioxide. The methanogenic bacteria can therefore also be referred to as anaerobic, chemolithoautotrophic, hydrogen-oxidizing bacteria; they obtain energy by the **oxidation of hydrogen to methane** and fix carbon dioxide in the course of an assimilatory reduction of carbon dioxide via acetyl-CoA and pyruvate.

The biotechnological importance of this group of bacteria resides in the properties of methane, which is an excellent energy carrier and which does not need to be distilled off from the fermentation charge after its formation, since it is volatile and substantially insoluble in the aqueous medium.

Formation of Acetate by the Reduction of Carbonate

The acetogenic bacteria are likewise to be regarded as anaerobic chemolithoautotrophic hydrogen-oxidizing bacteria which obtain their metabolic energy by anaerobic respiration (carbonate respiration). Although hitherto only two forms, *Clostridium aceticum* and *Acetobacterium woodii,* have been described, it may be expected that with diligent searching it will also be possible to isolate thermophilic and still more robust strains. The bacteria are probably involved in the formation of acetate in sewage tanks during the formation of methane and are responsible for their acidification (see Chapter 16).

Formation of Succinate by the Reduction of Fumarate

In the description of the fermentation process, succinate was put forward as a fermentation product without its being mentioned that the formation of succinate can be linked with an electron-transport phosphorylation process. Succinate is the product of the reduction of fumarate, which arises by the carboxylation of phosphoenol pyruvate.

This step, which is catalyzed by fumarate reductase, takes place in the membrane and can be linked with a phosphorylation. There are many bacteria, mainly among the facultatively anaerobic fermentative species, that make use of this efficient mode of energy production.

3.4.5 Basic Properties of Phototrophic Organisms

The elementary process of photosynthesis consists in the conversion of light energy into biochemically utilizable energy (see 3.2.4). In some groups of procaryotes and eucaryotes, photosynthetic electron transport also leads to the provision of reducing power in the form of $NADPH_2$. Among the organisms that are capable of using light as a source of energy for growth, i.e., are phototrophic, two major groups are to be distinguished.

a) The **purple bacteria** and the **green bacteria** operate an anoxygenic photosynthesis. In addition to light, they also rely on reduced hydrogen donors, such as hydrogen sulfide or hydrogen (H_2) or organic compounds and evolve no oxygen during photosynthesis.

$$H_2S + CO_2 \xrightarrow{\text{light}} \text{cell substance} + S$$

b) In contrast to these, the **cyanobacteria** utilize water as the hydrogen donor and evolve oxygen in the light:

$$H_2O + CO_2 \xrightarrow{\text{light}} \text{cell substance} + O_2$$

They operate an oxygenic photosynthesis.

Representatives of both procaryotes can easily be used in fermenters with light and some even without illumination and be employed for various purposes. With the aid of both groups of organisms it is possible to obtain biomass by utilizing light energy and carbon dioxide. They also serve to remove nutrient salts from the prepared water in the final stages of sewage purification.

Finally, they can be used as raw material for the manufacture of pigments, enzymes, and vitamins. Investigations being performed intensively have the aim of splitting water in light with the aid of isolated components or synthetic systems in order to obtain hydrogen as an important energy carrier.

3.5 The Impulse to Research

The comparative physiology of metabolism has led to a satisfactorily clear picture. Against the background of known relationships, it should not be difficult to use known organisms for biotechnological purposes and to profit from their activities. However, there are no grounds for settling back in a state of self-satisfaction and persisting in the assumption that we have a good idea of the metabolic plans of the known microorganisms and know their principles and there are no new types of metabolism and relationships to be discovered. The successes of research on microorganisms and their application are largely due to the investigation of a few model organisms and studies on fewer (mono)cultures. Practically no studies have been made on the metabolism of mixed cultures and in natural habitats. Furthermore, the physiology of metabolism has justifiably been oriented towards molecular biology and primarily to the easily studied metabolic processes. However, the biotechnologist has to deal with fermenter charges which frequently last for several days and in which the organisms reach their most productive phase in the second week. Under these conditions he comes across many phenomena which cannot be explained by our present knowledge of molecular biology. It is not only the short-term but also the slowly acting effects of the medium and modes of reaction of the microorganisms that must be studied.

In addition to this, out of the almost unimaginable number of bacteria, fungi, unicellular algae, and protozoa only a vanishingly small group has hitherto been studied intensively and used for biotechnological processes, and even if not every species may prove to be an extreme individualist, there are nevertheless sufficient combinations that must be investigated. Here, particular attention should be devoted to organisms adapted to extreme environmental conditions. According to the most recent findings available, only a small proportion of the organisms adapted to extremely high or low temperatures, hydrogen ion concentrations, oxygen concentrations, illumination situations, concentrations of poisons, and ionic strengths has been studied. Basic research should not be neglected, either, nor should a project be broken off if after five years' work it does not yet promise to yield a profit. If one may apply the old gardeners' saying in this form, an overemphasis on applied research at the expense of basic research makes rich sons but poor grandsons.

3.6   *Literature*

3.6.1   *Cited Literature*

Brock, T. D.: *Biology of Microorganisms,* 3rd Ed. Prentice-Hall, Englewood Cliffs 1979.
Kieslich, K.: *Microbial Transformation of Nonsteroid Cyclic Compounds.* Thieme-Verlag, Stuttgart 1976.
Pelczar, M. J., Chan, E. C. S., Krieg, N.: *Microbiology.* Mc Graw Hill Brook Comp., New York 1986.
Schlegel, H. G.: *Allgemeine Mikrobiologie,* 6th Ed. Thieme-Verlag, Stuttgart 1985.
Stanier, R. Y., Ingraham, J. L., Wheelis, M. L., Painter, P. R.: *The Microbial World,* 5th Ed. Prentice-Hall, Englewood Cliffs, New Jersey 1986.
Starr, M. P., Stolp, H., Trüper, H. G., Balows, A., Schlegel H. G. (eds.): *The Prokaryotes. A Handbook on habitats, isolation and identification of bacteria.* Vol. I and II. Springer-Verlag, Berlin 1981.
Sutherland, I. W., Ellwood, D. C., "Microbial exopolysaccharides – industrial polymers of current and future potential", *Soc. Gen. Microbiol. Symp.* **29,** 107–160, (1979).

Tornabene, T. G.: "Microbial formation of hydrocarbons". In: H. G. Schlegel, J. Barnea (eds.): *Microbial Energy Conversion.* Goltze-Verlag, Göttingen 1976, pp. 281–299.

3.6.2   *Further Reading*

a)   Basic Metabolism

Gottschalk, G.: *Bacterial Metabolism,* 2nd Ed. Springer-Verlag, Heidelberg 1986.
Jungermann, K., Möhler, H.: *Biochemie.* Springer-Verlag, Berlin 1980.
Karlson, P.: *Kurzes Lehrbuch der Biochemie,* 12th Ed. Thieme-Verlag, Stuttgart 1984.
Lehninger, A. L.: *Biochemistry, the Molecular Basis of Cell Structure and Function.* 2nd Ed. Worth Publishers, New York 1975.

b)   Fermentation Organisms and Other Anaerobes

Balch, W. E., Fix, G. E., Magrum, L. H., Woesse, C. R., Wolfe, R. S., "Methanogens: Reevaluation of a unique biological group", *Microbiol. Rev.* **43,** 260 (1979).
Gottschalk, G., Andreesen, J. R., "Energy metabolism in anaerobes", *Int. Rev. Biochem.* **21,** 85–105 (1979).
Gottschalk, G.: "The anaerobic way of life of prokaryotes". In: Starr, M. P. et al. (eds.): *The Prokaryotes: A Handbook on Habitats, Isolation and Identification of Bacteria.* Springer-Verlag, New York 1981.

c)   Metabolism of Aerobic Producing Agents

Aida, K., Chibata, I., Nakayama, K., Takinami, K., Yamada, H.: "Biotechnology of amino acid production". In: *Progress in industrial Microbiology* Vol. 24 (1986). Kondansha Ltd., Tokyo, 1986 – Elsevier Amsterdam–Oxford–New York–Tokyo.
Foster, J. W.: *Chemical Activities of Fungi.* Academic Press, New York 1949.
Iizuka, H., Natio, A.: *Microbial Transformation of Steroids and Alkaloids.* University of Tokyo Press, 1967.

Umbarger, H. E., "Amino acid biosynthesis and its regulation", *Annu. Rev. Biochem.* **47**, 533 (1978).

d)   Lithotrophic and Phototrophic Bacteria

Clayton, R. W., Sistrom, W. R. (eds.): *The Photosynthetic Bacteria*. Plenum Press, New York 1978.
Collins, V. G., "Isolation, cultivation and maintenance of autotrophs", *Meth. Microbiol.* **3B** (1969).

Hardy, R. W. F., Bottomley, F., Burns, R. C. (eds.): *A Treatise on Dinitrogen Fixation*. Wiley, New York 1979.

Schlegel, H. G.: "Mechanisms of chemo-autotrophy". In: O. Kinne (ed.): *Marine Ecology, a Comprehensive, Integrated Treatise on Life in Oceans and Coastal Waters*, Vol. II: *Physiological Mechanism*, Part 1. Wiley, London 1975, pp. 9–60.

Chapter 4

Secondary Metabolism

Hans Zähner

4.1 Introduction

The term secondary metabolism was coined by plant physiologists in order to cover those parts of the plant metabolism which are not generally distributed and to the products of which no immediate function could be ascribed. Since the same problems exist for microorganisms, the term has also been introduced into microbiology, although a division into general and special metabolisms would have given less occasion for misunderstandings.

There is no account of secondary metabolism covering **all its aspects:** on the other hand, reference may be made to recent accounts for sections of this field. Publications of Mann (1977) and Bu'Lock (1979) are devoted mainly to the biogenesis of **secondary metabolites.** Introductions to the subject of **antibiotics** have been written by Asselineau and Zalta (1973), Bérdy (1974, 1981), and Kurylowicz (1976), while Korzybski et al. (1978), Umezawa et al. (1967, 1978), and Glasby (1976) have attempted to draw up **complete lists.** The review in the "Handbook of Microbiology" (Laskin and Lechevalier, 1973) is not restricted to antibiotics.

The secondary metabolism of microorganisms has very many aspects – like the primary metabolism – which cannot all be treated uniformly in a single article. The main points presented here are directed to relationships with and differences from the primary metabolism.

Secondary metabolites are characterized in the ideal case by:

1. the specificity of their occurrence;
2. their wide variation;
3. by the appearance of chemical groups and structural units which are absent in the primary metabolism; and
4. the difficulty of recognizing a function of the metabolites for the producing agent.

4.2 Occurrence of Secondary Metabolites in Microorganisms

If the approximately 6000 secondary metabolites from microorganisms that have been described so far are classified according to their producing microorganism strains an extremely unequal distribution is found. Table 4-1 shows the distribution of antibiotics (1974/state). The percentage distribution would not change appreciably if the totality of secondary metabolites were included and not only the antibiotics were considered. More than 50% of all antibiotics described hitherto are formed by **actinomycetes,** particularly those of the genus Streptomyces. Among the other procaryotes there is still a relatively large number of antibiotics in the Bacillaceae and the Pseudomonadaceae (Leisinger and Margraff, 1979), but here the number of parent substances is already greatly restricted. Hitherto, no antibiotic of which the structure has been elucidated has been isolated from the widespread family of the Enterobacteriaceae. The distribution is also unequal in the case of the eucaryotes. Good producing organisms of secondary metabolites are the genera of Fungi Imperfecti – Penicillium, Aspergillus, Cephalosporium, Trichoderma, and Fusarium – and also some of the Basidiomycetes (Anke, 1978). On the other hand, so far there have been no confirmed observations on the secondary metabolites from true yeasts and Zygomycetes.

The question arises as to whether this unequal distribution is "true" or whether it is simulated by unequal treatment. Both aspects may play a part in the distribution such as is shown in Table 4-1. However, a quite substantial part of the unequal distribution is undoubtedly true. Among the procaryotes, for example, the genera Escherichia, Salmonella,

Table 4-1. Distribution of Antibiotics from Microorganisms (after Berdy, 1974, modified).

Groups of organisms	Production of antibiotics per group		Production of antibiotics within the groups	
	number	in %	number	in % of the group
Pseudomonadales	87	2.7		
Eubacteria including Bacillus	274	8.5	171	62.4
Actinomycetales including Streptomycetaceae	2078	64.7	1950	93.8
Fungi including Aspergillaceae including Basidiomycetes	772	24.1	242	31.3
			140	18.1
	3211	100		

and Shigella have been very well studied in relation to their metabolisms, and, in spite of this, no antibiotics have been described; the same observation applies in the field of eucaryotes for the true yeasts. On the other hand, the small number of antibiotics from Myxobacteria, Halobacteria, and Methanobacteria among the procaryotes and from the Myxomycetes and Acrasiomycetes among eucaryotes is probably to be ascribed to a still inadequate study as the result of certain difficulties in cultivation.

If the reasons for the true part of the unequal distribution – which, incidentally, can also be observed for the secondary metabolic products of the higher plants – are sought, one does not get beyond hypotheses. If an attempt is made to find common properties of the "good" producing microorganisms and then compares them with the "poor" ones, something like the following pattern is obtained:

a) The **"gifted" strains** of secondary metabolites are predominantly **soil-inhabiting saprophytes.** The soil as an ecological niche represents for the microorganisms a

rapidly changing environment – changing in relation to temperature, humidity (and therefore osmophily), and the supply of nutrients in quantity and composition. On the other hand, the "poor" strains often occur in ecological niches which are stabilized by external conditions (gut, milk, plant material, fruit juices, etc.). All microorganisms living predominantly as parasites or symbionts form relatively few secondary metabolites; they have available an environment stabilized by the host.

b) The good producing strains of secondary metabolites **form spores** (exospores in the case of the Actinomycetes, endospores in the case of the Bacillaceae, and conidia in the case of the Fungi Imperfecti); non-spore-forming bacteria are less well endowed, and the same applies to the true yeasts among the eucaryotes. Among species of Bacillus, a participation of antibiotics in spore formation has been conjectured. However, whether the secondary metabolites play a wide role in differentiation must remain an open question.

c) Among those microorganisms that are capable of the manifold formation of antibiotics, the regulation in the **intermediate metabolism** does not appear to be equally good for all the end-products. For example, the pool of individual amino acids in *Escherichia coli* appears to be regulated at a uniformly low level. This by no means applies to the streptomycetes. If the formation of a secondary metabolite requires a higher pool of a particular precursor, good regulation can mask the capacity for forming a secondary metabolite. In this case, microorganisms endowed with the capacity for synthesizing many secondary metabolites would be those that are incapable in relation to the regulation of the intermediate metabolism.

d) Those groups of microorganisms which are in a position to assimilate **unusual substrates** over a wide range (Actinomycetes, Pseudomonas species, Eurotiales) also form **many different** secondary metabolites. A broad palette of substrate-degrading enzymes is positively correlated with the capacity for forming secondary metabolites.

According to definition, secondary metabolites do not occur in all microorganisms and their formation may be order-, family-, genus-, species-, or strain-specific. The question of the **specificity** of the formation of the given secondary metabolites must be answered in very different ways according to the example selected. With some substances or groups of substances, the specificity is so pronounced that a true **chemotaxonomy** is possible. For other substances or groups of substances, as Nara et al. (1977) recommend, only pronounced concentrations of their occurrence in certain groups of families can be given. The second case is perhaps of general application if it is borne in mind that a statement concerning specificity is possible only after intensive study for years in various laboratories with quite different methods, and at the present time such comprehensive investigations have been carried out for only a very few groups. In individual cases, the formation of a given secondary metabolite is distributed pointwise in no recognizable pattern through the biological system. For example, β-nitropropionic acid (bovinocidin) occurs in strains of the genus Streptomyces and in *Aspergillus avenaceus*, while tryptanthrine is recognized as an antibiotic of *Candida lipolytica* and has been described as an alkaloid of a higher plant.

However, the number of true deviations from the rule of specificity is relatively small (Lechevalier, 1975); furthermore, of the approximately 30 deviations given in the publication mentioned, probably some would not stand up to a careful reexamination.

The **biosynthesis** of complicated antibiotics such as the aminoglycosides requires a highly specialized enzymatic apparatus which, according to the present state of research, is very much the same for the various aminoglycosides. The fact that various streptomycetes and also strains of Micromonospora are capable of forming aminoglycosides is not surprising, but the fact that we can find the same group of antibiotics with only slight deviations in strains of Pseudomonas and in Bacillus, as well, does not fit in with our current ideas. The appearance in genetically independent cases of the capacity for forming aminoglycosides is completely improbable in view of the complicatedness of the biosynthetic pathways required. The very early appearance of this capacity in evolution, even before the divergence of Actinomyces, Pseudomonas, and Bacillus can probably not be envisaged, either. Consequently, only the transfer of genetic information for the secondary metabolism to genetically remote organisms remains. Since the organisms Streptomyces, Bacillus, and Pseudomonas live in the same ecological niche, the soil, a transfer of genetic material is quite possible, and in this connection protoplast fusion, plasmids, phages, or yet other mechanisms can be envisaged. This apparently ready transfer of genetic information must, however, be subjected to more severe restriction in other cases. As an example, chartreusin, a simpler substance than the aminoglycosides, occurs only in numerous strains of the species *Streptomyces viridochromogenes* and has not yet been found in other streptomycetes, let alone in other microorganisms.

4.3 Variations in the Secondary Metabolism

It is always impressive to see in what rich variation microorganisms form secondary metabolites. Up to more than 50 variations of the same parent compound produced by a single microorganism have been described. The musical expression "variations on a theme" forces itself upon one, and so does the term "Nature's play impulse." The modern separation processes of organic chemistry, such as high-pressure liquid chromatography, today often permit the demonstration that compounds previously regarded as single substances are not so but consist of **mixtures of closely related components.** The impression is produced that secondary metabolites occur in almost infinite number.

For the **technical production** of a given metabolite the fact that most producing agents form a whole spectrum of related substances is often an obstacle and it is a case of seeking mutants or finding fermentation conditions in which the desired component is predominant.

However, the whole range of variations on a theme can be seen in its totality only if the

Table 4-2. Anthraquinones that can be derived from Endocrocin (after Anke et al., 1980).

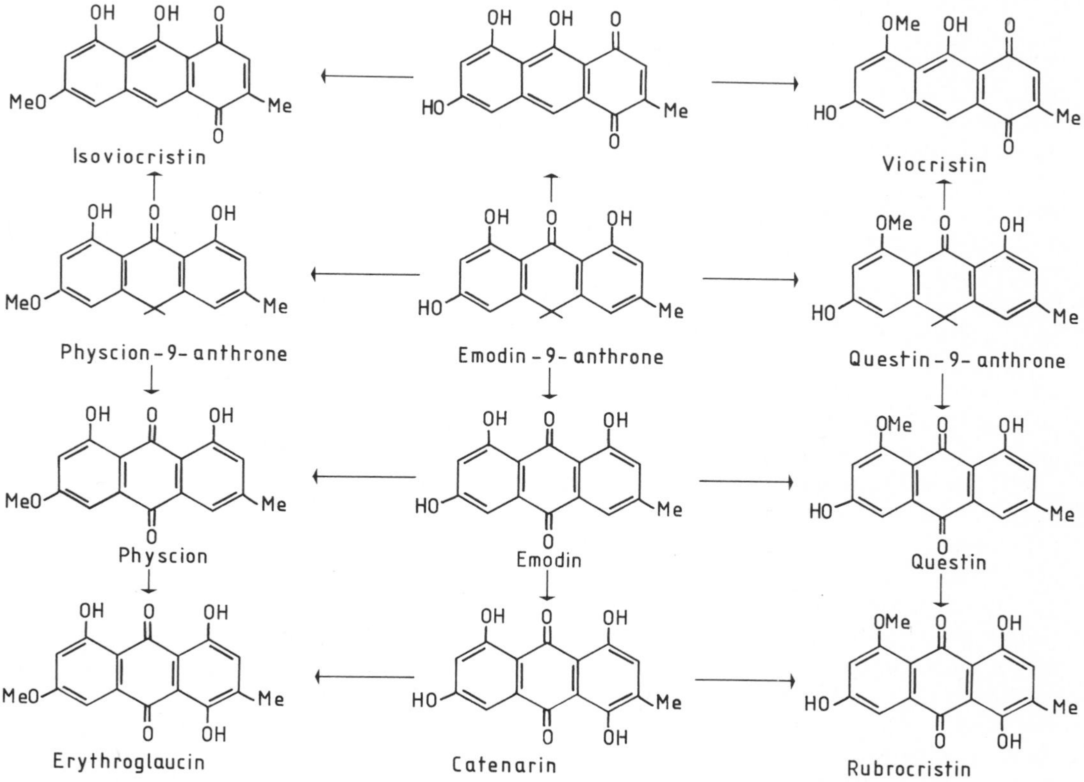

Isoviocristin — Viocristin

Physcion-9-anthrone — Emodin-9-anthrone — Questin-9-anthrone

Physcion — Emodin — Questin

Erythroglaucin — Catenarin — Rubrocristin

members from various microorganisms belonging to the same class of substances are reviewed. This is then equivalent to a puzzle game in which the still lacking members of all theoretically possible combinations must be found. Table 4-2 summarizes the **anthraquinones** that can be derived from endocrocin (Anke et al., 1980). What has been singled out here using the anthraquinones as an example can be shown for the overwhelming majority of the well-studied groups of secondary metabolites. Evolution takes place through an interplay of increasing variation by mutation and decreasing variation by selection. The part of the primary metabolism visible today hardly permits anything of the original variation to be recognized while, on the other hand, it is just the secondary metabolism that shows this side of evolution particularly clearly.

If the statement is made with no limitation that the primary metabolism is uniform and the secondary metabolism variable, a **broad transition region** is suppressed. The **lipids** in membranes vary particularly widely, and the mureins and pseudomureins of bacterial cell walls are all other than uniform. But the principle of uniformity is not even maintained in the area of the **coenzymes**; e.g., vitamin B_{12} and its analogs with various bases, and the variations in the ferredoxins and ubiquinones. The **iron transport compounds** – for which it is disputable whether they are to be included among the primary or secondary metabolisms – form a good example of the fact that compounds with the same function in the same microorganism may occur in rich variety; indeed many streptomycetes form a whole palette of sideramines. The iron transport compounds are, simultaneously, an example of the fact that the same function can be fulfiled by chemically quite different basic compounds. The assumption of a function does not automatically lead to an ending of variation nor automatically to the same basic compounds.

The surprising thing is **not** the occurrence of more than 100 variants in the actinomycins, over 200 in the anthracyclines, or more than 100 different iron-transport compounds but the **uniformity** of NAD, FAD, etc., throughout the whole biological system.

4.4 Special Chemical Groups and Basic Intermediates in the Secondary Metabolism

In the secondary metabolism a number of chemical groups, intermediates, and key substances occur which are absent from the primary metabolism. The secondary metabolism therefore does not merely represent a new combination of the structural units known from the primary metabolism. A selection of these features will be presented here with a few examples of each.

4.4.1 Covalently Bound Chlorine or Bromine

So far, more than 100 chlorine-containing metabolites have been described from the secondary metabolism of microorganisms, and these include the technically important **chloramphenicol** (I)[*], **griseofulvin** (II), **chlortetracycline** (III), and **pyrrolnitrin** (IV). If radioactive chlorine is added to the nutrient medium and the formation of labeled metabolites is checked, it is found that chlorine-containing metabolites are very much more numerous than could have been assumed on the basis of those described. Many chlorine-containing metabolites have hitherto been overlooked. In this connection we may start from the assumption that many chlorine-free sec-

---

[*] The Roman numerals denote the formulas of the compounds mentioned in the Appendix on p. 708.

ondary metabolites have chlorine-containing analogs in nature (Krauss, 1977). However, microorganisms are capable of chlorinating other metabolites which they do not themselves form (König et al., 1977). If chlorine or common salt in the nutrient solution is replaced by sodium bromide, in many cases the **brominated analogs** of the originally chlorinated compound are obtained. An extreme case of a brominated compound is probably **bromonitrin C** (V) with seven bromine atoms in the molecule (Ajisaka et al., 1972).

It is generally assumed that chlorine-containing compounds are usually difficult to degrade. If, however, substantially more chlorine-containing compounds occur in nature than was previously assumed, the question arises: what happens to these compounds? Likewise, more enzymes probably exist for the degradation of biogenic chlorine-containing compounds than was previously assumed, and our experience of the degradation of synthetic chlorinated hydrocarbons cannot be transferred to the natural materials.

4.4.2 Unusual Nitrogen Compounds

As unusual nitrogen compounds may be mentioned those containing nitro, nitroso, cyano, diazo, nitrilo, isonitrilo, and hydroxamic acid groups. Nitro groups are present in many secondary metabolites – at least 25 – including the commercial products **chloramphenicol** (I) and **pyrrolnitrin** (IV). The diazo-group-containing antibiotics **DON** (VI), **azaserine** (VII), and **alazopeptin** (VIII) possess a considerable antitumoral activity, but their toxicity prohibits practical use. The cyano-group-containing compounds **borrelidin** (IX), **toyocamycin** (X) and the nitrosamine-group-containing **alanosine** (XI) are highly toxic and the same applies to the isonitrile **xanthocillin** (XII) and the nitrile **isonitrin A** (Fujiwara et al., 1978) (XIII).

In comparison with the total number of secondary metabolites, these unusual nitrogen compounds are relatively rare but, on the other hand, compounds with hydroxamic acid groups are common. The overwhelming number of microorganisms form iron-transport compounds and the bulk of these are trihydroxamic acids or dihydroxamic acids. In the case of the procaryotes, the predominating representatives are the sideramines derived from lysine (the **ferrioxamines**, e.g., **ferrioxamine B** (XIV), **arthrobactin** (XV), **schizokinen** (XVI), etc.), while in fungi sideramines derived from ornithine predominate (**ferricrocin** (XVII), **coprogen** (XVIII), **fusigen** (XIX), etc.). A total of more than 80 iron-transporting compounds have been described which complex iron through hydroxamic acid groups.

This series of simple groups does not complete the series of unusual nitrogen compounds. We must also mention, for example, unusual heterocyclic compounds such as **emimycin** (XX) with two nitrogen atoms in the para positions of a six-membered ring.

4.4.3 Unusual Compounds Containing Phosphorus

The important phosphorus compounds in the primary metabolism are all esters of phosphoric acid, and a direct carbon-phosphorus bond plays no part in the intermediate metabolism. Astonishingly, in contrast to this, in the secondary metabolism phosphoric acid esters play a very small role so far as end-products are concerned while that of some other phosphorus compounds with phosphonic, phosphinic, and phosphonamidic groups is a large one. Other examples of compounds with a C—P bond that may be mentioned are **phosphonomycin** (XXI) which has been introduced into therapy, and **plumbemycin B** (Park et al., 1977) (XXII). This group also includes the new compounds of the type of FR 31564 (XXIII) that have recently been described, which are taken up by the same transport system as phosphonomycin (Okuhara et al., 1980; Iguchi et al., 1980). **Phosphinothricylalanylalanine** (Bayer et al., 1972) (XXIV) is, so far, the only example with a C—P—C bond. There is also only one example of the phosphoramides, **phosphoramidon** (XXV), an inhibitor of metallo-endopeptidases (Komiyama et al., 1975).

The question of why only a few phosphoric acid esters occur, or have been described, as end-products in the secondary metabolism may have various answers:

a) Esterases are very widespread and not particularly substrate-specific. The phosphoric acid esters of secondary metabolites formed are perhaps rapidly cleaved and therefore cannot be detected.

b) Phosphoric acids are hardly taken up by intact cells. Since in the search for new metabolites we have so far mainly used antibiotic tests with whole cells, these compounds have been overlooked.

c) The difficulty with which a phosphoric acid ester passes through a membrane possibly applies not only to entry into but also to exit from the cell. The compounds remain in the cell and are cleaved by esterases there.

4.4.4   Unusual Organometallic Compounds

Many iron-containing or specifically iron-complexing compounds occur in the secondary metabolism, most of which are to be ascribed to the transport of iron but otherwise exhibit all the characteristics of the secondary metabolism. The diversity of these sideramines and sideromycins (so far more than 100 different ones have been described) and their pronounced specificity in occurrence fit completely into the pattern of the secondary metabolism. **Ferrioxamines** (XIV) derived from lysine occur only in actinomycetes and some bacteria related to them (e.g., *Arthrobacter simplex*), while fungi, with the exception of the true yeasts and the zygomycetes, form sideramines that are derived from ornithine (see as an example **ferricrocin** (XVII) or **coprogen** (XVIII)). But here again there is one exception that infringes this principle; a strain of Streptomyces forms ferricrocin, a sideramine of the ferrichrome type.

Not all iron compounds in the products of the secondary metabolism can be ascribed to the transport of iron. **Ferroverdin** (XXVI), an iron complex with bivalent iron, can be ascribed not to the transport of iron but possibly, as Blinov et al. (1979) suggest, to the acceptance of iron from the transport compound. According to these authors, ferroverdin and related substances are much commoner than was previously assumed.

Magnesidin (XXVII) specifically complexes magnesium, while **YC 73** (fluopsin XXVIII) can be found both as an iron complex and as a copper complex. Specific copper-containing antibiotics are the **bleomycins** (XXIX) which today occupy an important place in the chemotherapy of tumors, and the **phleomycins** and **zorbamycins,** which belong to the same group.

4.4.5   Boron-Containing Metabolites

So far, only two boron-containing antibiotics have been described, **boromycin** (XXX) and **aplasmomycin** (Nakamura et al., 1977), which are closely related to one another and are both formed by streptomycetes. Whether these two boron-containing metabolites are only the first representatives of a large group or whether they are two rarities of "inorganic biochemistry" the next few years will show.

4.4.6   Unusual Amino Acids

All twenty of the amino acids occurring in proteins are α-L-amino acids. This also applies, with the exception of the β-alanine found in folic acid, to all amino acids of intermediate metabolism occurring as intermediate products of the biosynthesis of amino acids. Of these theoretically possible amino acids, only a quite small selection occurs in the intermediate metabolism. In the secondary metabolism, this pattern changes completely, and far more than 100 unusual amino acids occur in the free state or as structural components of peptides. In individual peptides, the proportion of unusual amino acids reaches more than 50%. Table 4-3 shows a small selection of amino acids from the secondary metabolism.

4.4.7   Unusual Ring Systems

The intermediate metabolism recognizes homo- or heterocyclic five- or six-membered rings which may be more or less heavily substituted or be linked with other rings. In addition to these, some larger ring

Table 4-3. Some Unusual Amino Acids from the Secondary Microbial Metabolism. (Among others, the numerous D- analogs of the L-amino acids that are common in the intermediate metabolism have not been included in the Table although these D-amino acids frequently occur in microbial polypeptides).

Name	Formula	Occurrence	Producing agent
Alanosine	$H_2N-CH-COOH$ $\vert$ CH_2 $\vert$ $HO-N-N=O$	free, antibiotic	*Streptomyces alanosinicus*
Aminodichlorobutyric acid	$H_2N-CH-COOH$ $\vert$ CH_2 $\vert$ $Cl-CH-Cl$	free, antibiotic	*Streptomyces armentosus*
Aminochlorodihydro-isoxazolylacetic acid	$H_2N-CH-COOH$ (ring) $Cl-\!=\!\!=\!N$, O	free, antibiotic	Streptomyces sp.
Azaleucine	$H_2N-CH-COOH$ $\vert$ CH_2 $\vert$ $H_3C-N-CH_3$	free, antibiotic	*Streptomyces neocaliberis*
Azaserine	$H_2N-CH-COOH$ $\vert$ CH_2 $\vert$ O $\vert$ $C=O$ $\vert$ CH $\Vert$ $N^{\oplus}$ $\Vert$ $N^{\ominus}$	free, antibiotic	Streptomyces species
O-Carbamyl-D-serine	$H_2N-CH-COOH$ $\vert$ CH_2 $\vert$ O $\vert$ $C=O$ $\vert$ NH_2	free, antibiotic	Streptomyces species
3-Chloro-3-(3-hydroxy-2-oxoazetidin-1-yl-methyl)alanine	$H_2N-CH-COOH$ $\vert$ CH_2 $\vert$ $Cl-CH$ $\vert$ (ring) $HO-\square=O$, $N-H$	dipeptide with Ala, antibiotic	Streptomyces sp.
3-Cyclohexenylglycine	$H_2N-CH-COOH$ (cyclohexenyl ring)	free, antibiotic	Streptomyces species
Diaminosuccinic acid	$H_2N-CH-COOH$ $\vert$ $H_2N-CH-COOH$	free, antibiotic	*Streptomyces rimosus*

Table 4-3. (continued)

Name	Formula	Occurrence	Producing agent
Dihydrophenylalanine	$H_2N-CH-COOH$ $\quad\quad\mid$ $\quad\quad CH_2$ (cyclohexadiene ring)	free, antibiotic	Streptomyces species
DON (6-diazo-5-oxo-L-norleucine)	$H_2N-CH-COOH$ $\quad\quad\mid$ $\quad\quad(CH_2)_2$ $\quad\quad\mid$ $\quad\quad C=O$ $\quad\quad\mid$ $\quad\quad CH$ $\quad\quad\parallel$ $\quad\quad N\oplus$ $\quad\quad\parallel$ $\quad\quad N\ominus$	free, and as Ala-DON-DON, and in duazomycins A and B	Streptomyces species
4-Oxalysine	$H_2N-CH-COOH$ $\quad\quad\mid$ $\quad\quad CH_2$ $\quad\quad\mid$ $\quad\quad O$ $\quad\quad\mid$ $\quad\quad(CH_2)_2$ $\quad\quad\mid$ $\quad\quad NH_2$	free, antibiotic	Streptomyces species
Phosphinothricin (PTS)	$H_2N-CH-COOH$ $\quad\quad\mid$ $\quad\quad(CH_2)_2$ $\quad\quad\mid$ $HO-P=O$ $\quad\quad\mid$ $\quad\quad CH_3$	as PTS-Ala-Ala, antibiotic	Streptomyces species
Phosphonomethionine sulfoximine	$H_2N-CH-COOH$ $\quad\quad\mid$ $\quad\quad(CH_2)_2$ $\quad\quad\mid$ $O-S-CH_3$ $\quad\quad\parallel$ $\quad\quad N$ $\quad\quad\mid$ $O-P-OH$ $\quad\quad\mid$ $\quad\quad OH$	as tripeptide with Ala-Ala, antibiotic	Streptomyces sp.
Rhizobitoxin	$H_2N-CH-COOH$ $\quad\quad\mid$ $\quad\quad CH$ $\quad\quad\parallel$ $\quad\quad HC$ $\quad\quad\mid$ $\quad\quad O$ $\quad\quad\mid$ $\quad\quad CH_2$ $\quad\quad\mid$ $H_2N-CH-CH_2OH$	bacterial toxin	*Rhizobium japonicum*
Tabtoxin	$H_2N-CH-COOH$ $\quad\quad\mid$ $\quad\quad(CH_2)_2$ $\quad\quad\mid$ $HO-\square=O$ $\quad\quad\mid$ $\quad\quad N-H$	wildfire toxin with Thr as dipeptide	*Pseudomonas tabaci*

Note: Streptomyces sp. denotes a species of the genus Streptomyces not more strictly specified. Streptomyces species denotes more than one species of the genus Streptomyces.

systems occur. The secondary metabolism recognizes a whole series of other ring systems such as, for example, small rings with three or four members (e.g., β-lactams – see the penicillins) or seven-membered rings, e.g., tropolones, such as sepedonin (XXXI) or large rings such as macrotetrolides (e.g., nonactin, XXXII), macrolides, ansamycins, etc..

We have still not exhausted the list with these seven groups of examples of unusual structural units. To do this we should also have to mention, for example, unusual sugars (branched sugars, dideoxysugars, dimethyl-aminosugars), unusual linkages of sugars, etc.

4.5 The Function of Secondary Metabolites

The occurrence of so many secondary metabolites with sometimes extremely complicated structures and without obvious functions is difficult to harmonize with our ideas of evolution as a continuous interplay between the expansion of variation by mutation and the limitation of variation by selection. This has led to a series of ideas and hypotheses concerning a possible function of the secondary metabolism. Some of these hypotheses will be presented briefly here.

4.5.1 Secondary Metabolism as Derailed Primary Metabolism

The biosynthesis of numerous secondary metabolites contains many individual steps which, apart from a few exceptions, resemble the enzymatic steps of the intermediate metabolism. If we assume that only one step brings about a true deviation from the intermediate metabolism and the resulting unusual product

is then subjected to further, normal transformations, we have an explanation of the diversity of the final products and nevertheless need only a very few special enzymes in the secondary metabolism. This hypothesis may be illuminating for many simple metabolites but is of no help in the case of complicated molecules such as **boromycin** (XXX) or **bleomycin** (XXIX).

4.5.2 Secondary Metabolites as "Biochemical Appendices"

According to this hypothesis, the secondary metabolites that can be detected today and currently have no function did have a function in an earlier stage of evolution but have lost it in the intermediate period in a comparable manner to the human appendix – an elegant hypothesis which cannot be confirmed or refuted.

4.5.3 Secondary Metabolites as Waste Products, Shavings from an Imperfectly Functioning Intermediate Metabolism

This hypothesis is based on the fact that in the intermediate metabolism, in spite of the high specificity of the reactions, a small proportion of "faulty" products arises, or the wrong substrates are converted into just such products. Since many reactions are arranged in cycles and these are run through several times, individual faulty products can accumulate even when they arise in only small amounts. Subsequent modification with normal steps would give the variation, and the specificities of the intermediate metabolism would be responsible for the unequal distribution. This hypothesis does not apply in all those cases where it must be assumed that complicated multienzyme complexes must be present for the secondary metabolism, e.g., in nonribosomal polypeptide synthesis or polyketide synthesis.

4.5.4   Secondary Metabolites as Products of Detoxification Mechanisms

It has been shown for individual secondary metabolites that they themselves are less toxic than some of the intermediate products, which has led to the thought of whether the secondary metabolism might not generally have the function of a detoxification process. However, in view of the toxicity of certain secondary metabolites, such as the actinomycins, for the producing cell it is impossible to ascribe any more general significance to this hypothesis.

4.5.5   Secondary Metabolites as Results of an Inhibited Growth

In many cases, it has been possible to show that the formation of a secondary metabolite does not take place in the growth phase proper nor during optimum growth. If, with a reduced supply of the true substrates, the enzymes use other substrates, even with a lower turnover rate, we should have an explanation of the variety of the secondary metabolism without at the same time having to demand a large number of special enzymes.

4.5.6   The Secondary Metabolism as a Playing Field of Biochemical Evolution

This hypothesis will be given in somewhat more detail (Zähner, 1978, 1979). The biological system has five important levels for the development of an organism:

Level 1: The intermediate metabolism.
This level is well known in relation to biochemistry and forms the main part of any biochemical textbook. If one disregards the archaebacteria, the intermediate metabolism is also relatively uniform throughout the whole biological system. The basic reactions of the intermediate metabolism, including the macromolecular synthesis of DNA, RNA, and protein, are probably the relatively oldest parts of evolution.

Level 2: Regulation of the intermediate metabolism.
Our knowledge of this part of the biological system is already substantially sparser; in particular, there are only few comparative studies on organisms that are fundamentally different enzymatically. What is known concerning the regulation of the biosynthesis of tryptophan, for example, indicates great differences in the same biosynthetic pathway in different organisms.

Level 3: Transport of substrates and metabolites.
Here, research is still at the very beginning, so that hardly any relevant statements can be made concerning the uniformity of the transport systems in different organisms.

Level 4: Differentiation.
Even to understand the simplest differentiation – e.g., the formation of spores in *Bacillus subtilis* – still presents difficulties. We are still very far removed from unitary ideas concerning differentiation that would be generally valid.

Level 5: Morphogenesis.
The appearance of certain forms can be explained satisfactorily where they are determined directly by the structure of the structural units, e.g., in the coats of viruses, but where this is not the case, e.g., for the mureins in relation to the form of the bacteria or in the formation of multicellular systems, there are hardly any starting points for a usable theory.

The fact that the five levels constructed here are **artefacts of our mode of thought** will probably be clear. In nature, these five levels are indissolubly linked with one another. The severe conditions of the fight for existence in nature form an extremely narrow framework for any change on any of the five levels. The necessity for maintaining reproduction at a competitive height no longer leaves any appreciable room between the expansion by mutation and its contraction by selection. We may now assume that at the side – again in our abstract representation of the situation – a free space exists, – almost a playground. In this free space a change in a metabolite has no direct consequence for any of the five levels, since the original metabolite had no function in this free space. Under the assumption that a new metabolite has **no adverse effects** on any of the five levels, here it can be varied in any desired way. Since the genetic information for the secondary metabolism, at least in Actinomyces, is present on extrachromosomal elements to a considerable but not precisely determined degree, and these elements can relatively easily be transferred from organism to organism, this biochemical free space also has a genetic background. Fig. 4-1 attempts to show the situation graphically.

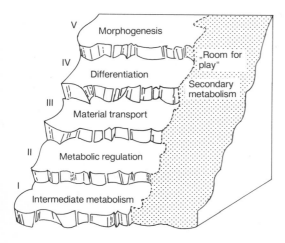

Fig. 4-1. The secondary metabolism and the levels of phylogenetic development.

If a compound should occur in this free space which offers **an advantage** for **one** of the five levels, this information can be taken over into the corresponding level. The genetic foundation is fixed by the integration of the extrachromosomal elements into the chromosome. A further genetic stabilization can take place by the fact that the genes that are necessary for the synthesis of a secondary metabolite are incorporated in an operon in a cluster.

The ready transmission of genetic information, e.g., in streptomycetes, would permit the situation that the given secondary metabolite does not necessarily find a function in **that particular** group of organisms in which it arose. This idea can be developed to a division of labor in evolution. New compounds arise in an organism with a pronounced secondary metabolism, and they can find a function in others, e.g., those with a small free space for the secondary metabolism.

From this point of view, the secondary metabolism would be the field for future development and not the "graveyard" of failed experiments.

If this hypothesis is more than a mere mental game, a whole series of secondary metabolites should have a function for the producing organism. This is certainly the case for the iron-transport compounds and probably also for some of the ionophoric antibiotics. The fact that the finding of a function is so difficult is understandable, since hitherto we have probably carried out the search mainly in the wrong place. The statement that, for example, a minus mutant of an antibiotic-producing agent grows as well as the wild strain says little unless it is checked whether the mutant does this under the most diverse conditions and up to the same stage of development. For example, a breakdown in the capacity for forming iron-transport compounds is expressed only under quite definite conditions. Hitherto we have sought the function of secondary metabolites mostly in the area of the intermediate metabolism and have not taken into account the much more extensively divided levels of regulation, transport, differentiation, and morphogenesis.

Using iron-transport compounds as an example, it can also be shown that the antibiotic effect of certain sideramines has nothing to do with the function of these substances for the producing cell. Of the more than 100 iron-transport compounds, only **nocardamin** (XXXIII) and desferritriacetylfusigen show an antibiotic effect, and this only in organisms which are incapable of removing iron from its complexes with these compounds. The antibiotic effect is only that of an elimination of iron (Anke, 1977) and there is no doubt that the function of these two compounds for the producing strain is again that of an iron-transport compound. If the cells gain an additional advantage from the antibiotic action of nocardamin or desferritriacetylfusigen, we should have to assume that these two sideramines were common or at least represent the main sideramines of the strains concerned. This is a very fine example of the randomness of an antibiotic effect postulated as long ago as 1971 by Turner.

Studies on the question of the function of a secondary metabolite immediately suggest themselves on the basis of this hypothesis. In this connection, the following points should be borne in mind:

a) The possible function must be sought on the levels of morphogenesis, differentiation, transport, and regulation rather than in the intermediate metabolism. Particular attention is also warranted by the area of spore formation, spore germination, and the resistance of spores.

b) The expected function will probably not express itself in an "all or nothing reaction," as in the case of the absence of a product of the intermediate metabolism. An increase in sensitivity to unfavorable conditions of growth, incompleted differentiation, an interrupted morphogenesis, or the failure of an inhibition of germination, for example, come into consideration.

c) A similar function need not be taken over by a chemically similar compound (chemically different but functionally equivalent compounds). This, also, can be demonstrated satisfactorily in the series of iron-transport compounds e.g., by a comparison of **enterochelin** (XXXIV), **ferricrocin** (XVII), **fusigen** (XIX), and **ferrioxamine B** (XIV).

d) Such investigations appear particularly stimulating where the occurrence of similar compounds is common and large groups of related substances exist, e.g.:

- Function of actinomycins, anthracyclines, and quinoxaline antibiotics in relation to the transcription of DNA in the producing cell;

- Function of the macrolides, aminoglycosides, etc., in relation to the biosynthesis of the proteins of the producing cell;

- Function of streptolydigins, tirandamycins, oleficin, and lipomycins for the magnesium economy of the producing cell;

- Participation of the tropolone antibiotics in the uptake of iron by the producing cell;

- Participation of the polyene antibiotics in the germination of spores or the inhibition of this process in the producing cell;

- Participation of ionophoric antibiotics in the formation or germination of spores;

- β-lactams in streptomycetes in relation to murein biosynthesis during differentiation and spore germination.

4.6   Biogenesis and Biosynthesis of Secondary Metabolites

The expressions biogenesis and biosynthesis are often used erroneously as synonyms, but the term **biogenesis** should be reserved for the origin of the carbon skeleton or of all the atoms of a molecule, i.e., for the question of structural units, and the term **biosynthesis** be reserved for the enzymatic part. Biogenesis is therefore in essence a problem of organic chemistry and biosynthesis one of biochemistry, although in both cases microbiology must perform the preliminary work. Before at least a large part of the biogenesis is known, it is pointless to look for the enzymes and before the enzymatic steps have been formulated it is impossible to handle the question of regulation. However highly biotechnology is interested in regulation with a view to the highest possible yields, it is pointless to call for investigations of regulation while the biogenetic and biosynthetic foundations are completely lacking. A parallel treatment involving genetic methods is the optimum.

The wealth of secondary metabolites calls for a principle of classification that makes them easy to survey. Classifications based on the producing organism or on biological action cannot be satisfactory. The best classification so far is based on the structural units, i.e., on biogenesis when one accepts the fact that many metabolites crop up at two or more points.

Table 4-4, which has been taken from Bu'Lock (1965) shows the **origin of the structural units** from the intermediate metabolism for large groups of secondary metabolites. This table might give rise to the false impression that the secondary metabolites contain exclusively structural units from one source, e.g., only amino acids, only sugars, or only acetate units. This is not the case: as a rule, a simple metabolite contains structural components from two or more sources. How differ-

Table 4-4. Classification of the Secondary Metabolites According to the Origin of the Structural Components.

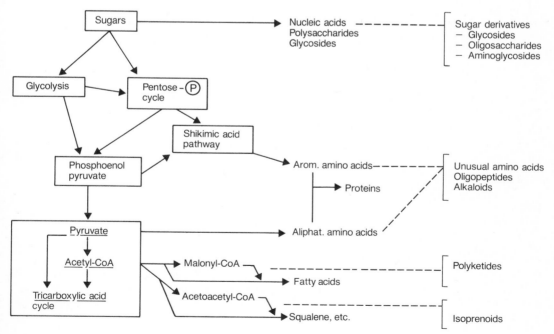

ent the origin of these may be is shown, for example, by **novobiocin** (Fig. 4-2). Part of the molecule is derived from glucose, part from mevalonic acid, and another part from shikimic acid, and the whole is modified further by methyl groups from methionine.

The **classification** of secondary metabolites **according to their biogenesis,** i.e., according to their linkage with individual parts of the intermediate metabolism, yields important information when it is a question of increasing the yield of a certain metabolite. The supply of precursors can be increased, for example, by an increased amount of nutrients or the appropriate control of fermentation, or else be deregulated by genetic methods in biosynthesis. If the supply of precursors is limiting for the amount of metabolites formed, this opens up a way of increasing yield.

Only the introduction of isotope technique (^{14}C, ^{3}H, ^{32}P) had first truly permitted research on biogenesis, and from 1952 it triggered off a veritable race in this field. If truly substantiated statements are to be made, isotope technique presupposes the specific degradation of the molecule in such a way that the radioactivity of each individual C-atom can

be determined directly or indirectly. While the elucidation of the structure of organic molecules was carried out substantially via degradation and the identification of the degradation products, good preliminary work was available for research on biogenesis in this field. Today, where the elucidation of structure is taking place more and more with the aid of purely spectroscopic methods on complete molecules or very large fragments, the foundations for a specific degradation are often completely lacking at the beginning of a biogenetic study. Today, the ^{14}C-isotope technique is being increasing replaced by ^{13}C-NMR spectroscopy. The biogenesis of many metabolites can be investigated without degradation by means of ^{13}C-NMR spectroscopy. Prerequisites for this are:

1. The existence of an interpretable ^{13}C-NMR spectrum of the metabolite.

2. An applicable hypothesis about possible structural units.

3. ^{13}C-Labeled structural units.

4. The presumable structural units or intermediate products must be capable of being taken up by intact cells and should not be metabolized further too rapidly.

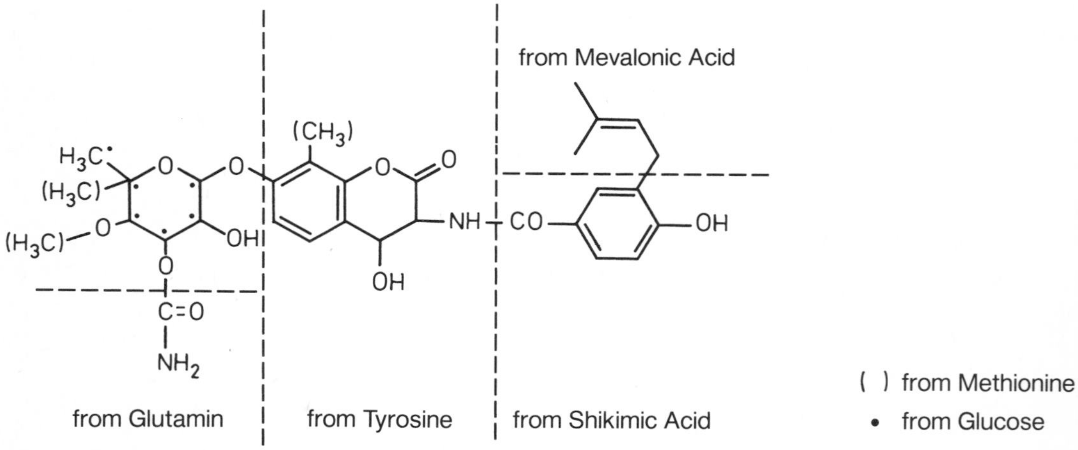

Fig. 4-2. Biogenesis of novobiocin.

The great advances in the methodological field should not blind us to the fact that without the satisfaction of these requirements biogenetic research is still a very laborious business even today.

Biogenetic research, regardless of whether is done through ^{14}C- or ^{13}C-labeling, yields only a little information on possible intermediate stages of biosynthesis and the sequence of the individual reactions. Although today we are in a position to give a plausible-seeming biogenesis for most secondary metabolites, in relation to biosynthesis we are only at the beginning. Even for **penicillin,** which has been worked on for 50 years, we can give no certain gapfree chain. As a rule, a complete elucidation of biosynthesis requires a very close cooperation between microbiologists, geneticists, biochemists, and organic chemists, which only rarely exists. The pathway to the elucidation of the biosynthesis of a complicated metabolite can be sketched somewhat as follows:

a) Elucidation of biogenesis with the aid of ^{13}C-NMR spectroscopy.

b) Isolation of mutants with defects in the synthesis of the metabolite, isolation of possible enrichment products, elucidation of their structures, and attempt to place the products found in a meaningful biosynthetic relationship.

c) Construction of a cellfree system for biosynthesis and checking whether the products isolated under b) are true intermediate products.

d) Filling up the gaps by hypothetical intermediate stages, synthesis of the presumable intermediate stages, and testing their incorporation in the cell-free system.

e) Seeking enzymes for the individual steps.

f) Investigations on the regulation of the individual enzymatic steps.

At the present time there is no simple example in which all the steps have been carried out logically and for the whole chain to its termination. The furthest advanced is the biosynthesis of nonribosomal polypeptides, the β-lactams, the tetracyclines, and some macrolides.

4.6.1 Polyketides

In 1953, Birch and Donovan proposed a head-to-tail linkage of acetate units as the biogenetic pathway to various secondary metabolites. The pathway was first shown exhaustively by Birch (1967), and a more recent review has been given by Bu'Lock (1979). **Polyketides** is the name given to secondary metabolic products which can be derived mainly or exclusively from poly(β-keto acids) $(-(CHRCO)_n-)$.

The subunits may be:
$-CH_2CO-$ acetate unit
$-CHMeCO-$ propionate unit
$-CHEtCO-$ butyrate unit and higher ones, i.e., all monocarboxylic acids that occur as CoA-derivatives in the intermediate metabolism. By far the most frequent are acetate units. So far as is known today, the formation of the poly(β-keto acids) takes place in substantial analogy with the synthesis of fatty acids (Fig. 4-3). A chain can be built by the repetition of this step. If complete reduction is carried out between the individual steps of chain lengthening, a fatty acid is produced; otherwise, a

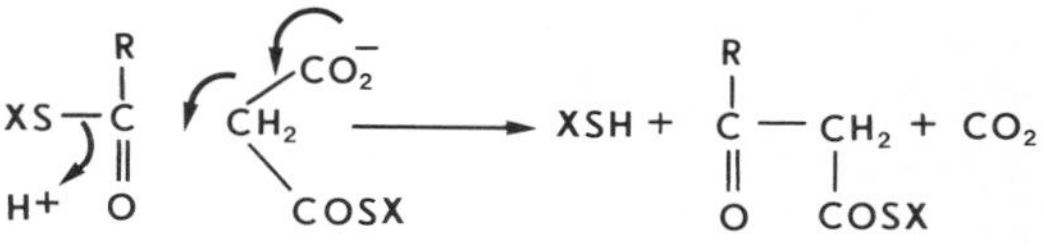

Fig. 4-3. Linkage of acetate units.

polyketide. The analogy with the synthesis of fatty acids is also expressed by the fact that the biosynthesis of the polyketides, like that of the fatty acids, is sensitive to **cerulenin** (XXXV). The presumable poly(β-keto acid) is unstable; only stabilized and multiply modified derivatives occur in the free form. The most common stabilization process is **ring formation**. Since the poly(β-keto acid) arising is not continuously cyclized and aromatized, a special step in enzymatic synthesis is assumed.

Figure 4-4 shows the origin of a simple polyketide constructed of four acetate units. The Figure, taken over from Bu'Lock (1979) is based on studies by Light and Hager (1968) and of Dimroth et al. (1970). The synthesis of this polyketide, 6-methylsalicylic acid, presumes a multienzyme complex. This probably applies to all the polyketides.

This basic principle, the synthesis of a poly-(β-keto acid) with stabilization and modification now permits an almost unlimited number of possibilities. Here the individual possibilities of variation can only be sketched and illustrated with a few examples.

Possibility of variation 1: The number of units linked to form a chain. Polyketides with four or more units are common. The largest polyketides contain up to 19 subunits, but the question whether these are synthesized as a single chain is open.

Possibility of variation 2: The degree of reduction in the chain. A continuous complete reduction of the chain in the course of synthesis leads to a fatty acid, and an incomplete or totally lacking reduction leads to a polyketide. The degree of reduction and the positions of the reduced sites give a very wide-ranging possibility of variation. The positions of the reduced sites probably also decide the type of cyclization or folding of the chain. The degree to which a chain is reduced can easily be determined by labeling the positions of the oxygen atoms originally in the chain and then carrying out a comparison with the number of oxygen atoms still present at these sites in the complete polyketide.

Possibility of variation 3: Dehydration in the partially reduced chain. Dehydration often leads to an aromatization that can also be found at different positions in isolated or conjugated systems. Examples of a dehydration with aromatization are the many anthraquinones of Table 2, and an example of

dehydration without aromatization is the formation of a polyene, e.g., **amphotericin B** (XXXVI).

Possibility of variation 4: Incorporation of units other than acetate in the chain, e.g., propionate or butyrate. Such deviations from a strict acetate scheme occur particularly in metabolites from actinomycetes. Usually only the starter molecule is modified, e.g., in ε-**pyrromycinone** (XXXVII), but often propionate units are also found within the chain. Erythronolide, the aglycone of **erythromycin** (XXXVIII) is constructed of one propionyl-CoA and six methylmalonyl-CoA units.

Possibility of variation 5: The nature and degree of cyclization. A chain, even one of a given length, can be cyclized in quite diverse ways, e.g., with the formation of a lactone, of a simple aromatic system, or of a complicated polycyclic system in which the polyketide can hardly be recognized any longer. However, a given ring system need not mean a chain of given length. The nature of the formation of rings is very probably determined by the position and degree of reduction in the chain.

Possibility of variation 6: The introduction of additional oxygen functions. Reduction leads to the elimination of oxygen functions which are then absent from positions where oxygen function would be expected from biogenetic considerations; conversely, in many polyketides we can find oxygen functions in unexpected positions which were introduced subsequently.

Possibility of variation 7: Introduction of C-methyl and O-methyl groups. In many cases, it has been shown that both O-methyl and also C-methyl groups arising from methionine are incorporated. For O-methyls this is probably the general case, but for C-methyls this must be checked in each individual case, since methyl groups may also arise from a C-3 fragment.

Possibility of variation 8: Subsequent chain modifications. The simplest case here is the decarboxylation of the terminal carboxy group, but there are also substantially more complicated changes, as in the case of chartreusin, where both carboxylation and the cutting out of a section of the chain take place later.

Possibility of variation 9: Introduction of chlorine or bromine atoms. Examples of this possibility of variation have already been mentioned in the section on unusual structural units. Polyketides of

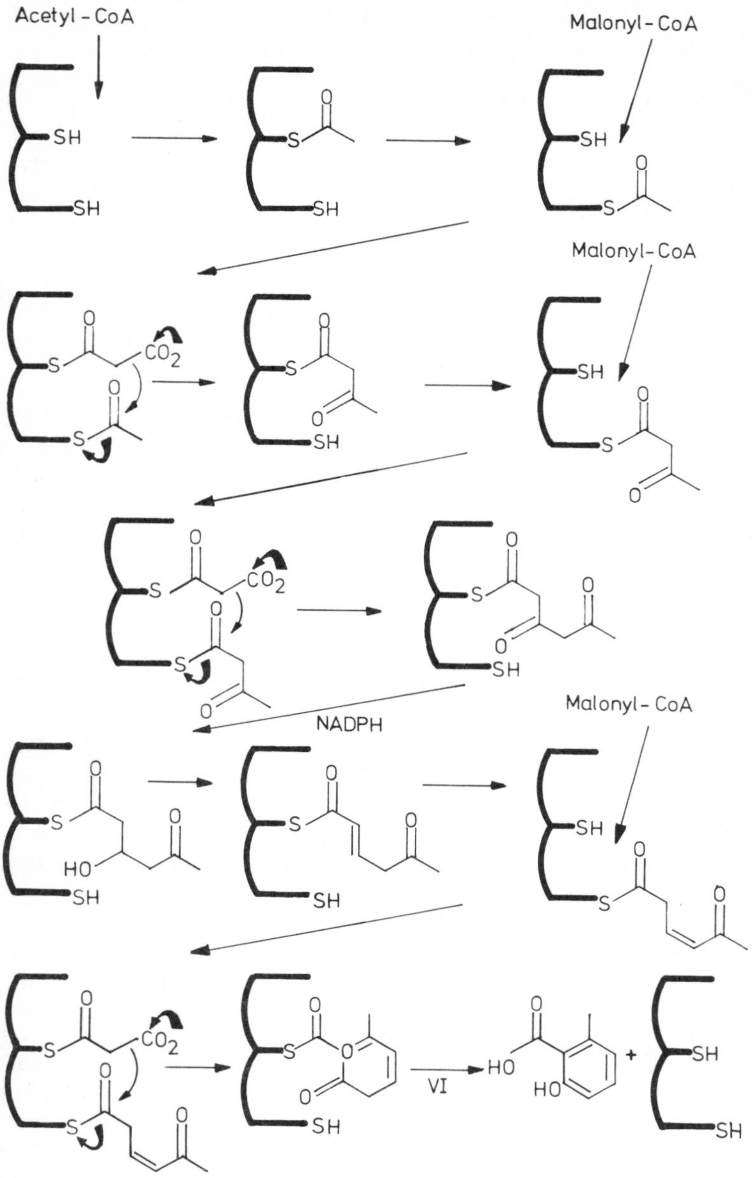

Acetyl - CoA

Malonyl - CoA

Malonyl - CoA

NADPH

Malonyl - CoA

VI

Fig. 4-4. Synthesis of 6-me-
thylsalicylic acid, a simple polyketide, according to
Bu'Lock, 1979.

practical importance that contain chlorine are **gri-seofulvin** (II) and **chlortetracycline** (III).

Possibility of variation 10: Combination of the polyketide moiety with other structural units. Particularly common are glycosides of polyketide agly-

cones; for example, in the macrolides [**erythromycin** (XXXVIII)], anthracyclines, and some polyenes [**amphotericin B** (XXXVI)]. Amino acids also appear in combination with presumable polyketides; for example, in **geldanamycin** (XXXIX) an alanine residue has been incorporated in the ring while in **ansa-trienin** (XL) (Weber et al., 1981) an alanine residue appears in the side chain. The possibilities of variation by combination with other structural units are almost unlimited.

Possibility of variation 11: Dimerization. Examples of this possibility are found particularly among the benzoquinones and anthraquinones; for example, **phenicin** (XLI) in the benzoquinone series or **skyrin** (XLII) in the anthraquinone series.

Because they include very numerous variants, even when several of these possibilities are mutually excluded, the eleven basic possibilities of variation given here lead to an almost astronomical number of possible polyketides. The fact that we know only a minute fraction of them can probably be explained both by our still extremely meager knowledge and also by the still very high selection pressure which takes care that only a small proportion occurs simultaneously in nature. A simple calculation can show, on the one hand, how high this selection pressure must be and, on the other hand, how minute our knowledge probably is.

Possibilities of variation:

Estimated minimum number of variants

1. Number of units	8
2. Degree and position of reductions	100
3. Extent and position of dehydrations	50
4. Other units (nature, number, positions)	50
5. Type of cyclization	8
6. Additional O-functions (number, positions)	50
7. C-Methyls, O-methyls (number, positions)	200
8. Subsequent chain modifications	4
9. Introduction of chlorine or bromine (number, positions)	50
10. Combination with other structural units	2000
11. Dimerization	2

This would give a theoretically possible number of 1.28×10^{17} combinations for polyketides. On the basis that 99.9% of these theoretically possible combinations exclude one another in practice, we still are left with a number of about 10^{14} possibilities. How many of them are present in nature today and how many have already been eliminated again or did not arise in the first place, is completely open. However, the fact is clear that we know only an extremely small fraction of the polyketides actually occurring in nature and that probably, more are being currently formed than we can handle.

4.6.2 Amino Acids as Structural Units of Secondary Metabolites

The number of secondary metabolites derived from amino acids that have been described is substantially smaller than that of the polyketides, which, however, is probably due more to the different level of knowledge than to the actual situation. Polyketides are often colored and often possess an antibiotic activity, which is frequently used as a criterion for the isolation of secondary metabolites. Secondary metabolites derived from amino acids are rarely colored and only a relatively small proportion of them possess antibiotic action. From the large field of amino acids as structural units of secondary metabolites, we shall consider five groups of questions:

a) Unusual amino acids

In addition to the proteinogenic amino acids, very many unusual amino acids occur as structural units of secondary metabolites. Table 4-3 shows a small selection of the more than 200 unusual amino acids that have been described either as free compounds or as parts of secondary metabolites. In numerous secondary products, the proportion of nonproteinogenic amino acids is more than 50%. Many of the unusual amino acids have been found in polypeptides and have not so far been confirmed as occurring in the free state. Here again, the reason is probably our technique of investigation. If an unusual amino acid exhibits no antibiotic effect either because it is not taken up by intact cells or because it possesses no activity in the cellfree system, the amino acid is easily overlooked in screening for antibiotics. A change in the screening procedure, e.g., to detection with ninhydrin, would show up a very large number of new amino acids, especially those which hitherto have been described only in peptides.

While the biogenesis and biosynthesis of the proteinogenic amino acids is well known, our knowledge on the origin of the unusual amino acids is scanty. It may be assumed for the D-analogs of the proteinogenic L-amino acids that they are formed by a racemase from the L-forms. For the case of dihydrophenylalanine, Floss (1980) showed that after the deviation from the normal biosynthetic pathway to phenylalanine at the prephenate stage, a whole number of steps are still necessary.

b) **The transformation of an individual amino acid into a secondary metabolite**

In the case of **psilocine** (XLIII) and **psilocybine** (XLIV) (Hofmann et al., 1959), it is not difficult to recognize the original tryptophan in the final secondary metabolites. Both substances are narcotics from Basidiomycetes. The example of lysergic acid from Claviceps strains likewise leads into the field of narcotics. Here one tryptophan molecule is linked with one mevalonic acid molecule and cyclized to a complicated ring system (Fig. 4-5). In a later step, e.g., in *Claviceps purpurea*, the lysergic acid is linked through a peptide moiety to form the pharmacologically important ergot alkaloids (for a summary, see Rutschmann and Stadler, 1978). Here, examples starting from tryptophan have been selected, but very many examples starting from other amino acids could be cited.

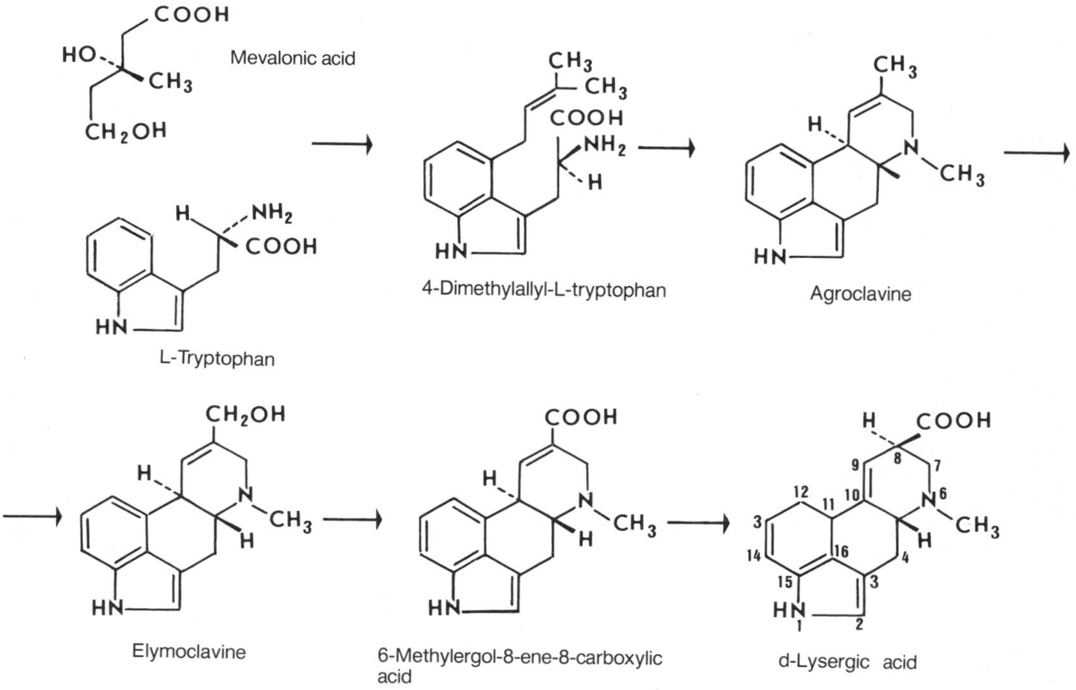

Fig. 4-5. Biogenesis of ergot alkaloids.

c) Synthesis of a secondary metabolite from a few amino acids

The number of secondary metabolites which are constructed of only a few amino acids is very large. Most still permit the original amino acids to be readily recognized, e.g., where a simple diketopiperazine is present or is still recognizable as in **aspergillic acid** (XLV) or **pulcherrimin** (XLVI). In other cases, the original amino acids can hardly be recognized. The β-lactam antibiotics penicillin and cephalosporin C occupy a middle position. Figure 4-6 summarizes the biosynthesis of the penicillins and cephalosporins that has been shown by the recent investigations

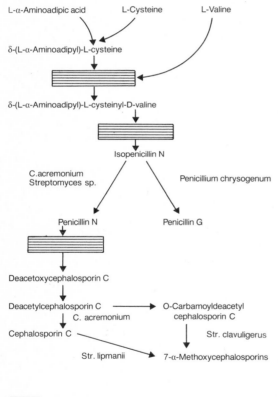

Fig. 4-6. Biosynthesis of penicillin and cephalosporin.

of O'Sullivan et al. (1979a, b, c) and of Sawada et al. (1979). The initial components, L-aminoadipic acid, L-cysteine and L-valine had already been long known as structural units. What is new is the proof, which presupposed a cell-free system, that a LLD-tripeptide (D-valine) is incorporated and must be regarded as a true intermediate stage. The change in configuration must take place before or directly during the formation of the tripeptide, since a LLL-tripeptide is not incorporated. How this happens is an open question, just like the mechanism of the ring expansion of penicillin N to cephalosporin and the cyclization of the tripeptide to isopenicillin N. A group at the Massachusetts Institute of Technology has recently succeeded in isolating and provisionally characterizing the enzymes involved in cyclization and ring expansion (Demain et al., 1982), so that the way to elucidating the mechanisms of these processes is now open. Surprising is the fact that, according to everything known today, the biosynthetic pathway to the cephalosporin skeleton in Cephalosporium strains is the same as in the cephalosporin-producing streptomycetes.

d) The nonribosomal synthesis of polypeptides

In the biosynthesis of proteins the ribosomal synthetic apparatus ensures that the information given by mRNA is correctly converted into the protein. The composition and the sequence of amino acids in the microbial polypeptides are also genetically determined, and yet the synthesis takes place by a nonribosomal pathway. Exhaustive accounts of the biosynthesis of polypeptides have been given by Katz and Demain (1977) and by Zimmer et al. (1979). The best-studied example is **gramicidin S** (XLVII). Its synthesis takes place in a total of 16 steps with two enzymes, 4-phosphopantetheine acting as carrier or acceptor of the amino acids. On the first enzyme, L-phenylalanine is activated and is converted into the activated D-phenylalanine, and on the second enzyme proline is activated and then the start, proper, of the polypeptide synthesis takes place in which the bound and activated D-phenylalanine is transferred from the first enzyme to the second enzyme and an enzyme-bound dipeptide arises which is then lengthened to the pentapeptide. Finally, two enzyme-bound pentapeptides are cyclized and the complete gramicidin S is liberated. So far, none of the polypeptide antibiotics from microorganisms have acquired great importance (bacitracin and tyrocidin are of subordinate importance, and even polymixin and colistin are used to only a small extent). For a number of polypeptides, e.g., the hexapeptide sideramines, a function for the producing strains has been established, and it has been shown to be probable for a number of others, e.g., ionophoric polypeptides. This explains how such a complicated synthetic apparatus could be retained in the course of evolution.

For a long time, a function in connection with the formation of spores was assumed for the **gramicidins.** Now that it has been shown that there are antibiotic-minus mutants which still sporulate normally, the question of a function of these compounds is again open, but a possible inhibition of the germination of the spores might be considered as a function.

While it is easy to imagine a connection between iron transport or ion selectivity and even – although improbably – between antibiotic action and polypeptide synthesis, in the case of the immunosuppressive **cyclosporins** (XLIII) no relationship between biological action outside the cell and function for the producing agent can be imagined.

e) **The linkage of polypeptides with other structural units**
The number of non-amino-acid structural units in polypeptides is large and extends over several chemical groups, e.g., fatty acids [an example is **polymyxin** (XLIX)], sugars [example are the **bleomycins** (XXVIII)], **polyamines** (examples are again the bleomycins), or heterocycles as in **actinomycin** (L) or the **quinoxaline** antibiotics (e.g., **echinomycin**). In the case of the **actinomycins** with the same chromophore there are a hundred variants, all differing in the amino acid moiety. In the case of the bleomycins, there is also a pronounced variation in the non-amino-acid moiety.

In the case of the polyketides, the almost unimaginable variation has been shown in de-

tail. The same can be said in the field of amino acids as structural units of secondary metabolites. Here again **the number of possible variants is unlimited** and here, also, we know only a quite small part of this variation. However, nature has not tried out all the possibilities and, finally, evolution has left us only a small fraction, and of this fraction, again, we known only a quite minute part.

4.6.3 Sugars as Structural Units of Secondary Metabolites

The number of sugars that occur as structural units of secondary metabolites is much larger than the number of sugars that are known from the intermediate metabolism. This applies particularly to many mono- and dideoxysugars, aminosugars, dimethylaminosugars, and aminouronic acids. Here again we find secondary metabolites that are derived from only a single structural unit, e.g., **nojirimycin** (LI) and **streptozotocin** (LII), and those which contain only a few sugars up to secondary metabolites which are pronounced oligosaccharides, such as the orthosomycins [one example being **avilamycin** (LIII), Keller-Schierlein et al., 1979]. In this series, also in addition to the usual glycosidic bonds unusual bonds occur [e.g., in **avilamycin** (LIII)].

Important representatives that include sugars as structural units are the aminoglycosides (see the special section), the macrolides, and the anthracyclines.

4.6.4 Mevalonic Acid as a Structural Unit of Secondary Metabolites

Representatives of secondary metabolites which are derived from mevalonic acid are very common. Examples containing only one mevalonic acid unit have already been mentioned [novobiocin (Fig. 4-2) and the ergot alkaloids (Fig. 4-5)]. Examples of metabolites constructed from several mevalonic acid units will not be mentioned here (terpenes) although in this series, as well, large variation in the secondary metabolism can again be shown.

isolated for other reasons but were later tested widely for general pharmacological properties, e.g., immunosuppressive action of the cyclosporins (Ruegger et al., 1976; Dreyfuss et al., 1976; Borel et al., 1976). Here a marked expansion of our knowledge is to be expected in the next few years (Demain, 1983).

4.7   Biological Effects of Secondary Metabolites Outside the Producing Cell

If one goes through the secondary metabolites from microorganisms that have been described above, the impression arises that most secondary metabolites possess antimicrobial activity. However, this is clearly due to the selection principle and does not agree with reality. In addition to the antibiotic properties very frequently described, numerous other biological activities are known. Activities have been found in microbial metabolites wherever a proper screening program has been performed. A good example is the large number of **enzyme inhibitors** that have been found in a corresponding program from the Institute of Microbial Chemistry in Tokyo (Umezawa, 1972, 1977). How frequent such inhibitors are has been confirmed by Frommer et al. (1979); they found inhibitors for α-glucosidases in 10% of all the streptomycetes tested. Widespread are compounds which are **toxic for warm-blooded animals** (for reviews, see Ajl et al., 1971 to 1972, and Mirocha et al., 1979), the mycotoxins being particularly important because of their carcinogenic action.

Other pharmacological activities of microbial metabolites have been found either on the basis of studies of native medicine (psychotropic agents, actions on the uterus) or in a screening of microbial metabolites that were

4.8   Literature

Ajisaka et al.: Japanese Patent 7214916 (1972), cited by Glasby, J. S.: *Encyclopaedia of Antibiotics*. J. Wiley and Sons, London 1976.

Ajl, S., Ciegler, A., Kadis, S., Montie, T. C. and Weinbaum, G. (eds.): *Microbial Toxins*, I–VIII. Academic Press, London 1971/1972.

Anke, H., "Desferritriacetylfusigen, an antibiotic from *Aspergillus deflectus*", *J. Antibiot.* **30,** 125–128 (1977).

Anke, H., Kolthoum, I. and Laatsch, H., "Anthraquinones of the *Aspergillus glaucus* group. II. Biological activities", *Arch. Microbiol.* V **126,** 231–236 (1980).

Anke, T., "Antibiotika aus Basidiomyceten", *Z. Mykol.* **44,** 131–141 (1978).

Asselineau, J. and Zalta, J. P.: *Les Antibiotiques*. Hermann, Paris 1973.

Bayer, E., Gugel, K. H., Hägele, K., Hagenmaier, H., Jessipow, S., König, W. A. and Zähner, H., "Phosphinothricin und Phosphinotricyl-Alanyl-Alanin", *Helv. Chim. Acta* **55,** 224–239 (1972).

Bérdy, J., "Recent developments of antibiotics research and classification of antibiotics according to chemical structure", *Adv. Appl. Microbiol.* **18,** 309–406 (1974).

Bérdy, J.: *CRC Handbook of Antibiotic Compounds*
Vol. I.   Carbohydrate Antibiotics.
Vol. II. Macrocyclic Lactone Antibiotics.
Vol. III. Quinone and Similar Antibiotics.
Vol. IV. Amino Acid and Peptide Antibiotics.
CRC Press, Florida 1981.

Birch, A. J., "Biosynthesis of polyketides and related compounds", *Science* **156,** 202–206 (1967).

Birch, A. J. and Donovan, F. W., "Studies in relation to biosynthesis. I. Some possible routes to derivatives of orcinol and phloroglucinol", *Austr. J. Chem.* **6**, 306–368 (1953).

Blinov, N. O., Blinov, I. N. and Khokhlov, A. S., "Viridimycins and actinoviridins. Antibiotics and pigments of the o-nitrosophenol group: their role in iron metabolism in Streptomycetes", Int. Symp. Antibiotics Weimar (1979) C-11.

Borel, J. F., Feuer, C., Gubler, H. U. and Stähelin, H., "Biological effects of cyclosporin A: A new antilymphotic agent", *Agents Actions* **6**, 468–475 (1976).

Bu'Lock, J. D.: *Biosynthesis of Natural Products.* McGraw-Hill, London 1965.

Bu'Lock, J. D.: "Polyketide biosynthesis". In: Barton, D. and Ollis, W. D. (eds.): *Comprehensive Organic Chemistry.* Pergamon Press, Oxford 1979, pp. 927–987.

Demain, A. L., "New applications of microbial products", *Science* **219**, 709–719 (1983).

Demain, A. L., Kupka, Y., Shen, Y. Q. and Wolfe, S., "Microbial synthesis of β-lactam antibiotics". In: *Trends in Antibiotic Research,* pp. 233–247, Jap. Antibiotics Research Association, 1982.

Dimroth, P., Walter, H. and Lynen, F., "Biosynthese von 6-Methylsalicylsäure", *Eur. J. Biochem.* **13**, 98–110 (1970).

Dreyfuss, M., Härri, E., Hofmann, H., Kobel, H., Pache, W. and Tscherter, H., "Cyclosporin A and C", *Eur. J. Appl. Microbiol.* **3**, 125–133 (1976).

Floss, H. G.: „Biosynthesis of some aromatic antibiotics". In: Corcoran (ed.): *Antibiotics,* IV. Springer, New York 1980.

Frommer, W., Junge, B., Müller, L., Schmidt, D. and Truscheit, E., "Neue Enzyminhibitoren aus Mikroorganismen", *Planta Med.* **35**, 195–217 (1979).

Fujiwara, A., Okuda, T., Tazoe, M., Miyamoto, C., Sekine, Y. and Fujiwara, M.: Studies on isonitrile antibiotics. *Ann. Meeting Agr. Chem. Soc.* (1978).

Glasby, J. S.: *Encyclopaedia of Antibiotics.* J. Wiley & Sons, London 1976.

Hofmann, A., Heim, R., Brack, A., Kobel, H., Frey, A., Ott, H., Petrzilka, Th. and Troxler, F., "Psilocybin und Psilocin, zwei psychotrope Wirkstoffe aus mexikanischen Rauschpilzen", *Helv. Chim. Acta* **42**, 1557–1572 (1959).

Iguchi, E., Okuhara, M., Kohsaka, M., Aoki, H. and Imaka, H., "Studies on new phosphoric acid antibiotics. Taxonomic studies on producing organisms of the phosphonic acid related compounds", *J. Antibiot.* **33**, 18–23 (1980).

Kamiya, T., Hemmi, K., Takeno, H. and Hashimoto, M.: Studies on new phosphonic acid containing antibiotics. *Abstr. 11th Internat. Congr. of Chemotherapy,* Boston (1979).

Katz, E. and Demain, A. L., "The peptide antibiotics of Bacillus: chemistry, biogenesis and possible function", *Bacteriol. Rev.* **41**, 449–474 (1977).

Keller-Schierlein, W., Heilman, W., Ollis, W. D. and Smith, Ch., "Die Avilamycine A und C: Chemischer Abbau und spektroskopische Untersuchungen", *Helv. Chim. Acta* **62**, 7–20 (1979).

König, W. A., Krauss, C. and Zähner, H., "6-Chlorgenistein und 6,3'-Dichlorgenistein", *Helv. Chim. Acta* **60**, 2071–2078 (1977).

Komiyama, T., Aoyagi, T., Takeuchi, T. and Umezawa, H., "Inhibitory effects of phosphoramidon on neutral metalloendopeptidases and its application on affinity chromatography", *Biochem. Biophys. Res. Commun.* **65**, 352–357 (1975).

Korzybski, T., Kowszyk-Gindifer, Z. and Kurylowicz, W.: *Antibiotics,* I–III. American Soc. Microbiol., 1978.

Krauss, Ch.: *Chlorhaltige Metabolite aus Streptomyceten. Chloractinomycin und Chlorisoflavone.* Dissertation, Tübingen 1977.

Kurylowicz, W. (ed.): *Antibiotics, a Critical Review.* Polish Medical Publishers, Warsaw 1976.

Laskin, A. I. and Lechevalier, H. A. (eds.): *Handbook of Microbiology,* Vol. III. Microbial Products. CRC Press, Cleveland 1973.

Lechevalier, H., "Production of some antibiotics by members of different genera of microorganisms", *Adv. Appl. Microbiol.* **19**, 25–45 (1975).

Leisinger, T. and Margraff, R., "Secondary metabolites of the fluorescent Pseudomonads", *Microbiol. Rev.* **43**, 422–442 (1979).

Light, R. J. and Hager, L. P., "Molecular parameters of 6-methyl-salicylic acid synthetase from gel filtration and sucrose density gradient centrifugation", *Arch. Biochem. Biophys.* **125**, 326–333 (1968).

Luckner, M., Nover, L. and Bohm, H.: *Secondary Metabolism and Cell Differentiation.* Springer-Verlag, Berlin 1977.

Mann, I.: *Secondary Metabolism*. Oxford University Press, 1977.

Mirocha, C. J., Pathre, S. V. and Christensen, C. M.: "Mycotoxins". In: Rose, A. H. (ed.): *Secondary Products of Metabolism*. Academic Press, London, New York 1979, pp. 468–522.

Nakamura, H., Itaka, H., Kitahara, T., Okazaki, T. and Okami, Y., "Structure of aplasmomycin", *J. Antibiot.* **30**, 714–717 (1977).

Nara, T., Kawamoto, I., Okachi, R. and Oka, T., "Source of antibiotics other than Streptomyces", *J. Antibiot.* **30**, 174–189 (1977).

Okami, Y., Okazaki, T., Kitahara, T. and Umezawa, H., "A new antibiotic, aplasmomycin, produced by a Streptomycete isolated from shallow sea mud", *J. Antibiot.* **29**, 1019–1025 (1976).

Okuhara, M., Kuroda, Y., Goto, T., Okamoto, M., Terano, H., Kohasaka, M., Aoki, H. and Imanaka, H., "Studies on new phosphonic acid antibiotics. I. FR – 900098, Isolation and characterization", *J. Antibiot.* **33**, 13–17 (1980). "III. Isolation and characterization of FR – 31564, FR – 32863, and FR – 33289", *J. Antibiot.* **33**, 24–28 (1980). "IV. Structure determination of FR – 33289, FR – 31564 and FR – 32863", *J. Antibiot.* **33**, 29–35 (1980).

O'Sullivan, J., Aplin, R. T., Stevens, C. M. and Abraham, E. P., "Biosynthesis of a 7-α-methoxycephalosporin. Incorporation of molecular oxygen", *Biochem. J.* **179**, 47–52 (1979 a).

O'Sullivan, J., Bleaney, R. C., Huddleston, A. and Abraham, E. P., "Incorporation of ^{3}H from δ-(L-α-amino[4,5-^{3}H]adipyl)-L-cysteinyl-D[4,4-^{3}H]valine into isopenicillin N", *Biochem. J.* **184**, 421–426 (1979 b).

O'Sullivan, J., Huddleston, A. and Abraham, E. P.: "Biosynthesis of penicillin and cephalosporins in cellfree systems". In: Baddiley, J. and Abraham, E. P. (eds.): *Penicillin Fifty Years after Fleming*. Royal Society London 1980, pp. 197–198.

Park, B. K., Hirota, A. and Sakai, H., "Structure of plumbemycin A and B, antagonists of L-threo-nine from *Streptomyces plumbeus*", *Agric. Biol. Chem.* **41**, 573–579 (1977).

Rüegger, A., Kuhn, M., Lichti, H., Loosli, H. R., Huguenin, R., Quiquerez, Ch. and Wartburg, A. v., "Cyclosporin A, ein immunsuppressiv wirksamer Peptidmetabolit aus *Trichiderma polysporum* (Link ex Pers.) Rifai", *Helv. Chim. Acta* **59**, 1075–1092 (1976).

Rutschmann, J. and Stadler, P. A.: "Chemical Background in Ergot Alkaloids and Related Compounds". In: Born, G. V. R. et al. (eds.): *Handbook of Experimental Pharmacology*, Vol. 49. Springer-Verlag, Berlin, Heidelberg, New York 1978, pp. 29–85.

Sawada, Y., Hunt, N. A. and Demain, A. L., "Further studies on microbial ring expansion of penicillin N", *J. Antibiot.* **32**, 1303–1310 (1979).

Umezawa, H.: *Enzyme Inhibitors of Microbial Origin*. Tokyo University Press, 1972.

Umezawa, H.: *Institute of Microbial Chemistry*. 1962–1977. Microbial Chemistry Foundation, Tokyo 1977.

Umezawa, H. (ed.): *Index of Antibiotics from Actinomycetes*.

Vol. I,   University of Tokyo Press, 1967.

Vol. II, University Park Press, Baltimore 1978.

Weber, W., Zähner, H., Zeeck, A., Russ, P. and Damberg, M., "Ansatrienins A and B, ansamycin antibiotics produced by a strain of *Streptomyces collinus*", *Zentralbl. Bakteriol. Parasitenk. Infektionskr. Hyg. Abt. 1 Orig. C* **2**, 122–139 (1981).

Zähner, H.: "The search for new secondary metabolites". In: Hütter, R., Leisinger, T., Nüesch, J. and Wehrli, W. (eds.): *Antibiotics and other Secondary Metabolites*. Academic Press, London 1978.

Zähner, H., "What are secondary metabolites?", *Folia Microbiol.* **24**, 435–443 (1979).

Zimmer, T. L., Frøyshov, Ø. and Laland, S. G.: "Peptide Antibiotics". In: A. H. Rose (ed.): *Secondary Products of Metabolism*. Academic Press, London, New York 1979, pp. 124–150.

Chapter 5

Plant and Animal Cell Cultures

Jochen Berlin and Jürgen Bode

5.1   Introduction

In the last few years, the interest of biotechnology in plant and animal cell cultures has dramatically expanded. The increasing importance of cell cultures can be recognized from the fact that in books on biotechnology space is being made more and more frequently for information on higher cells (Kurz and Constabel, 1979; Dougall, 1979; Kruse and Patterson, 1973; Mauersberger, 1971; Paul, 1973; Jacoby and Pastan, 1979) and that biotechnological symposia now always devote some sessions to biological and technological aspects of plant and animal cell cultures.

The aim of this chapter is to acquaint the reader with the nature, the maintenance, the problems, and the literature of plant and animal cell cultures. Many aspects must necessarily be left out of consideration. However, we hope that our choice gives the reader a clear overview of the present state, the possibilities, and the difficulties of using higher cells in biotechnology. Plant and animal cell cultures differ so greatly in their characteristics that the two systems are treated separately.

5.2   Plant Cell Cultures

5.2.1   General

The number of laboratories dealing with plant cell cultures has increased continuously in the last few years. In 1972, 940 scientists from 41 countries belonged to the "International Association for Plant Tissue Cultures". In 1980, the Association already had more than 2000 members in 63 countries. An International Congress for plant cell cultures is held by the group every four years. The programs of these congresses best reflect the fact that work with

plant cells is being performed for many different purposes. For example, plant cell cultures are an excellent tool for answering some basic biological questions. As we will show, answers to basic questions are as necessary as applied research for planning a broad biotechnological utilization of plant cell cultures in industry and agriculture. Commercial applications of cell cultures are seen, in particular, in the **production of important natural compounds** and in the **improvement of crop plants** (Hepner and Male, 1978). These two areas cannot be considered equally here; the product-oriented aspect of plant cell cultures will be emphasized more, since biotechnology – at least in the past – has dealt to some extent with fermentation and product recovery. The decision to favor product-oriented cell culture research does not mean that this area will become accessible to a broader commercial application earlier. On the contrary, at the present time it appears that the improvement of useful plants through cell culture technique may be achieved before the production of natural compounds from cell cultures at economically acceptable cost.

For two reasons it seems necessary to give an introduction into working with plant cell cultures before describing the biotechnological aspects. First, the field is uncharted territory for many biotechnologists, and, second, at the present time there is no collection of plant cell cultures from which definite lines can be obtained. Consequently, as a rule, in most cases one has to establish the required cell culture oneself.

5.2.2   Work with Plant Cell Cultures

Equipment of a Cell Culture Laboratory

Since plant cell cultures grow much more slowly than many microorganisms, the highest commandment in handling plant cell cultures is sterile working. A cell culture laboratory should therefore have available a clean bench with laminar air flow. Plant cell cultures should be maintained under constant conditions. Cultivation may take place in climatized chests, or still better, in climatized rooms. In most laboratories, plant cultures are maintained both on **agar media** and in **liquid media.** Suspension cultures must be shaken continuously on shaking machines for continuous operation (with an emergency power supply). The biosynthetic productivity of a culture is frequently affected by light. In order to test these effects on the cultures, different light fields should be available for such experiments. Anyone requiring detailed information on the construction and equipment of a cell culture laboratory may be referred to an article by Street (1977a).

Media for Plant Cell Cultures

The choice of medium is a decisive factor for setting up a culture (callus induction) and for the growth and biosynthetic productivity of a cell culture. The cells of most plants can be grown on definite **synthetic media.** Only in a few cases have additives such as yeast extract, casein hydrolysate, and coconut milk proved to be necessary (Gamborg et al., 1976). An outstanding position has been achieved by the **MS medium** according to Murashige-Skoog. All media for plant cell cultures contain mineral salts (major and trace nutrient elements), vitamins, sucrose, and growth regulators (phytohormones). A comparison of the compositions of the most important media has been made (Gamborg et al., 1976; see Table 5-1).

Setting Up of Cell Cultures

The numerous publications on the influence of media on growth processes may be regarded as guides for one's own procedure in establishing a culture (Street, 1976; Aitchison et al., 1977; King and Street, 1977). The opti-

mum conditions for a newly set up callus culture and for suspension cultures derived from it, however, must be determined in each case according to the question under investigation. Up to the present, plant cell cultures of **dicotyledons, monocotyledons, gymnosperms, ferns,** and **mosses** have been set up. It may therefore be assumed that in principle cell cultures of any plant can be established.

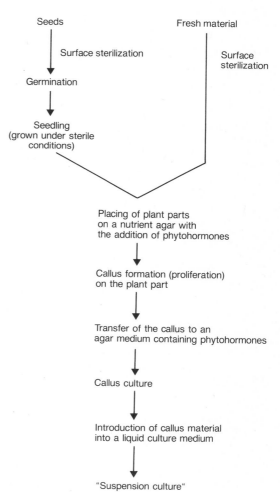

Fig. 5-1. The establishment of plant cell cultures.

Table 5-1. Composition of Two of the Media Most Frequently Used for Plant Cell Cultures (Gamborg et al., 1976).

	MS		B5	
Major elements	mg/L	mmol/L	mg/L	mmol/L
NH_4NO_3	1650	20.6		
KNO_3	1900	18.8	2500	25
$CaCl_2 \cdot 2\,H_2O$	440	3.0	150	1.0
$MgSO_4 \cdot 7\,H_2O$	370	1.5	250	1.0
KH_2PO_4	170	1.25		
$(NH_4)_2SO_4$			134	1.0
$NaH_2PO_4 \cdot H_2O$			150	1.1
Trace elements	mg/L	μmol/L	mg/L	μmol/L
KI	0.83	5.0	0.75	4.5
H_3BO_3	6.2	100	3.0	50
$MnSO_4 \cdot 4\,H_2O$	22.3	100		
$MnSO_4 \cdot H_2O$			10	60
$ZnSO_4 \cdot 7\,H_2O$	8.6	30	2.0	7.0
$Na_2MoO_4 \cdot 2\,H_2O$	0.25	1.0	0.25	1.0
$CuSO_4 \cdot 5\,H_2O$	0.025	0.1	0.025	0.1
$CoCl_2 \cdot 6\,H_2O$	0.025	0.1	0.025	0.1
$Na_2 \cdot EDTA$	37.3	100	37.3	100
$FeSO_4 \cdot 7\,H_2O$	27.8	100	27.8	100
Vitamins	mg/L		mg/L	
Inositol	100		100	
Nicotinic acid	0.5		1.0	
Pyridoxine · HCl	0.5		1.0	
Thiamine · HCl	0.1		10.0	
Glycine	2.0			
Sucrose		30		20
pH		5.7		5.5

Phytohormones

Indolylacetic acid, naphthylacetic acid, 2,4-dichlorophenoxyacetic acid, kinetin, in various concentrations – 10^{-7} to 10^{-5} mol/L

The starting material for the initiation of a cell culture may be any part of a plant. Depending on the plant material (pieces of stems, leaves, roots or cotyledons), the formation of calluses may proceed at different rates. Consequently, in the setting up of a culture, different parts of the plant should be tested as starting material. The plant material must previously be made germ-free. If seeds are available, these can be treated with 2 to 5% sodium hypochlorite solution or other antimicrobial agents for 10 to 60 min. After the sodium hypochlorite solution has been washed out with sterilized water, the seeds are placed on moist filter paper or on a weak agar medium for germination under sterile conditions. If no seeds are available as starting material, surface-sterilized fresh plant parts can be used to set up cultures. The seedlings or the sterile parts of older plants are cut into several small pieces under sterile conditions which are then placed on an agar for callus initiation. To induce calluses in an explant it is recommended first to carry out a trial with MS medium to which 2,4-dichlorophenoxyacetic acid (2,4-D) has been added in a concentration of 10^{-5} to 10^{-6} mol/L. 2,4-D promotes cell division and suppresses morphogenesis. If it is desired to establish a culture for studying morphogenesis, 2,4-D should be replaced by α-naphthylacetic acid, benzylaminopurine, or zeatin, individually or in combination (Gamborg et al., 1976). Callus formation is frequently observed first on the cut surfaces (wound points). The speed of callus formation depends greatly on the species of plant and the plant material and the process may last for between eight days and three months. Once the first calluses are visible on the explant, the subsequent procedure is governed by the problem under investigation. On the one hand, the calluses can be separated from the explant and cultivated further on fresh agar. Observation under the microscope shows that the primary calluses may still contain organized structures. If this morphological differentiation is not desired and does not disappear in the course of the next 3 to 4 passages, the concentration of 2,4-D in the medium should be raised. If suspension cultures are to be obtained as rapidly as possible, the explants should be cultivated with the calluses on a shaker in a liquid medium. In some cases, well-growing suspension cultures are obtained by this method only six weeks after the initiation of calluses.

Definition of Plant Cell Cultures

The term "plant cell culture" should be understood today in a narrower sense than previously. The culture of seedlings, embryos, and isolated plant organs (tissue culture) should be clearly distinguished from true cell cultures which have arisen by proliferation at wounded parts of plants. After some time, these callus cultures contain none of the original tissue of the intact plant. In ordinary use, the term "**callus cultures**" is used for cell cultures that have arisen by proliferation and are maintained on agar. **Suspension cultures** is the name generally given to cultures kept under submerged conditions in a liquid medium. By definition, however, the term suspension cultures should be limited to cell cultures consisting of individual cells and few-cell aggregates (clumps). The biochemical reasons why certain species of plants grow without difficulty as fine suspensions while other always reaggregate are unknown. The methods used hitherto for maintaining finer suspensions in such cases are not always successful (Street, 1976). Many established cultures are unsuitable or even unusable for fermentation just because of their behaviour in growth.

In setting up cultures anew, one must not assume beforehand that the various explants of a plant always lead to cultures with the same properties. The initial calluses may differentiate in the course of cultivation. To what extent the physiological state of the explant affects the development of the initial calluses and to what extent the later biosynthetic output is affected by this is unknown. The significance of the initial material for the capacity of a culture for organogenesis is, however, clear from many studies (Street, 1976; Green, 1978). Not only morphological differentiation but also the selection of different types of cells determine the further development of the culture. The situation seems to be even more complicated by the observation that plant cell cultures themselves generate genetic variability (somaclonal variation) (Larkin and Scowcroft, 1981). This may be an advantage for plant improvement as suggested by Larkin and Scowcroft or a disadvantage for the fer-

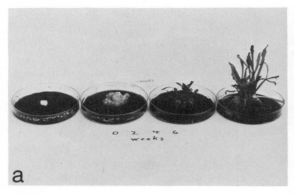

a

Fig. 5-2a. Establishment of *Cichorium intybus* cultures with subsequent regeneration. A piece picked out of the root (already sterile) forms a callus on a Murashige-Skoog medium (1 ppm of indolylacetic acid) after two weeks, and from this shoots differentiate after two further weeks.

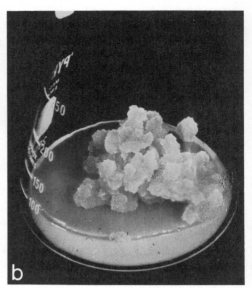

b

Fig. 5-2b. Callus culture of *Nicotiana tabacum* on a MS medium + 0.4 ppm of 2,4-dichlorophenoxyacetic acid. The culture was established in 1959 and since then has been subcultivated at four-week intervals.

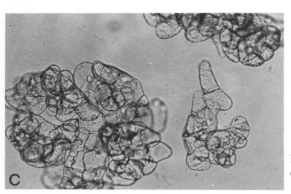

c

Fig. 5-2c. Cell aggregates of a TXD suspension culture *(Nicotiana tabacum)* at a magnification of 175 ×.

mentation by plant cells. Consequently, one may and must expect spontaneous changes even in cloned cell cultures (Tabata and Hiraoka, 1976). However, the overall stability of product formation by once-established cell lines or the case with which a producing cell strain can be recovered from a deteriorated culture shows that somaclonal variation is a manageable problem for product-oriented research. In spite of all the uncertainty over the importance of the primary explant it has clearly been shown that the biosynthetic potential of a culture does not depend on whether the explant was capable of a particular synthesis in the intact plant (Tabata and Hiraoka, 1976). The question of whether well-producing plants are of decisive importance for establishing well-producing cultures has not been definitely decided (Zenk et al., 1977; Roller, 1978). If possible, however, one should probably start from plants with a high productivity.

5.2.3 Biotechnological Application

In what areas can a biotechnological application of plant cell cultures be considered? Two completely opposite possibilities suggest themselves. On the one hand, one may attempt, through cell cultures, to achieve **fast multiplication** or **improvement** of cultivated plants. The biotechnological success of such experiments is recognized from the properties of the plants regenerated from the tissue or cell cultures. On the other hand, one may attempt to utilize the **biosynthetic capacities** of the morphologically dedifferentiated cells. Here, biotechnological success is measured by the yield of product and a cost analysis of the fermentation process.

Like any higher form of life, the intact plant is of great complexity. This means that only a vanishingly small part of the total genetic information is ever expressed in a given tissue or organ. In plant cell cultures, we have very greatly reduced the morphological and, as a necessary consequence, the biochemical complexity in comparison with the intact plant. It is known that the cells – at least those of a young culture – still contain all the genetic information, since it is sometimes possible to regenerate even from single cells intact plants which differ in no way from the mother plant. The first aim (regardless of whether the improvement of the plants or the production of natural materials is desired) must therefore be to differentiate the dedifferentiated cells into the desired directions. This differentiation is called in the one case **induction of organogenesis** and in the other case **induction of cytodifferentiation,** e.g., the biosynthesis of a natural product. At the present time there are no generally binding guidelines for achieving this aim. These must be worked out anew in each case for the various plant species or biosynthetic pathways. The induction of the desired differentiation must therefore in many cases be done purely empirically.

5.2.4 Agricultural Use of Plant Cell Culture Technique

Investigations with plant cell cultures which aim at restoring the intact plant, can be divided roughly into two groups: **vegetative mass multiplication** and **improvement of plant material** through the selection of cell lines with definite properties. The latter also includes the production of new plants, by the fusion of cells from two different plant species (hybrid plants) or by the incorporation of new genetic material into the plant genome. In addition, by the tissue culture techniques disease-free plants can be obtained even if the mother plants were infected.

Clonal Mass Multiplication

The clonal mass multiplication of plants goes back to investigations by Morel who multiplied orchids via meristem cultures (Rao, 1977). This method is generally used in the orchid industry today and explains the uniformity of the blooms of a given variety of orchid. The observations on **orchids** can be transferred to numerous other plants. The multiplication of many garden plants is carried out today via tissue cultures, since this procedure often takes place much faster than conventional multiplication. From one **lily bulb** 100 000 plants were obtained in six months. Several review articles deal with the possibilities of this expanding field, which is of great economic interest (Holdgate, 1977; Bonga, 1977; Murashige, 1978).

Production of Pathogen-free Plants

Many crop plants are likely to be attacked by fungi, bacteria and viruses, which often leads to lower yields. However, phytopathogenic germs penetrate into meristematic tissue relatively late. If cells are taken from the tip of a meristem culture of an infected plant before the germs have penetrated into the tip these cells can successfully be regenerated to intact pathogen-free plants. This economically important aspect of applied cell culture research has recently been discussed in detail by Walkey (1978).

Clonal mass multiplication and the production of pathogen-free plants are, therefore, two areas in which cell culture research has already led to practical application.

However, it must be emphasized that we are **not** dealing with cell cultures in the sense of the definition. Here, organized tissue is taken from a plant and is maintained in such a way that it does not dedifferentiate but multiplies with maintenance of its status and regenerates the intact plant. Clonal mass multiplication can also be envisaged as starting from a callus. Depending on the conditions of maintenance and the age of the culture, the uniformity of the plant material would then certainly no longer be guaranteed to the same extent.

Cell Culture Technique for Plant Breeding

Plant breeders have greatly improved the properties of crop plants by the development of new varieties in the past. Breeding programs are, however, time-consuming processes. The question arises of whether it is possible to find lines with improved properties faster and more purposefully by means of the cell culture technique. Here are some examples:

a) Obtaining Improved Plants by Chemical Selection

There are plant-specific pathogenic organisms which, when they attack a field, cause great loss of yield. The toxic action of the organisms is frequently produced by phytotoxins. Plants with natural resistance to given pathogenic organisms are generally resistant to the corresponding phytotoxin. Screening for phytotoxin resistance cannot be performed in a field trial but from callus and suspension cultures it is relatively easy to select phytotoxin-resistant cells from which in some cases intact resistant plants have been regenerated (Gengenbach et al., 1977; Heinz et al., 1977; Behnke, 1979). Field trials must show whether these lines are suitable for agriculture.

Selection trials are being carried out in cell cultures also for other resistances. Thus, lines resistant to analogues of amino acids and nucleic acids, to antibiotics, to herbicides, to sodium chloride, and to cold have been described (Widholm, 1977; Maliga, 1978; Gressel, 1979). In some cases the resistances were found in the regenerated plants but sometimes they had been lost again or were not inheritable. The chance of obtaining a desired "resistant" cell line is, on the whole, regarded as good. Chemical selection need not necessarily start from individual cells, since sensitive cells are slowly eliminated. The chance of regenerating a resistant line can hardly be estimated beforehand, since the expression and stability of the new trait in the regenerated plant are not guaranteed, and other valuable characteristics of the mother plant may have lost. Despite such obstacles, selection seems to be an interesting and promising field of cell culture technique (Chaleff, 1983).

b) Obtaining New Plants from Individual Cells

If it is desired to contribute to an increased genetic variability in a plant variety by mutation, by somatic hybridization, or by genetic transformation, selection must begin at the stage of the individual cell (or even protoplasts). Only in relatively few cases has it been possible to achieve regeneration from a single cell to the intact plant (Thomas and Wernicke, 1978). Investigations on Solanaceae (Petunia, Datura, Nicotiana, Solanum) show that individual cells can be regenerated to intact plants under certain conditions (Binding, 1974; Schieder, 1975; Vasil and Vasil, 1974). The culture of anthers for the production of haploids is also possible with greater success in Solanaceae than with other families. Thus, for this family a combination of somatic and conventional genetics for plant breeding is already available (Melchers, 1977). Wenzel et al. (1979) have suggested a breeding program for Solanum which, together with conventional steps, includes the culture of microspores and the fusion of protoplasts.

The production of **interspecific hybrids** by the fusion of the protoplasts of two species may be of great importance – for the pharmaceutical industry, *inter alia* – if their corresponding sexual hybrids do not form. Thus, various somatically induced Datura hybrids contained 20 to 25% more hyoscyamine and scopolamine than the sexually incompatible parents (Schieder, 1979). Somatic hybrid plants have been obtained not only by fusion of protoplasts within one species but also by fusions within a genus or family (Melchers et al., 1978; Krumbiegel and Schieder, 1979; Gleba and Hoffmann, 1979). In many other fusion products, the capacity for division was lost very early. Chromosome elimination or the loss of its capacity for regeneration has also been observed (Constabel, 1978).

A wider application of the production of plants via individual cell cultures appears possible at the present time only for Solanaceae (Keller and Stringham, 1978; Hoffmann, 1980). However, the advances of the last few years justify favorable predictions for other plant families as well (Binding et al., 1982).

c) Obtaining New Plants by Genetic Engineering

There have been numerous attempts to modify plant cells by the exogenous application of genetic material. The feeding of isolated DNA to plant cells is regarded as unpromising at the present time. The application of organelles of another species to a cell culture has likewise not led to convincing results. Great hopes are now placed on the transfer of genetic material through vectors such as plasmids. Certain plant tumors are produced by *Agrobacterium tumefaciens*. The tumor-inducing principle (TIP) located on a plasmid is integrated into the plant genome (Drummond et al., 1977; Lippincott, 1977). Since the first detection of this stable incorporation of a piece of bacterial plasmid

DNA into the nuclear genome of a plant cell this area has advanced spectacularly. To give an adequate idea of such a rapidly advancing area a review of its own would be necessary. Therefore only headlines can be given. It is believed that every dicotyledon can now genetically be transformed with *Agrobacterium tumefaciens*. It has been shown that newly acquired genetic information is not only stably maintained in regenerating plants but can also be inherited sexually (Otten et al., 1981). The small fragment (T-DNA) of the Ti-plasmid transferred to and incorporated in the plant genome has been well characterized, although not all of its functions are known (Bevan and Chilton, 1982; Joos et al., 1983). The T-DNA has now been modified in such way that the transformation of plant cells can be achieved even when the DNA-sequences coding for the tumor characteristics are no longer present in the fragment (Leemans et al., 1981; Matzke and Chilton, 1981). Only the borders of the T-DNA seem to be necessary to achieve incorporation into the plant genome (Zambryski et al., 1982). Modified Ti-plasmids have now successfully been used as host vectors to introduce desired new traits into a plant cell. Thus, the bacterial gene coding for kanamycin resistance has been transferred by this technique to Petunia cells and was expressed by these plant cells (Fraley et al., 1983). The gene for the storage protein phaseolin was transferred via a T-DNA vector from beans to tobacco plantlets and was expressed (Murai et al., 1983). Further improved vectors and the development of efficient promoters for better expression make this area the most promising one in modern plant biotechnology.

The practical implications for plant breeding of the successful selection for resistance of new somatic hybrids, as well as of genetically transformed cells, will depend upon the feasibility of regenerating plants. The moment when cell cultures will make a broad contribution to plant improvement is therefore difficult to estimate, since, in spite of all advances, the basic processes of morphogenesis still have not been elucidated (Thomas and Wernicke, 1978).

5.2.5 Use of Plant Cell Cultures in Industry

Even today, higher plants are suppliers of indispensible raw materials and drugs. Since it has been possible to maintain plant cells in a similar manner to microorganisms, discussion as to how far plant cell cultures can replace the intact plant as producers of natural material has not ceased. Before we venture on a scientific stocktaking of the present situation, we first should touch on the economic question. Optimistic estimates (Zenk, 1978) start from manufacturing costs of $ 500 per kg of natural material if in a 100-m^3 fermenter 1 g of substance is formed per liter of culture medium in 15 days. Other calculations – starting from previous accumulation yields of cell cultures – make the pure production costs jump to $ 5000 to 7000 per kg of natural material isolated (Hepner and Male, 1978). These widely differing cost calculations result from different evaluations of the chances of establishing good producing lines. The immense fermentation costs mean that it will probably hardly ever be possible to obtain a large number of important natural materials via cell cultures at a favorable cost. Only natural materials with a high market price can therefore be considered for production through cell cultures.

In the discussions on the feasibility of producing known natural materials via cell cultures, today many people push the cost comparison with field cultivation too much into the foreground. The present state of our knowledge of how to accumulate desired secondary products in a culture is so inadequate that the cost discussion is not yet meaningful. On the contrary, a cost analysis carried out.at the wrong time may be very detrimental to the field of operations. The fact that it is often impossible to induce the main product of the intact plant in a cell culture shows to what a small extent it has so far been possible to manipulate plant cells. Since we have hitherto succeeded in modifying the biosynthetic output of plant cells to only a very limited extent and since we can express only a small part of the information for the formation of secondary products under the usual culture conditions, new ways must be found in this area. Discussions concerning the economic potential of cell cultures will be profitable only when we can purposefully call up more information from the genetic potential – more than is possible today.

Then calculations will no longer lead to such different results. These remarks on the discussion of cost imply that basic investigations on the production of secondary materials in cell cultures are necessary and research in this area should not be limited only to expensive natural products.

Total Synthesis of Natural Products by Cell Cultures

A broad spectrum of natural products has already been detected in cell cultures (Nickell, 1980; Misawa and Suzuki, 1982; Barz and Ellis, 1981). The facts summarized in the cited papers show that in principle the synthesis of any natural product may be expected, since there are positive findings from almost every group of natural compounds (alkaloids, flavonoids, terpenoids). However, a review of the literature shows that most natural products accumulate in vanishingly small amounts. Nevertheless, a series of investigations, particularly in Japan, has given rise to patent applications and patents (Misawa, 1977) which, however, have not led to any industrial application (Misawa and Samejima, 1978) with perhaps one exception (Fujita et al., 1982). These authors claim that the production process of shikonins (naphthoquinones) by cell cultures of *Lithospermum erythrorhizon* can compete successfully with the conventional production process of extracting root material. In spite of many disappointing results concerning the accumulation of secondary products in cell cultures, one can state that plant cell cultures are capable in principle of forming considerable amounts of natural products. Cultures of *Coleus blumei* accumulate 15% of their dry weight as rosmarinic acid (Razzaque and Ellis, 1977). The anthraquinones in *Morinda citrifolia* make up 18% of the dry weight (Zenk et al., 1975). Cinnamoyl putrescines likewise reaches levels of about 10% in tobacco cultures (Berlin et al., 1982). In fermentations, between 2 and 4 g of these compounds per liter of culture medium have been obtained. Nearly all compounds found in high levels in plant cell cultures are rather unimportant from the economic aspect but they prove that quite high amounts of secondary products can accumulate in cell cultures. Considering such high levels of synthesis and accumulation, it may be assumed that in many other cases the correct conditions for high accumulation have not (yet) been found. The main problem, however, seems to be that often a morphological differentiation is required for expression of certain secondary metabolites. Today it is not possible deliberately to separate morphological from chemical differentiation. Differentiated cells grow rather slowly and therefore are hardly acceptable for fermentation processes.

Below, using as examples three important groups of plant drugs, we shall show the present state of research in this field and what possibilities exist for developing highly productive cell cultures.

a) Synthesis of **Cardiac Glycosides** in Cell Cultures

Cardiac glycosides are among the most important drugs that can be obtained only from plants. Cardiac glycosides have been isolated from numerous plants (Digitalis, Convallaria, Adonis, Cheiranthus, Thevetia, Strophanthus, Scilla, etc.). Digoxin, which is used in the treatment of cardiac insufficiency, is obtained from the Grecian foxglove *Digitalis lanata,* a plant which is grown mainly in the Balkans. The importance of digoxin justifies an attempt to obtain this substance from cell cultures. Cultures of Digitalis and other cardenolide-containing plants have therefore been thoroughly studied with respect to their productivity. Most of the cultures investigated contained no cardenolides, while in others, traces were detected which then substantially disappeared in the course of cultivation (dedifferentiation). Only differentiated tissue cultures contained measurable amounts of cardenolides (Garve et al., 1980; Lui and Staba, 1979; Hagimori et al., 1982). Attempts to establish highly productive suspension cultures by analytical screening with a sensitive radioimmunoassay have not so far been successful.

No doubt exists that Digitalis cultures are capable of forming cardenolides, at least initially. The justified hope therefore exists of maintaining the formation of cardenolides by means of a suitable program of media. The regeneration of callus tissue to intact plants leads to the original cardenolide pattern, which shows that the genetic potential for the synthesis is repressed in the cell culture. At the present time, leaf organ cultures accumulate the most digoxin with surprisingly good growth (Lui and Staba, 1979). As compared with intact plants, however, the content on a dry weight basis is 3 to 15 times smaller, depending on the age of the plant. Light appears to have a positive influence on the accumulation (Garve et al., 1980; Hagimori et al., 1982). Since illuminated cultures appear to be superior to dark cultures and in the intact plant the cardiac glycosides accumulate in the leaves, the question arises as to whether one should attempt a new selection from green, possibly even photoautotrophic, cultures (Hüsemann and Barz, 1977). The formation of chlorophyll in cell cultures implies not only a morphological but also a biochemical differentiation which could be important for such secondary products of a leaf. On the other hand chloroplasts are not essential for cardenolide formation (Hagimori et al., 1982).

b) Formation of *Morphinans* in *Papaver* Cultures.

The alkaloids **morphine** and **codeine** are still obtained at the present time from the latex juice of poppy capsules. **Thebaine** has gained in importance particularly because it can easily be converted by demethylation into codeine. Unlike morphine, thebaine is not habit-forming and cannot be converted directly into heroin (Nyman and Bruhn, 1979).

The thebaine content of *Papaver bracteatum* cultures was very low (20 to 60 µg/g dry weight in callus cultures) and decreased by a factor of at least 100 in the course of cultivation (Kamimura et al., 1976). Suspension cultures generally yielded still less thebaine. Somewhat higher levels were found under conditions promoting organogenesis (Kamimura et al., 1976; Staba et al., 1982). Many attempts have been made to establish cell cultures of *Papaver somniferum* producing morphinan alkaloids. However, no appreciable amounts of morphinan alkaloids have been reported. It is generally believed that callus cultures synthesize these alkaloids during the first passages; however, after repeated subculturing the biosynthetic route to morphinan alkaloids is switched off (Hodges and Rapoport, 1982a). Again, after morphogenesis this route is reexpressed (Schuchmann and Wellmann, 1982; Kamo et al., 1982). In *Papaver somniferum* and *Papaver bracteatum*, a correlation exists between the appearance of laticifer-like cells and morphinan

alkaloids in these cells (Kutchan et al., 1983). Papaver cell cultures seem to be a reasonable system for investigating why the accumulation of certain secondary metabolites requires specialized cells. This requires biochemical, molecular, and genetic studies. The first biochemical steps in this direction have been taken. The biosynthetic pathway to the isoquinoline alkaloids begins with the coupling of dopamine and 3,4-dihydroxyphenylacetaldehyde by S-norlaudanosoline synthase which has already been partially purified (Schumacher et al., 1983). Reticuline is regarded as the central intermediate and branching point. While $(-)$-(R)-reticuline is converted into protopine and other alkaloids, $(+)$-(S)-reticuline is converted by oxidative para-ortho coupling into salutaridine, which is then metabolized into thebaine, codeine and morphine. Salutaridine synthase, the key enzyme of morphine alkaloid biosynthesis has very recently been detected in *Papaver somniferum* (Hodges and Rapoport, 1982b). The main question is why this enzyme seems to be repressed under cell culture conditions (Furuya et al., 1978). Cultures of Papaveraceae and related families accumulate high levels of other reticuline-derived isoquinoline alkaloids e.g. sanguinarine, protopine, magniflorine, berberine, jatrorrhizine (Furuya, 1972; Fukui et al., 1982; Berlin et al., 1983). While the alkaloid patterns of cultures of the various Papaver genera often resembled one another, on redifferentiation the specific differences of the individual plants again came into effect. It must be assumed that the above-mentioned alkaloids are phylogenetically older and their formation is not associated with specialized cells (Böhm, 1978). According to this, the morphinans are compounds which require a quite specific cytodifferentiation. Papaver cell cultures will only be of biotechnological interest if we succeed in separating the cytodifferentiation that is evidently required from the chemical synthesis of the morphinan alkaloids. A success in this system would surely have great implications for the awaited breakthrough of the whole field.

c) *Indole Alkaloids in Catharanthus roseus*

The dimeric indole alkaloids vinblastine (vincaleucoblastine) and vincristine (leurocristine) from *Catharanthus roseus* are, at the present time, the most important plant antitumor agents with clinical application. In a crude extract, together with more than 70 other alkaloids, 0.0003 to 0.001% of vincristine is found. The importance of the two alkaloids and the small amounts in which they appear explain their high price and both would therefore be ideal candidates for production from cell cultures. These two compounds are also the reason why well-known cell culture laboratories in association with the industry have devoted themselves to *Catharanthus roseus*. Among the many other alkaloids in *Catharanthus roseus,* the alkaloids of the Corynanthe type, ajmalicine and serpentine, are of pharmaceutical importance because of their hypotensive action.

The first investigations on the formation of alkaloids in *Catharanthus roseus* indicated the presence of only small amounts of indole alkaloids (Carew, 1975). The work of Zenk and his colleagues (Zenk et al., 1977) completely changed the pattern that had previously existed. The group applied an improved strategy to the investigation which we must give here separately as an example. Their postulates ran as follows:

1. The search for a natural product can be successful only if a sensitive analytical test is available.

2. A medium must be found which permits the maximum production of desired metabolites.

3. From the heterogeneous cell population cells with high levels of the metabolite must be selected analytically.

4. Only particularly highly productive plants should be used as the starting material for callus induction.

Their investigations began with the development of radioimmunoassays for sensitive and rapid analysis. The productivities of a large numbers of cell colonies were checked in this way. In analogy to the formation of secondary products by microorganisms, different media conditions were used for growth and production. Using this strategy it was possible to select lines containing 1% of the dry weight as ajmalicine (0.8% as serpentine). Most of the selected lines, however, had to be kept under continuous selection pressure, since otherwise the production of alkaloids fell back to the level of unselected lines (Zenk, 1978). Other laboratories have now likewise succeeded in establishing cell cultures with high ajmalicine or serpentine contents (Roller, 1978). From our own experiences and those of a number of other cell culture laboratories it can be stated that Catharanthus cultures – even without any screening – almost always accumulate many monomeric indole alkaloids at low levels (Kutney et al., 1983; Kohl et al., 1982). By directed selection from this level there are no longer great difficulties today in finding relatively highly productive, but rather unstable, strains. Therefore, the best lines yielded only between 40 to 50 mg serpentine per liter of culture medium when grown in air-lift fermenters (Zenk et al., 1977; Smart et al., 1982).

In future, analytical selection must be supported by other methods. Experiments to increase the accumulation of secondary products by selecting stable biochemical variants have been initiated. The knowledge that a high activity of tryptophan decarboxylase (TDC) is one requirement for a good producing cell line has allowed us to select cell lines with increased TDC activity. This was possible by selecting for resistance to tryptophan analogues which are detoxified by TDC. Some of the resistant cell lines had not only increased TDC activity but also increased alkaloid levels (Sasse et al., 1983). In addition to selection, increased attention should be devoted to the composition of the media. By the use of media with low phosphate and nitrogen levels it has been possible to raise the level of alkaloids in cell cultures of *Catharanthus roseus* considerably (Knobloch and Berlin, 1980).

The investigations on *Catharanthus roseus* cultures were begun mainly because of the dimers, since they are the more important components of the Catharanthus plant from the medical and economic point of view. The presence of dimeric indole alkaloids in these cultures has not convincingly been proven up to now. Whether producing strains will be found by intensified screening is more than questionable. A specific radioimmunoassay is available for such investigations (Langone et al., 1979). However, the modified Polonovski reaction (Potier, 1980) has perhaps made the search for dimers no longer necessary today. It would be sufficient if monomers such as catharanthine and vindoline were present in good yield in the cultures. Today the presence of vindoline has not convincingly been demonstrated while catharanthine is present in many cell lines, at, however, rather low levels (Kutney et al., 1983). The next few years will show whether, by selection and optimization of the media, the yields of minor alkaloids of the cell cultures can be improved to the same extent as has been possible for the main alkaloids of the Corynanthe type. So far about 30 different indole alkaloids of the Corynanthe, Strychnos, Aspidosperma, and Iboga types have been isolated from cell cultures (Stöckigt and Soll, 1980; Kohl et al., 1982; Kutney et al., 1983).

Cell cultures of the three important groups of drug plants have so far accumulated the desired natural products either not at all, in very small amounts, or in amounts still inadequate economically. This result shows how little we know about the regulation of the synthesis of secondary products in cell culture. However, we should not discredit the **cell culture system** but seek for new methods of manipulating the secondary metabolism of the cell into a wanted direction. Since the results of the past were not sufficient to achieve the desired breakthrough, our institute is now trying to manipulate the cells by the techniques of genetic engineering. Our first steps in this area have been outlined recently (Berlin, 1984).

The account given so far relates to natural products the pharmacological and economic value of which is known. In cell cultures, many biosynthetic pathways take place in a manner not necessarily the same as in the intact plant (Butcher and Connolly, 1971). In this way, **new substances** with interesting pharmacological properties may possibly accumulate. An analysis of cell culture extracts should therefore not be limited to known substances. Every cell culture group having the opportunities for detailed chemical analysis of cell cultures will find a product spectrum which differs from that of the intact plant, and sometimes new compounds will be detected (Witte et al., 1983). When chemical analysis has been combined with biological tests, promising results have been reported (Misawa and Samejima, 1978; Arens et al., 1982). However the claim that plant cell cultures will become an important source of new pharmacological active compounds has not been proven and too high expectations are not justified by the published results.

Biotransformation by Cell Cultures

Plant cell cultures can metabolize a broad spectrum of exogenously applied compounds. The following reactions are the main ones that have been found: reduction, oxidation, hydroxylation, epoxydation, glycosidation, esterification, methylation, demethylation, and isomerization. The field has been discussed thoroughly in review articles (Furuya, 1978; Reinhard and Alfermann, 1980; Stohs, 1980). Biotransformation with plant cells must always be seen in competition with biotransformation by microorganisms. Consequently, from the economic aspect, reactions are interesting that are not performed by microorganisms. A reaction brought about by microorganisms extremely rarely is **glycosidation.** In contrast, plant cells glycosidate many exogenously applied compounds. The resulting water-soluble derivative can then be stored in the vacuoles. To what extent this reaction will lead to economically interesting compounds cannot be answered yet.

Biotransformation with intermediate stages of a biosynthetic pathway can be regarded as desirable from various points of view. As we will show later, intermediate products are frequently transformed into the end-product even when the culture is incapable of forming the end-product. In other cases, however, intermediates are not metabolized (Furuya et al., 1978) or are converted into metabolites that do not occur in nature (Romeike, 1975). The transformation of analogs of intermediates of biosynthetic pathways has not yet been studied thoroughly. New end-products could be expected. Certain reactions of biosynthetic pathways can also take place in cultures that cannot form such products biosynthetically. Thus, codeinone is converted into codeine by many cell cultures that are unable to synthesize morphinan alkaloids (Furuya et al., 1978). Harman alkaloids have been found in Phaseolus cultures after the additon of tryptamine (Veliky and Barber, 1975).

The biotechnologically most promising biotransformation is the 12-β-hydroxylation of methyldigitoxin. As already mentioned, **digoxin** is the most important naturally occurring cardiac glycoside. During extraction of digoxin from *Digitalis lanata* leaves considerable amounts of **digitoxin** also arise in the working up of drug material. Digitoxin, however, possesses an unfavorable therapeutic index. Early

attempts failed to convert the glycoside digitoxin into digoxin (12β-hydroxylation) with the aid of microorganisms, since the microorganisms hydroxylated only the aglycone. This failure with microorganisms and the lack of synthetic alternatives made experiments with plant cell cultures of interest. Exogenously added cardenolides are modified by many cell cultures (Reinhard and Alfermann, 1980). Here we shall consider in more detail only the pharmaceutically most important reaction, the 12β-hydroxylation of digitoxin to digoxin. Professor Reinhard's group (University of Tübingen) noticed during their first experiments with cell cultures of *Digitalis lanata* only a rather low activity for the 12β-hydroxylation reaction. To screen for strains with a better capacity they used β-methyldigitoxin as substrate, since digitoxin itself was not only hydroxylated but also subjected to other reactions. A piece of good luck was that methyldigitoxin was almost always metabolized to methyldigoxin which has long been marketed as a drug. Three groups of cell cultures were found: a) those which demethylated and glycosidated; b) those which hydroxylated at C-12 with simultaneous demethylation, acetylation, and glycosidation, and c) those which only hydroxylated at C-12 (*Digitalis lanata* and *Digitalis leucophaca*). By screening it has been possible to obtain strains performing the desired transformation to such an extent that an industrial application appears possible. A yield of 4 g of β-methyldigoxin can be obtained after 12 days in a 20-L airlift fermenter. Interestingly, the product accumulates in the medium, and not in the cells. The original culture gave a rate of conversion that was only 1/1000 of that of the current strains. The technical optimization of the process is under way. The example of the 12β-hydroxylation of digitoxin shows that certain enzymes of a biosynthetic pathway may be present in cell cultures even when the end-product itself is not formed. Very interesting from an economic point of view are reports that dimeric indole alkaloids can be transformed by plant cell cultures. Cell cultures of nonproducing *Catharanthus roseus* have been able to transform anhydrovinblastine into vinblastine (McLauchlan et al., 1983) and leurosine and catharine (Kutney et al., 1983). Further progress in the field of biotransformation does not depend only on the optimization of these processes but also on finding some other economically important reactions catalyzed by plant cell cultures.

Technological Aspects

We have been able to show that in some cultures secondary products accumulate in relatively large amounts. Even though these include practically no substances for which an industrial process is immediately in prospect, the question must nevertheless be put as to whether cell cultures can also be fermented on the large scale. The number of publications on the **fermentation of plant cells** in vessels larger than 10 L so far is very small. Plant cells differ substantially from microorganisms in two points. Plant cells are much larger than microorganisms and divide rather slowly (16 to 72 h). This latter necessarily leads to longer fermentation times. Due to their sizes and their large vacuoles plant cells are rather sensitive to shear stress. Consequently, sterility must be maintained over long fermentation periods and agitation of the cells must be done rather carefully. A scaling up from 10 to 1000 L may take 6 to 8 weeks depending on the culture. Despite these problems there is no question that the technical problems can be solved. For example, tobacco cells have been cultivated in 20,000-liter fermenters with 15 g dry weight/liter of culture medium (Hashi-

moto et al., 1982). Catharanthus and Lithospermum cells have been scaled up to 750 L in mechanically agitated fermenters (Fujita et al., 1982; Berlin et al., unpublished). Digitalis cells maintained their hydroxylating capacity in 200-liter airlift fermenters. It must therefore be assumed that the technological problems raised by plant cell cultures can be overcome more easily than the biological and biochemical difficulties that have been outlined. On the basis of our own experience over the last three years we recommend fermenters equipped with slowly moving impellers supported by adequate aeration from the bottom as suitable for many culture systems.

Growth and **production** are frequently in opposition. Then two-stage processes with a growth fermenter followed by a production fermenter are recommended (Fujita et al., 1982). In some cases, however, fed-batch fermentation may minimize this problem (Schiel et al., 1984). These authors showed that the negative effect of surplus phosphate (in the growth medium) on the production of cinnamoyl putrescines can be prevented without growth reduction by keeping the cells under phosphate limitation.

Like other biological organisms, plant cells can be entrapped in various materials (Prenosil and Pedersen, 1983; Lindsey et al., 1983). However, one problem characteristic of plant cells is that the products are mostly stored in the vacuoles. Immobilization of plant cells will therefore be helpful only if the products are released into the medium or viable "secreting" cells can be found. Immobilized cells of *Digitalis lanata* and Mucuna cells efficiently hydroxylate β-methyldigitoxin and L-tyrosine, respectively. The biotransformation products β-methyldigoxin and L-dopa are found in the culture medium (Alfermann et al., 1980; Wichers et al., 1983). Sometimes permeabilized cells have also been used successfully as "enzyme reactors" although they were no longer viable (Felix, 1982).

5.2.6 Summary

This brief review of the biotechnological aspects has clearly shown that a broad use of cell culture technique in the plant breeding sector is yet to come, just as in the field of the production of natural compounds. It is difficult to predict when a broad use of these techniques will be possible, since we do not adequately know the basic processes of differentiation and are incapable of controlling them. However, there are already encouraging examples in the field of plant breeding, in the field of biotransformation, and in total synthesis, so that even from the biotechnological standpoint it appears justified to continue in the elucidation of the mechanisms of differentiation and regulation by intensified basic research. To achieve the biotechnological goals envisaged, intensified basic research in all areas of plant cell metabolism is urgently needed.

5.2.7 Literature: Plant Cell Cultures

A Review Literature

[1] Alfermann, A. W. and Reinhard, E.: *"Production of Natural Compounds by Cell Culture Methods"*. Ges. f. Strahlen- und Umweltforschung, München 1978.
[2] Barz, W., Reinhard, E. and Zenk, M. H.: *Plant Tissue Culture and its Biotechnological Application*. Springer-Verlag, Berlin, Heidelberg, New York 1977.
[3] Fujiwara, A.: "Plant Tissue Culture 1982", *Proc. 5th Int. Congr. Plant Tissue Cell Culture,* Maruzen Press, Tokyo 1982.
[4] Reinert, J. and Bajaj, Y. P. S.: *Applied and Fundamental Aspects of Plant Cell, Tissue, and Organ Culture*. Springer-Verlag, Berlin, Heidelberg, New York 1977.
[5] Street, H. E.: "Plant tissue and cell culture". In: *Botanical Monographs* Vol. 11, 2nd Ed. Blackwell Scientific Publications, 1977.

[6] Thorpe, T. A.: *Frontiers of Plant Tissue Culture 1978*. University of Calgary, Alberta, Canada 1978.

B Special Literature
(The figures in square brackets relate to the review literature.)

Aitchison, P. A., Maclead, A. J. and Yeoman, M. M.: "Growth patterns in tissue (callus) cultures". In: [5], 267–308 (1977).
Alfermann, A. W., Schuller, I. and Reinhard, E., "Biotransformation of cardiac glycosides by immobilized cells of *Digitalis lanata*", *Planta Med.* **40**, 218–223 (1980).
Arens, H., Borbe, H. O., Ulbrich, B. and Stöckigt, J., "Detection of pericine, a new CNS-active indole alkaloid, from Picralima nitida cell suspension culture by opiate receptor binding studies", *Planta Med.* **46**, 210–214 (1982).
Barz, W. and Ellis, B. E., "Plant cell cultures and their biotechnological potential", *Ber. Dtsch. Bot. Ges.* **94**, 1–26 (1981).
Behnke, M., "Selection of potato callus for resistance to culture filtrates of *Phytophthora infestans* and regeneration of resistant plants", *Theor. Appl. Genet.* **55**, 69–71 (1979).
Berlin, J., "Plant cell cultures – a future source of natural products?", *Endeavour,* New Series, **8**, 5–8 (1984).
Berlin, J., Forche, E., Wray, V., Hammer, J. and Hösel, W., "Formation of benzophenanthridine alkaloids by suspension cultures of *Eschscholtzia california*", *Z. Naturforsch.* **38c**, 346–352 (1983).
Berlin, J., Knobloch, K.-H., Höfle, G. and Witte, L., "Biochemical characterization of two tobacco cell lines with different levels of cinnamoyl putrescines", *J. Nat. Prod.* **45**, 83–87 (1982).
Bevan, M. W. and Chilton, M.-D, "T-DNA of the Agrobacterium Ti and Ri plasmids", *Ann. Rev. Genet.* **16**, 357–384 (1982).
Binding, H., "Regeneration von haploiden und dihaploiden Pflanzen aus Protoplasten von *Petunia hybrida*", *Z. Pflanzenphysiol.* **74**, 327–356 (1974).
Binding, H., Nehls, R. and Jörgensen, J.: "Protoplast regeneration in higher plants". In: [3], 575–578 (1982).

Böhm, H.: "Regulation of alkaloid production in plant cell cultures". In: [5], 201–211 (1978).

Bonga, J. M.: "Applications of tissue culture in forestry". In: [4], 93–108 (1977).

Butcher, D. N. and Connolly, J. D., "An investigation of factors which influence the production of abnormal terpenoids by callus of *Andrographis paniculata*", *J. Exp. Bot.* **22**, 314–322 (1971).

Carew, D. P.: "Tissue culture studies of *Catharanthus roseus*". In: Taylor, W. I. and Farnsworth, N. R. (eds.): *The Catharanthus Alkaloids*. Marcel Dekker, New York 1979, pp. 193–208.

Chaleff, R. S., "Isolation of agronomically useful mutants from plant cell cultures", *Science* **219**, 676–682 (1983).

Constabel, F.: "Development of protoplast fusion product heterokaryocytes and hybrid cells". In: [6], 141–149 (1978).

Dougall, D. K., "Production of biologicals by plant cell cultures", *Adv. Exp. Med. Biol.* **118**, 135–152 (1979).

Drummond, M. H., Gordon, M. P., Nester, E. W. and Chilton, M.-D., "Foreign DNA of bacterial plasmid origin is transcribed in crown gall tumours", *Nature* **269**, 535–536 (1977).

Felix, H., "Permeabilized cells", *Anal. Biochem.* **120**, 211–234 (1982).

Fraley, R. T. and 13 co-authors, "Expression of bacterial genes in plant cells", *Proc. Natl. Acad. Sci. USA* **80**, 4803–4807 (1983).

Fujita, Y., Tabata, M., Nishi, A. and Yamada, Y.: "New medium and production of secondary compounds with the two-staged culture method". In: [3], 399–400 (1982).

Fukui, H., Nagakawa, K., Tsuda, S. and Tabata, M.: "Production of isoquinoline alkaloids by cell suspension cultures of *Coptis japonica*". In: [3], 313–314 (1982).

Furuya, T.: "Biotransformation by plant cell cultures". In: [6], 191–200 (1978).

Furuya, T., Ikuta, A. and Syono, K., "Alkaloids from callus tissue of *Papaver somniferum*", *Phytochemistry* **11**, 3041–3044 (1972).

Furuya, T., Nakano, M. and Yoshikawa, T., "Biotransformation of (RS)-reticuline and morphinan alkaloids by cell cultures of *Papaver somniferum*", *Phytochemistry* **17**, 891–893 (1978).

Gamborg, O. L., Murashige, T., Thorpe, T. A. and Vasil, I. K., "Plant tissue culture media", *In Vitro* **12**, 473–478 (1976).

Garve, R., Luckner, M., Vogel, E., Tewes, A. and Nover, L., "Growth, morphogenesis and cardenolide formation in long-term cultures of *Digitalis lanata*", *Planta Med.* **40**, 92–103 (1980).

Gengenbach, B. G., Green, C. E. and Donovan, C. M., "Inheritance of selected pathotoxin resistance in maize plants regenerated from cell cultures", *Proc. Natl. Acad. Sci. USA* **74**, 5113–5117 (1977).

Gleba, Y. Y. and Hoffmann, F., "Arabidobrassica, plant genome engineering by protoplast fusion", *Naturwissenschaften* **66**, 547–554 (1979).

Green, C. E.: "In vitro plant regeneration in cereals and grasses". In: [6], 411–418 (1978).

Gressel, J., "A review of the place of in vitro cell culture systems in studies of action, metabolism and resistance of biocides affecting photosynthesis", *Z. Naturforsch.* **34c**, 905–913 (1979).

Hagimori, M., Matsumoto, T. and Obi, Y., "Studies on the production of Digitalis cardenolides by plant tissue culture", *Plant Physiol.* **69**, 653–656 (1982).

Hashimoto, T., Azechi, S., Sugita, S., and Suzuki, K.: "Large scale production of tobacco cells by continuous cultivation". In: [3], 403–404 (1982).

Heinz, D. J., Krishnamurthi, M., Nickell, L. G. and Maretzki, A.: "Cell, tissue and organ culture in sugarcane improvement". In: [4], 3–17 (1977).

Hepner, L. and Male, C.: "Tissue culture – technological applications and significance for the future". In: *Important for the Future*. Unitar 1978, pp. 1–22.

Hodges, C. C. and Rapoport, H., "Morphinan alkaloids in callus cultures of *Papaver somniferum*", *J. Nat. Prod.* **45**, 481–485 (1982).

Hodges, C. C. and Rapoport, H., "Enzymic conversion of reticuline to salutaridine by cell-free systems of *Papaver somniferum*", *Biochemistry* **21**, 3729–3734 (1982).

Hoffmann, F., "Pflanzliche Zellkulturtechniken als Züchtungsschritt am Beispiel Raps", *Naturwissenschaften* **60**, 301–306 (1980).

Holdgate, D. P.: "Propagation of ornamentals by tissue culture". In: [4], 18–43 (1977).

Hüsemann, W. and Barz, W., "Photoautotrophic growth and photosynthesis in cell suspension cultures of *Chenopodium rubrum*", *Physiol. Plant* **40**, 77–81 (1977).

Joos, H., Inzé, D., Caplan, A., Sormann, M., Van Montagu, M. and Schell, J., "Genetic analysis of T-DNA transcripts in nopaline crown galls", *Cell* **32**, 1057–1067 (1983).

Kamimura, S., Akutsu, M. and Nishikawa, M., "Formation of thebaine in the suspension culture of *Papaver bracteatum*", *Agric. Biol. Chem.* **40**, 913–919 (1976).

Kamo, K. K., Kimoto, W., Hsu, A. F., Mahlberg, P. G. and Bills, D. D., "Morphinan alkaloids in cultured tissues and redifferentiated organs of *Papaver somniferum*", *Phytochemistry* **21**, 219–222 (1982).

Keller, W. A. and Stringham, G. R.: "Production and utilization of microscope-derived haploid plants". In: [6], 113–122 (1978).

King, P. J. and Street, H. E.: "Growth patterns in cell cultures". In: [5], 308–387 (1977).

Knobloch, K.-H. and Berlin, J., "Influence of medium composition on the formation of secondary compounds in cell suspension cultures of *Catharanthus roseus*", *Z. Naturforsch.* **35c**, 551–556 (1980).

Kohl, W., Witte, B. and Höfle, G., "Alkaloids from *Catharanthus roseus* tissue cultures, III", *Z. Naturforsch.* **37b**, 1346–1351 (1982).

Krumbiegel, G. and Schieder, O., "Selection of somatic hybrids after fusion of protoplasts from *Datura innoxia* and *Atropa belladonna*", *Planta* **145**, 371–375 (1979).

Kurz, W. G. W. and Constabel, F., "Plant cell cultures and their biosynthetic potential", *Microb. Technol.* **21**, 389–416 (1979).

Kutchan, T. M., Ayabe, S., Krueger, R, J., Coscia, E. M. and Coscia, C. J., "Cytodifferentiation and alkaloid accumulation in cultured cells of *Papaver bracteatum*", *Plant Cell Rep.* **2**, 281–284 (1983).

Kutney, J. P. and 12 co-authors, "Studies in plant tissue culture. The synthesis and biosynthesis of indole alkaloids", *Tetrahedron* **39**, 3781–3795 (1983).

Langone, J. J., D'Onofrio, M. R. and Van Vunakis, H., "Radioimmunoassay for the Vinca alkaloids vinblastine and vincristine", *Anal. Biochem.* **95**, 214–221 (1979).

Larkin, P. J. and Scowcroft, W. R., "Somaclonal variation – a novel source of variability from cell cultures for plant improvement", *Theor. Appl. Genet.* **60**, 197–214 (1981).

Leemans, J., Shaw, Ch., Deblaere, R., De Greve, H., Hernalsteens, J. P., Maes, M., Van Montagu, M. and Schell, J., "Site-specific mutagenesis of Agrobacterium Ti plasmids and transfer of genes to plant cells", *J. Mol. Appl. Genet.* **1**, 149–164 (1981).

Lindsey, K., Yeoman, M. M., Black, G. M. and Mavituna, F., "A novel method for the immobilisation and culture of plant cells", *FEBS Lett.* **155**, 143–149 (1983).

Lippincott, J. A., "Molecular basis of plant tumour induction", *Nature* **269**, 465–466 (1977).

Lui, J. H. C. and Staba, E. J., "Effects of precursors on serially propagated *Digitalis lanata* leaf and root cultures", *Phytochemistry* **18**, 1913–1916 (1979). .

Maliga, P.: "Resistance mutants and their use in genetic manipulations". In: [6], 381–392 (1978).

Matzke, A. J. M. and Chilton, M.-D., "Site-specific insertion of genes into T-DNA of the Agrobacterium tumor-inducing plasmid: An approach to genetic engineering of higher plant cells", *J. Mol. Appl. Genet.* **1**, 39–49 (1981).

McLauchlan, W. R., Hasan, M., Baxter, R. L. and Scott, I. A., "Conversion of anhydrovinblastine to vinblastine by cell-free homogenates of *Catharanthus roseus* cell suspension cultures", *Tetrahedron* **39**, 3777–3780 (1983).

Melchers, G., "Kombination somatischer und konventioneller Genetik für die Pflanzenzüchtung", *Naturwissenschaften* **64**, 184–194 (1977).

Melchers, G., Sacristan, M. D. and Holder, A. A., "Somatic hybrid plants of potato and tomato regenerated from fused protoplasts", *Carlsberg Res. Commun.* **43**, 203–218 (1978).

Misawa, M.: "Production of natural substances by plant cell cultures described in Japanese patents". In: [2], 17–26 (1977).

Misawa, M. and Samejima, H.: "Production of biologically active substances by plant tissue cultures". In: [6], 353–362 (1978).

Misawa, M. and Suzuki, T., "Recent progress in plant cell culture – research on the production of useful plant metabolites in Japan", *Appl. Biochem. Biotechnol.* **7**, 205–216 (1982).

Murai, N. and 10 co-authors, "Phaseolin gene from bean is expressed after transfer to sunflower via tumor-inducing plasmid vectors", *Science* **222**, 479–482 (1983).

Murashige, T.: "The impact of plant tissue culture on agriculture". In: [6], 18–26 (1978).

Nickell, L. G.: "Products". In: Staba, E. J. (ed.): *Plant Tissue Culture as a Source of Biochemicals.* CRC-Press, Boca Raton, Florida 1980, pp. 235–270.

Nyman, W. and Bruhn, J. G., "*Papaver bracteatum* – a summary of current knowledge", *Planta Med.* **35**, 97–117 (1979).

Otten, L., De Greve, H., Hernalsteens, J. P., Van Montagu, H., Schieder, O., Straub, J. and Schell, J., "Mendelian transmission of genes introduced into plants by the Ti plasmids of *Agrobacterium tumefaciens*", *Mol. Gen. Genet.* **183**, 209–213 (1981).

Potier, P., "Synthesis of the dimeric indole alkaloids from Catharanthus species (vinblastine group)", *J. Nat. Prod.* **43**, 72–86 (1980).

Prenosil, J. E. and Pedersen, H., "Immobilized plant cell reactors", *Enzyme Microb. Technol.* **5**, 323–331 (1983).

Rao, A. N.: "Tissue culture in the orchid industry". In: [3], 44–69 (1977).

Razzaque, A. and Ellis, B. E., "Rosmarinic acid production in Coleus cell cultures", *Planta* **137**, 287–291 (1977).

Reinhard, E. and Alfermann, A. W.: "Biotransformation by plant cell cultures". In: Fiechter, A. (ed.): *Advances in Biochemical Engineering* **16**, *Plant Cell Cultures* I. Springer-Verlag, Berlin, Heidelberg, New York 1980, pp. 49–84.

Roller, U.: "Selection of plants and plant tissue cultures of *Catharanthus roseus* with high content of serpentine and ajmalicine". In: [1], 95–104 (1978).

Romeike, A., "Investigations on esterification of tropine and tropic acid in tissue cultures of plants", *Biochem. Physiol. Pflanz.* **168**, 87–92 (1975).

Sasse, F., Buchholz, M. and Berlin, J., "Selection of cell lines with increased tryptophan decarboxylase activity", *Z. Naturforsch.* **38c**, 916–922 (1983).

Schieder, O., "Regeneration von haploiden und diploiden *Datura innoxia* Mesophyll Protoplasten zu Pflanzen", *Z. Pflanzenphysiol.* **76**, 462–466 (1975).

Schieder, O., "Höhere Erträge bei Arzneipflanzen durch künstliche Zellfusion", *Umsch. Wiss. Tech.* **79**, 545–546 (1979).

Schiel, O., Jarchow-Redecker, K., Piehl, G.-W., Lehmann, J. and Berlin, J., "Increased formation of cinnamoyl putrescines by fedbatch-fermentation of cell suspension cultures of *Nicotina tabacum*", *Plant Cell Rep.* **3**, 18–20 (1984).

Schuchmann, R. and Wellmann, E., "Somatic embryogenesis of tissue cultures of *Papaver somniferum* and *Papaver orientale* and its relationship to alkaloid and lipid metabolism", *Plant Cell Rep.* **2**, 88–91 (1983).

Schumacher, H.-M., Rüffer, M., Nagakura, N. and Zenk, M. H., "Partial purification and properties of (S)-norlaudanosoline synthase from *Eschscholtzia tenuifolia* cell cultures", *Planta Med.* **48**, 212–220 (1983).

Smart, N. J., Morris, P. and Fowler, M. W.: "Alkaloid production by cells of *Catharanthus roseus* grown in airlift-fermenter systems". In: [3], 397–398 (1982).

Staba, E. J., Zito, S. and Amin, M., "Alkaloid production from Papaver tissue cultures", *J. Nat. Prod.* **45**, 256–262 (1982).

Stöckigt, J. and Soll, H. J., "Indole alkaloids from cell suspension cultures of *Catharanthus roseus* and *C. ovalis*", *Planta Med.* **40**, 22–30 (1980).

Stohs, S. J.: "Metabolism of steroids in plant tissue cultures". In: Fiechter, A. (ed.): *Advances in Biochemical Engineering* **16**, *Plant Cell Culture* I. Springer-Verlag, Berlin, Heidelberg, New York 1980, pp. 85–108.

Street, H. E.: "Cell cultures: A tool in plant biology". In: Dudits, D., Farkas, G. L. and Maliga, P. (eds.): *Cell Genetics in Higher Plants.* Akademiai Kiado, Budapest 1976, pp. 7–38.

Street, H. E.: "Laboratory organization". In: [5], 11–30 (1977).

Tabata, M. and Hiraoka, N., "Variation of alkaloid production in *Nicotiana rustica* callus cultures", *Physiol. Plant* **38**, 19–23 (1976).

Thomas, E. and Wernicke, W.: "Morphogenesis in herbaceous crop plants". In: [6], 403–410 (1978).

Vasil, V. and Vasil, I. K., "Regeneration of tobacco and petunia plants from protoplasts and culture of corn protoplasts", *In Vitro* **10**, 83–96 (1974).

Veliky, I. A. and Barber, K. M., "Biotransformation of tryptophan by *Phaseolus vulgaris* suspension culture", *Lloydia* **38**, 125–130 (1975).

Walkey, D. G. A.: "In vitro methods for virus elimination". In: [6], 245–254 (1978).

Wenzel, G., Schieder, O., Przewozny, T., Sopory, S. K. and Melchers, G., "Comparison of single cell culture derived *Solanum tuberosum* plants and a model for their application in breeding programs", *Theor. Appl. Genet.* **55**, 49–55 (1979).

Wichers, H. J., Malingré, T. M. and Huizing, H. J., "The effect of some environmental factors on the production of L-dopa by alginate-entrapped cells of *Mucuna pruriens*", *Planta* **158**, 482–486 (1983).

Widholm, J. M.: "Selection and characterization of biochemical mutants". In: [2], 112–124 (1977).

Witte, L., Berlin, J., Wray, V., Schubert, W., Kohl, W., Höfle, G. and Hammer, J., "Mono- and diterpenes from cell cultures of *Thuja occidentalis*", *Planta Med.* **49**, 216–221 (1983).

Zambryski, P., Depicker, A., Kruger, K. and Goodman, H. M., "Tumor induction by *Agrobacterium tumefaciens:* Analysis of the boundaries of T-DNA", *J. Mol. Appl. Genet.* **1**, 361–370 (1982).

Zenk, M. H.: "Impact of plant cell culture on industry". In: [6], 1–14 (1978).

Zenk, M. H., El-Shagi, H. and Schulte, U., "Anthraquinone production by cell suspension cultures of *Morinda citrifolia*", *Planta Med. Suppl.* 79–101 (1975).

Zenk, M. H., El-Shagi, H., Arens, H., Stöckigt, J., Weiler, E. W. and Deus, B.: "Formation of indole alkaloids serpentine and ajmalicine in cell suspension cultures of *Catharanthus roseus*". In: [2], 27–43 (1977).

5.3   Animal Cell Cultures

5.3.1   General

During the last 20 years, the prerequisites for the **maintenance and propagation of animal cells in culture** have been worked out systematically. The present state of development is characterized by the fact that the cultivation of animal cells has been established in many laboratories and clinics in order to deal with biochemical, physiological, and morphological questions. Thus, cell culture techniques are firmly established in **diagnostic virology** (Moffat, 1968), in the **analysis of oncogenic** (Diamond, 1978) **and cytostatic substances** (Salmon et al., 1980), in **amniocentesis** (Valenti, 1973), in **ageing research** (Hayflick, 1979), for the **mapping of genes** (Kucherlapati et al., 1974), and for **studies on differentiation** (Ahmad et al., 1978) and of **cell-cycle related events** (Tobey et al., 1977). Since most types of animal cells are suitable for in-vitro cultivation, the present annual demand of 280 millions of experimental animals worldwide will be reduced as further developments become available (Wassermann, 1982).

Besides diagnosis and basic research, mammalian cells are of increasing importance for the **production of a variety of pharmaceutically important macromolecules.** Extensive efforts are currently being undertaken to transfer animal cells from the laboratory to the production level. To promote such developments, the NSF (National Science Foundation of the USA) has founded two cell culture centers in 1975 at the Massachusetts Institute of Technology, Cambridge, and at the University of Alabama in Birmingham. Detailed progress reports from these plants are published regularly (Lynn and Acton, 1975; Acton et al., 1979; Zwerner et al., 1981; Crespi et al., 1981).

The **cultivation of cells on a large technical scale** started with BHK (baby hamster kidney) cells which were adapted to growth in suspension in 1962 and have been used industrially since 1967 in the United Kingdom, Italy, Germany, Spain, Denmark, and France, particularly for the production of foot-and-mouth disease vaccines. Girard (1977) has reported the construction of a factory in which every year 500000 liters of cell suspension are processed in 3000 liter fermenters. More advanced processes are already based on fermenters with a capacity of up to 10000 liters (Boge, 1982).

A large range of other substances, such as **hormones, enzymes, antibodies** and **cytokines** are on the threshold of industrial manufacture. Because of its tremendous current interest, the developments relating to **interferon** have proceeded furthest and will be reported in greatest detail below as they represent a clear example of the rapid advance that is possible today as the result of directed development in such systems.

Animal cell culture deals with the study of parts of organs, tissues or individual cells in vitro. The starting point for such a culture is an **explant**; as long as this retains its structure and its function one speaks of an **organ or tissue culture.** If the organization of a tissue is destroyed by mechanical, chemical, or enzymatic action, transition to a **true cell culture** is complete.

Cells or tissue taken from an organism forms the **primary culture.** The term **"cell line"** is applied to the generations obtained after the first subcultivation and all subsequent ones. One should speak of a "cell strain" only when, by selection or cloning, cells with specific stable properties have been obtained (marker chromosomes, marker enzymes, resistances, antigens). A cell line can become a **continuous (permanent) cell line** by "culture alteration." Continuous cell lines possess the potential for an unlimited subcultivation in vitro.

In the present state of our knowledge, it is impossible to determine the moment when the transition to continuous cell line has taken place. However, a common criterion, is, an at least 70-fold subcultivation (passage) at intervals of about three days. The result of culture alteration was formerly generally called "transformation"; however, this term should now be used only in those cases in which the alteration can be ascribed unambiguously to the introduction of foreign genetic material.

5.3.2 Experimental Work with Animal Cell Cultures

Equipment of a Cell Culture Laboratory

The same rules for sterile working apply in laboratories for animal cell cultures as in laboratories for plant cell cultures. Some important details will be discussed below.

Diploid cells require for their growth a solid substrate with a defined surface charge. These demands are satisfied by glass, but in its cleansing detergents must be avoided and be replaced, for example, by polyphosphates (House, 1968). Recently, one-way polystyrene equipment which has been subjected to treatments that adjust the desired negative charge density has increased in importance (Maroudas, 1973). This has already been taken into account in commercial "tissue-culture grade" flasks and dishes; in contrast, polystyrene "bacteriological-grade" vessels are unsuitable. For cultivating cells at reduced levels of serum proteins, the coating of vessels with poly-D-lysine has been recommended (Ham and McKehan, 1979).

The cell lines that are processed at the present time are derived mostly from warm-blooded animals and require a cultivation temperature of 37°C. Climatized rooms are frequently considered too complex for this purpose and have the added disadvantage that practically only closed systems can be operated since otherwise the partial pressure of carbon dioxide necessary for a controlled metabolism would not be ensured. Such demands are satisfied best by incubators with an adjustable supply of carbon dioxide and also, recently, oxygen.

Almost all the nutrient media used for animal cultures contain thermolabile components, so that it is impossible to sterilize by autoclaving. Instead, high-pressure filtration through membrane filters with pore widths of about 0.2 μm is used. Such procedures can be carried out in clean benches with a horizontal, laminar airflow which offer the best protection against contamination from outside. For working with dangerous substances and also for handling primate cell cultures reference may be made to the US safety standards which require sterile boxes, with a vertical curtain of laminar air (Barkley, 1979).

In contrast to plant material, the cryopreservation of animal tissues and cells can usually be solved satisfactorily. For the critical temperature interval between +20 and −70°C, programmable apparatuses have been developed, but the graduated use of refrigerators in combination with insulating materials fulfils the same purpose (Paul, 1980; Adams, 1980). For long-term preservation, temperatures below −70°C are required, and for this purpose Dewar vessels with liquid nitrogen or more sophisticated "liquid nitrogen refrigerators" are available. The procedure requires a cryoprotective reagent. 10% glycerol is the preferred additive except for those cells that are permeated too slowly and may require a cytotoxic agent like 7.5% dimethyl sulfoxide. An alternative for the cryoprotection of critical lymphoid cells using 10% polyethyleneglycol (PEG 20000) has also been developed (Voigt and Maurer, 1981).

Methods of Cultivation

Safety regulations formulated first in 1967 in the USA required the cultivation of exclusively normal, diploid cells for the manufacture of biologicals for human medicine. It was felt that the dangers arising from the utilization of permanent or transformed cell lines could not be appreciated since cancerous cells of this type could be affected by tumor-inducing principles of unknown origin (reviewed by Hillman, 1978). These restrictions have had a considerable impact on technical developments during recent years since primary cells and the diploid cell lines derived from them grow exclusively on charged surfaces and cannot be adapted to suspension culture. In the near future, cell culture technology may take a completely different direction since the use of permanent cell lines is now seriously considered by WHO provided that a number of tests is performed and that the amount of DNA initially present is reduced at least 10^8 fold (van Wezel et al., 1981; Bundesgesundheitsamt, personal communication, 1983). The first product fulfilling such requirements (lymphoblastoid interferon) was approved for human clinical trials in 1981 (Mizrahi, 1983).

Traditionally animal cells are kept successfully in ordinary laboratory glass vessels or culture bottles with useful surfaces of up to 160 cm². The use of the whole inner surface of 600 to 1500 cm² is permitted by **roller culture bottles** that can be rotated in special incubators at 2 to 4 rpm. A further development envisages the semiautomatic exchange of media (Smith and Kozoman, 1973). With this arrangement, on inoculation with 4×10^5 cells/mL in 100 mL of medium a yield of 8×10^8 cells per flask can be obtained within six days. Corbeil (1977) used roller flasks with an inserted glass tube for a further tenfold increase in the useful surface; bottles with polyester spirals have been described by House (1973). A series of commercial culture chambers based on rotating spirals or stacks of plates has been described in a review (Keay and Burton, 1979). Their surface offers the equivalent of up to 100 roller bottles. More recently, Bioferon (Laupheim, Germany) and Nunc (Roskilde, Denmark) cooperatively developed a **multitray battery system** that is now available. It features an effective surface of 6000 cm² (WS-system) or 24000 cm² (BWS-system) corresponding to 2.5 and 10 liter of culture medium, respectively. With the corresponding peripheral equipment a semiautomatic operation is possible yielding 4 to 16×10^8 fibroblast cells per batch (Joester and Pakos, 1982).

Knazik (NIH) has developed a culture system using two types of **permeable capillaries** for supplying cells with components of the medium and gas and the concomitant removal of waste products. Although the arrangement cannot be scaled up significantly, it represents an optimum simulation of natural cell environments permitting anchorage-dependent cells to grow as a mass at densities not attained by any other technique (1×10^8 per mL of vessel volume). The apparatus has been used efficiently for the recovery of diffusible cell products up to $M_r = 5000$ (hormones) since solutes are exchanged continously. A somewhat related system "IL 410" is based on gas-permeable FEP-Teflon tubes shaped to form a reel. The reels are parts of a **medium-perfusion system** allowing continous changes of medium. IL 410 lends itself to automation and to scale-up. The properties of these techniques have been compared with the more conventional ones and it is concluded that the efficacy of culturing can be increased significantly by careful adjustments of the microenvironments, particularly by an optimum supply of oxygen (review by Jensen, 1981).

The harvesting of anchorage-dependent cells, i.e. their recovery from the charged support, requires the use of **lytic enzymes.** Trypsin is the most widely used, frequently in combination with 0,02% EDTA. Pancreatin is also used, and information has recently been given about a new neutral bacterial protease (Boehringer Information Service). Since damage to the cells by this enzyme appears to be negligible, increased use is to be expected in future (Matsumura et al., 1975).

Maintaining cells in suspension would offer great technological advantages. Among the diploid cells, however, only the lymphocytes, which are already present in the organism in the suspended state, are suitable for this. In many cases, continuous cell lines, especially those of tumor cells can be adapted for growth in suspension.

On the laboratory scale, the magnetically driven **spinner bottle** in sizes up to about 2 liters is the most common type of apparatus. In order to prevent the cells from adhering to the glass walls, these must be siliconized by coating them with a solution of silicone in isopropanol at 100 to 150°C. In addition, a tendency to aggregation may be suppressed by calcium (II) ion-free so called **"spinner media"** or by the addition of a protease (Matsumura et al., 1975). For the protection of cells against damage in agitated and especially in serum-free media, polymers such as methylcellulose (Methocel 15cps), carboxymethylcellulose, polyvinylpyrrolidone, Dextran 50000, Ficol 400 and polyglycols (the polyol Pluronic F-68) are added in concentrations of 0.1 to 2%. The critical factor in this cultivation technique is frequently the rapid dying-off at cell densities below 1×10^5 cells/mL or after the stationary phase has reached at 1 to 4×10^6 cells/mL.

For industrial purposes, glass spinner bottles with capacities up to 12 L, and also the conventional **fermenters for bacterial cultures** with pH and p_{O_2} control are used; modifications which procide for pH regulation by the feed of carbon dioxide are customary (Lynn and Acton, 1975; Zwerner et al., 1981). A list of fermenters recommended for culturing cells at bench scale and at industrial scale has been given by Mizrahi (1981). Himmelfarb's "spin filter" system is regarded as a substantial further development (Keay and Burton, 1979). Since in this the medium is withdrawn continuously through a magnetically driven cylindrical filter and can therefore be regenerated, extraordinary cell densities (10^7 to 10^8 cells/mL) can be achieved. Pollard and Khosrovi (1978) have referred to the advantages of a continuous fermenter equipped with a system of tubes in which the shear forces are substantially reduced by laminar flow. In future apparatuses, gas-permeable tube materials could permit a continuous exchange of gas and material.

The use of the so-called **"microcarrier technique"** offers an elegant possibility of keeping under the conditions of a suspension culture even those cells that require a substrate. These include, in the first place, the pharmaceutically important primary cells and the diploid cell lines. Advantages are also offered, however, for continuous cell lines, since with this method media can be regenerated and dead (i.e., nonadherent) cells can be removed by simple means. A review of 1979 (which is continuously updated by Pharmacia) gives a list of 60 different types of cells which have been successfully cultivated on carriers (Hirtenstein et al., 1979) and it appears as if this applies to all animal cells except those of lymphoid origin.

The microcarrier concept originated from observations by van Wezel, according to which DEAE-Sephadex A50 beads are accepted as substrates by animal cells. Systematic investigations by Levine et al. (1979) later showed that the charge density of DEAE-Sephadex (6.5 meq/g) lies far above a sharp optimum of 1.5 to 2 meq/g. The preparation of carriers optimized in this respect has been described (Thilly and Levine, 1979). Products based on cross-linked dextran (Pharmacia, Flow) or polyacrylamide (Bio Rad) are now commercially available. The dextran type is manufactured in three grades. Being a descendant of DEAE-Sephadex, type 1 is uniformly charged throughout the particles. It has the intrinsic disadvantage that it acts as an ion-exchanger binding many anionic medium components. Type 2 has only surface charges accessible to cells, and it has less stringent medium requirements and facilitates the detachment of cells by trypsin. Type 3, finally, is the most suitable for certain sensitive cells as it is coated with a quasi-natural substrate (denatured collagen). It permits cell detachment using collagenase, which appears less detrimental to biological membranes than other enzymes.

Used in typical amounts of 3 to 5 mg/mL, microcarriers offer a surface of 18 to 30 cm^2 per mL, i.e., a 75-mL culture would offer the effective surface of a large roller bottle or even more. With an inoculation density of five cells per bead or 1 to 5×10^5 cells/mL final concentrations in such cultures are to be expected which approach those of a suspension culture (5×10^6 cells/mL).

Most apparatuses for suspension cultures are suitable for the performance of microcarrier cultures, glass and metal vessels being siliconized. On the laboratory scale, spinner bottles rotated at 40 to 100 rpm are widely used; roller bottles with speeds of rotation of 8 to 10 rpm are somewhat inferior. If volumes of more than one liter are to be processed, fermenters with controlling devices for temperature, pH, p_{O_2}, and p_{CO_2} may be recommended. Although none of the present fermenter systems has been designed specially for this purpose, satisfactory results are obtained with them. An example is the culture of kidney cells in Bilthoven units of several 100 L in Holland.

Growth curves can be plotted and physiological parameters followed simply by taking aliquots from a microcarrier suspension; so far hardly any use has been made of this possibility in basic research. Furthermore, the method opens up new possibilities for cell synchronization (Mitchell and Wray, 1979) and the identification of humoral interactions between different cell types in an elegant co-cultivation system (Davies and Kerr, 1982).

For subcultivation, in the normal case the cells must be detached from the microcarrier, which requires fairly high concentrations of enzymes (0.25% trypsin or 0.1 to 1% collagenase). Reports according to which a continuous performance of the process is possible by **bead-to-bead transfer** probably relate only to special types of epithelial cells. Medium modifications permitting this cultivation technique have been described (Crespi et al., 1981).

Since the marketing of microcarriers commenced only in 1978, the most detailed instructions for their use are still to be found in the manufacturers' brochures. Some aspects are dealt with in the articles by Thilly and Levine (1979), Mered et al. (1980) and Crespi et al. (1981).

Media

All media for animal cell cultures contain at least the following components: a hexose (glucose or galactose), the 13 amino acids to be regarded as essential, 7 to 8 vitamins of the B series, choline, inositol, and inorganic salts. Such an isotonic nutrient solution can be used for the maintenance of many types of cells but it will not promote proliferation. What we are discussing here is the class of "minimal media" (Eagle's BME and MEM; DME, i.e., Dulbecco's modification of BME; McCoy's 5 A; and Leibovitz's L 15*), which have been proposed for use in combination with blood serum. Efforts have been made for a long time to replace serum by components of known structure. The following formulations were drawn up from this point of view but they are nevertheless generally used in combination with serum, since they maintain a limited growth only with a few continuous cell lines: M 199, NCTC 109 and 135, Waymouth's MB 752/1, and Ham's F 10 and F 12. The 12 media mentioned are made up by most manufacturers as liquid concentrates or as solids and are therefore available as handy bases for supplementation by specific additives. A list with 49 media and their possibilities of use is given by Ham and McKeehan (1979).

At the present time, the addition of 5 to 20% of a homologous or heterologous serum is still standard although great efforts are being made to circumvent this component, as it is the most variable and expensive additive.

Growth-promoting components have been found, particularly, in the group of α- and β-globulins. The level of γ-globulins in the serum of older animals inhibits growth, so that the use of fetal serum appears to be advisable; this component may, however, make up 75 to 95% of the cost of a medium. According to Inglot (1975), it is possible specifically to precipitate γ-globulins and also any bacteria and viruses that may be present with 6% polyethyleneglycol, so that increasing use is being made of this process, particularly at the production level (Mizrahi, 1980).

Certain properties of sera (promotion of cell attachment and proliferation, inhibition

---

* BME = Basal Medium Eagle; MEM = Minimum Essential Medium; DME = Dulbecco's Modification of MEM; McCoy 5 A: see McCoy et al., 1959; L = Leibovitz. For the compositions of these media see Ham and McKeehan, 1979.

of proteases) can be imparted by substitutes. Two concepts are followed here:

1. The composition of fully-defined media, which are necessarily composed of many more components than serum-containing media and which are much more expensive. In particular, the addition of growth factors (FGF, fibroblast growth factor; EGF, epidermal growth factor; NGF, nerve growth factor, etc.) and hormones (glucagon, hydrocortison, estradiol, prostaglandins, etc.) must be adapted to the respective cell type, as cells remain responsive to the stimuli experienced in vivo (Barnes and Sato, 1980). A list dating from August 1979 includes 35, exclusively permanent, cell lines which could be adapted to chemically defined media (Keay, 1979).

2. The design of cheap media suited for large-scale production. These nutrients usually require the addition of poorly-defined serum-substitutes like lactalbumin hydrolysate, yeast extracts, peptones or other natural products. Typical examples from this group are made up from only 20 to 30 components.

A medium which in some aspects falls in between these groups has been developed by Wissler (1981). It contains 94 defined components and is now used routinely for the large scale cultivation of lymphocytes. Whether this medium sustains the growth of non-lymphoid cells is currently being investigated.

Certain growth substances are synthesized and secreted by cells in culture themselves – a fact that is made use of in the **"conditioning"** of media. An elimination of these CSA (colony-stimulating activity) factors in the case of a complete change of medium is shown by the interruption of proliferation, so that only a partial (or continuous) exchange or a regeneration by rapidly degraded components should be performed. Table 5-2 gives a glimpse of the sequence in which essential components of a MEM medium are exhausted by hydrolysis or preferential consumption. The sequence shown here

Table 5-2. Loss of some Components of MEM Medium + 10% of Serum after Incubation at 37°C for Six Days in the Presence and in the Absence of Diploid Human Lung Fibroblasts (MRC-5 Cells). (After figures due to Lambert and Pirt, 1975).

Component	MRC-5 cells (% loss)	Incubated control (% loss)
Glucose	79	0
Cystine	74.5	5.5
Glutamine	73.0	42.0
Leucine	36.0	1
Threonine	53.0	8
Isoleucine	33	0
Methionine	33	6
Pyridoxine	30.5	0.5
Folic acid	29.6	11.1
Lysine	26	8
Tryptophan	23.5	10
Arginine	21	11
Nicotinamide	21	3
Inositol	20	1.6
All others less than 20%		

must be taken into account in the formulation of regeneration mixtures but it may vary according to the type of cell.

The better the metabolic features of a cell type are known, the sooner will it be possible to promote desired components and to suppress other in mixed cultures. Thus, the loss of specific synthetic powers of a cell culture is ascribed, *inter alia,* to the displacement of epithelial cells by more readily adaptable fibroblasts. These connective tissue cells are an undesirable accompaniment in primary cultures from organs but they have some properties that can be utilized in the design of media in order to limit their growth (Berman et al., 1979; Gilbert and Migeion, 1975; Sun et al., 1979; Kaneko and Goshima, 1982).

In addition to the nutritional requirements, the **pH optimum** (6.9 to 7.8) should be known for each cell line. According to observations due to Ceccarini (1975), in this way up to half the serum can be saved. In the past, for pH

control use was made of the equilibration of 5% of carbon dioxide in the air space with 2.2 g of sodium hydrogen carbonate (NaHCO$_3$) per liter of medium (Earle's salts). Recently, use has been made of nontoxic organic buffers, e.g., HEPES (N-2-hydroxyethylpiperazine-N'-2-ethanesulfonic acid) (pK 7.3 at 37°C) in combination of up to 850 mg NaHCO$_3$/L and a concentration of 2% of carbon dioxide in the external space, not least because the traditional concentration of carbon dioxide is above the optimum (Ham and McKeehan, 1979).

The use of **antibiotics** in media is disputed, but a mixture of 20 to 200 units of penicillin/mL and 10 to 100 µg of streptomycin/mL is added almost as routine and helps against the majority of **bacteria**. Antibiotics with action on **fungi** and **mycoplasmas** have been discussed exhaustively (Paul, 1980; Perlman, 1979). For contamination tests, reference may be made to the matter supplied by the media manufacturers. A routine test for **mycoplasmas** must definitely be advised, particularly since convenient methods of detection based on fluorescent dyes have been developed (Chen, 1977). Mycoplasmas do not lead to the immediate death of the cells but to fundamentally different nutritional requirements and cell properties; according to estimates, 60% of all cell lines are contaminated by these organisms.

The Setting Up of a Cell Culture

In 1925, on the recommendation of the Oncological Council and the National Cancer Research Institute a cell bank was founded in the USA (American Type Culture Collection, ATCC, Rockville, Maryland). The association publishes two catalogs, of which the volume "Strains II" (1979) lists 400 cell lines and 400 species, including about 200 human fibroblast lines with special genetic features. The sources of the cell lines are also described with their markers, the number of passages, the feeding conditions, the survival rate, the growth rate, the plating efficiency, morphology, density of a monolayer, and sterility.

The "Human Genetic Mutant Cell Repository" was established in 1972 at the Institute for Medical Research in Camden, New Jersey. The Repository establishes, characterizes and distributes cell cultures from patients with biochemical genetic disorders and chromosomal aberrations.

Since 1977, the ESACT (European Society of Animal Cell Technology) committee has been actively investigating the possibility of founding a "Cell Bank" in Europe. A single center similar to the ATCC was considered unrealistic in monetary and political terms. In 1980 the "European Federation of Cell and Virus Collections" (EFCVC) was formed which is considering the setting up a European Databank of cell lines used in various laboratories within the European Federation.

Meanwhile, primary cells and cell lines can be purchased from a number of firms in Europe (Flow Laboratories, Deutsche Bio Mérieux, Seromed). Some of these have been established by the firms themselves and others have been obtained from the ATCC. Cells are usually supplied as a monolayer culture which is incubated at 37 °C for 24 hours before reinoculation. Long-distance transport may also be performed in frozen ampuls which upon receipt should be brought to 37 °C as rapidly as possible and diluted to a tenfold volume to lower the concentration of cryoprotective reagents like DMSO (dimethyl sulfoxide) to less harmful levels. Subsequently cells have to be recovered by centrifugation and seeded into flasks containing fresh medium.

For **establishing one's own primary cultures** reference may be made to a series of monographs and articles (Merchant et al., 1965; Paul, 1980; Kaighn, 1974). The methods given in these publications can be divided into three groups which are generally used in combination:

- mechanical comminution of a tissue;
- chemical breakdown by chelating agents such as EDTA; and
- treatment with enzymes.

The most common enzyme for this purpose is a crude trypsin preparation with trace activities due to chymotrypsin, elastase, DNase, etc. Enzymes such as collagenase, pronase, and hyaluronidase have not found the same broad use but they are important in combination with trypsin. The advantages of dispase, a bacterial protease have been pointed out (Matsumara et al., 1975).

After such pretreatments, the "coverslip" method can be used for fibroblasts in order to supply a fragment of tissue between microscope slides with plasma or medium. On incubation, an exuberant growth of cells takes place, which can be removed from the glass support and transferred into a monolayer culture.

Organs with small proportions of connective tissue (liver, kidneys) can be perfused with an enzyme-EDTA mixture and thereby be broken down immediately after they have been dissected out or even *in situ* (van Wezel et al., 1978). After mechanical dissection, pieces of tissue or individual cells can then be transferred to culture bottles. Even embryonic and cancer-like tissues are susceptible to mild processes, since they contain a weak matrix. For other, differentiated, tissues, more intensive methods are necessary in order to degrade intercellular material (fiber proteins, mucopolysaccharides).

Cancer cells can be regarded as being already transformed and may be converted directly into a continuous cell line (Fig. 5-3). Diploid normal cells first pass through the phase of active division steps, after which they degenerate. Frequently, colonies with a higher rate of division remain or arise in a degenerating cell population because of selection, adaptation, mutation, or transformation. Usually, such a "culture alternation" can be correlated with

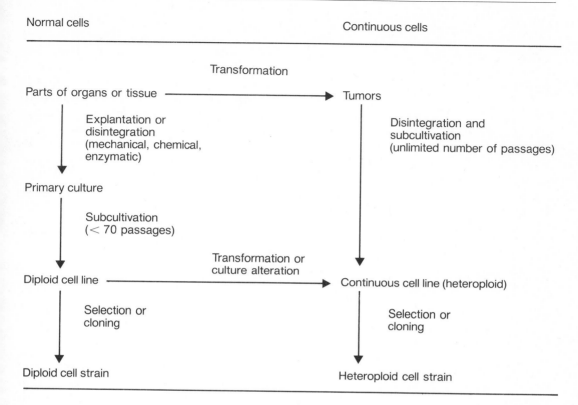

Fig. 5-3. Relationships between types of tissue and types of cells.

chromosomal aberrations (polyploidy, heteroploidy, aneuploidy). A number of established continuous cell lines owe their origin to this mechanism.

Treatments with oncogenic chemicals, transformation by viruses, or the fusion of the primary cells with cancer cells is suitable for the deliberate conversion of diploid primary cells into continuous cells. A review has been given by Pastan (1979).

5.3.3 Technological Uses of Animal Cell Cultures

Animal cells produce macromolecules of medical interest that are not available by

chemical methods. The only available source of such substances previously was urine, animal tissue or even human tissue when human-specific molecules such as growth hormones were required. At the present time, possibilities of continuous production based on cell lines are being developed for them; in many cases, these processes have to compete with technologies derived from the possibilities of genetic engineering in bacteria and yeasts. The most important commercial utilization of animal cell cultures at the present time is still the multiplication of viruses for the **manufacture of vaccines,** which offers considerable technological advantages over conventional production, e.g., in incubated eggs. In addition to this, there is a series of substances which are on the verge of being manufactured on the larger scale. However, their number is still manageable at the present time so that a discussion according to groups of substances appears to be indicated.

The Production of Virus Vaccines

Viruses require a living substrate for their multiplication. Previously, duck embryos or organ cultures from animal nerve and kidney tissue were used for the manufacture of virus vaccines. Such explants consist of different types of cells with different demands on the medium and have the added disadvantage that comprehensive sterility tests must be carried out before their use. Furthermore, tissues from the kidneys of wild apes frequently contain simian viruses (SV 5, SV 40) or their constituents. Side reactions were not infrequent after the administration of such vaccines (Aoki et al., 1975). The setting up of characterized cell cultures under sterile conditions gave a decisive advance.

The best conditions for the multiplication of viruses are generally afforded by unaltered diploid cells, diploid cell lines may be superior to explanted tissues.

An important exception is the continuous cell line BHK 21, which was derived from the kidneys of one-day **golden hamsters** (baby hamster kidney). After continuous multiplication for 84 days, the clone BHK 21 that had undergone a culture alteration was found. However, deviations from the diploid chromosome number in this line are relatively rare (ATCC No. CCl 10). BHK 21 cells can be multiplied in suspension and are used, for example, by Burroughs Wellcome on the scale of nore than 1000 L for the manufacture of a foot-and-mouth disease vaccine for veterinary medicine.

In **human medicine** only **vaccines from normal cells** with minimum deviations from the diploid chromosome set and a finite lifetime should be used. Such a cell line, WI 38, was set up in 1961 from the lung tissue of a human embryo; the tenth passage of these cells is currently available (ATCC No. CCL 75). WI 38 cells can pass through about 50 doublings before they degenerate. After the thirteenth population doubling, they are infected by viruses for the manufacture of vaccines. In this way it has been possible, in Prague, to obtain a vaccine from type 4 adenovirus, which has undergone intensive clinical investigation (Tint et al., 1969). At Mérieux (Lyon), WI 38 cells have been used to multiply rubella viruses, and the corresponding vaccine, obtained by inactivation by β-propiolactone, has been tested on volunteers in the United Kingdom (Aoki, 1975).

Normal diploid cells can be cultivated only on surfaces, so that in the past there have been severe problems in passing to the technical scale. Assistance was given here by the introduction of the **microcarrier technology.** Information on the production of **foot-and-mouth viruses** in a microcarrier system has come from Iffa-Mérieux (Lyon). The weekly production of the fermenter used corresponds to 600 to 900 roller bottles, and in this figure the somewhat lower yield of virus on microcarriers has already been taken into account. MEM medium with 5% of calf serum is used for the cultivation of porcine kidney cells. At the end of the growth phase, this medium is decanted from the microcarriers and replaced by serum-free medium. The infection with viruses is carried out at a cell concentration of $2.5 \times 10^6/$ mL. After the lysis of 90% of the cells, the microcarriers are allowed to settle and the viruses are obtained from the supernatant (Meignier et al., 1979).

The production of **polio vaccines** by the replication of the virus on simian kidney cells has been carried out for a long time at the Rijksinstituut voor de Volksgesondheit in Bilthoven (the Netherlands). In the past, an extensive subcultivation was avoided since secondary cultures were often destroyed by the presence of **simian viruses,** but is in prospect after the establishment of a primate center. It was possible to reduce the number of monkeys needed for the vaccine requirements of the Netherlands from 4751 animals in 1965 to 531 animals in 1976. These improvements are due to the introduction of perfusion techniques for obtaining primary cells and the replacement of bottle cultivation by the microcarrier technique.

After becoming attached to the support, the primary cells are grown for 7 to 8 days with no change of medium, which leads to a tenfold increase in their number. In this phase sterility tests and chromosome analyses can be carried out on aliquots. Three days after infection by **polio virus,** the culture is ready for the preparation of the vaccine by concentration, chromatography (Sepharose-6B and DEAE-Sephadex), and inactivation (formaldehyde). Similar processes have been used for the manufacture of rabies vaccine via dog kidney cells; the activity of the end-product corresponded to that of a vaccine from diploid human cells (van Wezel et al., 1978). The scale of production has been expanded by the Dutch group from 200 to the current 650 liters.

At the present time one of the primary efforts in the industrial production of viral vaccines is being dedicated to the development of serum-free media to avoid allergic reactions as a result of a repeated vaccination, to prevent the contamination of cell cultures by foreign viruses, e.g., from the bovine respiratory tract, and, finally, to eliminate dependence on the supply of serum (Boge, 1981).

Viral Pesticides

Pollard and Khosrovi (1978) proposed the production of viruses that are pathogenic for insects and can therefore be used for **insect control.** As the substrate a continuous insect cell line from *Tricoplusca ni,* kept in suspension in a tube flow-through reactor, was used. A cost analysis of the method showed that it could already compete with existing processes.

Cell Surface Antigens

The production of antigens at a large scale is performed for several purposes. Either these molecules are needed for a detailed **investigation of their structure and function** or they are used **to raise antibodies against themselves** which may then be used for **therapeutic and diagnostic purposes.** Finally, they can **serve as a vaccine,** for instance as an alternative to inactivated virus. The efforts put into the production of antigens by cell culture techniques have hardly been discouraged by the dramatic advances in recombinant DNA technology which make it possible to synthesize the desired molecules in bacteria (e.g., Hepatitis B and foot-and-mouth-disease viral antigens in 1981). Many important structures cannot be obtained from engineered bacteria and others have not been characterized sufficiently to permit an isolation of the genetic information.

Milligram quantities of **histocompatibility** (H2k) and **differentiation-specific** (Thy-1) **antigens** have been isolated at the cell culture center in Birmingham (Alabama) from murine lymphoblastoid cells. Going beyond the laboratory scale, these cells have been grown in a 12 L modified bacterial fermenter and then at the 200 L scale.

The work described by Barstad et al. (1977) demonstrated that the transformed BW 5147 cells showed a dramatically increased antigen expression compared to that of normal cells and this was attributed to their increased surface area. 3.1×10^{12} cells (3 kilograms) were isolated, corresponding to 60000 thymus equivalents of Thy-1 and more than 15000 spleen equivalents of H2k, produced at a fraction of the cost of 15000 mice.

Antilymphocyte serum (ALS) is an immune serum that is used as an alternative to proliferation-inhibiting medicaments after organ transplants in order to weaken the immune defense. In the past it was mostly enriched lymphocytes that were used as immunizing material, but these were frequently impure so that the antiserum obtained with them in the animal was also directed against other blood constituents. As an alternative, surface antigens from cultivated continuous human lymphoma or leukemia cell lines, which lead to the synthesis of far more specific antibodies, are used today. This possibility goes back to the fact that the surface antigens of lymphoid cell lines remain stable in spite of radical changes in their chromosome structure and they also occur in higher densities (Moore, 1972).

Since no lytic cell culture systems are available for the propagation of pathogenic **Herpes viruses,** alternatives had to be devised. Herpes simplex virus (HSV) in common with several other viruses induces **viral antigens** on the plasma membrane of the cells it infects. Vesicles of plasma membrane have been recovered from Vero cells and have been found to trigger an immune response (Thornton et al., 1981). Antigens of Epstein-Barr virus (EBV) could be induced in transformed lymphoblastoid cells by the application of tumor-promoting phorbol esters and this principle appears to hold for all oncogenic Herpes viruses (zur Hausen, 1981). It is hoped that these new concepts can efficiently be used for the production of vaccines in cases where a DNA-free product is required due to safety regulations or where no alternatives are at hand.

Parasites are uni- or multicellular organisms surviving in their hosts without being attacked by the immune system and this is due to their incorporation of host-specific antigens. *Schistosoma mansoni* has a snail as an intermediate host and therefore utilizes its antigens. In the Behringwerke AG (Marburg) it has been shown that mollusk cell cultures can serve as a **source of antigens** which may then be used to protect the final, warm-blooded, host from schistosomiasis (bilharziasis).

Monoclonal (Monospecific) Antibodies

Until recently, it was impossible to obtain reproducibly defined **antibodies** against certain **antigens.** It has been estimated that the immune response of a mouse against a determinant group in the antigen contains 5 to 10 different antibodies and these represent only a fraction of the total repertory in the order of 800 to 1000 possible varieties. The composition of the antibodies will vary correspondingly from animal to animal. Attempts to manufacture antisera against tumor-specific antigens were likewise made more difficult by the fact that antibodies were always present that reacted with all the cells of the organism. Since the pioneer work of Köhler and Milstein (1975) this problem has been solved in principle. These authors showed that it is possible to stabilize antibody-synthesizing spleen cells by fusion with myeloma cells and to maintain the desired properties of the initial cells in some of the resulting hybrid cells **(Hybridomas).**

Myeloma cells are derived from bone-marrow tumors and therefore have the potential for unlimited division. The cell line necessary for the process no longer produces antibodies itself, since otherwise, in combination with the spleen cells, a series of hybrid molecules would arise. In addition, by selection a situation has been achieved in which these cells, because of the defect in HGPRT (hypoxanthine guanine phosphoribosyl transferase) or TK (thymidine kinase), are no longer capable of synthesizing DNA from hypoxanthine and thymidine. Roughly, the experiment comprises the following steps:

– Injection of an antigen into a mouse or rat; after this, the lymphocytes of the spleen are induced to produce antibodies.

– Spleen cells are isolated and are fused with myeloma cells in the presence of polyethyleneglycol (PEG 1500). Because of their differentiated state, the remaining spleen cells will die, while myeloma cells and cell hybrids will survive because of their tumor-like properties.

– Selection for hybridoma cells in HAT (hypoxanthine-aminopterin-thymidine) medium; aminopterin blocks the principal pathway of DNA synthesis and makes the cells dependent on hypoxanthine/thymidine. The remainder of the myeloma cells die.

– Some of the remaining hybridomas will provide the required synthetic ability. Their isolation is carried out by cloning and, recently, also by electronic sorting processes (FACS, fluorescence-activated cell sorter).

To multiply the cell clones obtained, the usual culture techniques are available; with these, however, the concentration of antibodies rarely exceeds 50 µg/mL. Consequently, attempts have also been made to inject hybridomas into mice, where these have a tumorgenic action as transformed cells. The growing tumor retains the synthetic capacity of the initial cells and permits the isolation of 20 mg of antibodies per mL of blood; these contain only 5 % of foreign γ-globulins.

For future applications it appears indispensable that large-scale culturing systems be developed that operate with serum-free media to avoid the major source of protein contamination (Murakami et al., 1982).

Monoclonal antibodies become increasingly important in **affinity chromatography** and will thus enter biotechnology with great prospects for industrial purification and isolation processes. They have already established themselves as superior **tools for cell typing** and in a number of **fluorescent and radioimmunoassays.** Finally, their potential role as a **passive vaccine** in therapy has been recognized and even been demonstrated in certain diseases. Only a few illustrative examples will be mentioned below.

Affinity chromatography: Secher and Burke (1980) demonstrated the use of suitable screening methods to obtain a specific antibody to one minor constituent in a protein mixture (leukocyte interferon). This antibody could then be used for affinity chromatography, permitting a 5300-fold enrichment of the desired compound with a yield of 97 %. In principle, it is possible to start another round of the procedure with the purified protein in order to obtain antibodies of a higher specificity for an even more efficient purification procedure.

Cell typing: An investigation of the complex antigenic structures on cell surfaces has now become feasible as hybridoma techniques do not necessarily require their separation prior to immunization. Histocompatibility testing will be an obvious area of application. T-lymphocytes have already been classified in subsets on the basis of their antigenic markers. Following organ transplants, highly significant changes of these subsets have been monitored and graft rejection could reliably be predicted (Cosimi, 1981). Monoclonal antibodies have proven to be valuable tools for the identification of tumor-specific antigens on melanoma, neuroblastoma, teratocarcinoma and leukemia cells. Schlom et al. (1980) have shown that B-lymphocytes in patients with breast cancer are already primed by the antigens shed from the tumor cells. They have generated human monoclonal antibodies from human-mouse hybridomas which could subsequently be used to stain tissue sections with the immunoperoxidase technique. Antibodies against certain antigens shed by tumor cells are also being used increasingly for early diagnosis and for monitoring the response to anti cancer drugs.

Immunotherapy: Some of the antibodies used for T-cell monitoring by Cosimi et al. (1981) could also be used for immunotherapy, permitting the control of graft rejection. Other examples of interest deal with the application of murine monoclonal antibodies in the treatment of leukemia and lymphoma (reviewed by Ritz and Schlossmann, 1982). Although these antibodies were of non-human origin, unwanted immune responses were rarely observed, which fact may be ascribed to the purity of the preparations. Nevertheless, the production of human monoclonal antibodies remains a primary goal. Sometimes this can be achieved by interspecies (mouse × human) hybridization (Schlom, 1980), but human chromosomes may be lost preferentially from these hybridoma cells. Since a continous human B-cell line with the appropriate markers is now available (Croce et al., 1980), utilization of human hybridomas may become routine in the near future.

Monospecific antibodies have a reduced capability of fixing complement. Although binding to all tumor cells occurs, not all cells will thereby be eliminated (Ritz and Schlossmann, 1982). To support their action, monoclonal antibodies may be used as vehicles (**"immunotoxins"**) with which cytotoxic agents are delivered directly to tumor cells (Edwards and Thorpe, 1981). They may therefore become the "magic bullets" foreseen by Paul Ehrlich during his attempts to find new cures for human disease.

The new generation of **immunoassays:** Pure monoclonal antibodies cannot be used for certain conventional immunological procedures, such as the double diffusion assay, because they can only cross-link antigens to dimers rather than forming an insoluble lattice. On balance, they have some revolutionary practical advantages like their biosynthetic labeling capability by growing cells in media with radioactive labeled amino acids. Various modifications of two-site assays have been described in which one site of an antigen is used for its specific attachment to a solid support and the second for the attachment of a labeled antibody. Alternatively, the sites can be used to fix two enzymes in close proximity which enables them to generate a chromophor or fluorophor that is directly measured (Thompson, 1982). The very recent development of "hybrid hybridomas" producing bi-specific antibodies may revolutionize the ELISA (enzyme-linked immunosorbent assay) test which has hitherto required a specific antibody *and* an anti-antibody carrying the enzyme. Both functions can now be accomodated in a single molecule (Milstein, 1983).

Future prospects: in principle, it should be possible to construct monoclonal antibodies against antibodies which are themselves specific for hormones or enzyme substrates. This could lead to a technology of biologically active molecules with invaluable applications as hormone or inhibitor substitutes.

Two institutions, the Salk Institute in La Jolla (California) and the Institute of Medical Research in Camden (New Jersey) have undertaken the distribution of hybridoma cultures, which have been deposited with scientists there. Several companies (Sera Lab, New England Nuclear, Organon) have started the distribution of monoclonal antibodies and several diagnostic hormone (pregnancy) and virus (antigen and antibody) test kits are already available.

Cellular Mediators (Cytokines) and Humoral Mediators

Many cell types are involved in an immune response. Besides B-cells, the antibody-producing cells, and T-cells which are responsible for the cell-mediated immunity, macrophages, T-helper cells and many others are parts of a complex network where they communicate via several dozens soluble factors ("cytokines"), particularly **lymphokines** (lymphocyte-derived) and **monokines** (macrophage-derived).

T-Helper cells are the most prominent cells for the production of lymphokines. There are four principal ways by which these glycoproteins can be produced from them by cell culture techniques: **stimulation of lymphocytes** from buffy coat or spleen cells by nonspecific stimulators such as plant lectins, production using certain **continous tumor cell lines,** and synthesis by **immortalized lymphocytes** that have been obtained by hybridoma techniques (Sonneborn et al., 1981). While the first technique is still used most often (an early account is found in a review by Moore, 1972) the others will increase in importance.

A factor **"interleukin 2"** [formerly "T-cell growth factor"; for nomenclature see J. Immunol. **123**, 2928 (1979)] is attracting the greatest current interest. Its synthesis is triggered antigen-specifically in vivo but, once synthesized, it has an antigen-nonspecific proliferative and differentiating action upon cytotoxic T cells (CTL) which, in turn, communicate with natural killer (NK) cells via interferon-γ. Since CTL and NK cells are the most important in cellular immunity, interleukin 2 shows great promise as an agent through which the immune response can be regulated by a direct application in certain immune deficiency diseases or indirectly by growing antibodies and using them for the intermediate suppression of unwanted responses.

In the Federal Republic of Germany, a cooperative project on lymphokines and interferons is supported by the BMFT (Ministry of Research and Technology). Within the framework of this program a large-scale production of interleukin 2 is being performed at the GBF (Gesellschaft für Biotechnologische Forschung, Braunschweig), currently at the 10 L scale (cf. Bödeker, 1984). The clinical use of a highly purified preparation from this source has been reported.

Another lymphokine, the macrophage migration inhibition factor (MIF) is being obtained on the gram scale in the Organon laboratories (Oss, Netherlands). MIF takes part in allergic reactions and antibodies directed against MIF are used for their control.

A variety of **cellular and humoral factors,** formerly known as "mediators of inflammation" and "wound hormones", has been isolated by Wissler (1982) starting from porcine blood. A 50-fold repetition of a typical 200 L batch was used to obtain 10^{14} leukocytes (50 kg) which were subsequently cultured at a 1000 L scale to yield mg quantities of several mediators. Among these, the angiotropins, i.e., protein cytokines promoting the vascularization of tissues, may become important in wound treatment. Antibodies directed against them may become useful to prevent the vascularization of tumorous tissue.

Chalones are those substances which arrest the cell cycle of differentiated cells in the G1 phase. In cancer cells, this mechanism is put out of action. Chalones are tissue-specific peptides or peptide-factors upon the injection of which the regression of a number of tumors has been reported. Since tumors bind the mitotic regulators less well than normal tissues, another idea is also being followed: a region of tissue arrested in G1 would, with a lowering of the chalone concentration, selectively release the tumor cells into the S-phase, where these could be destroyed by a number of known S-phase poisons. Houck (1976) gives a review of the production of chalones, particularly from lymphocytes and he also gives a critical discussion of the use of this class of substances in cancer treatment. A more recent progress report has been given by Maurer (1982).

Interferons

The term "interferon" comprises three groups (IFN-α, -β and -γ) of species-specific cytokines which have in common an inhibitory action upon the multiplication of viruses in cells more or less adjacent to the affected ones. Because interferons have acted as pacemakers in the development of tissue culture technologies they are treated separately here.

Today, the **antiviral action of interferons** is well understood and interferon therapy is about to become routine in viral diseases like herpes zoster and virus encephalitis (Hofschneider and Obert, 1983). Without doubt, the greatest impact on interferon research has been made by some early findings that interferons may **inhibit tumor growth** through a chalone-like action in the G1 phase of the cell cycle, by activating the immune system (macrophages and natural killer cells) and possibly by affecting putative tumor viruses. Although the use of interferon in cancer therapy has been somewhat discouraged by toxic side effects of even the most highly purified preparations at the required concentrations (Scott et al., 1981), our present state of knowledge and technology is mostly due to its potential benefit in this area.

The current classification of interferons into IFN-α, IFN-β and IFN-γ (J. Immunol. **125**, 2353, 1980) roughly corresponds to the previous terms leukocyte, fibroblast, and immune interferon. Recombinant DNA techniques have so far shown that the α-family consists of 21 members of higly related species while only one sequence each has been identified for β- and γ-interferons. The formation of α- and β-interferons is induced by a viral infection which may be mimicked by a segment of double-stranded RNA. Being a lymphokine, γ-interferon is either induced by specific antigens or (for production purposes) by non-specific mitogens.

Until recently, the bulk of **α-interferon** has been obtained by the process of Cantell et al. (1974) from buffy coats (leukocyte pellets) which are available as a waste product from blood banks. The leukocytes can be brought into suspension (10^7 cells/mL) and induced to secrete interferon with Newcastle-disease or Sendai virus. This process can also be carried out in serum-free media which has advantages in the subsequent purification process (Rubinstein et al., 1979).

For a sum of $ 2.4 million the American Cancer Society (ACS) in 1978 acquired 4×10^{10} units of α-interferon, 30% of the annual production of the Public Health Laboratory in Helsinki, for clinical tests on 150 cancer patients. In 1980 this sum was increased by $ 3.4 millions for the continuation of studies and for technological improvements.

The specific disadvantages of the leukocyte system are:

1. The risks of contamination with viruses;
2. The limited capacity of the cell for division; and
3. The simultaneous synthesis of immunoglobulins which interfere with the application of the product has led to the development of alternative cell systems.

Continuous lymphoblastoid cell lines have the advantage of **unlimited subcultivatability.** The most important of these cell lines at the present time, Namalva, was established from the Burkitt tumor of an African child of this name, adapted to media with a low serum content, and deposited in the ATCC (No. CRL 1432).

A number of organizations — pharmaceutical companies as well as governmental institutions — are currently involved in developing processes for the large-scale production of lymphoblastoid (α-type) interferon (see contributors to Methods Enzymol. **78**, 1981, edited by S. Pestka). Important aspects to be considered for fermentation have been discussed in detail (Mizrahi, 1981). The Wellcome Foundation (Beckenham, U.K.) has reported production on the 1000 L scale (Johnston et al., 1979), already sufficient to satisfy a U.K. Medical Research Council sponsored trial in myelomatosis. Agreements with the Sumitomo Chemical Company have permitted the introduction of the Wellcome technology in Japan.

Like most transformed cell lines, Namalva first showed a very low interferon yield of 10 to 200 units/10^6 cells while 20 000 units can be obtained from the same number of diploid cells (Fig. 5-4). This made the conclusion obvious that the transformation is accompanied by **defects in the biosynthetic apparatus.** One of these defects could be traced to the molecular level (Bode et al., 1982, and references therein) and may be remedied by butyrate. In vitro, butyrate is suitable for stabilizing the low, and at the same time highly fluctuating, yields of interferon at a 10- to 60-fold higher level, which is comparable to that of diploid cells (Fig. 5-4). In the fermentation process, increases by a factor of 5 have been reported (Bodo, 1981).

Namalva cells carry two segments of the genome of the carcinogenic Epstein-Barr virus. Interferon from this source could therefore be approved for human clinical trials only after fulfilling strict regul-

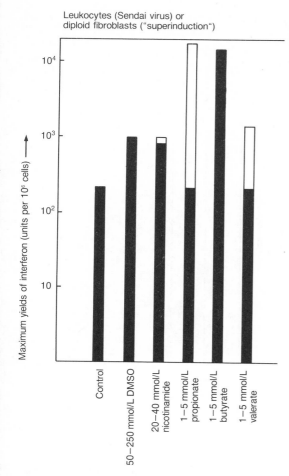

Leukocytes (Sendai virus) or
diploid fibroblasts ("superinduction")

Fig. 5-4. Increase in the yield of interferon by substances which permit a partial redifferentiation of the transformed cells. After results due to Adolf and Swetly (1979).

ations which comply with the guidelines published by the USA Food and Drug Administration (Petricciani, 1981). The most efficient purification step for interferon from this source, i.e. the application of affinity chromatography using monoclonal antibodies, has already been reported above (Secher and Burke, 1980). It is the most important step on the way to the pure product with about 10^9 units per mg of protein.

To date, the most common producers of **β-interferon** are still diploid fibroblasts, particularly the FS-4 cell line, which has a limited life span corresponding to about 30 passages.

Between 1974 and 1980, eleven institutions entered the field of the mass production of IFN-β (listed by van Damme and Billiau, 1981). The Searle and Abott Laboratories have expanded their production capacities in the expectation that the current costs of $ 50 for 10^5 units of interferon can be halved. Since April 1980, Searle interferon has been clinically tested on 30 cancer patients. In Germany, Bioferon (Laupheim), with the support of the BMFT, has developed a technology for producing IFN-β ("Fiblaferon"). The procedure is being developed further by using liquid two-phase systems developed at the GBF (Braunschweig) as an initial step in the large-scale purification process. Since 1978, 300 patients have been treated with Fiblaferon, and the results have clearly demonstrated that IFN-β has a spectrum of action differing from IFN-α (Hofschneider and Obert, 1982).

Fibroblasts of the FS-4 type require a charged support for their growth, a disadvantage when scaling up production of biologicals. While Bioferon has refined the application of multitray-systems (Joester and Pakos, 1982), a substantial improvement has also been reported by using the microcarrier system (Giard et al., 1979). In their hands, a 1 liter culture is capable of replacing at least 100 roller bottles. Utilizing their system in conjunction with a "superinduction" scheme, the cost-determining volume yields approached the levels obtained in suspension cultures (Fig. 5-5). Simultaneously, the time of liberating the maximum amount of interferon was reduced from 24 to 4 hours as a result of the altered cellular microenvironments. It has been reported that further refinements of the process could lower the manufacturing costs to 1/20 of the present level.

As for α-interferon, transformed continous cell lines also exist for the β-type. One of the best available strains, MG 63, was obtained from the osteosarcoma of a boy and has been deposited with the ATCC (CRL 1427). Probably because of polyploidy, MG 63 is superior

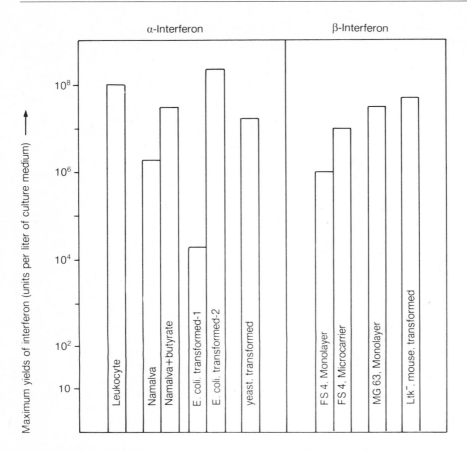

Fig. 5-5. Volume yields of α-interferons in suspension cultures from leukocytes, lymphoplastoid cells, transformed bacteria and yeasts and of β-interferon from monolayer and microcarrier cultures of fibroblast-like cells. After results due to Billiau et al. (1977), Derynck et al. (1980), Giard et al. (1979), Hauser et. al. (1982), Hitzemann et al. (1981), and Nagata et al. (1980).

in its output even to normal diploid cells (Fig. 5-5). The production of 4 to 8 × 10^8 units weekly of IFN-β in a pilot plant at the Rega Institute (University of Louvain, Belgium) has been reported (van Damme and Billiau, 1981).

Among oncologists, there is an increasing interest in **γ-interferon,** which is produced by B- or T-lymphocytes. Although yields are low on a per-cell basis, there are indications that

IFN-γ is 50 to 100 times more active than the other interferons in destroying tumor cells (Mizrahi, 1983) and a synergistic action of γ- and β-interferons has also been observed (Fleischmann et al., 1979). IFN-γ is currently being produced in short-term cultures of freshly isolated leukocytes and the techniques involved are closely related to the conventional ones used for IFN-α. The large-scale production of human immune interferon has been described by several groups (Mizrahi, 1983).

The manufacture of interferons presents one of the greatest current challenges for scientists of various disciplines (cell culture, protein laboratory synthesis, DNA synthesis, genetic engineering). There is hardly any other field that is being revolutionized to such an extent by the advent of **recombinant DNA techniques.**

The first report in this direction goes back to Weissmann and coworkers who succeeded in coupling one of the IFN-α genes with the *E.coli* genome to bring about interferon synthesis in bacteria (Nagata et al., 1980). The initial yield of 20 interferon units per mL (corresponding to two active molecules, probably of prointerferon, per bacterial cell) was far too low to compete with the existing processes but it was raised to 250 000 units in the very same year (Goeddel et al., 1980). Later on, cloned yeast cells became available as an alternative source. Today, large quantities of interferon from recombinant technologies are being supplied (Searle, Biogen, Dupont) for human clinical trials.

This success is, however, due to two particular properties of the IFN-α molecule. First, it is highly resistant to proteolysis and also to the procedures required for its liberation from the bacterial plasma and/or periplasmatic space. Second, its biological activity does not appear to depend on **glycosylation steps,** which cannot be performed correctly by bacteria; it is still a matter of discussion whether the major components of IFN-α are glycosylated at all (Bocci, 1983).

In contrast, the production of IFN-β in *E.coli* appears extremely difficult, although it is being exploited by Genentech and Cetus. The synthesis of 5000 IFN-β molecules per bacterial cell has been demonstrated (Taniguchi, 1980) but the recovered activity is rather modest (100 units per mL). There is agreement now that production of IFN-β in bacteria is not straightforward and that eucaryotic cells

are required to produce correctly glycosylated, fully active, interferon of this type. Considering this, the report by Hauser et al. (1982) that at least 50 copies of **the IFN-β gene** have successfully been **cloned into mouse Ltk⁻ (thymidine kinase negative) cells** by a thymidine kinase cotransformation technique and have been induced to a considerable level (Fig. 5-5) comes as a breakthrough. It combines the specific advantages of a mammalian cell (secretion of a correctly modified glycoprotein directly into the medium; repeated inducibility) with the advances of genetic engineering (high number of gene copies, unlimited possibilities of varying sequences), opening up an entirely new field for cell culturing technologies.

Since the mechanism of interferon induction is beginning to be understood, there is also hope that animal cells with a constitutive (not needing induction) production of interferon will become available in the near future. This goal may be aided by totally synthetic genes for the major types of interferon which are already at hand.

As for IFN-γ, the situation appears closely related to IFN-β. Gene expression has been achieved both in engineered *E.coli* and in monkey cells (Gray et al., 1982) but it was possible to recover only 8 to 80 active molecules per bacterial cell. IFN-γ is the most labile among the interferons and probably possesses two glycosylation sites. Therefore the animal cell system may prove superior also in this case.

According to estimates of American investment firms, interferon could achieve a market of $ 750 millions in the USA within three to five years and one of as much as $ 200 millions worldwide. Interferon would therefore in the foreseeable future advance into the order of magnitude of the antibiotics market (annually $ 15 thousand millions worldwide). In the USA, the proportion of interferon in cancer therapies could rise to 2/3 ($ 170 millions) and it could replace about half the conventional steroid treatments in chronic inflammations such as arthritis (\$ 300 millions). In the field of viral diseases, it could open up a market of \$ 270 millions.

Polypeptide Hormones

Classical studies in this field used the GH (growth hormone) strain of rat cells which was established in 1965 from a hypophyseal tumor (Yasumara et al., 1966). Clonal strains of this origin (ATCC, No. CCL 82 and 82.1) have retained their levels of production of prolactin and growth hormone, respectively, during 75 passages, 1 liter of suspension yielding 1 mg of hormone per day. This demonstrates that tumor cells may retain some differentiated functions opening the way to a technical application of such systems.

The species specificity of many polypeptide hormones makes it necessary to develop highly productive strains of human origin, of which, however, only a few have so far been described. Thus, **calcitocin**-secreting cell lines from thyroid tumors ceased their growth after a few months. A cell line "BeWo" (ATCC No. CCL 98) from a placental tumor is available which efficiently secretes **human chorionic gonadotropin** (HCG). It represents the only bulk producing source for a human hormone that has been established *in vitro*. A cell line from a kidney carcinoma secreting **erythropoietin** has not acquired the same importance since the optimum conditions for cultivation have yet to be worked out (Ogle, 1978).

The availability of both human insulin and human growth hormone from engineered bacteria has discouraged the corresponding attempts to establish human cell lines for *in vitro* production purposes. However, a solution has been suggested for achieving a physiological way of administering insulin. The proposal is based on the observation that protection of grafted cells with artificial membranes prevents immune rejection while permitting the diffusion of insulin. Hollow fiber systems have been constructed that enclose beta cells in order to obtain an artificial pancreas that senses and responds to glucose levels (Puchinger et al., 1982; Rolly et al., 1982). Clearly, much basic research has to be done before these systems can be used in human medicine but already today they appear as a realistic alternative to electromechanical devices including a glucose sensor, an information processor, and an insulin delivery mechanism.

Enzymes

A number of enzymes are used therapeutically. In order to circumvent problems of immunity, it is preferable to use homologous enzymes which, again, are basically available through cell culture techniques. As in the case of the hormones, however, only the first beginnings can be reported in this field.

Urokinase (plasminogen activator) is a medically important protease for the treatment of thromboses and embolisms. Previously, 1500 L of urine had to be worked up for a single dose. Findings that this fibrinolytic substance can be obtained from kidney cell cultures from human fetuses have promoted the development of technological processes for its isolation and have now made clinical application possible (Lewis, 1979). The production of urokinase from a continuous line of porcine kidney cells (LLC-PK$_1$; ATCC, No. CL 101) has been patented by the Lilly Research Laboratories (US Patent 3 904 480, 1975).

5.3.4   Prospects

After a phase of active basic research, processes and cell lines are available today which permit products to be obtained from cells of animal and human origin. While in the past species-specific proteins and peptides for human clinical use could be isolated only from human glands, serum or urine, the advance of new cell culture technology is now opening up entirely new sources. On the one hand, mammalian cells can be **used directly** for the production of the required compound by **fermentation** processes. Alternatively, they may play an **intermediate role** for obtaining the **genetic message** of interest to be used for recombinant DNA technologies with bacteria or eucaryotic cells as recipients. The best prospect for obtaining a correctly processed and postsynthetically modified protein are given if the **gene is introduced into an immortalized cell** of the type which in the living organism secretes the desired products. Signal sequences will be recognized by such a cell which will then deliver the molecule to the medium from where it can be recovered under quasi-physiological conditions.

McLimans (1976) has predicted that animal cells will achieve and even surpass the importance of bacteria in the industry. Cell factories for the manufacture of blood cells are just as conceivable as the production of transplants or artificial organs. The present report has shown that a considerable part of his predictions has already been realized. Some of the crucial hurdles in the mass cultivation of animal cells have already been taken. Before the introduction of membrane-perfusion and, particularly, of microcarrier systems, the microenvironments of cells growing on glass or plastic surface could be controlled only inadequately (Jensen, 1981; Feder and Tolbert, 1983). With microcarriers, cultivation of anchorage-dependent cells can be reduced to the principles of suspension culture, so that a transfer from the laboratory scale to the production scale no longer requires the development of radically different concepts. While the pharmaceutical industry is promoting such developments rapidly, details are hardly available.

My thanks are therefore due to Dr. McLimans (Roswell Park Memorial Cancer Institute, Buffalo,

N.Y.), Dr. R. T. Acton (Cell Culture Center, University of Alabama, Birmingham), Dr. van Wezel (Rijksinstituut voor de Volksgesondheit, Bilthoven), Dr. J. Clark (Pharmacia, Uppsala) and Dr. Meignier (Iffa-Mérieux, Lyon) for valuable information and data which have greatly facilitated the writing of this chapter.

5.3.5   Literature: Animal Cell Cultures

There are several standard text in the field which are referred to extensively in the above article. These books permit a detailed insight into the current state of cell culture techniques and therefore are quoted separately under A.

A   Review Literature

[1] Acton, R. T. and Lynn, J. D.: *Cell Culture and its Application*. Academic Press, New York 1977.
[2] Jakoby, W. B. and Pastan, I. H., *Methods Enzymol.* **58** (1979).
[3] Kruse, P. F. and Patterson, M. K.: *Tissue Culture, Methods and Applications*. Academic Press, New York 1973.
[4] Adams, R. L. P.: *Cell Culture for Biochemists*. Elsevier/North-Holland, 1980.
[5] Paul, J.: *Zell- und Gewebekulturen*. deGruyter, Berlin, New York 1980.
[6] BMFT[(German) Federal Ministry for Research and Technology]-Statusseminar: Tierische Zellkulturen, Bonn 1982.

B   Special Literature
(The figures in square brackets relate to the review literature.)

Acton, R. T., Barstad, P. A. and Zwerner, R. K.: "Propagation and scaling-up of suspension cultures". In: [2], 211–221 (1979).
Adolf, G. R. and Swetly, P., "Interferon production by human lymphoblastoid cells is stimulated by inducers of friend cell differentiation", *Virology* **99**, 158–166 (1979).
Ahmad, F., Russel, T. R., Schultz, J. and Werner, R.: *Differentiation and Development*. Academic Press, New York 1978.

Allen, G. and Fantes, K. H., "A family of structural genes for human lymphoblastoid (leukocyte-type) interferon", *Nature* **287**, 408–416 (1980).

Aoiki, F. Y., Tyrrell, D. A. S. and Hill, L. E., "Immunogenicity and acceptability of a human diploid cell culture rabies vaccine in volunteers", *Lancet* **1975**, 660–662.

Barkley, W. E.: "Safety considerations in the cell culture laboratory". In: [2], 36–43 (1979).

Barnes, D. and Sato, G., "Methods for growth of cultured cells in serum-free medium", *Anal. Biochem.* **102**, 255–270 (1980).

Barstad, P. A., Henley, S. L., Cox, R. M., Lynn, J. D. and Acton, R. T., "Production of milligram quantities of H-2k and Thy-1 alloantigens by large-scale mammalian cell culture", *Proc. Soc. Exp. Biol. Med.* **155**, 296–300 (1977).

Berman, J., Perantoni, A., Jackson, H. M. and Kingsbury, E., "Primary epithelial cell culture of adult rat kidney, enhancement of cell growth by ammonium acetate", *Exp. Cell Res.* **121**, 47–54 (1979).

Bocci, V., "What is the role of carbohydrates in interferons?", *Trends Biochem. Sci.* **8**, 432–434 (1983).

Bödecker, B. G. D., Lehmann, J., v. Damme, J., Kappmeyer, H., Gassel, W. D., Havemann, K., Schwulera, U., Rühl, F. and Mühlradt, P. F., "Production of five human lymphokines (granulocyte-macrophage colony stimulation factor, interferon-γ, interleukin-2, macrophage cytotoxicity factor, and macrophage migration inhibitory factor) from Con A stimulated lymphocyte cultures in bioreactors", *Immunbiology,* in press.

Bode, J., Hochkeppel, H. K. and Maaß, K., "Links between the effects of butyrate on histone hyperacetylation and regulation of interferon synthesis in Namalva and FS-4 cell lines", *J. Interferon Res.* **2**, 159–166 (1982).

Bodo, G., "Procedures for large-scale production and partial purification of human interferon from lymphocyte (Namalva) cultures", *Methods Enzymol.* **78**, 69–75 (1981).

Boge, A.: "Entwicklung von chemisch definierten Kulturmedien zur industriellen Stoffproduktion". In: [6], 421–425 (1982).

Cantell, K. and Hirvonen, S., "Preparation of human leukocyte interferon for clinical use", *Tex. Rep. Biol. Med.* **35**, 138–144 (1977).

Ceccarini, C., "Effect of pH on plating efficiency, serum requirement and incorporation of radioactive precursors into human cells", *In Vitro* **11**, 78–86 (1975).

Chen, T. R., "In situ detection of mycoplasma contamination in cell cultures by fluorescent Hoechst 33258 Stain", *Exp. Cell Res.* **104**, 255–262 (1977).

Corbeil, M. B., Marchess, F. and Trudel, M., "Efficient large-scale cell-culture system using media circulation and roller bottle principle", *In Vitro* **13**, 177 (1977).

Cosimi, A. B., Colvin, R. B., Burton, R. C., Rubin, R. H., Goldstein, G., Kung, P. C., Hansen, W. P., Delmonico, F. L. and Russel, P. S., "Use of monoclonal antibodies to T-cell subsets for immunologic monitoring and treatment in recipients of renal allografts", *New England J. Med.* **305**, 308–313 (1981).

Crespi, C. L., Imamura, T., Moi Leong, P., Fleischaker, R. J., Brunengraber, H. and Thilly, W. G., "Microcarrier culture: applications in biologicals production and cell biology", *Biotechnol. Bioeng.* **23**, 2673–2689 (1981).

Croce, C. M., Linnenbach, A., Hall, W., Steplewski, Z. and Koprowski, H., "Production of human hybridomas secreting antibodies to measles virus", *Nature* **288**, 488–489 (1980).

v. Damme, J. and Billiau, A., "Large-scale production of human fibroblast interferon", *Methods Enzymol.* **78**, 101–119 (1981).

Davies, P. F. and Kerr, C., "Co-cultivation of vascular endothelial and smooth muscle cells using microcarrier techniques", *Exp. Cell Res.* **141**, 455–459 (1982).

Diamond, L., O'Brian, T. G. and Rovera, G., "Tumor Promoters: Effects on proliferation and differentiation of cells in culture", *Life Sci.* **23**, 1979–1988 (1978).

Edwards, D. C. and Thorpe, R. E., "Targeting toxins – the retiarian approach to chemotherapy", *Trends Biochem. Sci.* **6**, 313–316 (1981).

Feder, J. and Tolbert, W. R., "The large-scale cultivation of mammalian cells", *Sci. Am.* **248** (1), 24–31 (1983).

Fleischmann, W. R., Georgiades, J. A., Osborne, L. C. and Johnson, H. M., "Potentiation of interferon activity by mixed preparations of fibroblast and immune interferon", *Infect. Immun.* **26**, 248–253 (1979).

Giard, D. J., Loeb, D. H., Thilly, W. G., Wang, D. I. C. and Levine, D. W., "Human interferon production with diploid fibroblast cells grown on microcarriers", *Biotechnol. Bioeng.* **21**, 433–442 (1979).

Gilbert, S. F. and Migeon, B. R., "D-Valine as a selective agent for normal human and rodent epithelial cells in culture", *Cell* **5**, 11–17 (1975).

Girard, H. C.: "Problems encountered in large-scale cell production plants". In: [1], 111–128 (1977).

Goeddel, D. V., Yeverton, E., Ullrich, A., Heyneker, H. L., Miozzari, G., Holmes, W., Seeburg, P. H., Dull, T., May, L., Stebbing, N., Crea, R., Maeda, S., McCandliss, R., Sloma, A., Tabor, J. M., Gross, M., Familletti, P. C. and Pestka, S., "Human leukocyte interferon produced by *E.coli* is biologically active", *Nature* **287**, 411–416 (1980).

Gray, P. W., Leung, D. W., Pennica, D., Yelverton, E., Najarian, R., Simonsen, C. C., Derynck, R., Sherwood, P. J., Wallace, D. M., Berger, S. L., Levinson, A. D. and Goeddel, D. V., "Expression of human immune interferon cDNA in *E.coli* and monkey cells", *Nature* **295**, 503–508 (1982).

Ham, G. and McKeehan, L.: "Media and growth requirements". In: [2], 44–93 (1979).

Hayflick, L., "Cell Biology of Aging", *Fed. Proc. Fed. Am. Soc. Exp. Biol.* **38**, 1847–1850 (1979).

zur Hausen, H.: "Wege zur Antigenproduktion pathogener Herpesviren". In: [6], 365–372 (1981).

Hauser, H., Gross, G., Bruns, W., Hochkeppel, H. K., Mayr, U. and Collins, J., "Inducibility of human β-interferon gene in mouse L-cell clones", *Nature* **297**, 650–654 (1982).

Hillmann, M. R., "Line cell saga – an argument in favor of production of biologicals in cancer cells", *Adv. Exp. Med. Biol.* **118**, 47–58 (1978).

Hirtenstein, M., Clark, J., Lindgren, G. and Vretblad, P., "Microcarriers for animal cell culture: a brief review of theory and practice", *Dev. Biol. Stand.* **46**, 109–116 (1980).

Hofschneider, P. H. and Obert, H.-J., "Stand klinischer Interferonstudien in der Bundesrepublik Deutschland", *Münch. Med. Wochenschr.* **124**, 911–914 (1982).

Houck, J. C.: *Chalones.* North Holland, 1976.

House, W., "Control measures in cell culture laboratory", *Lab. Pract.* **17**, 587–590 (1968).

House, W.: "Bulk culture of cell monolayers". In: [3], 338–344 (1973).

Inglot, A. D., "Use of polyethylene glycol-treated calf serum for cell cultures in virus and interferon studies", *Acta Virol.* **19**, 250–254 (1975).

Jensen, M. D., "Production of anchorage-dependent cells – problems and their possible solutions", *Biotechnol. Bioeng.* **23**, 2703–2716 (1981).

Joester, K. E. and Pakos, V.: "Produktion von Fibroblasten-Interferon". In: [6], 59–77 (1982).

Johnston, M. D., Christofinis, G., Ball, G. D., Fantes, K. H. and Finter, N. B., "A cell culture system for producing large amounts of human lymphoblastoid interferon", *Dev. Biol. Stand.* **42**, 189–192 (1979).

Kaighn, M. E., "Birth of a culture", *J. Nat. Cancer Inst.* **53**, 1437–1442 (1974).

Kaneko, H. and Goshima, K., "Selective killing of fibroblast-like cells in cultures of mouse heart cells by treatment with a Ca ionophore, A 23187", *Exp. Cell Res.* **142**, 407–416 (1982).

Keay, L. "Serum-free media for animal cell culture", *Process Biochem.* **14**, 28–32 (1979).

Keay, L. and Burton, C. W., "Recent advances in the technology of animal cell production", *Process Biochem.* **14**, 17–21 (1979).

Köhler, G. and Milstein, C., "Continous cultures of fused cells secreting antibodies of predefined specificity", *Nature* **256**, 495–497 (1975).

Kucherlapati, R. S., Creagan, R. P. and Ruddle, F. H.: "Progress in human gene mapping by somatic cell hybridization". In: Busch, H. (ed.): *The Cell Nucleus,* Vol. II. Academic Press, 1974, pp. 209–222.

Lambert, K. and Pirt, S. J., "The quantitative requirements of human diploid cells for amino acids, vitamins and serum", *J. Cell Sci.* **17**, 397–411 (1975).

Levine, D. W., Wang, D. I. C. and Thilly, W. G., "Optimization of growth surface parameters in microcarrier cell culture", *Biotechnol. Bioeng.* **21**, 821–845 (1979).

Lewis, L. J., "Plasminogen activator (urokinase) from cultured cells", *Thromb. Haemostasis* **42**, 895–900 (1979).

Lynn, J. D. and Acton, R. T., "Design of a large

scale suspension culture facility", *Biotechnol. Bioeng.* **17,** 659–673 (1975).

Mc Coy, T. A., Maxwell, M. and Kruse, P. F., "Amino acid requirements of the Novikoff hepatoma in vitro", *Proc. Soc. Exp. Biol. Med.* **100,** 115–123 (1959).

McLimans, W. F., Gailani, S. and Horng, C. B.: "Perspectives of mass culture and the mammalian cell". W. Alton Jones Cell Science Center Workshop (1976).

Maroudas, N. G., "Adhesion and spreading of cells on charged surfaces", *J. Theor. Biol.* **49,** 417–424 (1973).

Matsumura, T., Yamanaka, T., Hashizuma, S., Irie, T. and Nitta, K., "Tissue dispersion, cell harvest and fluid suspension culture by use of bacterial neutral protease", *Jap. J. Exp. Med.* **45,** 377–382 (1975).

Maurer, H. R.: "Das Lymphozyten-Chalon: Isolierung, Reinigung und Testung sowie potentielle pharmazeutische Bedeutung". In: [6], 271–289 (1982).

Meignier, B., Mongeot, H. and Faure, H.: *Foot and mouth disease virus production on microcarrier-grown cells.* House Publication Iffa Mérieux, Lyon 1979.

Merchant, D. J., Kahn, R. H. and Murphy, W. H.: *Handbook of Cell and Organ Culture.* Burgess, 1965.

Mered, B., Albrecht, P. and Hopps, H. E., "Cell growth optimization in microcarrier culture", *In vitro* **16,** 859–865 (1980).

Milstein, C. and Cuello, A. C., "Hybrid hybridomas and their use in immunohistochemistry", *Nature* **305,** 537–539 (1983).

Mitchell, K. J. and Wray, W., "Mitotic cell population obtained from a microcarrier culturing system", *Exp. Cell Res.* **123,** 452–455 (1979).

Mizrahi, A., Reuveni, S., Traub, A. and Minai, M., "Large-scale production of human lymphoblastoid (Namalva) interferon", *Biotechnol. Lett.* **2,** 267–271 (1980).

Mizrahi, A., "Production of human lymphoblastoid interferon", *Methods Enzymol.* **78,** 54–68 (1981).

Mizrahi, A., "Production of human interferon – an overview", *Process Biochem.* **8,** 9–12 (1983).

Moffat, M. A. J., "Cell culture in diagnostic medical virology", *Lab. Pract.* **17,** 576–582 (1968).

Moore, G. E., Hasenpusch, P., Gerner, R. E. and Burns, A. A., "A pilot plant for mammalian cell culture", *Biotechnol. Bioeng.* **10,** 625–640 (1968).

Moore, G. E., "Cultured human lymphocytes", *J. Surg. Oncol.* **4,** 320–352 (1972).

Murakami, H., Masui, H., Sato, G. H., Sueka, N., Chow, T. P. and Kano-Sueoka, "Growth of hybridoma cells in serum-free medium: Ethanolamine is an essential compound", *Proc. Natl. Acad. Sci. USA* **79,** 1158–1162 (1982).

Nagata, S., Traira, H., Hall, A., Johnsrud, L., Streuli, M., Ecsödi, J., Boll, W., Cantell, K. and Weissmann, C., "Synthesis in *E.coli* of a polypeptide with human leukocyte interferon activity", *Nature* **284,** 316–320 (1980).

Ogle, J. W., Lange, R. D. and Dunn, D. R., "Production of erythropoietin in vitro: A review", *In Vitro* **14,** 945–950 (1978).

Pastan, I. H.: "Cell transformation". In: [2], 368–370 (1979).

Perlman, D.: "Use of antibiotics in cell culture media". In: [2], 110–115 (1979).

Petricciani, J. C.: "Points to be considered in the production and testing of interferon intended for investigational use in humans. Manuscript published by the Dept. of Health, Education and Welfare, Bethesda 1980, pp. 104–114.

Pollard, R. and Khosrovi, B., "Reactor design for fermentation of fragile tissue cells", *Process Biochem.* **13,** 31–37 (1978).

Puchinger, H., Müller, U. and Erhardt, "Insulinbiosynthese mit Pankreaszellen in Membranperfusionssystemen". In: [6], 25–35 (1982).

Ritz, J. and Schlossmann, S. F., "Utilization of monoclonal antibodies in the treatment of leukemia and lymphoma", *Blood* **59,** 1–11 (1982).

Rolly, H., Pünter, J. and v. Kalinowski, H.: "Untersuchungen zur Kultivierung insulinproduzierender B-Zellen". In: [6], 37–50 (1982).

Rubinstein, M., Rubinstein, S., Familetti, P. C., Miller, R. S., Waldman, A. A. and Pestka, S., "Human leucocyte interferon: Production, purification to homogeneity, and initial characterization", *Proc. Natl. Acad. Sci. USA* **76,** 640–644 (1979).

Salmon, S. E., Alberts, D. S., Meyskens, F. L., Durie, B. G. M., Jones, S. E., Soehnlen, B., Young, L., Chen, G. H. S. and Moon, T. E.: "Clinical correlations of in-vitro drug sensitivity". In: *Cloning of Human Tumor Stem Cells.* Alan R. Liss, New York 1980, pp. 223–253.

Schlom, J., Wunderlich, D. and Teramoto, Y. A., "Generation of human monoclonal antibodies reactive with human mammary carcinoma cells", *Proc. Natl. Acad. Sci. USA* 77, 6841–6845 (1980).

Scott, G. M., Secher, D. S., Flowers, D., Bate, J., Cantell, K. and Tyrell, D. A. J., "Toxicity of interferon", *Clin. Res.* 282, 1345–1348 (1981).

Secher, D. S. and Burke, D. C., "A monoclonal antibody for large scale purification of human leukocyte interferon", *Nature* 285, 446–448 (1980).

Smith, R. E. and Kozoman, F.: "Device for automatic rapid harvest of roller culture supernatant fluid", *Appl. Microbiol.,* 25, 1008–1010 (1973).

Sonneborn, H. H., Schwulera, U., Lohmann-Mattes, M. L., Otz, U. and de Weck, A. L.: "Gewinnung und Reinigung von Lymphokinen aus Lymphozytenkulturen humanen Ursprungs für Diagnostik und Therapie". In: [6], 91–113 (1982).

Sun, N. C., Sun, C. R. Y., Tennant, R. W. and Hsie, A. W., "Selective growth of some rodent epithelial cells in a medium containing citrulline", *Proc. Natl. Acad. Sci. USA* 76, 1819–1823 (1979).

Taniguchi, T., Guarente, L., Roberts, T. M., Kimelman, D., Douhan, J. and Ptashne, M., "Expression of human fibroblast interferon gene in *Escherichia coli*", *Proc. Natl. Acad. Sci. USA* 77, 5230–5233 (1980).

Thilly, W. G. and Levine, D. W.: "Microcarrier culture: A homogenous environment for studies of cellular biochemistry". In: [2], 184–194 (1979).

Thornton, B., Griffiths, J. B. and Walkland, A., "Herpes simplex virus vaccine using cell membrane-associated antigen in an animal model", *Abstr. Joint IABS-ESACT Meeting, Heidelberg* (1981).

Thompson, R. J., "Are monoclonal antibodies the end of radioimmunoassay?", *Trends Biochem. Sci.* 7, 418–420 (1982).

Tint, H., Stone, J. L., Minecci, L. C. and Rubin, B. A., "Type 4 adenovirus vaccine, live, prepared in human diploid cell system for oral administration", *Prog. Immunobiol. Stand.* 3, 113–122 (1969).

Tobey, R. A., Walters, R. A., Hohmann, P. G., Hildebrand, C. E. and Gurley, L. R.: "Sequential biochemical events in the cell cycle". In: [1], 5–22 (1977).

Valenti, C.: "Diagnostic use of cell cultures initiated from amniocentesis". In: [3], 617–622 (1973).

Voigt, W. D. and Maurer, H. R., "Kryokonservierung von Lymphozyten unter Verwendung von Polyethylenglykolen hohen Polymerisationsgrades", *Blut* 43, 257–264 (1981).

Wassermann, O.: "Anwendung von Zellkulturen in der Toxikologie als Ergänzung zu Tierversuchen". In: [6], 429–447 (1982).

van Wezel, A. L., van Steenis, G., Hannik, C. A. and Cohen, H., "New approach to the production of concentrated and purified inactivated polio and rabies tissue culture vaccines". *Dev. Biol. Stand.* 41, 159–168 (1978).

van Wezel, A. L., van der Marel, P., van Beveren, C., Verma, I. and Salk, J., "Detection and elimination of cellular nucleic acids in biologicals from continous cell lines", *Abstr. Joint IABS-ESACT Meeting, Heidelberg* (1981).

Wissler, J. H.: Vollsynthetisches Zellkulturmedium. D.O.S. DE 31 105 599 (1981), pp. 1–23.

Wissler, J. H.: "Biotechnik der Gewinnung leukozytärer Entzündungsmediatoren und Wundhormone". In: [6], 293–303 (1982).

Yasumura, Y., Tashjian, A. H. and Sato, G. H., "Establishment of four functional clonal strains of animal cells in culture", *Science* 154, 1186–1189 (1966).

Zwerner, R. K., Cox, R. M., Lynn, J. D. and Acton, R. R., "Five year perspective of the large-scale growth of mammalian cells in suspension culture", *Biotechnol. Bioeng.* 23, 2717–2735 (1981).

Chapter 6

Bioreactors

Karl Schügerl and Wolfgang Sittig

6.1   Introduction

In a bioreactor, the **transformation of raw materials into desired products** is carried out by the enzyme systems of living microorganisms or by isolated enzymes.

The cells continuously strive by modifying their environment to achieve and maintain the **optimal conditions** for their growth. In a bioreactor, this tendency of the cells is assisted. The reactor has the task of ensuring the **supplying of the cells** with the means for growth or for the production of metabolites, i.e., of guaranteeing as far as possible the optima of the temperature and the pH and a sufficient supply of substrate, nutrient salts, vitamins, and oxygen (see Chapters 2 and 3).

The optimum conditions for the selected strain must be determined experimentally. This is carried out in the laboratory, frequently in shake cultures (Fig. 6-1). However, these have the disadvantage that their pH value and the concentration of dissolved oxygen cannot, as a rule, be controlled. Consequently, only the optimum **temperature and composition of the nutrient solution** and the **supplementation of the substrate** in them can be determined. The optimization of the **pH** and of the **concentration of dissolved oxygen** in the medium is generally carried out in small **laboratory reactors** which should be provided with a pH control and, if possible, with stirrer speed and gas flow measurement.

To find the optimum conditions for the enzyme reactions, the same laboratory units can be used as for fermentations. The **products** of these biochemical reactions must be separated from the medium, purified, and, if necessary, processed further. The unconverted or unconsumed components of the medium and the intermediate products and by-products must be utilized elsewhere or be disposed of without harming the environment.

The total manufacturing process must be carried out in such a way that when all the boundary conditions are satisfied the product is competitive with respect both to **quality** and **price**. Since, in general, an increase in the production capacity of a unit low-ers both the product-specific investment costs and the variable costs, attempts are made to erect large **single-line units.** In the case of fermentation products, this economic drive leads to large fermenters. This requires knowledge on the design of large reactors. The information obtained in small units is not adequate for large scale design, since the fluid dynamics, the transport processes, and even the behavior of the cells may change considerably (e.g., by an intensification of turbulence) when the size of the unit is increased. For these reasons, the **laws** that operate in the geometric enlargement of a reactor should be known. Because of the absence of this information, **pilot plants** have to be constructed which subdivide the large step of this "scaling-up" procedure between laboratory and production units in order to reduce the risk involved in the design of the production unit.

Most of the information that is discussed below was obtained on **small pilot plants.** Only a few results from industrial demonstration plants have been published.

In process engineering, the passage from the model to the production unit can often be facilitated with the aid of **similarity theory.** In general, this theory can be used to only a limited extent in chemical and biochemical reactors, since when the unit is enlarged the geometric similarity is not necessarily matched by that of fluid motion and mass transfer of the individual transport processes. If, however, a single parameter is rate-determining, similarity theory can be very helpful in the calculation of reactors.

Similarity theory deals with the criteria which permit a calculation of the performance of a system on the large scale based on small scale model experiments. For each elementary process, the process-determining factors can be comprised within a characteristic number which must remain constant during the enlargement of the reactor if the similarity between the laboratory and the pilot reactors (or between the pilot and production reactors) in relation to this process is to be preserved. If this similarity exists, the results that were obtained on laboratory or pilot reactor scale can be used for the production reactors, also.

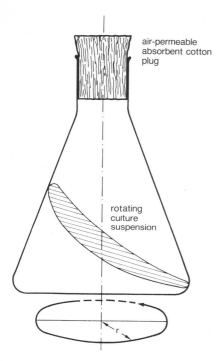

air-permeable absorbent cotton plug

rotating culture suspension

Fig. 6-1. Erlenmeyer shaking flask. $2r$ = amplitude of shaking; volumes 50 to 2000 mL; degree of filling ⩽ 20%.

In order to reduce the number of variables these quantities are brought together according to definite rules to form dimensionless characteristic numbers (dimensional analysis). The results found in the laboratory or pilot reactor are then correlated by a combination of these characteristic numbers.

In this handbook, also, use is made of similarity theory and dimensional analysis by correlating the results as the products of the relevant characteristic numbers.

Before the mode of operation (discontinuous, continuous, semicontinuous), the type, the size, and the operating conditions of the reactor are deter-

mined, a preliminary choice must be made of the mode of operation and of the type of reactor, which are predetermined by the organisms used, the media, the characteristics of the biochemical process, and the site. The mode of operation and the type of the reactors for enzymatic transformations are affected by a comparatively small number of properties (molecular mass, stability) of the enzyme. To discuss these questions quantitatively, some basic concepts must first be defined.

6.2 Basic Concepts

6.2.1 Batch Operation

The cultivation begins at time $t = 0$ and is stopped at time $t = t'$. At first the proliferation of the cells takes place under nonlimiting conditions. After a higher cell density is reached, it passes into substrate- (nutrient- or oxygen-) -limited operation.

Particularly for oxygen, which is consumed very rapidly, a continuous supply to the medium must be guaranteed so that its concentration does not fall (see Table 6-1).

6.2.2 "Extended Culture" Operation

The term "extended culture" describes the mode of operating a reactor in which the concentration of the limiting substrate is kept constant by supplying it continuously (see Table 6-1).

6.2.3 Continuous Operation

A continuous stream of nutrient solution is supplied to the reactor and this is matched by the discharge of a harvesting stream of approximately the same magnitude. A steady

Table 6-1. Basic Concepts.

Conditions	Rate of growth		Consumption of substrate		Productivity	
Batch, unlimited	$r_X = \dfrac{dx}{dt} = \mu_m \cdot X$	[1]	$-r_S = -\dfrac{dS}{dt} = \dfrac{1}{Y_S}\dfrac{dX}{dt} = \dfrac{1}{Y_S}\mu_m \cdot X$	[2]	$PR = \dfrac{dX}{dt} = \mu_m \cdot X$	[3]
substrate-limited	$\mu = \mu_m \cdot \dfrac{S}{K_S + S}$	[4]	$-r_S = \dfrac{1}{Y_S}\cdot \mu_m \cdot \dfrac{S}{K_S+S}\cdot X$	[5]	$PR = \mu \cdot X$	[6]
oxygen-limited	$\mu = \mu_m \cdot \dfrac{C_{O_2}}{K_O + C_{O_2}}$	[4a]	$-r_{O_2} = \dfrac{1}{Y_O}\cdot \mu_m \cdot \dfrac{C_{O_2}}{K_O+C_{O_2}}\cdot X$	[5a]	$PR = \mu \cdot X$	
Extended culture, substrate-limited	$\mu = \mu_m \cdot \dfrac{S}{K_S + S}$	[7]	$q_S = \dfrac{dX}{dt}\cdot\dfrac{1}{Y_S}$	[8]	$PR = \dfrac{dX}{dt} = q_S \cdot Y_S$	[9]
Continuous, unlimited	$\mu = \mu_m$	[10]	$D(S_0 - S_1) = \dfrac{1}{Y_S}\mu_m \cdot X_1$	[11]	$PR = \mu_m \cdot X_1 = D \cdot X_1$	[12]
substrate-limited	$\mu = \mu_m \cdot \dfrac{S_1}{K_S + S_1}$	[13]	$D(S_0-S_1) = \dfrac{1}{Y_S}\cdot \mu_m \cdot \dfrac{S_1}{K_S+S_1}\cdot X_1$	[14]	$PR = \mu_m \cdot \dfrac{S_1}{K_S+S_1}\cdot X_1$	[15]
oxygen-limited	$\mu = \mu_m \cdot \dfrac{C_{O_2}}{K_O + C_{O_2}}$	[13a]	$D(S_0-S_1) = \dfrac{1}{Y_S}\cdot \mu_m \cdot \dfrac{C_{O_2}}{K_O+C_{O_2}}\cdot X_1$	[14a]	$PR = \mu_m \cdot \dfrac{C_{O_2}}{K_O+C_{O_2}}\cdot X_1$	[15a]

r = rate of growth of the cells (g L^{-1} h^{-1})
X = concentration of the dry biomass (g L^{-1})
μ = specific rate of growth (h^{-1})
t = time of cultivation (h)
K = Monod's saturation constant (g L^{-1})
PR = productivity (g L^{-1} h^{-1})

Y = yield coefficient (g g^{-1})
S = substrate conc. (g L^{-1})
C_{O_2} = oxygen conc. (g L^{-1})
q_S = rate of feed of substrate (g L^{-1} h^{-1})

S = substrate
X = cell mass
O = oxygen
m = maximum

state is reached with a theoretically constant cell density and constant concentrations (see Table 6-1).

6.2.4 Production of Heat During Cell Growth

During the growth of the cells, the following amount of heat is generated

$$Q_z = \frac{1}{Y_{kJ}} \mu X \quad \left(\text{in } \frac{kJ}{h \, L}\right) \tag{6-16}$$

where Y_{kJ} is the heat yield coefficient (in $g \, kJ^{-1}$):

$$Y_{kJ} = \frac{Y_S}{\Delta H_S - Y_S \Delta H_X} \tag{6-17}$$

ΔH_S and ΔH_X are the heats of combustion of the substrate or of the cells, given in $kJ \, g^{-1}$.

The energy demand and the production of heat for cultivation can be estimated satisfactorily (Solomons, 1964; Lewis, 1976).

6.2.5 Stirring Power

In **ungassed liquids,** the relations given in Table 6-2 apply. The Reynolds numbers (Re) are different for vessels with and without baffles.

The constants given were determined by a model experiment. The knowledge of the stirring power demand of an ungassed medium is important for the operation of the bioreactor during sterilization and also for enzyme reactors.

Calculation of Viscosity

In non-Newtonian liquids, the representative viscosity η_r is frequently used:

$$\eta_r = \frac{\tau_S}{\left(\dfrac{du}{dx}\right)} \tag{6-18}$$

here: τ_S is the shear stress and $\left(\dfrac{du}{dx}\right)$ the mean shear gradient.

For calculation of the mean shear gradient the following two approximations are most frequently used: the Metzner-Otto relation (Metzner and Otto, 1957):

$$\left(\frac{du}{dx}\right) = k^* \, n \tag{6-19}$$

where k^* is an empirical constant ($k^* \sim 11$) which depends only slightly on the type of stirrer and on d/d_T (Metzner et al., 1961), or the Calderbank–Moo-Young relation (Calderbank and Moo-Young, 1959):

Table 6-2. Calculation of Stirring Powers without Aeration.

Region	Re	Power P	Power number
Laminar	$\leqslant 10$	$k_1 \cdot n^2 \cdot d^3 \cdot \eta$ [18a]	$Ne \sim Re^{-1}$
Transitional			$Ne \sim Re^{-1/3}$
Turbulent with baffles	$\geqslant 10^2$	$k_2 \cdot n^3 \cdot d^5 \cdot \rho$ [18b]	$Ne = K_2$
Turbulent without baffles	$\geqslant 5 \cdot 10^4$		$Ne = K_2$

$$\left(\frac{du}{dx}\right) = k^* n \left(\frac{4m}{3m+1}\right)^{\frac{m}{1-m}} \qquad (6\text{-}20)$$

From Eq. 6-20 for η_r we obtain:

$$\eta_r = \frac{K}{(k^* n)^{1-m}} \left(\frac{3m+1}{4m}\right)^{m} \qquad (6\text{-}21)$$

The constants K and n are obtained from the rheological behavior according to the **Ostwald-de-Waele model**:

$$\tau_S = K \left(\frac{du}{dx}\right)^{m} \qquad (6\text{-}22)$$

Here:

K = consistency factor (for Newtonian liquids, $K = \eta$), and

m = flow index (for Newtonian liquids, $m = 1$; for pseudoplastic liquids, $m < 1$; for dilatant liquids, $m > 1$).

6.2.6   Oxygen Transfer

In order to maintain specific growth rate according to equation 6-4a the concentration of dissolved oxygen, C_{O_2}, must be kept from falling by the continuous introduction of oxygen into the medium.

The oxygen transfer rate, *OTR*, is given by:

$$OTR = k_L a \, (C^*_{O_2} - C_{O_2}) \qquad (6\text{-}22a)$$

$C^*_{O_2}$ = saturation concentration of oxygen.

The maximum oxygen transfer rate is achieved when C_{O_2} has fallen to a critical value below which the cells can no longer be sufficiently supplied by the dissolved oxygen

$$(OTR)_{max} = k_L a (C^*_{O_2} - C_{O_{2k}}) \qquad (6\text{-}22b)$$

$C_{O_{2k}}$ = critical concentration of dissolved oxygen.

Since the rate of cell growth is low in comparison with the speed of the establishment of equilibrium between the concentrations of oxygen in the gas and the liquid, the system can be regarded as in a quasi-steady state.

We therefore have:

$$(OTR)_{max} = k_L a (C^*_{O_2} - C_{O_{2k}}) = \mu_m \frac{X}{Y_{O_2}} \qquad (6\text{-}22c)$$

If the demand is higher, limitation by oxygen transport sets in. Here the productivity is given by 6-9:

$$PR = \frac{dX}{dt} = \mu_m X = Y_{O_2} (OTR)_{max} \qquad (6\text{-}22d)$$

Under these conditions the following expression applies for the rate of consumption of substrate (oxygen limiting, substrate not limiting):

$$-k_S = -\frac{dS}{dt} = \frac{1}{Y_S} \frac{dX}{dt} = \frac{Y_{O_2}}{Y_S} k_L a (C^*_{O_2} - C_{O_{2k}}) \qquad (6\text{-}22e)$$

In aerated liquids, the gas throughput is denoted by q_G. In stirred tanks, the gas throughput referred to the volume of the liquid q_G/V is used, and in columns the gas throughput referred to the cross-section of the column A,

$$q_G/A = w_{SG}, \qquad (6\text{-}23)$$

where w_{SG} is called the superficial gas velocity since the liquid is not taken into account.

In **stirred vessels** with well-mixed liquid and gas phases, the **volumetric mass transfer coefficient** $k_L a$ can be calculated directly from the oxygen transfer rate (*OTR*) by means of Eq. 6-22a:

$$k_L a = \frac{OTR}{\Delta C_{O_2}} \qquad (6\text{-}24)$$

Here, ΔC_{O_2} is the driving oxygen concentration difference between the saturation concentration and the actual concentration in the culture solution:

$$\Delta C_{O_2} = C^*_{O_2} - C_{O_2} \qquad (6\text{-}25)$$

In **column reactors,** $C^*_{O_2}$ and C_{O_2} are position-dependent. Consequently, the local gas and liquid oxygen concentrations are required to determine k_L.

In gas/liquid reactors with height-constant cross-section the following expression applies for the **gas void fraction** ε_G:

$$\varepsilon_G = \frac{V - V_L}{V} = \frac{H - H_L}{H} = \frac{V_G}{V} \qquad (6\text{-}26)$$

Here,

V is the volume of the aerated layer;
V_L is the volume of the gas-free liquid;
V_G is the volume of the gas;
H is the height of the aerated layer; and
H_L is the height of the gas-free liquid.

The **specific interfacial area** between the gas and liquid phases is given by

$$a = \frac{A'}{V_L} = \frac{6\varepsilon_G}{d_s(1-\varepsilon_G)}, \qquad (6\text{-}27a)$$

$$a^* = \frac{A'}{V_L} = \frac{6\varepsilon_G}{d_s} \qquad (6\text{-}27b)$$

if the bubbles are of approximately spherical shape.

Here:

A' is the gas-liquid interfacial area in the reactor;
V_L is the volume of the liquid in the reactor;
V is the volume of the mixture;
d_s is the Sauter bubble diameter

$$d_s = \frac{\sum n_i d_{Bi}^3}{\sum n_i d_{Bi}^2} \qquad (6\text{-}28)$$

n_i is the number of bubbles with diameter d_{Bi}

With static gassing devices, it is possible to calculate the **size of the primary bubbles** with the aid of the balance of forces (Kumar and Kuloor, 1970).

According to Davidson and Schüler (1960):

$$V_B = \left(\frac{15\,\eta_L q_G}{2\rho_L q}\right)^{3/4}\left(\frac{4\pi}{3}\right)^{1/4} \qquad (6\text{-}29)$$

These relations can also be applied to non-Newtonian liquids (Krishnamurthi et al., 1968), e.g., the Davidson-Schüler model gives relation 6-30 for liquids the rheological behavior of which can be described by the Ostwald-de-Waele model:

$$V_B = \left(\frac{9\,X_m k}{2^m g}\right)^{\frac{3}{1+3m}}\left(\frac{4\pi}{3}\right)^{\frac{1}{1+3m}}\left(\frac{1+4m}{3}\right)^{-\frac{3m}{1+3m}}\left(q_G\right)^{\frac{3m}{1+3i}} \qquad (6\text{-}30)$$

For X_m and the drag coefficient C_D for spherical bodies the following relation applies:

$$C_D = \frac{24\,X_m}{Re} \qquad (6\text{-}31)$$

Where X_m is a constant (for Newtonian liquids, $X_m = 1$):

$$Re = \frac{\rho\,d^m u^{2-m}}{k} \qquad \text{(Reynolds number)}$$

The dynamic equilibrium bubble size can also be derived from the balance of forces (Calderbank, 1967) by using the Kolmogorov theory for isotropic turbulence (Davies, 1972):

$$d_e = C_1\frac{\sigma^{0.6}}{\rho^{0.2}(P/V_L)^{0.4}} \qquad (6\text{-}32)$$

where d_e is the diameter of a bubble in the dynamic equilibrium; C_1 is a constant; and P/V_L is the specific power input.

The **homogenizing** or **mixing time** denominates the time that is necessary to achieve a desired degree of homogeneity. During the mixing process, the local concentration of the component A, C_A, varies as a function of the time and place. The deviation from the finally reached concentration $C_{A,t} = C_{A,\infty} - C_{A,t}$ can be related to the total change $C_{A,\infty} - C_{Ao}$, which gives a relative deviation (e.g., 5%, Hiby, 1978). The mixing time θ that is necessary for the deviation to fall below 5% or to achieve a mixing quality of 95% is denoted, for example, by θ_{95}. Measurements of the mixing time in fermenters have been reported by Einsele (1976).

Particularly in continuous cultures, the mixing time can affect productivity (Solomons, 1963). Relation 6-12 hold true only when the mixing time is substantially shorter than the mean residence time of the medium in the reactor. If this condition is not satisfied, 6-12 no longer applies. We then have the inequality

$$\mu X_1 > D X_1 = PR \qquad (6\text{-}12a)$$

6.3   Selection of the Reactor

6.3.1   Characteristics Predetermined by the Nature of the Organism Used

The mode of operation of a reactor depends substantially on the **stability of the strain.** For instance, only strains that are sufficiently stable can be used in continuous operation (Aiba et al., 1973; Righelato, 1976).

The operating conditions are decisively affected by whether the organism is **aerobic** or **anaerobic** (Bailey and Ollis, 1977). In the breeding of aerobic organisms, an adequate amount of dissolved oxygen must always be available in the medium. Since the solubility of oxygen in the medium is very low (Schumpe and Deckwer, 1979), it must be supplied continuously. This is usually done by the dispersion of air in the medium. The higher the degree of dispersion (in low-viscosity media) or the more favorable the degree of dispersion (in high-viscosity media, because of the long residence time of very small bubbles), the higher is the oxygen transfer rate into the medium (Motarjemi and Jameson, 1978), and the better are the cells supplied with oxygen).

The **size** and **shape of the cells** also have a considerable influence on the type of reactor and its operation (Miura, 1976; Atkinson and Ur-Rahman, 1979). Spherical cells are usually smaller and less sensitive to shear than filamentous organisms. The former need a higher degree of dispersion of the air than filamentous mycelia. Small dimensions ensure a high surface-to-volume ratio and a high rate of uptake of substrate, and therefore also rapid growth. Aerobic cells with high rates of growth exhibit high rates of oxygen consumption.

Filamentous organisms only grow at the end of the threads. This leads to a low rate of growth and to a low oxygen demand. Since such cells are often sensitive to shear (Midler and Finn, 1966; Taguchi, 1971), high dispersing forces may cause damage. In fact, they would disperse not only the gas phase but also the filamentous organisms themselves.

The **formation of mycelium** and **agglomeration** of the organisms have a considerable effect on the choice of reactor. Agglomerates of cells have a low surface-to-volume ratio, a low rate of uptake of substrate, and a low rate of growth (Miura, 1976; Atkinson and Ur-Rahman, 1979; Phillips, 1966). The low rate of oxygen uptake permits the use of reactors which disperse the air to only a slight or moderate degree.

Cells that form agglomerates are easier to separate from the media (Aiba and Nagatani, 1971) and return to the reactor in order to raise the cell density. In many reactors (e.g., in high tower reactors) the cell density diminishes considerably with increasing height. When the medium outlet is placed at the head of the reactor, only a small amount of cell mass is removed from the tower (Smith et al., 1978).

In this way the residence time of the cells in the reactor can be considerably extended without increasing the residence time of the medium. Agglomeration of the cells therefore permits the **continuous operation** of a metabolite-producing reactor without the retention of the cells by special separating devices (e.g., centrifuges, filters) (Smith and Greenshields, 1974).

Cell agglomerates may have different morphologies. These depend not only on the strain but also on the conditions of shear in the reactor. With low mechanical stress, many filamentous organisms (e.g., mold fungi) form voluminous agglomerates interlocking with one another which lead to a high apparent viscosity of the medium (Charles, 1978; Metz et al., 1979). These agglomerates are often sensitive to shear stress. When the mechanical stress is increased, the same organisms may form pellets. This leads to a marked reduction in the apparent viscosity of the medium.

Many organisms tend to grow on **surfaces**. In the case of metabolite-producing organisms or of sewage treatment, these properties may be desirable if continuous operation is required. If this property is highly pronounced, surface reactors may be used (see Section 6.5). In general, film formation is not desirable. If cells show a tendency to grow on surfaces, the formation of stagnant regions at the surface must be avoided by a suitable reactor design.

6.3.2 Characteristics Predetermined by the Properties of the Medium

The choice of the strain generally determines not only the culture medium but also exerts a pronounced influence on the choice of reactor.

The **physical properties** of the substrate used differ: gaseous (e.g., methane), liquid and water-soluble (e.g., methanol, ethanol) (Präve, 1977; Laskin, 1977), solid and water-soluble (e.g., glucose, lactose), liquid and water-insoluble (e.g., gas-oil and paraffin) (Präve, 1977; Einsele and Fiechter, 1971; Litchfield, 1977), and solid and sparingly soluble or insoluble in water (e.g., starch, cellulose). Each physical state exerts a considerable influence on the reactor to be selected (see. 6.7.5). Since, for example, methane and air can form an explosive mixture, reactors with large interconnected gas volumes should not be used. Liquid and water-soluble substrates offer no difficulties. In the case of volatile substrates, cocurrent flow with little axial mixing or multistage units should be used in order to minimize losses in the waste gas. The aeration of oil-in-water emulsions has been thoroughly studied (MacLean, 1977). The presence of higher paraffins has a reducing effect on the oxygen transfer rate. In general, surface reactors are unsuitable for the fermentation of oil emulsions. If a solid, water-soluble substrate is used in batch operation, a highly viscous medium is often present initially. Special reactors (e.g., stirred tanks with helical stirrers) can be used for highly viscous media. The presence of hard solids (e.g., calcium carbonate in the *Penicillium chrysogenum* culture medium) or a fibrous substrate (e.g., pretreated straw) narrow the choice of reactor. Fine long threads in dilute suspensions lower the flow resistance, and large particles or fibrous materials may block openings (e.g., two-phase nozzles). In this case inserts with constrictions must be avoided. Special two-phase nozzles have been developed for these media (e.g., sewage) (Zlokarnik, 1979).

On the other hand the **biokinetic effects** of the substrate or the products also affect the choice of reactor. In the case of substrates showing inhibition or repression of growth (Wang et al., 1979), the process is carried out either in semicontinuous operation with sustained feed of the substrate ("extended culture" or "fed batch culture") or in a continuous culture. In the case of products that induce inhibition or repression effects in relatively high concentration (e.g., glucose and cellobiose with *Trichoderma viride,* ethanol with *Saccharomyces cerivisiae*), it is desirable to use a multistage arrangement.

The use of **difficultly sterilizable** (heat-sensitive) components of the medium requires special measures and, frequently, separate sterilization of these materials.

The influence of the medium on the coalescence of bubbles has repercussions on the construction of the dispersing devices and on the reactor itself (Zlokarnik, 1978; Schügerl et al., 1977). When **coalescence-suppressing media** are used it is desirable to apply high rates of energy dissipation in a dispersing device (two-phase nozzle, single stirrer) with a locally limited effect (Schügerl, 1978) and, even, bubble removal by physical means. In such media, the small bubbles so formed are fairly stable. In media with coalescence-enhancing properties (e.g., when antifoaming agents are used), the rate of energy dissipation must be as uniform as possible throughout the reactor. In fact, the small bubbles formed by effective gassing devices grow very rapidly by coalescence if they come into a region of low energy dissipation.

The **rheological behavior** of the medium has a very great influence. Low-viscosity media present no problems whatever with respect to mixing time and oxygen transfer rate, provided that no extremely fast-growing organisms or very large units are involved. An increase in viscosity may have various causes, which may arise together:

a) High concentration of substrate (particularly with batch operation at the beginning of cultivation);

b) The secretion of highly viscous products, e.g., pullulan and xanthan (Margaritis and Zajic, 1978), particularly in batch operation at the end of the formation of product; and

c) The morphology of the organisms (see section 6.2.1) (in batch operation at the end of the growth phase).

When substrate or product is responsible for the high viscosity, the medium frequently has a Newtonian behavior. A high apparent viscosity due to the morphology of the organisms is almost always associated with a non-Newtonian behavior. The reasons for the adverse influence of a high viscosity on the mixing process and on the oxygen transfer rate are thoroughly discussed in (Schügerl 1981).

Any formation of foam during cultivation interferes considerably with the operation of the plant, since the waste gas entrains the cell-containing foam and this blocks the waste-gas filter. Another consequence is a drastic loss of material from the fermenter (Sittig and Heine, 1977).

There are several methods for preventing excess foaming:

a) It may be possible to perform the process in such a way that **no formation of foam takes place.** For example, a high oxygen transfer rate eliminates oxygen transport limitation and makes the process substrate-limited. Under certain circumstances, this may reduce foam formation, particularly when it is caused by dissolved proteins which are liberated from dying and lysing cells.

b) The formation of foam is reduced by the use of antifoaming agents. Simultaneously, however, the coalescence behavior of the bubbles in the medium is changed. The medium then has a coalescence-promoting nature, which must be taken into account in the selection of the reactor. Likewise, mass exchange may be hindered by an enrichment of the (insoluble) antifoaming agent at the gas-liquid interface.

c) The foam can be destroyed by **mechanical aids** after it is formed. This can be done either by a foam destroyer incorporated at the waste gas outlet or by a suitable construction of the reactor (e.g., by rapid circulation of the liquid in so-called draught tube reactors). These measures do not combat the causes of the appearance of foam but only prevent its gaining the upper hand.

6.3.3 Characteristics Predetermined by the Parameters of the Biochemical Process

A fundamental factor influencing the choice of reactors in the cultivation of aerobic organisms is the specific **oxygen transfer rate** in the medium. In the case of continuous fermentations, the processes are never carried out in the regime of unlimited growth, since here a reactor is unstable. Furthermore, a large amount of expensive substrate is not used properly. When a substrate which does not itself contain oxygen (e.g., paraffins) is used, the yield referred to oxygen Y_{O_2} is lower and the oxygen demand is higher. As a simplified rule, with increasing concentration of oxygen chemically bound in the substrate Y_{O_2} rises and the oxygen demand falls.

The rates of growth and of product formation are **temperature-dependent.** Consequently, the cultivation and the formation of product are usually carried out at controlled temperatures. To facilitate the removal of the process heat from the reactor to the cooling water, the highest possible temperatures and hence the use of thermophilic organisms is favorable. As the volume of the reactor is increased, a limit is reached at which the heat produced cannot be removed solely via the cooling jacket of the reactor. In this case, additional heat exchangers located inside or outside the reactor must be used.

The **pH** of cell cultivation is determined by the pH optimum for the desired reaction (Pirt,

1975; Rehm, 1980). The lowest possible pH is favorable in order to suppress any infection by other organisms.

6.3.4 Characteristics Predetermined by the Site

The choice of reactor depends on the production site. A number of factors are:

- Raw materials supply and costs (e.g., sugar in the form of starch, molasses, sugar syrup);

- trading facilities for product and raw materials;

- availability and qualification of manpower;

- market features (stable sales – single product plant; variable sales – flexible plant);

- cost and availability of energy and cooling water (under certain circumstances it is better to operate a larger fermentation volume at lower productivity in order to save energy);

- working and safety regulations;

- regulations limiting environmental pollution; and

- the possibility of an economical use of by-products such as, for example, the cell mass (Litchfield, 1971).

All these aspects affect the choice of the reactor system and its performance.

6.4 Submerged Reactors and their Characterization

While in surface reactors the culture adheres to solid surfaces and is supplied with oxygen from the gas phase to the continuously wetted solid surface, the gas-liquid exchange is maintained in submerged reactors by dispersing the gas phase in the liquid through the continuous input of energy.

Submerged reactors can be divided into three groups according to the nature of the energy input:

– Reactors with mechanically moved internal members (mechanical stirrers);

– reactors with forced convection of the liquid (by pumps); and

– reactors with pneumatic operation (by compression of the air).

6.4.1   Power Input by Mechanically Moved Internal Devices

Mechanically Stirred Reactors

Mechanically stirred reactors consist of a cylindrical container with a height-to-diameter ratio $H/d_T = 1$ to 3 and are often provided with **baffles** in order to avoid the formation of vortices. In general, four baffles with a width of $0.1\ d_T$ are arranged symmetrically with respect to the stirrer shaft. Their wall distance is at least $0.02\ d_T$. The heat is transferred either by a double jacket, by helical or winding coils, or by both. Mixing and dispersion are brought about by a coaxial stirrer which also increases heat transfer.

In practice, numerous types of stirrer are used.

Typical **stirrers for low viscosity media** are: marine-propeller and pitched-blade turbine stirrers, which cause axial fluid motion, and flat-blade (Rushton) turbines and impellers, which produce radial fluid flow. In **liquids of mean viscosity,** use is made of the multistage-impulse-countercurrent (MIG) stirrer, which causes axial flow with radial components, and cross paddle-gate and paddle agitators, which produce tangential to radial flow.

In highly **viscous media,** helical stirrers which bring about axial motion and anchor and "multiple-rod" stirrers (Steel and Maxon, 1966; Swallow et al., 1978), which have a tangential action, are used. The mode of action of flat-blade turbines has been described by Biesecker (1972) and Brauer (1979), of MIG stirrers by Weihrauch (1968, 1972), and Kipke (1977), and of blade stirrers by Karwat (1959), and Miller (1974).

The power consumption and gas absorption in stirring vessels fitted with flat-blade turbines have been investigated by numerous authors (Michel and Miller, 1962; Zlokarnik, 1973; Loiseau et al., 1977; Judat, 1977).

In these investigations, the effects of the number of blades, the height of the internal members, the ratio of the diameters of stirrer and vessel d/d_T, and an eccentric arrangement of the stirrer were also determined.

The investigations cited above were carried out mainly with water. Distilled water has coalescence-promoting properties, while solutions of salt and alcohol have a coalescence-suppressing nature (see section 6.3.2). Tap water is coalescence-suppressing if it possesses a high degree of hardness and coalescence-promoting when it is soft. Consequently, the conditions of investigations that were carried out with tap water are not well defined. The influence of dissolved salts on the behavior of a mechanically stirred system, particularly on mass transport, have likewise been studied (see section 6.3.3) (Hassan and Roberts, 1977; Prasher, 1975).

The influence of the rheological behavior of highly viscous media on the power demand and on the mixing time have also been discussed in numerous publications (see section 6.3.2) (Metzner et al., 1961; Höcker and Langer, 1977; Henzler, 1978a and b). Only a few groups have reported on heat transfer (Steiff, 1978; Kipke, 1979) and mass transfer (see section 6.3.2) in highly viscous media.

Low-Viscosity Media

– Power input

The best known relationship for the change in power with the rate of gassing is due to Michel and Miller (1962) (see Table 6-3). According to this, the power uptake of a stirred unit falls with an increase in the supply of gas. The constants of the equation change with the properties of the system, so that different formulas are obtained for foaming and non-foaming media.

Table 6-3. Equations recommended by Miller and Michel (1962) and Loiseau et al. (1977).

$$P = C \left(\frac{P_o^2 \, n \, d_i^3}{q_G^{0.56}} \right)^m = C \, M^m$$

$C = 0.69$, $m = 0.45$ for $M < 2 \cdot 10^3$
$C = 1.88$, $m = 0.31$ for $M \geqslant 2 \cdot 10^3$ for foaming media
$C = 0.83$, $m = 0.45$ for nonfoaming media

Ranges of validity:
for foaming media $\qquad 2 \leqslant P \leqslant 100$
$\qquad\qquad\qquad\qquad\quad 10 \leqslant M \leqslant 106$
and for nonfoaming media $\quad 10 \leqslant P \leqslant 150$
$\qquad\qquad\qquad\qquad\qquad 1 \leqslant M \leqslant 10^5$

P (in aerated systems); P_o (in nonaerated systems) [W], n [s^{-1}], d_i [m], q [m^3 s^{-1}]

Judat (1977) developed correlations on the basis of similarity theory for description of the power uptake as a function of the geometry and the intensity of gassing of stirred tanks for flat-blade turbines with 6, 12, 18, and 24 blades, for perforated disk and for propeller stirrers. With increasing size of the stirrers, the Froude number – the ratio of the inertial force to gravitation – gains importance. The influence of the distance of the stirrer from the bottom is only moderate. An eccentric ar-

rangement of the stirrer in the vessel leads to a higher power demand. Since the best utilization of the energy exists just below the flooding point, Fig. 6-2 correlates the gas throughput number applying to this situation with the Froude number. Flat-blade turbines with a large number of blades have the highest gas loading capacity. The efficiency of stirrers can be characterized by a combination of coefficients introduced by Judat. Figure 6-3 shows a comparison of various types of stirrers. Flat-blade turbines with a large number of blades have the highest and propeller and perforated disk stirrers the lowest efficiency.

– Mixing time characteristic, θn

According to Zlokarnik (1972), by plotting a modified power factor $P d \rho^2 / \eta^3$ as a function of a modified mixing coefficient $\theta \eta / d^2 \rho$ it is possible to obtain a **borderline for stirrers** which describes the energetically most favorable conditions. Unsatisfactory stirrers give curves which run above that plotted in the diagram. An extension of this concept for the turbulent region was carried out by Mersmann et al. (1975). By plotting on a double-logarithmic scale, straight boundary lines are obtained which the stirrers investigated here do not reach. The following relation can be derived from this boundary line for a mixing homogeneity of 99%:

$$n\theta = 6.7 \, (d/d_T)^{-5/3} \, Ne^{-1/3} \qquad (6-33)$$

This equation applies to propeller, blade, gate, pitched-blade, and INTERMIG (double-ended MIG; Kipke, 1979) stirrers. The power necessary for homogenization depends very greatly on the quality of mixing. For example, to raise the quality of mixing from 95 to 98% at constant mixing time, the power of the stirrer must be doubled (Henzler, 1978).

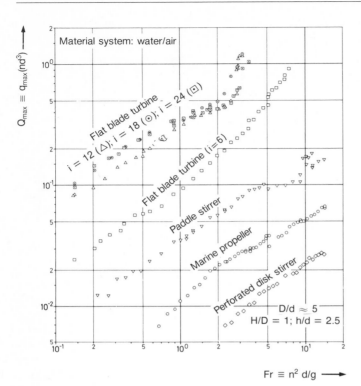

Fig. 6-2. Flooding characteristic Q_{max} (Fr) of various stirrers (tap water/air system); $i=$ number of blades (adapted from Judat, 1977).

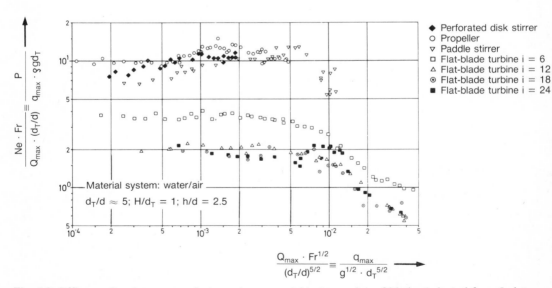

Fig. 6-3. Efficacy of various types of stirrers (tap water/air); $i=$ number of blades (adapted from Judat, 1977).

Table 6-4. Equation for Calculating the Heat-Transfer Coefficient in Aerated Stirred Tanks with Flat-blade Turbines According to Steiff (1978).

$$St_G = 0.137 (Re_G \ Fr_G \ Pr_L^2)^{0.33 - (0.73 + 0.167 \cdot 10^{-5} Re)} \cdot (Re + 1000) \ 0.047 \left(\frac{\eta_W}{\eta}\right)^{-0.42}$$

Range: $w_{SG} < 8.5$ cm s^{-1} $n < 16.7$ s^{-1}

$0.6 < \eta < 88$ mPa s $0.19 < d_T < 0.7$ m, $1 \leqslant h/d_T \leqslant 3$, $d_T/d_i = 3$

$$St_G = \frac{\alpha}{\rho \ C \ w_{SG}} \quad \text{Stanton number for the gas}$$

$$Re_G = \frac{w_{SG} \ d_i}{\nu} \quad \text{Reynolds number for the gas}$$

$$Fr_G = \frac{w_{SG}^2}{d_i \ g} \quad \text{Froude number for the gas}$$

The index W = at the wall

– Heat transfer in gassed stirred vessels

To calculate the transfer of heat during the un-gassed sterilization phase the relations well-known from the literature can be used which have been reviewed by Steiff (1978). The equation which he has developed for flat-blade turbines applies both for cooling and for heating via the wall of the vessel and a cylindrical coil (Table 6-4).

– Volumetric mass transfer coefficient, k_La

In the quantitative treatment of mass transfer it is important to take coalescence-promoting or -inhibiting properties into account (see Section 6.3.2). For a flat-blade turbine Robinson and Wilke (1973) proposed a relation in which the constants depend on the ionic strength of the solution (Table 6-5).

As can be seen from Table 6-5, the exponents increase with the ionic strength:

k_2 from 0.4 to 0.9, and k_3, from 0.35 to 0.40.

In the presence of hydrocarbons, k_La changes with the kind of compound and its

Table 6-5. Equations for Calculating the Volumetric Mass Transfer Coefficient in Aerated Stirred Tanks with Six-Flat-Blade Turbines According to Robinson and Wilke (1973).

$$k_La = k_1 \left(\frac{P}{V_L}\right)^{k_2 k_3} w_{SG} \cdot \xi$$

$$\xi = \frac{\rho^{0.553} \ D_L^{2/3}}{\sigma^{0.6} \ \eta^{1/3}} \quad \text{(dimensionless)}$$

D_L (cm^2 s^{-1}), σ (N cm^{-1}), η (mPa s), w_{SG} (cm s^{-1})

$\Gamma \geqslant 0.40 : k_1 = 1275, \quad k_2 = 0.9, \quad k_3 = 0.40$

$0 \leqslant \Gamma \leqslant 0.40$:

$$k_2 = 0.40 + \frac{0.826 \ \Gamma}{0.274 + \Gamma}$$

$k_3 \sim 0.35 + 0.1 \ \Gamma$

Range of validity:

$43 \leqslant k_La \leqslant 1537$ h^{-1}
$0.114 \leqslant w_{SG} \leqslant 0.457$ cm s^{-1}
$31.6 \leqslant P/V_L \leqslant 17950$ W m^{-3}

concentration. The increase in k_La as a function of the concentration of various hydrocarbons has been shown graphically in Hassan and Robinson's paper (1977).

Zlokarnik has proposed a relation for coalescence-promoting media (see Section 6.3.2) that is valid for flat-blade turbines and hollow stirrers in the range of $3 \cdot 10^4 < (P/q)^* < 1 \cdot 10^7$:

$$k_La' \sim (P \cdot q)^{0.5} \qquad (6\text{-}34)$$

Hassan and Robinson (1977) have proposed further relations for calculating the relative gas content in stirred vessels with flat-blade turbines.

Highly Viscous Media

– Power input

In the calculation of the power input in highly viscous non-Newtonian media, it is convenient to define a representative viscosity which is effective in the stirred vessel under investigation (Metzner et al., 1961) (see Section 6.2.5).

In Fig. 6-4, some power number functions $Ne=f(Re)$ have been plotted for aqueous solutions of carboxymethylcellulose (CMC), for five different stirrers. For gassed stirred tanks, it is desirable to plot Ne as a function of the gas throughput factor $Q = \dfrac{q_G}{n\,d_i^3}$ (Zlokarnik, 1973), the Froude number $Fr = \dfrac{n^2\,d_i}{g}$ being chosen as parameter. The course of these functions depends on the type of stirrer and on the rheological behavior of the liquid (Höcker and Langer, 1977). According to another plot, Ne is represented as a function of the Galilei number $Ga = \dfrac{g\,d_i^3\,\rho^2}{\eta_r^2}$ and Q as a parameter at constant Froude number (Fig. 6-5).

In the region of the horizontal branch of the curve $Ne=f(Ga^{0.5})$ the dispersion of the gas phase becomes more and more ineffective with increasing viscosity, since the stirrer is increasingly flooded and large trails of gas form behind the blades. Complete flooding is reached as soon as all the curves run into a single line. Figure 6-6 shows such a flooded stirrer in a polyacrylamide (PAA) solution. The flooding can be substantially shifted to higher gas flow rates by a suitable design of the stirrer.

– Heat transfer

The results of investigations of heat transfer in highly viscous gassed stirred tanks are not sufficient for the determination of quantitative relationships (Steiff, 1978; Kipke, 1979).

– Volumetric mass transfer coefficient k_La

The number of high viscosity investigations is small (Henzler, 1978). The results of the measurements have been represented in different ways. Perez and Sandall (1974) and Yagi and Yoshida (1975) have developed equations holding only for media of medium viscosity (Table 6-6).

Henzler (1978) has found a convenient relation which is based on the measurements of Yagi and Yoshida (1975), Höcker and Langer (1977), and Kipke (1979) (Table 6-7).

Experiments carried out with fermentation liquors during cell growth or metabolite production can be regarded as only qualitative with respect to the dependences on the Ne number, the dimensionless mixing time, and the volume-related transfer coefficient on the most important operating parameters. Nevertheless, they give useful information for the operation of the corresponding bioreactors (Steel and Maxon, 1966; Margaritis and Zajic, 1978).

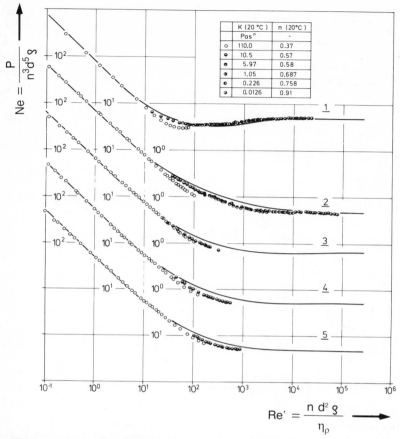

	K (20 °C)	n (20°C)
	Pa s^n	-
○	110.0	0.37
◐	10.5	0.57
◑	5.97	0.58
◔	1.05	0.687
◕	0.226	0.758
◒	0.0126	0.91

$$Ne = \frac{P}{n^3 d^5 \varrho}$$

$$Re' = \frac{n\, d^2\, \varrho}{\eta_\rho}$$

Fig. 6-4. Power characteristics in aqueous CMC solutions at $H/d_T = 1$
1) Flat-blade turbine; 2) dispersing disk; 3) MIG-4; 4) MIG-6; 5) MIG-7 (adapted from Höcker, 1979).

Mechanically Stirred Draught Tube Reactors

In baffled mechanically stirred reactors, regardless of the type of stirrer used, complex liquid flow takes place which can be described by loops of different geometries (Fig. 6-7). In the draught tube (and stirred loop) reactors, the highly stochastic flows of a stirred tank are so directed by the use of a coaxially arranged cylinder (draught tube) that a well-defined circulation flow is formed (Fig. 6-8).

The behavior of draught tube reactors has been investigated in detail in the last few years. They are operated in such a way that either the draught tube is covered by the liquid (completely filled state of operation) or the tube projects from the liquid surface (overflow operation).

Reactors in the completely filled state of operation have been investigated, particularly, by Fiechter (1978). A comparison of these two states of operation has been made by Keitel (1978).

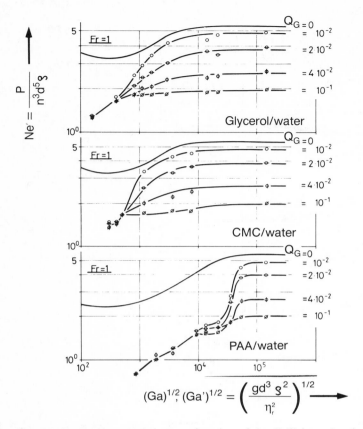

$$(Ga)^{1/2}, (Ga')^{1/2} = \left(\frac{gd^3 \, \varsigma^2}{\eta_r^2}\right)^{1/2} \longrightarrow$$

Fig. 6-5. Power characteristics as a function of the Galilei number for different aeration numbers Q_G. Flat-blade turbine, glycerol/water, CMC/water, and PAA/water solutions (adapted from Höcker and Langer, 1977).

Table 6-6. Equation for Calculating the Sherwood Number According to Yagi and Yoshida (1975).

$$Sh' = 0.06 \, Re'^{1.5} \, Fr^{0.19} \, Sc_r^{0.5} \left(\frac{\eta_r \, w_{SG}}{\sigma}\right)^{0.6} \left(\frac{n \, d_i}{w_{SG}}\right)^{0.32} [1 + 2 \, De^{0.5}]^{-0.67}$$

$$Sh' = \frac{k_L a \, d^2}{D_L} \qquad Re' = \frac{n \, d^2 \rho}{\eta_r} \qquad \eta_r = \frac{\tau_S}{11 \, n}; \qquad D_e = \lambda^* n$$

λ^* characteristic time determined from the function $\eta_r/\eta_O = f(\mathrm{d}u/\mathrm{d}x)$:

$$\lambda^* = \left(\frac{\mathrm{d}u}{\mathrm{d}x}\right) \, \eta_r/\eta_O = 0.67 \qquad \eta_O = |\eta| \, \frac{\mathrm{d}u}{\mathrm{d}x} \to 0$$

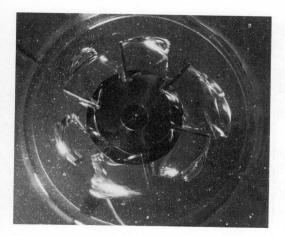

Fig. 6.6. Gas trails behind the blades of a flat-blade turbine with the supply of gas stopped (adapted from Höcker and Langer, 1977).

The power uptake is lower in overflow operation than in the completely filled state of operation. A comparison of the *Ne* values in the draught tube reactor with those in conventional stirred tanks showed that reactors with draught tubes take less power than those without draught tubes.

Without gassing, *Ne* does not depend on *Re* if propeller stirrers are used. This behavior is known to be typical for propeller stirrers (Judat, 1977).

– Gas content

In Fig. 6-10, the gas void fractions ε_G are shown as a function of the stirrer speed for stirred tanks ($H/d_T = 1$ and 2) and for a

Table 6-7. Equation for Calculating $k_L a$ According to Henzler (1978).

$$k_L a \, \frac{V_L}{q_G} = k_1 \left(\frac{P}{q_G} \right)^{*k_2} k_3 \, Sc$$

k_1	k_2	k_3	Sc_{min}	Sc_{max}	$(P/q)^*_{min}$	$(P/q)^*_{max}$	Medium
0.082	0.6	−0.3	$8 \cdot 10^3$	$1.5 \cdot 10^5$	$2 \cdot 10^3$	$2 \cdot 10^5$	CMC solutions
0.045	0.5	−0.3	$4 \cdot 10^2$	$1.5 \cdot 10^6$	10^3	$2 \cdot 10^6$	glycerol and glucose solutions
0.0125	0.6	−0.17			10^3	$2.5 \cdot 10^5$	millet gruel gel

– Power input

While with conventional stirred tanks the power input is a function only of the gas throughput coefficient *Q*, in the case of the overflow regime, the curves for different gas flow rates do not coincide (Fig. 6-9). In the completely filled state of operation, *Ne* is almost constant for different values of *Q*. In overflow operation, *Ne* falls with increasing speed of rotation.

draught tube reactor ($H/d_T = 2$). It can be deduced from the plot that higher gas contents are achieved in the stirred tank and the influence of the stirrer speed is greater than in the corresponding draught tube reactor. The influence of the gas flow rate is approximately the same in the two types of reactor.

– Mixing time θ

In Fig. 6-11, the mixing time θ (s) for a com-

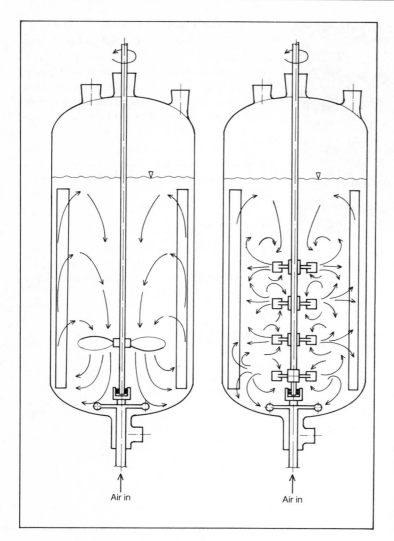

Fig. 6-7. Liquid flow in baffled tanks in the case of an axially-conveying marine propeller stirrer and a radially-conveying flat-blade disk stirrer (adapted from Zlokarnik, 1972).

pletely filled reactor is shown as a function of the specific stirring power P/V_L in ungassed water and in 2% carboxymethyl-cellulose (CMC) solution. According to this, the mixing times no longer change from about 3 kW/m³ in water and from about 10 kW/m³ in CMC solution. As was to be expected, the mixing time in highly viscous CMC solution is longer than in water.

– Volumetric mass transfer coefficient $k_L a$

Keitel (1978) measured the values of $k_L a$ in different liquids for completely filled and overflow operation with flat blade turbines

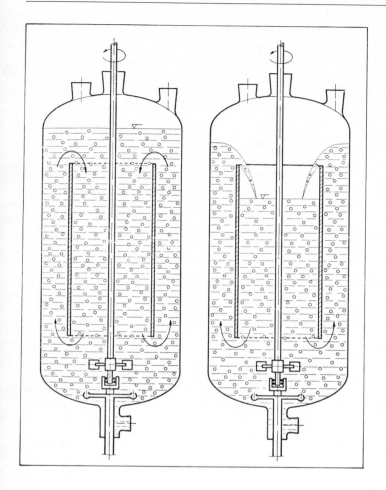

Fig. 6-8. States of flow when operating with complete filling (on the left) and with overflow (on the right) (adapted from Keitel, 1978).

and marine propeller stirrers. The equations that he recommends are given in Table 6-8.

In Fig. 6-12, the $(k_L a)^*$ values as functions of $(P/V)^*$ are compared with one another for draught tube reactors (1) and stirred tanks (2), with flat blade turbines (BT) in coalescence-promoting media, and also for stirred vessels with hollow stirrers (HS) (3) and with injector nozzles (4) in coalescence-suppressing media.

For **coalescence-promoting media,** higher $(k_L a)^*$ values are obtained with a draught tube than without it.

This must be ascribed to the fact that the directed flow of the liquid reduces the probability of collision and, hence, the coalescence of the bubbles. Particularly high $(k_L a)^*$ values are achieved with short draught tubes and with overflow operation. In the latter, the surface aeration gives a significant contribution to $(k_L a)^*$ (Keitel, 1978).

Propeller stirrers achieve an optimum circulation within the draught tube but can be used only at low rates of gassing. Here, they are energetically more favorable than **flat**

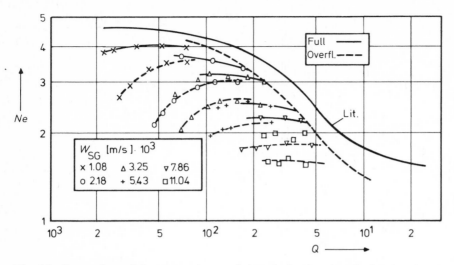

Fig. 6-9. Comparison of the power characteristics of stirred tank and stirred tank loop reactors (adapted from Keitel, 1978; Lit.: Zlokarnik, 1973).

Table 6-8. Equations for Calculating $k_L a$ in Stirred Tank Loop Reactors According to Keitel (1978).

$$(k_L a)^* = C_i \left(\frac{P}{V}\right)^{*k_1} \left(\frac{q}{V}\right)^{*k_2} \left(\frac{d_i}{d_T}\right)^{k_3}$$

Stirrer type	k_1	k_2	k_3	$(P/V)^*_{max}$	$(P/V)^*_{min}$	$(q/V)^*_{max}$	$(q/V)^*_{min}$
Flat-blade turbine full	0.38	0.84	0	0.7	$1.1 \cdot 10^{-2}$	$1.5 \cdot 10^{-4}$	$2.5 \cdot 10^{-6}$
Flat-blade turbine overflow operation	0.48	0.66	0	0.7	$1.1 \cdot 10^{-2}$	$1.5 \cdot 10^{-4}$	$2.5 \cdot 10^{-6}$
Propeller full	0.58	0.68	0.71	35	0.75	10^{-5}	$3 \cdot 10^{-6}$
Propeller overflow operation	0.48	0.88	1.05	35	0.75	10^{-5}	$3 \cdot 10^{-6}$

Constant C_i	Flat-blade turbine		Propeller	
	Overflow	Complete filling	Overflow	Complete filling
Water	0.05	0.54		
0.08 mol/L NaCl	—	0.73		
0.5 mol/L NaCl	0.19	1.81	1.8	0.1
0.27–1% CMC	0.09	0.64		
0.27–0.82 mol/L isopropanol	0.17	1.42		

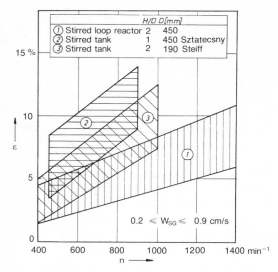

	H/D	D[mm]	
① Stirred loop reactor	2	450	
② Stirred tank	1	450	Sztatecsny
③ Stirred tank	2	190	Steiff

$0.2 \leqslant W_{SG} \leqslant 0.9$ cm/s

Fig. 6-10. Comparison of the gas holdup of a stirred tank and of a stirred tank loop reactor for water/air. The measurements of Sztatecsny and Steiff are given for comparison (adapted from Keitel, 1978; Steiff, 1976; Szatecsny, 1975).

blade turbines, which are to be preferred at higher rates of gassing and must be ar-ranged underneath the draught tube. A compact form of this reactor (Fig. 6-13) which must be operated in the completely filled state and was optimized to give the best mixing time θ has been used success-fully in the continuous cultivation of *S.cerevisiae* and of *T.cutaneum* (Fiechter, 1978).

Mechanically Stirred Loop Reactors

In contrast to the mechanically stirred draught tube reactors which are constructed with $H/d_T = 1$ to 2, the mechanically stirred loop reactors are slender ($H/d_T \sim 5$ to 15).

A special construction of mechanically operated loop reactors has been described by Katinger (1973).

A propeller forces the liquid downwards which is gassed by an injector nozzle. The two-phase system so formed first flows downwards in a draught-tube and then, at the end of the tube, rises in the annular space. The medium is degassed in an enlargement of the outer tube, and in the degassed state it again flows past the propeller.

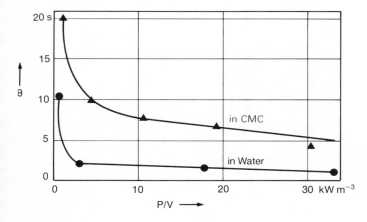

Fig. 6-11. Mixing time θ as a function of the specific stirred power P/V at different viscosities. Completely filled reactor (adapted from Karrer, 1978).

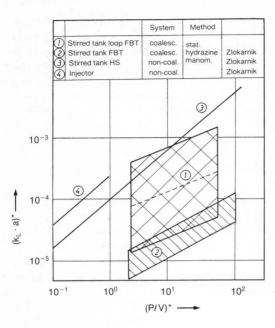

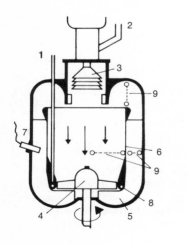

		System	Method	
①	Stirred tank loop FBT	coalesc.	stat.	
②	Stirred tank FBT	coalesc.	hydrazine	Zlokarnik
③	Stirred tank HS	non-coal.	manom.	Zlokarnik
④	Injector	non-coal.		Zlokarnik

Fig. 6-12. Comparison of the sorption characteristics of different types of stirrers (FBT = flat-blade stirrer; HS = hollow tube stirrer) and liquid media. Zlokarnik's results have been included here (adapted from Keitel, 1978; Zlokarnik, 1978).

Mechanically Stirred Gas-aspiring Reactors

Through an air-supply tube, the hollow stirrer automatically sucks in gas from the space above the surface of the liquid and distributes it finely in the liquid. No vortices are formed. The suction effect of these stirrers is brought about by the low pressure that arises in the flow of the liquid behind the stirrer blades. Numerous designs of hollow stirrers are known. Investigations performed hitherto with hollow tube stirrers (Topiawala and Hamer, 1974; Joshi and Sharma, 1977; Zlokarnik, 1970) indicate that the four-tube stirrer is the most effective.

– Power input

With hollow stirrers, as well, Michel and Miller's relation can be used satisfactorily (Joshi and Sharma, 1977).

– Gas throughput

Zlokarnik (1970) gives the following relationship:

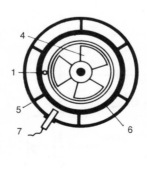

Fig. 6-13. Completely filled reactor, side view and plan view:
(1) air inlet; (2) air outlet; (3) foam separator; (4) propeller; (5) baffles; (6) draught tube; (7) pH and oxygen probe; (8) sparger; (9) measuring points for propeller anemometer (adapted from Karrer, 1978).

$$\left(Q\,\frac{d_i}{d_T}\right)^{-1} = 10\left(Fr\,\frac{d_i}{H}\right)^{-2.37} + 1.05 \qquad (6\text{-}35)$$

Ranges of validity:

$$0.05 \leqslant \left(Q\,\frac{d_i}{d_T}\right) \leqslant 1$$

$$0.06 \leqslant \left(Fr\,\frac{d_i}{H}\right) \leqslant 8$$

- Volumetric mass transfer coefficient, $k_L a$

Equations have been given by Zlokarnik (Table 6-9).

Table 6-9. Equations for Calculating $k_L a$ in Stirred Tanks with Hollow-tube Stirrers According to Zlokarnik (see 6.3.2).

Coalescence-suppressing
$(k_L a)^* = 1.1\cdot 10^{-4}\,(P/V)^{*0.8}$
$10^{-5} \leqslant (k_L a)^* \leqslant 2\cdot 10^{-3}$
$5\cdot 10^{-2} \leqslant (P/V)^* \leqslant 50$

Coalescence-promoting
$k_L a\,(q/V_L)^{-1} = 1.5\cdot 10^{-2}\,(P/q)^{*0.5}$
$2 \leqslant k_L a\,(q/V_L)^{-1} \leqslant 50$
$3\cdot 10^4 \leqslant (P/q)^* \leqslant 10^7$

The use of gas-aspiring hollow stirrers of special design for the manufacture of vinegar has been treated by Ebner. With a specific power input of 2.77 kW/m³, a specific exchange surface of 2315 m²/m³ was achieved in a unit with a liquid charge of 80 m³ (Frings aerator, type 12000) (Ebner, 1973).

Stirred Cascade Reactor

Stirred cascade reactors are column reactors in which several sections arranged above one another are formed by intermediate plates. In these sections, mixing and the dispersion of gas are intensified by the movement of various mixing members. Two types of reactors can be distinguished:

- Reactors with rotating mixing members (Brauer et al., 1979; Falch and Gaden, 1969; Páca and Grégr, 1977);

- Reactors with axially moving mixing members (Brauer and Sucker, 1978).

Páca and Grégr (1977) have cultivated yeast in a reactor with rotating mixer members. Brauer and Sucker (1978) use a reactor with axially moving mixing members in order to treat sewage.

Paddle Wheel Reactors

By relatively slow rotation, the horizontally arranged paddle wheel built into the vessel produces a forced spray of the liquid phase in the gas space (Zlokarnik, 1975). Without compressed air, up to 50% utilization of oxygen is achieved at a high concentration of biomass (Faust et al., 1976). In a 6 m³ pilot plant at $n = 30$ rpm a productivity of 10 kg of dry biomass per hour was achieved. The apparatus is recommended for simple processes in developing countries (see Section 6.3.2).

6.4.2 Power Input by Liquid Circulation with an External Pump

Mechanical energy is imparted to the liquid in order to mix it and to disperse the gas phase in it.

The dispersion of gas can take place by various methods:

a) with the aid of two-phase nozzles;
b) by means of a plunging jet;
c) by means of a combination of liquid pump and gas compressor.

In a **two-phase nozzle,** the gas is entrained and dispersed by a jet of liquid accelerated to 5 to 100 m/s. The performance can be made more effective when the two-phase nozzle is combined with momentum exchange tube in which, because of the high local power input, a particularly high degree of dispersion can be achieved (Sinn et al., 1970). The total energy input consists of the liquid energy and that of the gas fed to the annular nozzle under pressure. The **mechanism of gas dispersion** has been investigated by Jackson (1964), by Kürten and Maurer (1977), and also by Hallensleben et al. (1977), and a turbulent dispersion theory has been applied successfully.

High-speed photographs of the momentum exchange tube show that the dispersion of the gas takes place in the field of shear between the fast liquid jet and a stream of liquid sucked in slowly. The gas issues from the gas nozzle in large bubbles which, in the momentum exchange tube, through the breakdown of the driving jet into drops are pre-

liminarily dispersed very rapidly. Further dispersion then takes place in accordance with the laws of local turbulence. The design of these nozzles depends on whether they are operated without or with a gas pressure head. Well known two-phase nozzles are the BASF nozzle (Sinn et al., 1970) and the Bayer nozzle (Zlokarnik, 1979) (Fig. 6-14). The latter has been further developed for the gassing of sewage. The Hoechst radial flow nozzle is used particularly for the laminar gassing regime.

A combination of the input of energy by a liquid pump and gas compression is realized in the **Vollmüller-Walburg nozzle** (1971). The gas can be sucked into an annular distributor (perforated ring, sintered ring) located in the narrowest part of a Venturi nozzle by the low pressure existing there. The input of gas can be increased by subjecting the gas to pressure.

A combination of nozzle and downward flow is realized in the **Waagner-Biró reactor.**

Another possibility of increasing the efficacy of the input of gas consists in preventing the influence of the coalescence of the bubbles by the continuous formation of new bubbles. For this purpose, the li-

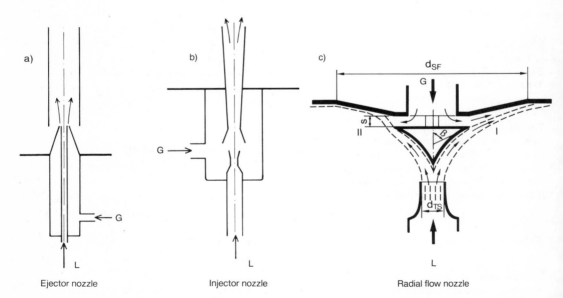

Fig. 6-14. Schematic representation of two-phase nozzles (G = gas; L = liquid; d_{SF} = diameter of the shear field; d_{DJ} = diameter of the driving jet; β = angle of deviation; s = slit width; I = gas overpressure; II = gas underpressure) (adapted from Schügerl, 1977).

quid is caused to flow in countercurrent to the gas in a multistage appararus (Voigt and Schügerl, 1978). Here the energy introduced by the pumped liquid serves to maintain the countercurrent flow.

Plunging Jet Reactors

Plunging jet reactors were first developed for the aeration of highly loaded sewage and were later also used for the production of yeast (Liepe et al., 1978; Schreier, 1975).

In these units, the gas is dispersed by the free jet from the nozzle or a slot impinging perpendicularly on the surface of the liquid (with a velocity of 8 to 12 m/s).

The jet impinges on the surfaces, breaks through it, and penetrates into the liquid volume. The identity of the jet is retained so long as it is surrounded by a mantle of the entrained gas. The breakdown of this mantle leads to the formation of small close-packed bubbles which move in the liquid downwards and sidewards, so that the swarm of bubbles forms a cone. By exchange of momentum, the surrounding liquid is entrained and is mixed with the two-phase jet (van de Sande and Smith, 1976; Suicu and Smigelschi, 1976).

The energy of the liquid jet is supplied by feed pumps which sometimes pump the liquid back through a heat exchanger into the nozzle tube. They must be capable either of eliminating the amount of very small bubbles of gas that have not separated out or of their trouble-free pumping together with the liquid.

By suitable design, gas entrainment ratios q_G/q_L of up to 2.5 have been achieved. In an optimum unit, the free jet of liquid reaches to the bottom of the reactor. The optimum falling height of the free jet is in the range of 6 to 9 m. The specific power demand is very high, but it is reduced with increasing the liquid charge and size of the unit to 8 kW/m^3. With 8 kW/m^3 a $k_L a$ value of 0.30 s^{-1} can be achieved (Lafferty et al., 1977).

Jet Loop Reactor

Jet loop reactors are tower reactors with a moderate slenderness ratio $(5 < H/d_T < 20)$ in which the liquid phase is returned from the outlet of the reactor to the inlet. Recycling can take place through a draught tube within the reactor proper or through a loop arranged outside the reactor. Most jet loop reactors work with the phases in cocurrent. The driving jet is produced by a circulating pump. Liquid velocities of about 20 m/s are reached in the nozzle. By imparting its impact the jet from the nozzle entrains the liquid contents of the reactor and circulates it. In this way, an internal liquid loop arises.

In another arrangement, the two-phase system is passed through a long tower reactor, degassed in a cyclone, and returned by a pump.

The jet loop reactors with draught tube, i.e., with an internal loop, have been investigated by Blenke et al. (1979) thoroughly.

When a two-phase nozzle is used, the influence of the gas flow rate q_G and of the velocity of the driving jet can be determined separately (Fig. 6-15). An increase in q_G raises ε_G considerably. Yet the driving jet has a stronger influence on the gas content, particularly at low gassing levels. At high rates of gassing and velocities of the driving jet the gas content is reduced through an increase in H/d_T, due to the more pronounced coalescence of the bubbles.

The specific interfacial area (a) of a reactor has been measured by the catalytic oxidation of an aqueous sulfite solution. It therefore applies only to coalescence-inhibiting media. In these media the influence of the velocity of the driving jet on ε_G is more pronounced than in coalescence-promoting media. At high velocities of the driving jet and high rates of gassing, the relative gas content reaches very high levels (up to 70%). With this limitation, Fig. 6-16 shows the specific interfacial area as a function of the superficial velocity of the gas, w_{SG}, and the specific jet power input, P_L/V. It can be

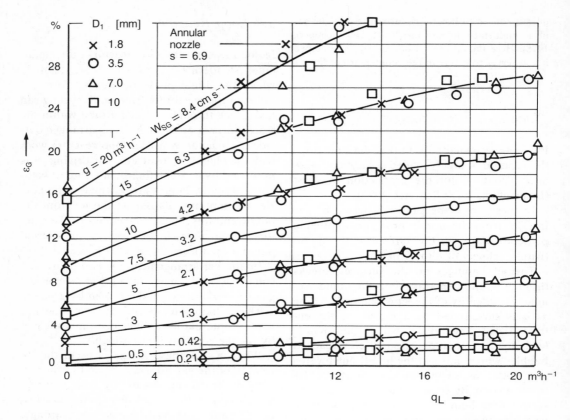

Fig. 6-15. Mean gas holdups as functions of the flow rates of gas and liquid in an ejector nozzle (acc. Fig. 6-14a) (adapted from Blenke, 1979; Hirner, 1974).

seen that an increase in the gas throughput q_G at a low superficial gas velocity w_{SG} greatly increases the specific interfacial area, particularly at high driving jet power inputs. This pronounced dependence of the specific interfacial areas on W_{SG} and P_L/V decreases at higher gas flow rates and jet power inputs.

Jet loop reactors have been used for the **mass cultivation of yeast** on paraffin (Birckenstädt et al., 1977), and for the **cultivation of bacteria** (Präve, 1972; Faust, 1979).

Immersed Slot Reactors

In the immersed slot reactors, the potential energy of the circulated liquid is converted into **kinetic energy** in a down flow channel. In order to make this conversion as complete as possible, the liquid is accelerated by a slot-shaped constriction of the down flow channel (with an oblong cross-section). At the narrowest point, where the velocity reaches its high-

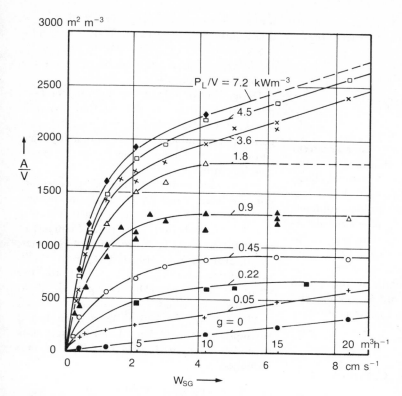

Fig. 6-16. Specific interfacial area in the jet loop reactor as a function of the superficial gas velocity for various specific jet power inputs P_L/V; sulfite system (adapted from Blenke, 1979).

est value and the static pressure its lowest value, air is sucked in through holes located there and is dispersed. The downward flow entrains the bubbles so formed to the bottom of the channel, where they rise through the reactor and finally leave the liquid (Müllner, 1973). The liquid is circulated by a pump.

The specific oxygen transfer rate depends on the height of filling of the reactor. With increasing height of filling, the energy-related oxygen transfer rate rises. In pilot plants, efficiencies of up to 4 kg oxygen/kW theoretical pumping power have been reached.

Circulation Nozzle Reactors

In circulation nozzle reactors, the metabolism of the cells is claimed to be accelerated by a brief pressure oscillation in the range of 20 to 0.3 bar (Intermag, 1970). With such high pressure heads, high liquid velocities (50 to 150 m/s) are reached in the nozzle. A high pressure head is produced before the nozzle which falls to the lower value in the narrowest part of the nozzle for a brief period. Downstream from this narrowest point the pressure rises again. A brief fall in pressure, for example, from 5 bar to 0.3 to 0.4 bar for a period of about 1 µs doubles the rate of growth of brewers' yeast cells.

Perforated-Plate or Sieve-Plate Cascade Reactors

These include the **multistage countercurrent bubble columns** in which the liquid level in the stages is determined by overflow pipes. Such units have so far been rarely used in bioreactors. The relative gas content and the volumetric mass transfer coefficient have been determined in model media of low and high viscosities. The smaller the diameter of the holes and the free cross-sectional area of the perforated plates and the height of the mixed phase, the higher are ε_G and $k_L a$ (Voigt and Schügerl, 1979). In the cultivation of yeast, this increases productivity.

6.4.3   Power Input by Compressed Gas

All those reactors in which the dispersion of the compressed gas at the bottom of the vessel is carried out by static gas distributors (perforated plates, sintered plates, etc.) belong to this group. The bubbles formed rise in the liquid because of their buoyancy and leave the two-phase system at the head of the column. The formation of bubbles at static distributors is treated in section 6.2.6.

Single-Stage Bubble Columns

A reactor of this type consists of a slender column containing a gas distributor at its base. Its construction is therefore very simple. Even when the liquid (at a low velocity) and the gas are fed to the reactor in cocurrent flow it be-

longs – according to the above definition – to this group. Review articles facilitate orientation (Gerstenberg, 1979; Mersmann, 1977; Deckwer, 1977). Highly viscous systems are treated in section 6.3.2.

Depending on the gas throughput, the two-phase flow exists in different fluid-dynamic states: at a low gas throughput there is homogeneous or laminar flow, and at a high gas throughput the heterogeneous or turbulent state prevails.

Investigations with **biological systems** are comparatively rare: the production of beer and vinegar, the cultivation of yeasts (Chapter 10) (Kloud and Sterbacek, 1972; Schügerl et al., 1978), of bacteria (Lehmann and Hammer, 1978), of mold fungi (Figett and Smith, 1978), cell cultures (Katinger et al., 1979), and the treatment of sewage (Diesterweg et al., 1978) have been described.

The following relations have been found for **liquid mixtures** (alcohol and salt solutions in a column with $d_T = 14$ cm, $H = 391$ cm) (Schügerl et al., 1977).

For the mean gas void fraction

$$\varepsilon_G = 0.91 \left(\frac{w_{SG}}{\sqrt{g}\, d_s} \right)^{1.19} \tag{6-36}$$

Range of validity:

$$0.2 \leqslant \varepsilon_G \leqslant 0.70; \quad 0.02 \leqslant \left(\frac{w_{SG}}{\sqrt{g}\, d_s} \right) \leqslant 1$$

For the volumetric mass transfer coefficient $k_L a$

$$k_L a = 0.0023 \left(\frac{w_{SG}}{d_s} \right)^{1.58} \tag{6-37}$$

Range of validity:

$$0.01 \leqslant k_L a \leqslant 1\,\mathrm{s}^{-1}; \quad 3 \leqslant \left(\frac{w_{SG}}{d_s} \right) \leqslant 45$$

The Sauter mean diameter, d_s depends on the type of gasser and the gas throughput (diameter of the primary bubbles), on the medium (rate of coalescence), and on the specific power input. Schügerl uses the dynamic equilibrium bubble diameter, d_e, which applies at a large distance from the gasser. In Schügerl et al. (1977) d_s values are given graphically for various types of gassing devices, gas flow rates, and media. With increasing column height, $k_L a$ falls. It must be pointed out that there may be considerable differences between the $k_L a$ values that exist in the nutrient medium (without cells) and those that are measured during cell growth. Moreover, in bubble-column bioreactors the $k_L a$ values are position-dependent. They are larger in the neighborhood of the gasser than at great distances from it (Buchholz et al., 1980).

b) Air-lift loops with **external** circulation (Fig. 6-17C) consist of two columns: that with the larger diameter (tower) is gassed, and the liquid flows back in the column with the smaller diameter (loop).

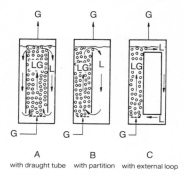

Fig. **6-17.** Air-lift loop reactors (G = gas, L = liquid) (adapted from Weiland, 1978).

Single-Stage Air-Lift Tower Loop Reactors

In an air-lift tower loop reactor, the circulation of the liquid is due to the difference in the densities of the mixed phases in the aerated tower and the nonaerated downcomer regions. The greater the difference in densities (or the gas contents) of the phases and the higher the column, the greater is the rate of circulation. The theory and optimization of the air-lift pump have been treated in numerous publications; e.g., Chakravarty (1976). In practice, several basic constructions are used (Fig. 6-17):

a) Air-lift loop with **internal** circulation

The tower reactor is divided into two regions by means of a coaxial draught tube (Blenke, 1979) or by a vertical plane partition. Only one of the regions is gassed, the other serving as loop.

Loop reactors with a coaxial draught tube but with propeller drive or jet drive have already been treated under 6.4.1 and 6.4.2, respectively.

Air-lift tower loop reactors are very common. Numerous investigations and applications are known (Pilepp et al., 1977; Hines, 1978; Müller et al., 1978; Sittig and Faust, 1980). In spite of the manifold use of this type of reactor, so far no relations have been published for calculating the volumetric mass transfer coefficient. It has only been stated that the **energy demand** for a loop reactor is about 1/5 of that of a conventional stirred vessel when this is used in the production of biomass (Präve, 1977).

The draught tube is frequently modified by additional baffles or dispersing members, e.g., according to Kuraishi et al. (1972).

Loop reactors with a **vertical plane partition** are used both for the treatment of sewage (Hines et al., 1975) and also for the production of SCP (single-cell protein).

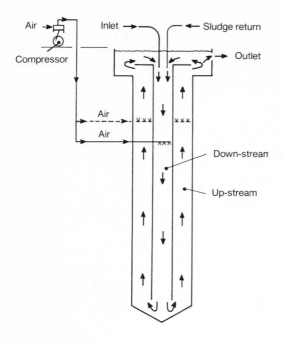

Fig. 6-18. "Deep shaft" reactor (adapted from Hines et al., 1975).

Reactors for sewage treatment include the "deep shaft" loop reactors in which the gassing of the liquid is stated not to be carried out from the bottom of the reactor but at about mid-height (mid-depth) of the downcomer (Fig. 6-18). Circulation is started by the gassing of the riser. Then the liquid in this shaft flows upwards. In the transition to the steady state, the liquid flowing downwards in the other shaft (downcomer) is gassed by nozzles directed downwards. The gassing of the riser can then be stopped. In steady-state operation, fresh gas is introduced only into the downcomer. The total gas buoyancy in the riser is then sufficient to overcome the force of buoyancy of the bubbles in the downcomer.

The depth of such reactors is considerable (50 to 150 m). In a reactor 60 m deep, an oxygen transfer rate of 10 kg O_2/h m^3 is reached at a relatively low specific power input. An air-lift loop reactor with external circulation has been used for the production of biomass (Cow et al., 1975).

If a narrow tube is used for the external downcomer, the rate of circulation is considerably reduced. Yeast (Schügerl et al., 1978; Buchholz et al., 1980), bacteria (Adler, 1980), and mold fungi have been cultivated, and the penicillin fermentation has been studied, in such reactors (König et al., 1982).

– Liquid velocity

In an air-lift tower loop reactor with external circulation and a mixing height of about 10 m, the following relations have been found for the superficial liquid velocity w_{SL} (Weiland, 1978):

$$w_{SL} = 1.15 \ w_{SG}^{0.414} \tag{6-38}$$

Range of validity:

$$0.002 \leqslant w_{SL} \leqslant 0.5 \text{ m s}^{-1}$$
$$0.005 \leqslant w_{SG} \leqslant 0.5 \text{ m s}^{-1}$$

– Relative gas content

In the same reactor, the following expression was found for the gas content with sintered-plate aeration and an ionic strength of 0.1:

$$\varepsilon_G = 55.8 \cdot w_{SG}^{0.725} \tag{6-39}$$

and with perforated-plate aeration, regardless of the ionic strength:

$$\varepsilon_G = 62.3 \cdot w_{SG}^{0.803} \tag{6-40}$$

Range of validity:

$$1 \leqslant \varepsilon_G \leqslant 12\%; \quad 0.005 \leqslant w_{SG} \leqslant 0.14 \text{ m s}^{-1}$$

– Mixing time θ

The air-lift tower loop reactor on the 1-m³ scale is a slow mixing apparatus. As compared with stirred reactors of the same operating capacity, approximately ten times the mixing time is necessary to achieve the same degree of mixing. However, with increasing size of the reactor the mixing times approach one another.

– Volumetric mass transfer coefficient $k_L a$

In air-lift tower loop reactors, the achievable $k_L a$ values are lower than those that can be obtained in the corresponding bubble-column reactors (Weiland, 1978). An influence of the type of gasser and the composition of the medium on $k_L a$ exists, but it is less pronounced than in bubble-column reactors.

Multistage Bubble Columns with Gas and Liquid in Cocurrent

Two types of units are treated here:

a) bubble columns divided into several sections by perforated plates (also called tower reactors), and

b) bubble columns that are provided with static mixers.

E.coli and yeast have been cultivated (Prokop et al., 1969) and sewage has been treated (Hsu et al., 1975) in **bubble columns with perforated plates.** A multistage bubble column with draught tubes has been used for the mass cultivation of yeast and bacteria (Kuraishi et al., 1979).

A mixed sewage culture has been grown in **columns with static mixers.**

The introduction of perforated plates or static mixers considerably reduces the intensity of the ax-ial mixing of the liquid. The use of perforated plates as stage separators considerably increases ε_G and $k_L a$, particularly at higher gas flow rates. The same applies to the static mixers. Probably because of the **numerous design variables** (hole diameter, free cross-sectional area, distance apart and number of the perforated plates, number and type of inserts, and the composition of the medium), no generally valid relation for calculating the operating parameters has so far been published in the literature. Only a few special relations for calculating the beginning of jet formation and the minimum gassing density to avoid weeping are known (Ruff et al., 1976).

6.5 Surface Reactors and their Characterization

Regarded historically, surface reactors were the first fermentation systems to be used. Since submerged reactors require the continuous supply of energy to maintain the gas-liquid interface, while surface cultures do not or to a substantially smaller degree, depending on the system, a renaissance of surface processes cannot be excluded.

6.5.1 Solid Nutrient Substrates

The use of microbial cultures on solid nutrient substrates is carried out predominantly in the laboratory (Oppermann, 1967) in the **search** for and **maintenance** of **strains.** Nutrient solutions treated with a gelling agent set at 50 to 45 °C and are inoculated with, for example, spores at the ambient temperature. The colonies forming after incubation permit the selection of suitable microorganisms. Through the composition of the medium it is possible to select the **conditions of growth** in such a way that unsuitable strains are substantially inhibited at the germination stage. Aeration is carried out by a supply of sterile filtered air.

Solid nutrient substrates are also used for the **cultivation of higher fungi forming fruiting bodies.** In addition to the (trivial) method of inoculating forest soil with fungal spores, e.g., for the cultivation of truffles, the cultivation of mushrooms on horse manure compost (Hunter, 1961) has achieved economic importance (see Chapter 9, p. 325). The cultivation of edible fungi directly on logs should also be mentioned as a nontechnical solid nutrient substrate process.

6.5.2 Fluidized Bed Reactors

Moebus et al. (1981) describe the fermentation of glucose to yield ethanol in a fluidized bed consisting of yeast granules. The fluidizing gas at the same time keeps the granules in motion and dries them.

6.5.3 Agitated Solid Bed Reactors

Deschamps (1981) reported a fermentation of cassava chips by Saccharomyces in a baker's kneader at a mean dry material concentration of 25 to 50%.

6.5.4 Tray Reactors

The growth of microorganisms on solid nutrient substrates is controlled by the rate of diffusion in the solid. This obstacle can be overcome by the introduction of **"fermentation tray processes"** in which a **liquid** is used in place of the jelly-like nutrient medium. The application of these processes is limited to such cultures as can float on the surface. What is aimed at is the formation of a closed mycelial coating under which the liquid can be changed several times as soon as the substrate has become exhausted.

The apparatus that was used at the beginning of the development of this process consisted of shallow Roux bottles which had to be harvested manually (Prescott and Dunn, 1959). They are still used in the laboratory field. For industrial production, fermentation trays (Fig. 6-19) arranged one above the other in sterilizable pressure vessels are employed so that filling, sterilization, and inoculation can be carried out automatically (Kretzschmar, 1955). By the introduction of fresh nutrient solutions as a lower layer, the apparatus can be used in a fed-batch mode of operation. Mass transfer can be varied within narrow limits by controlling the composition of the gas atmosphere.

An interesting variant of such "tray reactors" has been described by Kybal and Vlcek (1976), who have proposed the use of sterilized inflatable plastic cushions that can be filled with nutrient solution, be inoculated, and be aerated through gas-proof tube connections.

6.5.5 Packed-bed Reactors

As a rule, packed-bed reactors are operated in most cases with a continuous gas atmosphere. The nutrient solution is evenly distributed over the packing through a feed device. In these reactors there is no significant change in pressure over their height. They are used mainly in the sewage area, the packing usually being slag or, if the simultaneous absorption of harmful materials is required, activated carbon. Beech shavings are often used as the packing for vinegar fermentations (Ebner, 1976).

The flow of air is usually brought about by the fact that it is warmed by the heat of fermentation and, hence, rises in countercurrent flow to the nutrient solution. The microorganisms settle as a "biological film" on the packing. In principle a growth

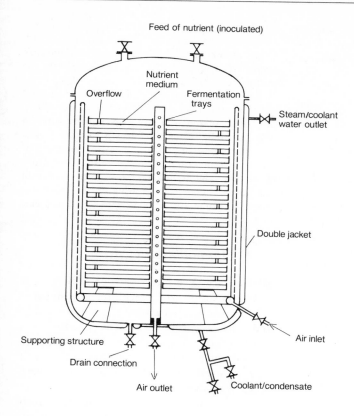

Feed of nutrient (inoculated)

Overflow

Nutrient medium

Fermentation trays

Steam/coolant water outlet

Double jacket

Supporting structure

Drain connection

Air inlet

Air outlet

Coolant/condensate

Fig. 6-19. Tray fermenter, sterilizable and coolable. Filling from the top to the bottom via overflow.

in suspension is equally possible. Atkinson and Ur-Rahman (1976) have given figures for the calculation of the moistened surface, the film thickness of mixed cultures, and the mass transfer in packed fermenters with hollow sphere packing and with Biopac®. The bulk of the data for calculation exists for chemical reactions and absorption procedures (Groto et al., 1976; Blass and Kurtz, 1977). A review of the principles of cocurrent reactors has been given by Hofmann (1975). According to him, the mass transfer coefficient is in the same order of magnitude as for freely rising bubbles. The velocity of the gas in the packing cannot be varied very greatly since it exerts a direct influence on the holdup of the liquid. The gas exchange coefficient k_G amounts to about 3 to $8 \cdot 10^{-4}$ ms^{-1}, and is, to an approximation, independent of the flow conditions. On the other hand, the liquid coefficient depends on the density of irrigation: $k_s \sim w_L^{0.6}$. The mass transfer surface depends on the rate of irrigation:

$a \sim q_L^{0.31}$ to $q_L^{0.5}$. This correlation also applies for the case in which microorganisms have settled on the packing.

6.5.6 Film Reactors

Frequently, instead of packings consisting of bodies of regular (or even irregular) structure, vertically arranged bundles of tubes or channels upon which the nutrient solution is distributed from above are used. The air for incubation is, as a rule, fed in at the bottom so that **countercurrent flow conditions** exist. Film reactors differ from the packed-bed reactors treated in the preceding passage, above all, by the fact that the velocity of the gas phase can be varied within wide limits and the hydrodynamics and mass transfer conditions can be defined better. Hikita et al. (1976) and Blass (1977) have given the mass transfer figures for tubes.

In essence, mass transfer increases with the differential velocity between the liquid and gas phases at the film surface:

$Sh_L = 0.71 \, Re^{0.4} \, Sc^{0.5} \, Ga^{-0.05}$ for $Re_L \leqslant 75$
$Sh_L = 1.69 \, Re^{0.2} \, Sc^{0.5} \, Ga^{-0.05}$ for $75 \leqslant Re_L \leqslant 400$
$Sh_L = 0.16 \, Re^{0.6} \, Sc^{0.5} \, Ga^{-0.05}$ for $Re > 400$

An arrangement of trapezoidal channels formed from plastic foil has been studied by Sittig (1977).

Here, for the gas-liquid mass transfer coefficient in water he found $k_L = 3 \cdot 10^{-4} \, m^{-1}$ at a superficial air velocity of 0.18 ms^{-1}. The operation of such units for the purification of highly loaded sewage is treated in more detail in Chapter 16.

6.5.7   *Immersing Surface Reactors*

By the term **immersing surface reactors,** should be understood all those apparatuses which ensure the supply of substrate and oxygen by the regularly repeated immersion of surfaces coated with the microbial culture into a nutrient solution and the passage of the wetted surfaces into the atmosphere. For the cells, similar conditions exist to those in film reactors. A considerable number of experimental fermenters works by this principle. In the simplest case they consist of horizontal drums immersed in a nutrient solution to the extent of 30 to 50% of their periphery, as has been described by Gorbach (1962), for example. Moser (1973) has studied the residence-time characteristics of the liquid phases as a function of the speed of rotation.

Phillips et al. (1979) have given the oxygen mass transfer figures for a horizontally rotating internally filled hollow cylinder. To a first approximation these rise linearly with the frequency of immersion and the pressure of the gaseous atmosphere. For the rate of mass transfer it is unimportant whether the wetted surface forms an inner or an outer wall. Other variants are used in the form of Caudron's (1979) "biodisque" or as "oxygen ditches" for the purification of sewage. The "Tauchwickel" ("immersion coil") an apparatus according to Engelbart (1969) consisting of a bundle of tubes wound helically on a horizontal drum scoops nutrient solution into each tube on immersion. On rotation, this is kept in the bottom part of the coil by the force of gravity and runs along the helix, wetting the surface of the tubes and driving out the air in front of it. In this way, the organisms growing on the inner surface of the tube are supplied with liquid and aerated.

6.5.8   *Immobilized Cells*

All "surface fermenters" which supply cells settled on solid surfaces with feeds of nutrient solution and gas work basically with immobilized cells. Atkinson regards the phenomenon as a method of preventing the washing out of the cells in continuous fermentation even at high dilution rates (Atkinson and Davies, 1972). With this method it is possible to lower the ratio of the necessary production of cell mass to the amount of substrate converted. Atkinson has expanded the method by introducing particles upon which the mycelium can grow into submerged reactors. The particles can be retained in the fermenter by means of sieves or centrifugal separators. Howell and Atkinson (1976) give a method of calculation based on a double-Monod kinetics by means of which the **ideal film thickness** can be calculated. According to Sittig (1977) an improvement in mass transfer can also be achieved by the introduction of specifically heavy particles upon which no organisms settle into upflow bubble columns. More recent endeavors to use fixed cells, i.e., cells enclosed in a suitable matrix, can help to achieve a breakthrough to the indisputable advantage of the "microbial film" system (Klein et al., 1978).

6.6 Comparison of Reactors

The wealth of reactor designs can be referred to basic types. Only a small amount of substantiated re-

sults, that, when supplemented by estimated values, can give points of reference for the choice of reactor can be filtered out from the literature available. Table 6-10 gives a representation of reactor variants that have become known, which is supplemented in the Appendix, p. 699, with the **maximum apparatus**

Table 6-10. Types of Reactors.

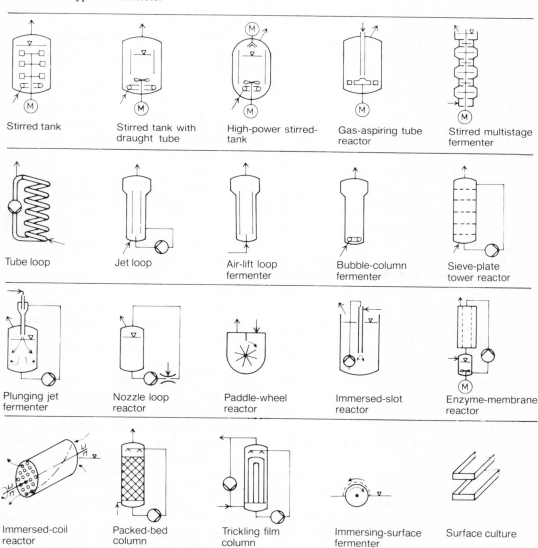

Stirred tank	Stirred tank with draught tube	High-power stirred-tank	Gas-aspiring tube reactor	Stirred multistage fermenter
Tube loop	Jet loop	Air-lift loop fermenter	Bubble-column fermenter	Sieve-plate tower reactor
Plunging jet fermenter	Nozzle loop reactor	Paddle-wheel reactor	Immersed-slot reactor	Enzyme-membrane reactor
Immersed-coil reactor	Packed-bed column	Trickling film column	Immersing-surface fermenter	Surface culture

volumes, the **total power inputs** (gas compression and mechanical energy), and the **achievable** or **reported oxygen transfer rates** that have been described for fermenters. In order to make the possible limitation of the range of use clearly apparent, the possible viscosity range of the medium has been estimated. The input rates given must obviously be reduced for the higher viscosities.

will be developed further, including, possibly, surface reactors. The use of fixed cells and enzymes will increasingly change or even replace fermentation processes. Here, presumably, the conversion of raw materials not used at the present time will form an important economic factor.

6.7   Reactors in Industry

6.7.1   Present State of the Art

Although the discussion of reactors is generally in a state of flux because of the increase in the cost of energy, nevertheless, as before, **aerated stirred apparatuses** occupy the first rank as the most used fermentation reactors (Paschke, 1978). Vessel volumes of up to 400 m^3 for antibiotics, stirrer powers of up to 5 kW/m^3, and viscosities of up to 2 Pa s mark the present state of the art. Dominating materials are stainless chromium-nickel steels. Design pressures range to 4 bar gauge. The stirrer drives used are multistage disk or turbine stirrers which can be exchanged if required. Bubble columns are used for the production of steroids, and bubble columns or gas-inducing aerator systems for the production of acetic acid, SCP, bakers' yeast. Review of bioreactors have been given by Sittig (1983) and Schügerl (1978, 1982, 1983).

6.7.2   Trends of Further Development

There is no doubt that in future designs the economic optima will be displaced more strongly towards **energy-saving systems.** The trend to more and more concentrated and therefore more viscous nutrient solutions will be stopped. Alternative nonstirred reactors

6.8   Practical Advice on the Choice of Reactor

Depending on the size of the production to be planned, the number of fermenter units should not fall below a minimum. In general, the plants must be capable of being used for the manufacture of **more than one product** so that an **economic utilization** of them is ensured. As Sittig and Heine (1977) have shown, the volume of investment for the fermentation proper changes only inconsiderably from product to product, while the harvesting process changes to an extraordinary degree.

As experience shows, even when the plant is used for a single product a flexible design comprising considerable reserves for the flows of material and the drives must be recommended: new strains of microorganisms with higher productivity will be bred and used which require more concentrated and therefore more viscous nutrient solutions, produce more waste heat, and need larger aeration flows. According to Oldshue (1970), the overwhelming number of all production plants have been used up to the limit of their output reserve. Because of the modern possibilities of **power control,** the installation of reserves affects the consumption of energy only insignificantly. The criteria for the choice of gas-liquid contact apparatuses in the chemical industry are given by Nagel et al. (1978), while Euzen et al. (1978) have drawn a comparison between mechanically stirred, air-lift, and loop fermenters which, however, only covers total volumes of up to 1000 L. According to this, for culture broths of low viscosity loop and air-lift systems are recommended. Lainé and Kuoppamäki (1979) have investigated the development of alternative stirred-tank fermenters and have come to the conclusion that draught tube fermenters or propeller fermenters are energetically more favorable than flat-blade turbine systems.

6.9   Literature

Adler, I.: *Reaktionstechnische Untersuchungen an Blasensäulen-Bioreaktoren*. Dissertation, Universität Hannover 1980.

Aiba, S., Humphrey, A. E. and Millis, N. F.: *Biochemical Engineering*, 2nd Ed. Academic Press, New York 1973.

Aiba, S. and Nagatani, M., "Separation of cells from culture media", *Adv. Biochem. Eng.* **1**, 51–54 (1971).

Atkinson, B. and Davies, I. J., "The completely mixed microbial film fermenter", *Trans. Inst. Chem. Eng.* **50**, 208–216 (1972).

Atkinson, B. and Rahmann, A. M. E., "Wetted area, slime thickness and liquid phase mass transfer in packed bed biological film reactors (trickling filters)", *Trans. Inst. Chem. Eng.* **54**, 239–250 (1976).

Atkinson, B. and Ur-Rahman, F., "Effect of diffusion limitations and floc size distributions on fermentor performance and interpretation of experimental data", *Biotechnol. Bioeng.* **21**, 222 (1979).

Bailey, J. E. and Ollis, D. F.: *Biochemical Engineering Fundamentals*. McGraw-Hill, New York 1977.

Biesecker, B. B.: *Begasung von Flüssigkeiten mit Rührern*. VDI-Forschungsheft **554** (1972).

Birckenstaedt, J. W., Faust, U. and Sambeth, W., "Production of SCP from n-paraffin. Process and products", *Process Biochem.*, Nov. (1977).

Blass, E., "Gas/Filmströmung in Rohren", *Chem. Ing. Tech.* **49**, 95–105 (1977).

Blass, E. and Kurtz, R., "Der Einfluß grenzflächenenergetischer Größen auf den Zweiphasen-Gegenstrom durch Füllkörpersäulen", *VT Verfahrenstech.* **11**, 44–48 (1977).

Blenke, H., "Loopreactors", *Adv. Biochem. Eng.* **13**, 121–124 (1979).

Blenke, H. and Schumm, W., "Örtliche Sauerstoffkonzentration im Schlaufenreaktor und ihre Bedeutung für die Berechnung der Phasengrenzfläche", *VT Verfahrenstech.* **14** (12), 797–803 (1980).

Brauer, H., "Power consumption in aerated stirred tank reactor systems", *Adv. Biochem. Eng.* **13**, 87 (1979).

Brauer, H. and Sucker, D., "Abwasser-Reinigung in einem Hochleistungsreaktor", *Chem. Ing. Tech.* **50**, 876 (1978).

Buchholz, H., Luttmann, R., Zakrzewski, W. and Schügerl, K., "Comprehensive study on the cultivation of yeast in a tower bioreactor", *Chem. Eng. Sci.* **35**, 111 (1980).

Calderbank, P. H., "Mass transfer in fermentation equipment", *Biochem. Biol. Eng. Sci.* **1**, 101–180 (1967).

Calderbank, P. H. and Moo-Young, M. B., "The prediction of power consumption in the agitation of non-Newtonian fluids", *Trans. Inst. Chem. Eng.* **37**, 26 (1959).

Caudron, D., "L'épuration des eaux usées par biodisques", *Tech. Eau Assainissement* **392/393**, 39–47 (1979).

Chakravarty, M., Singh, D. H., Baruah, J. N. and Tyengar, M. S., "Liquid velocity in a gas-lift column", *Indian Chem. Eng.* **16**, 17 (1974).

Charles, M., "Technical aspects of the rheological properties of microbial cultures", *Adv. Biochem. Eng.* **8**, 1–62 (1978).

Cow, J. S., Littlehailes, J. D., Smith, S. R. L. and Walter, R. B.: "SCP production from methanol". In: Tannenbaum, S. R. and Wang, D. I. C. (eds.): *Single Cell Protein*, Vol. II. MIT Press, 1975.

Davidson, J. F. and Schüler, B. O. G., "Bubble formation at an orifice in a viscous liquid", *Trans. Inst. Chem. Eng.* **58**, 144 (1960).

Davies, J. T.: *Turbulence Phenomena*. Academic Press, New York 1972.

Deckwer, W. D., "Gas/Flüssig-Reaktoren", *Fortschr. Verfahrenstech.* **15**, 303 (1977).

Deschamps, F., "Aliments fermentés enrichis en protéines", *Proc. Int. Symp. SCP,* Paris 1981.

Diesterweg, G., Fuhr, H. and Reher, P., "Die Bayer-Turmbiologie", *Industrieabwässer* 7–13 (1978).

Ebner, H.: "Über den Einsatz von selbstsaugenden Belüftern in Großfermentern". In: *3. Symposium Technische Mikrobiologie.* Inst. f. Gärungsgewerbe und Fermentationstechnik, Berlin 1973.

Ebner, H.: "Essig". In: *Ullmanns Encyklopädie der technischen Chemie,* Vol. **11.** Verlag Chemie, Weinheim 1976.

Einsele, A., "Charakterisierung von Bioreaktoren durch Mischzeiten", *Chem. Rundsch.* **29,** 25–53 (1976).

Einsele, A. and Fiechter, A., "Novel energy and carbon sources. Liquid and solid hydrocarbons", *Adv. Biochem. Eng.* **1,** 161–194 (1971).

Euzen, J. P. et al., "Comparison of the performance of various fermentors and selection criteria", *Chem. React. Eng.* **2,** 153–162 (1978).

Falch, E. A. and Gaden, E. L., "A continuous multistage tower fermentor, I and II", *Biotechnol. Bioeng.* **11,** 927 (1969) and **12,** 465 (1970).

Faust, U., "Process results from SCP-pilot plant based on methanol", *Dechema Monogr.* **83,** 125 (1979).

Faust, U., Knecht, R. and Wengeler, W. (Uhde GmbH), DOS 2454443 (1976).

Fiechter, A., "Specification of bioreactors. Requirements in view of the reaction and scale of operation", *Dechema Monogr.* **82,** 17 (1978).

Figett, M. and Smith, E. L.: "Microbial solids behavior in tower fermenters". In: *1st European Congress on Biotechnology,* Interlaken 1978, part **2,** 1–92 (1978).

Gerstenberg, H., "Blasensäulen-Reaktoren", *Chem. Ing. Tech.* **51,** 208 (1979).

Ghose, T. K., "Cellulose biosynthesis and hydrolysis of cellulosic substances", *Adv. Biochem. Eng.* **6,** 39–76 (1977).

Gorbach, G., "Die kontinuierliche Dünnschichtfermentation", *Fette, Seifen, Anstrichm.* **71** (2), 98–104 (1962).

Goto, S., Watabe, S. and Matsubara, M., "The role of mass transfer in trickle bed reactors", *Can. J. Chem. Eng.* **54,** 551–555 (1976).

Hallensleben, J., Buchholz, R., Lücke, J. and Schügerl, K., "Blasenbildung und -verhalten im dynamischen Bereich", *Chem. Ing. Tech.* **49,** 663 (1977).

Hassan, I. T. M. and Robinson, C. W., "Oxygen transfer in mechanically agitated aqueous system containing dispersed hydrocarbon", *Biotechnol. Bioeng.* **19,** 661 (1977 a).

Hassan, I. T. M. and Robinson, C. W., "Stirred-tank mechanical power input requirement and gas hold up in aerated aqueous phases", *A.I.Ch.E.J.* **23,** 48 (1977 b).

Henzler, H. J.: "Begasen höherviskoser Flüssigkeiten". In: *Verfahrenstechnische Fortschritte beim Mischen, Dispergieren und bei der Wärmeübertragung in Flüssigkeiten,* Düsseldorf, Dec. 4–5, p. 91. Gesellschaft für Verfahrenstechnik und Chemieingenieurwesen (1978 a).

Henzler, H. J.: *Untersuchungen zum Homogenisieren von Flüssigkeiten oder Gasen.* VDI Forschungsheft **587** (1978 b).

Hiby, J. W.: "Definition und Messung der Mischgüte in flüssigen Gemischen". In: *Verfahrenstechnische Fortschritte beim Mischen, Dispergieren und bei der Wärmeübertragung in Flüssigkeiten,* Düsseldorf, Dec. 4–5, p. 7. Gesellschaft für Verfahrenstechnik und Chemieingenieurwesen (1978).

Hikita, H. et al., "Mass transfer into turbulent gas streams in wetted-wall columns with cocurrent and countercocurrent gas-liquid flow", *J. Chem. Eng. Jpn.* **9** (5), 362–366 (1976).

Hines, D. A., "The large scale pressure cycle fermenter configuration", *Dechema Monogr.* **82,** 55 (1978).

Hines, D. A., Bailey, M., Onsby, J. C. and Roesler, F. C., "The ICI deep shaft aeration process for effluent treatment", *I. Chem. E. Symp. Series No.* **41,** D1 (1975).

Höcker, H. and Langer, G., "Zum Leistungsverhalten begaster Rührer in Newtonschen und nicht-Newtonschen Flüssigkeiten", *Rheol. Acta* **16,** 400 (1977).

Hofmann, H., "Hydrodynamik, Transportvorgang und mathematische Modelle bei Rieselreaktoren", *Chem. Ing. Tech.* **47,** 823–868 (1975).

Howell, J. A. and Atkinson, B., "Influence of oxygen and substrate concentration on the ideal film thickness and the maximum overall substrate uptake rate in microbial film fermenters", *Biotechnol. Bioeng.* **86,** 15–35 (1976).

Hsu, K. H., Erickson, L. E. and Fan, L. T., "Oxygen transfer to mixed cultures in tower systems", *Biotechnol. Bioeng.* **17,** 499 (1975).

Hunter, W.: *Champignonanbau.* Parey Verlag, Berlin 1961.

Intermag Getränke-Technik AG: *Verfahren und Vorrichtung zur Beschleunigung von Lebensvorgängen bei Mikroorganismen,* Patent Application, Aarau (1970).

Jackson, M. L., "Aeration in Bernoulli types of devices", *A.I.Ch.E.J.* **10,** 836 (1964).

Joshi, J. B. and Sharma, M. M., "Mass transfer and hydrodynamic characteristics of gas inducing type of agitated contactors", *Can. J. Chem. Eng.* **55,** 683 (1977).

Judat, H., "Das Dispergieren von Gasen mittels schnellaufender Rührertypen", *Fortschr. Verfahrenstech.* Abt. B **15** (1977).

Karwat, H., "Verteilung von Gasen in Flüssigkeiten durch Rührer", *Chem. Ing. Tech.* **31,** 588 (1959).

Katinger, H. W. D.: "Simulierung, Differenzierung und Bestimmung physikalischer Fermentationsparameter in Rezirkulationssystemen". In: *3. Symposium Technische Mikrobiologie,* Inst. f. Gärungsgewerbe und Fermentationstechnik, Berlin 1973.

Katinger, H. W. D., Schreier, W. and Krömer, E., "Bubble column reactor for mass propagation of animal cells in suspension culture", *Ger. Chem. Eng.* **2,** 31 (1979).

Keitel, G.: *Untersuchungen zum Stoffaustausch in Gas- und Flüssig-Dispersionen in Rührschlaufenreaktor und Blasensäule.* Dissertation, Universität Dortmund 1978.

Kipke, K.: "Begasen von nicht-Newtonschen Flüssigkeiten". In: DFVLR, Keune, H. and Scheunemann, R. (eds.): *Bioreaktoren.* BMFT-Statusseminar "Bioverfahrenstechnik". Braunschweig-Stöckheim 1977.

Kipke, K., "Rühren von dünnflüssigen und mittelviskosen Medien", *Chem. Ing. Tech.* **51,** 430 (1979).

Klein, J. et al., "Formation of 6-APA from Penicillin G by immobilized cells of *Escherichia coli,* ATCC 11, 1+5", *Dechema Monogr.* **82** (1978).

Kloud, J. and Sterbacek, Z., "Ein Beitrag zur diskontinuierlichen Kultivation von Futterhefe in einer Blasensäule", *Chem. Tech.* **24,** 688 (1972).

König, B., Schügerl, K., Seewald, Ch., "Strategies for penicillin fermentation in tower loop reactor", *Biotechnol. Bioeng.* **24,** 259–280 (1982).

Kretzschmar, H.: *Hefe und Alkohol.* Springer Verlag, Berlin, Heidelberg, New York 1955.

Krishnamurthi, S., Kumar, R. and Kuloor, N. R., "Bubble formation in viscous liquids under constant conditions", *Ind. Eng. Chem. Fundam.* **7,** 549 (1968).

Kumar, R. and Kuloor, N. R., "The formation of bubbles and drops", *Adv. Chem. Eng.* **8** (1970).

Kuraishi, M., Terao, I., Ohkouchi, H., Matsuda, N. and Nagai, I., "SCP-Process development with methanol as substrate", *Dechema Monogr.* **83,** 111 (1979).

Kürten, H. and Maurer, B.: "Gasdispergierung im turbulenten Scherfeld". In: Brauer, H. and Molerus, O. (eds.): *Partikel Technologie,* Vol. **47,** 47, Nürnberg 1977.

Kybal, J. and Vlcek, V., "Simple device for stationary cultivation of microorganisms", *Biotechnol. Bioeng.* **18,** 1713–1718 (1976).

Lafferty, R. M., Moser, A., Steiner, M. and Saria, A.: *Tauchstrahl-Schlaufenreaktor.* Vortrag auf der Dechema-Jahrestagung 1977.

Lainé, J. and Kuoppamäki, R., "Development of the design of large-scale fermentors", *Ind. Eng. Chem. Prod. Res. Dev.* **18,** 501–506 (1979).

Lehmann, J. and Hammer, J.: "Continous fermentation in tower fermentor". In: *1st European Congress on Biotechnology,* Interlaken 1978, part **2,** 1–73 (1978).

Lewis, C. W., "Energy requirement for single cell protein production", *J. Appl. Chem. Biotechnol.* **26,** 568 (1976).

Liepe, F., Jagusch, L., Stephan, W. and Ringpfeil, M., "The present state and the perspective of development of industrial high performance fermentors for aerobic fermentations", *Dechema Monogr.* **1,** 78 (1978).

Litchfield, J. H., "Food industry wastes: technological aspects of disposal and utilization", *Chem. Eng. Progr. Symp. Ser.* **67** (108), 164 (1971).

Litchfield, J. H., "Use of hydrocarbon fractions for the production of SCP", *Biotechnol. Bioeng. Symp.* **7,** 77 (1977).

Loiseau, B., Midoux, N. and Charpentier, J. C., "Some hydrodynamics and power input data in mechanically agitated gas-liquid contactors", *A.I.Ch.E.J.* **23**, 931 (1977).

MacLean, G. T., "Oxygen transfer in aerated systems with two liquid phases", *Process Biochem.* **12**, 22 (1977).

Margaritis, A. and Zajic, J. E., "Mixing, mass transfer and scale-up of polysaccharide fermentations", *Biotechnol. Bioeng.* **20**, 939 (1978).

Meister, D., Post, T., Dunn, I. J. and Bourne, J. R., "Design and characterization of a multistage, mechanically stirred column absorber", *Chem. Eng. Sci.* **34**, 1367 (1979).

Mersmann, A., "Auslegung und Maßstabsvergrößerung von Blasen- und Tropfensäulen", *Chem. Ing. Tech.* **49**, 679 (1977).

Mersmann, A., Einenkel, W. D. and Käppel, N., "Auslegung und Maßstabsvergrößerung von Rührapparaten", *Chem. Ing. Tech.* **47**, 953 (1975).

Metz, B., Kossen, N. W. F. and von Suijdam, I. C., "The rheology of mould suspensions", *Adv. Biochem. Eng.* **11**, 103 (1979).

Metzner, A. B. and Otto, R. E., "Agitation of non-Newtonian fluids", *A.I.Ch.E.J.* **3**, 3 (1957).

Metzner, A. B., Feehs, R. H., Ramos, H. L., Otto, R. E. and Tuthill, J. D., "Agitation of viscous Newtonian and non-Newtonian fluids", *A.I.Ch.E.J.* **7**, 3 (1961).

Michel, B. J. and Miller, S. A., "Power requirements of gas-liquid agitated systems", *A.I.Ch.E.J.* **8**, 262 (1962).

Midler, jr. M. and Finn, R. K., "A model system for evaluating shear in the design of stirred fermentors", *Biotechnol. Bioeng.* **8**, 71 (1966).

Miller, D. N., "Scale up of agitated vessel gas-liquid mass transfer", *A.I.Ch.E.J.* **20**, 445 (1974).

Miura, Y., "Transfer of oxygen and scale-up in submerged aerobic fermentation", *Adv. Biochem. Eng.* **4**, 3 (1976).

Moebus, O., Teuber, M. and Reuter, H., "Growth of *Saccharomyces cerevisiae* in form of solid particles in a gaseous fluidized bed", *Mitt. Bundesanstalt für Milchforschung,* Kiel 1981.

Moser, A., "Verweilzeitcharakteristik eines gerührten Rohrfermenters", *VT Verfahrenstech.* **7**, 198-201 (1973).

Motarjemi, M. and Jameson, G. J., "Mass transfer from very small bubbles. The optimum bubble size for aeration", *Chem. Eng. Sci.* **33**, 1415 (1978).

Müller, G., Sell, G., Bauer, A. and Leistner, G., "Abwasserreinigung in einem Bio-Hochreaktor", *Chem. Tech.* **7**, 257 (1978).

Müllner, J. (Waagner-Biro GmbH): "Verfahren und Einrichtung zur Behandlung von Flüssigkeit und Trüben". Austrian Patent 319864 (1973).

Nagel, O., Hegner, B. and Kürten, H., "Kriterien für die Auswahl und die Auslegung von Gas/Flüssigkeits-Reaktoren", *Chem. Ing. Tech.* **50** (12), 934-944 (1978).

Oldshue, J. Y., "The case for deep aeration tanks", *Chem. Eng. Prog.* **66** (1), 73-78 (1970).

Oppermann, A., *Zentralbl. Bakteriol. Parasitenk. Infektionskr. Hyg. Abt. 1 Orig.* **2**, 4 (1967).

Páca, J. and Grégr, V., "Growth characteristics of *Candida utilis* on volatile substrate in a multistage tower fermentor", *Biotechnol. Bioeng.* **19**, 539 (1977).

Paschke, M., "Bioreaktoren, ein Überblick", *GIT Fachz. Lab.* **2 Z**, 987-988 (1978).

Perez, J. F. and Sandall, O. C., "Gas absorption by non-Newtonian fluids in agitated vessels", *A.I.Ch.E.J.* **20**, 770 (1974).

Phillips, D. H., "Oxygen transfer into mycelial pellets", *Biotechnol. Bioeng.* **8**, 456 (1966).

Phillips, K. L., Sallans, H. R. and Spencer, J. F. T., "Oxygen transfer in fermentations", *Ind. Eng. Chem.* **5** (9), 749-754 (1961).

Pilepp, E., Scheffler, U. and Schmidt-Mende, P.: "Entwicklung eines Bioreaktors nach dem Umlaufprinzip unter besonderer Berücksichtigung der Meß- und Regeltechnik". In: Keune, H. and Scheunemann, R. (eds.): *Bioreaktoren.* BMFT-Statusseminar "Bioverfahrenstechnik". Braunschweig-Stöckheim 1977.

Pirt, S. J.: *Principles of Microbe and Cell Cultivation.* Blackwell Scientific Publishers, Oxford 1975.

Präve, P., "Die Nutzung des mikrobiellen Lebensraumes – Moderne Entwicklungen biologischer Technologien", *Angew. Chem.* **89**, 211 (1977).

Prasher, B. D., "Mass transfer coefficients and interfacial areas in agitated dispersions", *A.I.Ch.E.J.* **21**, 407 (1975).

Prescott, S. C. and Dunn, C. G.: *Industrial Microbiology.* McGraw-Hill, New York 1959.

Prokop, A., Erickson, L. E., Fernandez, J. and Humphrey, A. E., "Design and physical characteristics of a multistage, continuous tower fermentor", *Biotechnol. Bioeng.* **11**, 945 (1969).

Rehm, H. J.: *Industrielle Mikrobiologie,* 2nd Ed. Springer-Verlag, Berlin, Heidelberg, New York 1980.

Righelato, R. C., "Selection of strains of *Penicillium chrysogenum* with reduced penicillin yields in continuous cultures", *J. Appl. Chem. Biotechnol.* **26**, 153 (1976).

Robinson, C. W. and Wilke, C. R., "Oxygen absorption in stirred tanks. A correlation for ionic strength effects", *Biotechnol. Bioeng.* **15**, 755 (1973).

Ruff, K., Pilhofer, T. and Mersmann, A., "Vollständige Durchströmung von Lochböden bei der Fluid-Dispergierung", *Chem. Ing. Tech.* **48**, 759 (1976).

Schreier, K., "Neuer Hochleistungsfermenter nach dem Tauchstrahlverfahren", *Chem. Ztg.* **99**, 328 (1975).

Schügerl, K.: *Entwicklung von Bioreaktoren für die industrielle Praxis in der Biotechnologie.* Forschung Aktuell. Biotechnologie. Umschau Verlag, Frankfurt 1978.

Schügerl, K., "Oxygen transfer into highly viscous media", *Adv. Biochem. Eng.* **19**, 71 (1981).

Schügerl, K., "New bioreactors for aerobic processes", *Int. Chem. Eng.* **22**, 591 (1982).

Schügerl, K., "Apparatetechnische Aspekte der Kultivierung von Einzellern in Turmreaktoren", *Chem. Ing. Tech.* **55**, 123–134 (1983).

Schügerl, K., Lücke, J., Lehmann, J. and Wagner, F., "Application of tower bioreactors in cell mass production", *Adv. Biochem. Eng.* **8**, 63–131 (1978).

Schügerl, K., Oels, U. and Lücke, J., "Bubble column bioreactors", *Adv. Biochem. Eng.* **7**, 1–84 (1977).

Schumpe, A. and Deckwer, W. D., "Estimation of O_2 and CO_2 solubilities in fermentation media", *Biotechnol. Bioeng.* **21**, 1075 (1979).

Sinn, R., Herrmann, G., Nagel, O., Schring, H. and Hornberger, P.: "Verfahren und Vorrichtung zum Vermischen von Gasen und Flüssigkeiten mit einem flüssigen Medium". DOS 1557018 (1970).

Sittig, W., "Biochemical Reactors", *Fortschr. Verfahrenstech.* **21**, 397–421 (1983).

Sittig, W., "Untersuchungen zur Verbesserung des Stoffaustausches in Fermentern", *VT Verfahrenstech.* **11**, 12 (1977b).

Sittig, W. and Faust, U., "Methanol as carbon source for biomass production in a loop reactor", *Adv. Biochem. Eng.* **17** (1980).

Sittig, W. and Heine, H., "Erfahrungen mit großtechnisch eingesetzten Bioreaktoren", *Chem. Ing. Tech.* **49**, 595–605 (1977).

Smith, E. L. and Greenshields, R. N., "Tower-Fermentation systems and their application to aerobic processes", *Chem. Eng. (London)* **281**, 28 (1974).

Smith, E. L., James, A. and Fidgett, M.: "Fluidization of microbial aggregates in tower fermenters". In: *Engineering Foundation Fluidization Symposium,* Cambridge 1978. Cambridge University Press 1978.

Solomons, G. L., "Mixing and scale-up characteristics of an *Aspergillus* culture broth", *Contin. Cultiv. Microorg. Proc. Symp. 2nd 1962* (publ. 1964).

Steel, R. and Maxon, W. D., "Dissolved oxygen measurements in pilot- and production-scale Novocain fermentations", *Biotechnol. Bioeng.* **8**, 9 (1966a).

Steel, R. and Maxon, W. D., "Studies with a multiple-rod mixing impeller", *Biotechnol. Bioeng.* **18**, 109 (1966b).

Steiff, A.: "Wärmeaustausch in Rührkesseln bei mehrphasigen Systemen". In: *Verfahrenstechnische Fortschritte beim Mischen, Dispergieren und bei der Wärmeübertragung in Flüssigkeiten,* Düsseldorf, Dec. 4–5, 1978. Gesellschaft für Verfahrenstechnik und Chemieingenieurwesen (1978).

Suicu, G. D. and Smigelschi, O., "Size of the submerged biphasic region in plunging jet systems", *Chem. Eng. Sci.* **31**, 1217 (1976).

Swallow, B., Finn, R. K. and Einsele, A.: "Design of aerated fermentors for non-Newtonian liquids". In: *1st European Congress on Biotechnology,* Interlaken 1978, part **1**, 21 (1978).

Taguchi, H., "The nature of fermentation fluids", *Adv. Biochem. Eng.* **1** (1971).

Topiwala, H. H. and Hamer, G., "Mass transfer and dispersion properties in a fermentor with a gas-inducing impeller", *Trans. Inst. Chem. Eng.* **52**, 113 (1974).

van't Riet, K., Boom, J. M. and Smith, J. M., "Power consumption, impeller coalescence and recirculation in aerated vessels", *Trans. Inst. Chem. Eng.* **54,** 124 (1976).

van de Sande, E. and Smith, J. M., "Jet break-up and air entrainment by low velocity turbulent water jets", *Chem. Eng. Sci.* **31,** 219 (1976).

Voigt, J. and Schügerl, K., "Begasung nieder- und hochviskoser Fermentations-Modellmedien in mehrstufigen Gegenstrom-Blasensäulen", *Chem. Ing. Tech.* **50,** 721 (1978).

Voigt, J. and Schügerl, K., "Absorption of oxygen in countercurrent multistage bubble columns. I.", *Chem. Eng. Sci.* **34,** 1221 (1979).

Vollmüller, H. and Walburg, R.: "Blasengröße bei der Begasung mit Venturidüsen". In: *Gemeinsame Tagung der VTG und ICE über "Blasen und Schäume"*, Nürnberg 1971. VDI-Berichte Nr. **182** (1972).

Wang, D. I. C., Cooney, C. L., Demain, A. L., Dunnill, P., Humphrey, A. E. and Lilly, D. M.: *Fermentation and Enzyme Technology*. John Wiley and Sons., New York 1979.

Weihrauch, W., "Mehrstufen-Impuls-Gegenstromrührer", *VT Verfahrenstech.* **2,** 243 (1968).

Weihrauch, W., "Selbstsaugende Begasung mit dem MIG-Rührsystem", *VT Verfahrenstech.* **6,** 35 (1972).

Weiland, P.: *Untersuchungen eines Airliftreaktors mit äußerem Umlauf im Hinblick auf seine Anwendung als Bioreaktor.* Dissertation, Universität Dortmund 1978.

Yagi, H. and Yoshida, F., "Gas absorption by Newtonian and non-Newtonian fluids in sparged agitated vessels", *Ind. Eng. Chem. Prod. Res. Dev.* **14,** 488 (1975).

Zlokarnik, M., "Rohrrührer zum Ansaugen und Dispergieren großer Gasdurchsätze in Flüssigkeiten", *Chem. Ing. Tech.* **21,** 1310 (1970).

Zlokarnik, M.: "Rührtechnik". In: *Ullmanns Encyklopädie der technischen Chemie,* Vol. **2,** 4th Ed. Verlag Chemie, Weinheim 1972.

Zlokarnik, M., "Rührleistung in begasten Flüssigkeiten", *Chem. Ing. Tech.* **45,** 689 (1973).

Zlokarnik, M., "Der Schaufelradreaktor – ein spezieller Reaktortyp für Reaktionen im System gasförmig/flüssig", *VT Verfahrenstech.* **9,** 442 (1975).

Zlokarnik, M., "Sorption characteristics for gas-liquid contacting in mixing vessels", *Adv. Biochem. Eng.* **8,** 133–151 (1978).

Zlokarnik, M., "Sorption characteristics of slot injectors and their dependency on the coalescence behaviour of the system", *Chem. Eng. Sci.* **34,** 1265 (1979).

6.10   Explanation of the Symbols

A	Cross-section area of empty tube	(m^2)
$a = A'/V_L$	Specific interfacial area referred to the liquid volume, Eq. (6-27 a)	$(m^2\,m^{-3})$
$a^* = A'/V$	Specific interfacial area referred to the volume of the mixed phase, Eq. (6-27 b)	$(m^2\,m^{-3})$
A'	Gas-liquid interfacial area	(m^2)
c	Specific heat of the medium	$(kJ\,kg^{-1}\,K^{-1})$
C	Constant	
C_D	Drag coefficient	$(-)$
C_{O_2}	Concentration of dissolved oxygen	$(g\,L^{-1})$
$C_{O_2}^*$	Concentration of dissolved oxygen at saturation	$(g\,L^{-1})$
$C_{O_{2k}}$	Critical concentration of dissolved oxygen	$(g\,L^{-1})$
d	Diameter	(m)
d_T	Diameter of the tank	(m)
D	Rate of dilution	(h^{-1})
D_L	Molecular coefficient of diffusion of oxygen in the medium	$(m^2\,h^{-1})$
d_i	Diameter of the stirrer	(m)

d_e	Dynamic equilibrium bubble diameter	(m)
d_s	Sauter bubble diameter	(m)
ε	Gas void fraction, Eq. (6-26)	(-)
Fr	Froude number of stirrer $= \dfrac{n^2 d}{g}$	(-)
Ga	Galilei number $= \dfrac{g d^3 v^2}{\eta_r^2}$	(-)
g	Gravitational constant	(m s^{-2})
H	Height of the layer of mixed phase	(m)
H_L	Height of the layer of liquid	(m)
K	Fluid consistency index, Eq. (6-22)	(Pa s^n)
K_s, K_o	Saturation constants of the substrate and of oxygen	(g L^{-1})
k	Constant	(-)
k_L	Mass transfer coefficient through the gas/liquid interface	(m s^{-1})
$k_L a$	Volumetric mass transfer coefficient	(s^{-1}), (h^{-1})
$(k_L a)^*$	$= k_L a (v/g^2)^{0.33}$	
m	Flow behavior index, Eq. (6-22)	(-)
Ne	Newton number $P/n^3 d^5$	(-)
OTR	Oxygen transfer rate	(kg m^{-3} h^{-1})
P_G	Power input into the gassed system	(kW)
P_o	Power input into the ungassed system	(kW)
P_L	Power input of the driving jet	(kW)
Pr	Prandtl number of the medium $= \dfrac{\eta c}{\lambda}$	
PR	Productivity	(kg m^{-3} h^{-1})
$(P/V)^*$	Specific power input $(P/V_L)\,[\rho (g v^4)^{0.33}]^{-1}$	(-)
$(P/q)^*$	$(P/q_G)\,[\rho (g v)^{0.67}]^{-1}$	(-)
Q	Aeration number $q_G/n d^3$	(-)
Q_z	Production of heat during cell growth, Eq. (6-16)	(kJ h^{-1})
q_G	Gas flow	(m^3 h^{-1})
q_L	Liquid flow	(m^3 h^{-1})
q_s	Substrate feed rate, Eq. (6-8)	(kg h^{-1})
$(q/V)^*$	$(q/V_L)\,(v/g^2)^{0.33}$	(-)
Re	Reynolds number for the stirrer $= n d^2/v$	(-)
r_X	Rate of cell growth, Eq. (6-1)	(g L^{-1} h^{-1})
$-r_s$	Rate of consumption of substrate, Eq. (6-2)	(g L^{-1} h^{-1})
$-r_o$	Rate of consumption of oxygen, Eq. (6-3)	(g L^{-1} h^{-1})
S	Substrate concentration	(g L^{-1})
Sc	Schmidt number $Sc = \dfrac{v}{D_L}$; $Sc_r = \dfrac{v_r}{D_L}$	(-)
Sh	Sherwood number for mass transfer $Sh = \dfrac{k d}{D_L}$	(-)
t	Time of cultivation	(h)
u	Velocity of shear	(m s^{-1})
du/dx	Shear gradient, Eq. (6-19)	(s^{-1})
V	Volume of the mixed phase	(m^3)
V_L	Volume of the liquid	(m^3)
w_{SG}	Superficial gas velocity q_G/A	(m s^{-1})
w_{SL}	Superficial liquid velocity q_L/A	(m s^{-1})

X	Concentration of biomass	(g L^{-1})
Y_s	Substrate yield coefficient, Eq. (6-2)	(g g^{-1})
Y_o	Oxygen yield coefficient, Eq. (6-3)	(g g^{-1})
Y_{kJ}	Heat yield coefficient, Eq. (6-16)	(g kJ^{-1})
α	Heat-transfer coefficient	$(\text{kJ m}^{-2}\,\text{h}^{-1}\,\text{K}^{-1})$
Γ	Ionic strength	(g L^{-1})
ε_G	Gas void fraction	$(-)$
η	Dynamic viscosity of the medium	$(\text{Pa s}) =$
		(N s m^{-2})
θ	Mixing time	(s)
λ	Coefficient of thermal conductivity	$(\text{kJ m}^{-1}\,\text{h}^{-1}\,\text{K}^{-1})$
μ	Specific growth rate of the cells	(h^{-1})
$v = \eta/\rho$	Kinematic viscosity of the medium	$(\text{m}^2\,\text{s}^{-1})$
ρ	Density of the medium	(kg m^{-3})
σ	Surface tension of the medium	(N m^{-1})
τ	Mean residence time	(h)
τ_s	Shear stress	(N m^{-2})
ξ	Dimensionless number characterizing the properties of a liquid	$(-)$

Indices

1	In a well-mixed reactor	k	Critical value
B	Bubbles	L	Liquid
o	In the inflow	O_2	Oxygen
m	Maximum value	S	Substrate
r	Representative magnitude	X	Cell mass
G	Gas		

Chapter 7

Biological Regulation and Process Control

Armin Fiechter, Marinus Meiners, and
Dieter Andreas Sukatsch

7.1 Introduction

The basis of any biotechnological process is the growing or resting cell and its constituents (organelles, enzymes). The metabolic processes that are to be utilized for economic purposes in biotechnology are catalyzed by specific catalysts (= biocatalysts = enzymes) the activities of which are subject to certain control mechanisms.

A simple bacterial cell such as *Escherichia coli* has available more than 1000 to 2000 enzymes (actual or potential) which may make up as much as 70% of the total cell weight. In using them, the practical man is therefore employing a complex system he is quite incapable of viewing in its totality. Consequently, in process development he is usually forced to carry out empirical procedures and with his technical measures (design and performance of the process) acts on biological regulations of which he knows only an overall result.

Process control must start from the biological facts and utilize them for technical application. The metabolism of added substrates takes place via about 20 steps and yields about 20 amino acids, four deoxyribonucleotides, four ribonucleotides, about ten vitamins, and several fatty acids, from which more than 1000 proteins, three types of RNA (RNA = ribonucleic acid) DNAs (DNA = deoxyribonucleic acid) (+ plasmids), mucopeptides, polysaccharides, and lipids must be synthesized. In procaryotes, these processes may take place in 15 to 20 min (= one generation time), the coordination of the activities of the catalytic elements ensuring that undesired overproductions do not occur.

It is interesting that the regulation of enzyme activity takes place according to principles similar to those applied in technology (closed action cycle, Figs. 7-1a and b).

The organization and treatment of the material is adapted to the **special use,** and the total complex is constructed on the basis of the methods of measurement. This procedure takes into account the fact that measurement technique primarily follows independent tasks and aims precisely within the biotechnological process. Thus, the information obtained by **measurement** concerning the instantaneous state of operation of the process leaves open the question of whether and what useful application is made of the information obtained. Within the framework of process analysis, this application is limited to the search for the functional relationships of the process in order, in this way, to find the structures and acting relationships between the variables of state and to understand the principles of the biological system better. In the first place, therefore, this analysis follows the aim of broadening our knowledge on the interaction of the organisms with their environment.

On the basis of this knowledge, it is then possible to affect the features of the process in a desired manner by **control** or **regulation.** Here, the possibilities of the **controlled performance of the process** must be made use of by establishing and maintaining the optimum environmental conditions for the growth of the organisms and for the formation of products by them.

On the various levels of process study and directed action on the occurence of the process, the **process computer** is an effective aid. In association with process analysis this can bring into prominence the particular possibilities of a rapid **concentration of information.** When improved instrumentation is taken into account, it can readily be seen that these tasks are not trivial, and the desired information is often available only after the various process magnitudes have been combined. In addition to these tasks from the field of data processing and analysis, development has the aim of an increasing use of the computer in process control and regulation. In this connection it must be expected that even complex control strategies will be capable of being realized to an increased degree. From the point of view of

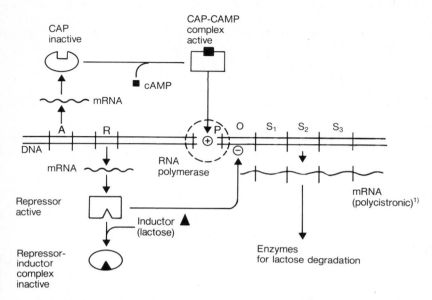

Fig. 7-1a. Substrate induction (derepression) of protein synthesis.

The induction of enzyme protein synthesis by the substrate already present forms the regulatory mechanism that is to be found mainly in degradative (= catabolic) metabolic pathways. The induction takes place at the transcription level.

Classical Jacob-Monod operon model in procaryotes. Catabolic pathway: cleavage of lactose for the inclusion of the resulting monoses in glycolysis. Inductor = lactose = substrate; a substance that inhibits the binding of the repressor to the operator gene.

A   activator gene (gene product: mRNA for CAP = catabolite activator protein)
R   regulator gene (gene product: mRNA for repressor protein)
P   promotor gene (binding site for CAP-cAMP and RNA polymerase)
O   operator gene (binding site for repressor protein)
S_1–S_3 structural genes (gene product: mRNA for lactose-degrading enzyme proteins)
CAP   catabolite activator protein, product of the activator gene
cAMP   cyclic adenosine monophosphate.

The function of the repressor protein is decisive:

Active: the repressor binds to the operator gene and blocks ($\ominus$) the transcription of the structural genes.

Inactive: Combination with the substrate (lactose) inactivates the repressor. The repressor-inductor complex does not bind to the operator gene and transcription of the structural genes can start. Therefore without lactose as the substrate of a catabolic pathway the excessive production of the enzymes that are necessary for its degradation is prevented.

A prerequisite for transcription is the binding of the RNA polymerase to the promotor gene. Fig. 1 a shows the important role of cAMP in this reaction. The combination of CAP with cAMP results in the formation of an active complex, CAP-cAMP. This complex binds to the promotor gene and thereby permits ($\oplus$) the binding of the mRNA polymerase ($\bigcirc$) to this region.

In addition to **substrate induction,** in certain cases **substrate inhibition** may also occur but this is not active at the transcription level (see Cleland, 1979).

---

[1] polycistronic mRNA: *one* mRNA molecule contains the information for *several* protein molecules

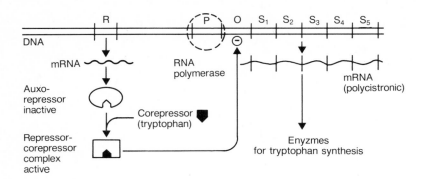

Fig. 1b. Repression of protein synthesis.

The repression of enzyme protein synthesis by the product which results from the action of these enzymes forms the regulatory mechanism that is to be found in synthetic (=anabolic) metabolic pathways. The repression takes place at the transcription level.

Classical Jacob-Monod operon model in procaryotes. Anabolic pathway: synthesis of the amino acid tryptophan. Corepressor = tryptophan = end product; a substance that permits the binding of the auxorepressor to the operator gene.

R   regulator gene (gene product: mRNA for auxorepressor protein)
P   promotor gene (binding site for RNA polymerase)
O   operator gene (binding site for repressor-corepressor complex)
S_1–S_5 structural genes (gene product: mRNA for tryptophan-synthesizing enzyme proteins).

The function of the repressor protein is decisive:

Active: By combination of the corepressor (the end product tryptophan) with the inactive auxorepressor the active repressor-corepressor complex is formed. This complex binds to the operator gene and blocks ($\ominus$) the transcription of the structural genes. Tryptophan as the end product of an anabolic pathway can therefore prevent excessive production of the enzymes which are necessary for its synthesis.

Inactive: The auxorepressor does not bind to the operator gene and transcription of the structural genes can start.

control techniques, the possibility of the **mathematical formulation** of individual biological or chemical-engineering process steps is also of particular importance. In this way, the process computer can finally make a contribution to the utilization of increasing knowledge concerning regulation phenomena within the cell for an improved performance of the process.

An **optimization** can be carried out on the basis of earlier knowledge (off-line) but, in the present state of the art, on-line calculations, made possible by the availability of modern digital computers, can also be used. Consequently, the interrelationship of the techniques of measurement, control, and computing must be studied.

The **number** of **process quantities** and **parameters** in fermentation is very large. For the description of microorganisms, biologists use about 100 different magnitudes, and in technical processes with microorganisms physical, chemical, and process-engineering magnitudes are involved in still greater number, so that the complex system of a fermentation cannot be calculated or described totally even

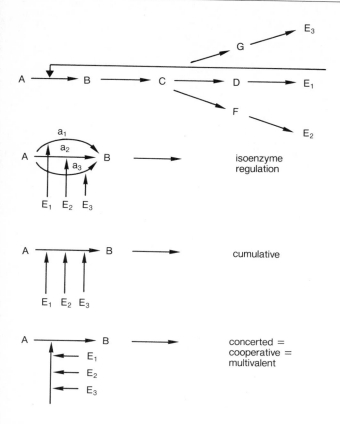

Fig. 1c. Inhibition of enzyme activity.

In anabolic metabolic pathways, regulation at the level of enzyme function by the end product of a synthetic sequence = **feedback regulation** is frequently observed. In the case of negative feedback, in the first line the first enzyme of the sequence is regulated; the following steps are switched off. This realizes an economic principle with respect to enzyme function. In the case of branched anabolic pathways, several end-products ($E_1 \ldots E_3$) may participate in the regulation of the first step. Depending on organization, end products act as effectors individually on individual isoenzymes ($a_1 \ldots a_3$) or, when a single enzyme is present, they act on this together. Their action may be cumulative or concerted.

Cumulative action of the effectors arises when the individual effector causes only partial repressional inhibition. All end products of the branches in the pathway are therefore necessary for complete blockage.

Concerted (multivalent, cooperative) feedback occurs when the enzyme (of the first stage) can be regulated to a significant extent, if at all, only by a simultaneous excess of several effectors. The molecular mechanism consists of inhibition.

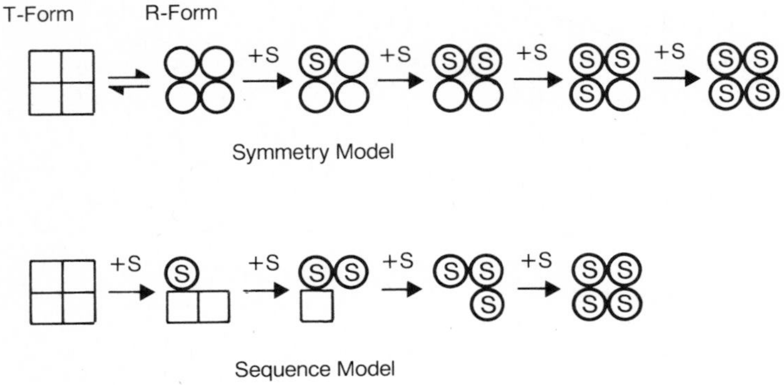

T-Form   R-Form

Symmetry Model

Sequence Model

Fig. 1d. Symmetry model and sequence model.

Substrate binding and inhibition are based on changes in enzyme conformation.

As an example of a change in conformation, the figure 1 d shows the autoregulation of so-called sigmoid enzymes in which the activity curve as a function of the substrate concentration is S-shaped (sigmoid). This regulation can be explained by the symmetry model or by the sequence model.

In the **symmetry model,** the sigmoid saturation by the substrate arises by the fact that an oligomeric enzyme is present in two forms each with sterically identical subunits (T-form = tensed; R-form = relaxed). Here, because of the binding of the substrate to the R-Form, with increasing concentration of the substrate the equilibrium between the two forms is displaced progressively in favor of the R-form. The conformational change therefore takes place symmetrically. No unsymmetrical oligomers occur. **Activators bind to the R-form and inhibitors to the T-form.**

A sigmoid saturation by the substrate arises in the **sequence model** by virtue of the fact that an enzyme exhibits several substrate-binding sites or consists of several subunits each having one binding site. These binding sites influence one another by the fact that the occupation of the first site by the substrate facilitates the occupancy of the second site, and this, in turn, that of the third site. Thus, unsymmetrical oligomers arise with sterically dissimilar subunits. **Activators promote** the conversion of subunits with a low affinity into ones with a high affinity, while **inhibitors oppose** this process. Frequently, in addition to the enzyme substrate, other effectors (ions, ATP, NADH, etc.) are also capable of bringing about the activation or inactivation of the subunits.

in an approximation. Limits are still set to the determination of measurements in biotechnology by technical factors, so that many process magnitudes can be measured

– not at all,
– not sufficiently accurately, or
– not on-line (and therefore not frequently enough).

Biotechnology, as a scientific technology, is still a very young field. In measurement and control technique, experience and, to a large extent, apparatus, have been taken over from chemical process engineering. In some measuring processes, adaptations have already been made to the particular features of biotechnology but other methods have been very incompletely used in biotechnology, in many cases. This applies particularly to control technique. Again, methods can be taken over from other sciences and applied to fermentation technique; e.g., from medicine.

In a bioprocess, four types of process magnitudes can be distinguished:

a) Control magnitudes (manipulated variables, input magnitudes)

b) magnitudes of state (measurements)

c) magnitudes of quality (optimization magnitudes, output magnitudes)

d) Characterization magnitudes (parameters)
   - theoretical parameters (physical, chemical, biological model)
   - experimental parameters (experimental process identification).

a) **Control magnitudes** are process magnitudes that can be predetermined externally as required, i.e., that can be adjusted independently of the process as, for example, flow rates, dosages, and speeds of rotation, and they are therefore also called manipulated magnitudes because the process can be manipulated with them. As control magnitudes they can always be used in a control circuit where they then depend, by feedback, on the variable magnitudes of the process and the process itself. In the diagram to represent the process (see Fig. 7-2), they are shown as input magnitudes. Table 7-1 gives the most important input magnitudes of a bioprocess.

b) **Magnitudes of state** describe the state of the process, and they depend on the process and the input magnitudes of the process. An example is the partial pressure of oxygen, which depends

Table 7-1. Manipulated Variables in Bioprocesses.

Stirrer speed
Air throughput
Concentration of oxygen in the feed air
Flowthrough (chemostat)
Cooling and heating flows (possibly electrical heating)
Coolant inlet temperature
Dosages: acid/alkali
         substrates
         salts
         antifoaming agent
         other

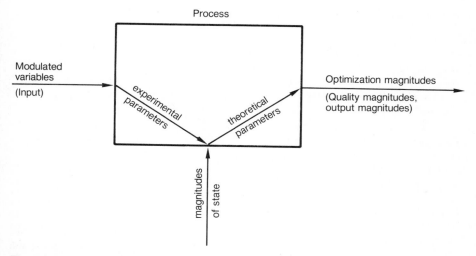

Fig. 7-2. Systematic representation of the process magnitudes.

not only on the consumption of oxygen by the organisms but also on the supply of air, the speed of the stirrer (as a manipulated variable), and on other magnitudes of state. Further examples are the pH, the temperature, and the concentrations of all the important constituents in the liquid and in the gas. The temperature depends on the conversion of energy by the organisms, on the input of energy through the stirring system and the air throughput, on thermal radiation, and, of course, on the flow of coolant and the temperature of the coolant. It can be seen from these examples that the relationship can be reversed when control measures are applied. Thus, the temperature may be predetermined so that the controller changes the flow of coolant until the desired level, within certain limits, is reached.

The most important magnitudes of state of the process are summarized in Table 7-2.

The multiplicity of the organic compounds that appear as substrates and main products and also as by-products and intermediates must be borne in mind. Apart from a few exceptions, it has so far been possible to determine their concentrations only by off-line analysis. In recent years, the mass spectrometer has been introduced for the determination of some compounds. Simple chemical methods of detection can be automated, e.g., by the use of auto-analyzers. Measuring probes based on semiconductor technology have been marketed for the determination of alcohol concentrations, and hydrogen probes work similarly. If the high state of semiconductor technology is taken into account, a large potential of development with good marketing prospects in fields other than biotechnology, as well, appears to exist here.

c) In addition to the measurable magnitudes, magnitudes making statements on the **quality of the process** are important to describe the process; these include magnitudes such as: growth, productivity, consumption, yield, etc. These magnitudes can be calculated from the values under a) and b) if, together with the measurements from b) the changes with time are included. For example, from the change in a concentration and the dosage it is possible to calculate the consumption of a substance.

Table 7-2. Important Magnitudes of State of a Bioprocess.

Liquid phase
Temperature in the fermenter, coolant outlet temperature
pH
Redox state
Pressure
Partial pressure of oxygen
Partial pressure of carbon dioxide
Substrate concentration, misc. (Alcohols, sugars, org. acids, vitamins, enzymes, ATP, NADH, etc.)
Salt concentration, misc.
Biomass
Product concentrations
By-product concentrations
Intermediate product concentrations
State of filling
Proportion of gas
Bubble size
Phase-boundary surface
Viscosity
Surface tension
Density

Gas phase
Oxygen concentration
Carbon dioxide concentration
Concentration of volatile substrates
Concentration of liquid products
Proportion of foam

Biomass
Amounts of carbon (C), nitrogen (N), oxygen (O), and hydrogen (H)
Concentration of protein
Concentration of DNA
Concentration of RNA
Fixed enzymes

By means of a balance calculation, the consumption of oxygen and the consumption of carbon dioxide can be determined from a knowledge of the air throughput and the proportions of oxygen and carbon dioxide in the air fed and discharged. Yields can be calculated by dividing consumption and production. A special case is the respiratory quotient.

The fact that these magnitudes can be calculated from differentials of the magnitudes of state shows that they represent new information and are therefore important for process control and operation and will certainly become more important in the future.

The quality variables are, in the sense of a description of the process (see Fig. 7-2), output magnitudes of the process. The most important output magnitudes are listed in Table 7-3, and in addition to this there are various combinations and extensions, e.g., due to multiplications of cost for economic criteria.

d) **Characterization magnitudes** are auxiliary magnitudes which describe the correlation of various

Table 7-3. Quality Magnitudes of a Bioprocess.

Growth	
Product formation	
By-product formation	
Oxygen consumption (Q_{O_2})	
Carbon dioxide production (Q_{CO_2})	
Consumption and production of heat	
Substrate consumption	1
Substrate consumption	2
Salt consumption	1
Salt consumption	2
Foam formation	
Yield	Biomass/substrate
Yield	Biomass/oxygen
Yield	Biomass/energy
Yield	Product/substrate
Yield	Product/oxygen
Yield	Product/energy
Yield	Product/ATP
Yield	Product/salts

Respiratory quotient $RQ = Q_{CO_2}/Q_{O_2}$
Various components/biomass
Maintenance variables: e.g.: Substrate, oxygen
Economic magnitudes by multiplication of the technical quality magnitudes by cost factors

process magnitudes. They give no new information but are meaningful for a description of the process. They are based on model ideas:

- **Theoretical models** can be developed from generally recognized principles of physics, chemistry, and biology, and the parameters then contain a physical, chemical, or biological meaning or interpretation. Taken together they promote an understanding of the process and are especially suitable for extrapolations, e.g., for scaling-up.

- **Kinetic model equations** define the relationship between magnitudes of state and quality variables. They can be derived from biological and chemical laws. Typical characterization magnitudes are the constants in Monod-type models.

- The **process-engineering characterizing magnitudes** include the well-known dimensionless characteristics and coefficients for describing the transport of mass and energy such as the $k_L a$ value for the transfer of oxygen from the gas phase into the liquid phase and conversely. These magnitudes are important both for scaling-up considerations and also for the adjustment of regulators.

- **Experimental models** can be derived from general mathematically formulated laws; the parameters have no physical meaning but are determined solely from experiment without the use of prior knowledge. They are meaningful for the technical manipulation of the process, e.g., for regulation.

It is often advantageous to combine experimental and theoretical models, e.g., in order to estimate process magnitudes that cannot be measured by means of an experimental theoretical law from magnitudes that have been measured, as for example, the biomass from the consumption of oxygen, of alkali, or of acid, etc.

Figure 7-2 shows a schematic representation of the process magnitudes in the form of a box diagram in which the manipulated variables are shown as **input magnitudes** and the quality variable as **output magnitudes,** while the **magnitudes of state** play an intermediary role and describe the process.

7.2 Characteristics of the Biological Control Cycle

7.2.1 Structure

Biotechnical production processes – apart, perhaps, from steroid syntheses – are usually designed as one-step processes. In principle, the synthesis of a desired by-product takes place by the metabolic transformation of the initial substance (substrate) via various intermediate steps (Demain, 1971). Here, the intermediate products, for their part, may act as effectors on other part-steps and in this way control whole metabolic sequences.

Since the biological situation is based in the final account on the genetic code, the **constructional elements of a biological control cycle** consist of genes, metabolic sequences, the enzymes, and whole structural parts (compartmentization).

With all the common features in the structure and function of living cells, it must not be overlooked that for the individual categories of them there are, nevertheless, **substantial differences.** This relates not only to the more highly developed formation of the cell organelles in the case of the eucaryotes but also to superposed regulation mechanisms that may become active in the association of cells. Even though, in the processes that have been introduced today, single-cell systems occupy the foreground, it must not be forgotten that even the simplest eucaryote cells have available regulatory enzymes that are also typical for higher forms of life.

An example of this type is **calmodulin,** which obviously has a key function in cell regulation (Cheung, 1980). This is a protein composed of 148 amino acid residues, among which the acidic types are strongly represented while cysteine, hydroxyproline, and tryptophan are completely absent. The carboxy groups of the acidic structural units are responsible for the reversible binding of calcium ions. The absence of the last-mentioned amino acids results in a tertiary structure of high flexibility since, as has been demonstrated, the protein is capable of interacting with other proteins, including adenylate cyclase, phosphodiesterase, phosphorylase kinase, NAD kinase (NAD = nicotinamide-adenine dinucleotide), and calcium-ATPase (ATP = adenosine 5′-triphosphate; ATPase = ATP-cleaving enzyme). The calcium-binding protein probably also takes part in the regulation of many other cell processes (guanyl cyclase, calcium-dependent protein kinase, phospholipase A_2, the breakdown of microtubules, etc.).

Since linkage of the hormone and nervous systems by calmodulin takes place with the participation of calcium ions (Ca^{2+}), and cyclic adenosine 3′,5′-monophosphate (cAMP), it cannot be excluded that these ions are also involved in the regulation of cyclic adenylates, and, therefore, of transcription, in single-cell organisms, as well.

As the examples of calmodulin and the action of phosphate in the synthesis of antibiotics show, the classical ideas on enzyme regulation (see Fig. 7-1) are by no means capable of providing all the desirable foundations for the systematic development and performance of processes. Additional knowledge of molecular biology is necessary for this purpose. In spite of these limitations, in the individual case considerable initial possibilities exist for the rational treatment of a biological process.

Catabolism

The catabolic pathways serve for the uptake of the molecules of the substrate and its preparation for inclusion in the following sequences that provide structural units and energy for synthesis. In correspondence with the most important classes of raw materials, a cell has at its disposal suitable initial sequences such as glycolysis for carbohydrates or an oxidation sequence for hydrocarbons. Such **primary sequences** are normally weakly regulated and are catalyzed by constitutive enzymes. Occasionally, steps are excepted from this rule that serve for the preparation of the substrate for uptake (e.g., β-galactosidase). A general regulation of the catabolic steps is frequently performed by **allostery** which leads to small time constants in the kinetic behavior. A typical example of this is the allosteric inhibition of phosphofructokinase, which catalyzes an irreversible step of glycolysis (Goldhammer and Paradies, 1979). On the other hand, strong regulatory effects are observed in the uptake (and sometimes also in the excretion) of poorly assimilable carbon compounds. When high apparent K_S figures appear, therefore, it must first be checked whether this is due to the absence of suitable enzymes or to non-permissive regulation effects.

Anaplerotic Sequences

Anaplerotic sequences have the aim of making up those metabolic pathways which suffer losses through the formation of energy and through synthetic reactions. Many types of cells therefore have at their disposal the possibilities of incorporating small molecules with the nature of intermediate metabolites, such as acetate, ethanol, or lactate. The corresponding enzymes are made available in accordance with the principles of adaptation. Derepression and induction imply increased time constants. A typical example is the glyoxylic acid shunt.

Anabolism (Synthetic Sequences)

Cell components such as proteins, DNA, RNA, lipids, and structural and reserve carbohydrates are synthesized from preformed structural units. Complicated regulatory situations often exist here. In the case of branched metabolic pathways such as are present, for example, in the synthesis of amino acids, complex regulatory interactions can be observed. Mechanisms come into operation which bring about a relative decrease in formation (repression) by the product of the sequence ("feedback inhibition"). The formation of smaller or greater relative amounts of an enzyme always leads to a rise in the time constants (see 7.2.3 and also Chapter 12).

Since 20 amino acids are involved in the synthesis of proteins, this synthetic step for the existence of the cell is difficult to review from the regulatory aspect. The systematic testing of the actual regulatory situation is therefore difficult and requires the use of special processes, such as the chemostat pulse technique (Kuhn, 1979).

In technical application, the formation of the largest possible amount of the desired product is required, which, under certain circumstances, means a **biological overproduction** for the cell. This is made possible by genetic and regulatory measures. Constitutivity of the inducible enzymes, hyperproduction and an increase in the gene copy number can be achieved by mutation or genetic manipulation. Regulation can be affected by the addition of inducers or a decrease in the concentration of repressor (e.g., the glucose effect). In the manufacture of antibiotics, for example, phosphorus plays an important role which has been described by Martin (1977) and Martin and Demain (1980). In particular, phosphates promote the primary metabolism and inhibit the formation of product precursors; they possibly bring about displacement of activity in the hexose monophosphate pathway (HMP) in favor of glycolysis (EMP = Embden-Meyerhof pathway) and thereby limit the synthesis of an inducer (e.g., tryptophan) of the secondary metabolite sequences. The correlation between cell growth and product formation therefore represents the fundamental aspect of model formation which is the basis of any systematic performance of a process.

The anabolic sequences are frequently regulated by their end-product(s) according to the principle of a closed action cycle. Here it is primarily the enzyme (or the isoenzymes) of the first step that is affected (see Fig. 7-1). **Repression** and **inhibition** are the most important mechanisms on which the concept of regulation is based.

7.2.2 Gene Expression

Every metabolic potentiality is laid down in the genetic code. Gene expression leads to a predetermined number of enzyme copies. It can be affected by genetic measures. Together with **activity regulation,** it is responsible for the quantitative formulation of a given metabolic step (see Fig. 7-1). Types of cells such as human or animal cells, have available comparatively few enzyme copies in their sequences that are decisive for growth. The technical manufacture of cell products that are formed only in extremely small amounts (hormones, interferons) is difficult for this reason.

Consequently, the tendency exists for transplanting the codes responsible for such substances into procaryotic cells in order to combine the desired properties of the rapid growth of the synthetic system with the synthesis of the desired product. In individual cases it has been possible to solve both part-problems of manipulation ("genetic engineering") – the transfer of the genes together with their effective expression – successfully.

7.2.3 Regulation of Enzyme Activity

Principles

The cell has a whole number of regulatory mechanisms available in order to cope with the various tasks of metabolism and the changing influences of the environment. **Short-term** tasks arise in the switching on and off of certain metabolic pathways in order to coordinate and integrate the various processes of cell activity (growth, formation of products and energy, lysis). The enzyme-controlled chemical activation and inactivation mechanisms based on physical interactions, such as autoregulation or allosteric regulation represent mechanisms directed for short-term tasks. **Long-term** changes in the enzyme pattern take place with the synthesis and lysis of proteins (formation of relatively larger and smaller amounts).

The rate of catalysis depends on four independent parameters, namely:

1. the concentration of the substrate $[S]$ (in mol/L);

2. the affinity of the enzyme for the substrate* K_m (in mol/L);

3. the activity of the enzyme k_2 (in min^{-1});

4. the concentration of the enzyme $[E]_{tot}$ (in mol/L); the following relation applying:

$$v = \frac{k_2 [E]_{tot} [S]}{K_m + [S]}$$

v is the rate of catalysis (in mol/L).

The equation applies to single-substrate and multi-substrate reactions as well when the concentrations of the other substrates (S_2, S_3 ...) are constant. In other cases, complicated, usually unmanageable, kinetics arise.

Microbial growth can therefore be described by kinetic considerations in which the specific rate of growth μ to some extent represents the integral of regulation.

___

* K_m is the saturation constant of the Michaelis-Menten equation.

Monod was the first to show that μ (in $\min^{-1}$) represents a function of the available amount of substrate provided that all the other components of the medium are present in excess and inhibitors are absent (μ_{max} is the maximum specific growth rate):

$$\mu = \mu_{max} \frac{[S]}{K_S + [S]}$$

Here K_S corresponds formally to the saturation constant K_m of the Michaelis-Menten equation and likewise forms an integrated value. In a continuous experimental arrangement, the relationship between the availability of the substrate and the specific rate of growth is given directly by the relevant relation:

$$D = \frac{F}{V} \equiv \mu$$

rate of dilution   spec. growth rate

F is the feed rate (in mL/min); V is the actual volume (in mL).

Table 7-4 shows the relationships between the four parameters and the mechanisms relating to them.

It can be seen from this summary that parameters 1 to 3 involve mechanisms which do not change the amount of enzyme protein present but do control its activity.

Allosteric enzymes can bind two ligands of different forms in different sites. These sites react conformationally: the inhibitor displaces the equilibrium in the direction of the inactive conformation of the enzyme, and the substrate displaces it in the opposite direction toward the active form.

Great possibilities in the regulatory process arise from the high sensitivity of the enzymes to small **changes in the concentration of the substrate.** The binding of the first molecule of the substrate or of the end product raises the affinity of the enzyme for additional molecules by changing the conformation of its subunits.

The ability of certain enzymes to oscillate between two conformations, however, means much more than simple regulation of the enzyme action. Such **conformational changes** play a key role in the operon repressor reaction and, probably, in many other processes, especially in eucaryotic systems, such as the actions of hormones and neurotransmitters, membrane transport, nervous activity, muscular contraction, cell motility, and interaction between antibodies and cells.

Allostery therefore means a second possibility of information transfer at the molecular level. This possibility does not arise from a code function as in the case of DNA for molecular patterns but from **concentration sensitivity** and, which must not be overlooked, the impressed time behavior determined by the protein structure.

The **regulation of the amount of enzymes** is carried out by the cell at the **transcription** and **translation** levels. Repression and derepression (induction) are described by the operon model, significant differences existing for pro- and eucaryotes [e.g., half-value time of the messenger RNA (mRNA)]. **Proteolysis** takes place at the existing enzyme; it is likewise a controlled process which leads to complete or partial disappearance of the enzyme (limited proteolysis).

In bacteria, yet other mechanisms of gene regulation have been discovered, e.g., proteins that activate operons instead of repressing them. Recently, a coupling of transcription and translation has actually been found which ends the formation of a messenger prematurely if the presence of adequate amounts of end products shows that it is not necessary. cAMP and other substances actually exert a pleiotropic action, since instead of a single operon they affect a whole class of operons.

This class is of special interest as a model for complete cascades of gene regulations during differentiations in higher organisms. However, even now there has been no adequate explanation of details of transcription such as, for example, the binding of regulatory enzymes to the DNA of the operator.

It must therefore be considered that these regulatory processes take place with very small amounts of effectors; for example, repressor protein exists as fewer than 10 copies per cell.

The new synthesis and proteolysis of enzymes lead to pronounced regulatory effects. However, they need not necessarily represent the only mechanisms but can definitely be combined with others. A typical example of the combined action of different mechanisms is the so-called **glucose effect** which, it is true, is called catabolite repression but in fact in-

Table 7-4. Summary of Important Regulation Mechanisms.

Parameter	Mechanisms	Level of Actions
1. Substrate concentration, $[S]$ (enzyme saturation)	Autoregulation – **hyperbolic** function of S and v (noncooperativity) – **sigmoid** function of S and v (cooperativity)	Posttranslational
2. Enzyme affinity, K_m Physical modification	Isosteric competitive product inhibition (change of $K_m = K$ type) Interaction of – enzyme with inorganic ions – enzyme with metabolites – enzyme with other proteins	
Chemical modification	**Activation-inactivation**	Posttranslational
3. Enzyme activity, k_2 Physical modification	Allosteric regulation (change of $v_{max} = V$ type) Interaction of – enzyme with inorganic ions – enzyme with metabolites – enzyme with other proteins	
Chemical modification	**Activation-inactivation**	Posttranslational
4. Enzyme concentration, $[E]$ Synthesis	Controlled protein synthesis: **Induction-repression** – substrate induction – end-product repression	Transcription
Degradation	**Controlled proteolysis**	Posttranslational

volves a whole regulatory system. For practical purposes, catabolite repression (e.g., glucose repression) and catabolite inactivation represent two complex mechanisms which cannot be explained only by classical ideas of the operon model for transcription.

Substrate Repression and Product Inhibition

In biology, substrate and product can act as effectors of decisive regulatory effects. These consist, above all, in a lowering of the reduction kinetics or a decreased formation of the desired product.

Regulatory effects of the substrate are generally termed **substrate repression** without the mechanisms upon which they are based having been elucidated in detail. A typical example is **glucose repression,** which is generally understood as catabolite repression. The so-called glucose effect has long been known and has been observed in many cases with bacteria, yeasts, and the cells of warm-blooded animals. It normally appears in a reversal of the metabolism and can lead to the formation of metabolites that are not formed under the conditions of derepression. In mixtures with carbon substrates, the glucose effect may lead to the situation in which the accompanying substrates are assimilated only when the glucose has been substantially metabolized (diauxic effect). This two-stage growth has been investigated in a binary mixture of substrates by Monod and has contributed decisively to the development of the operon theory. This aspect of the glucose effect is discussed in more detail in the following section on catabolite repression.

In this classical pattern of diauxic growth glucose appears as that sugar which is metabolized fastest. However, the knowledge that its presence triggers off a whole group of regulatory effects on enzymes that are not involved in the uptake of the other "disadvantaged" sugars is important. Extended experiments with glucose-sensitive strains of yeast have shown that, at least in these types of cells, all the enzymes of the tricarboxylic acid cycle, of the glyoxylic acid cycle, and the terminal transport of electrons are involved. Diauxic growth behavior can then therefore occur even in media which contain glucose as the sole source of carbon (Fig. 7-3). Here, in the first growth phase an intermediate metabolite (e.g., ethanol) is accumulated which, after the exhaustion of the glucose, again

serves as a substrate for growth and therefore leads to the diauxic pattern (Fiechter et al., 1981). Important is the observation that glucose does not decrease the maximum possible rate of growth, but leads only to a smaller yield of biomass at the expense of the formation of ethanol. In the practice of the manufacture of bakers' yeast the disadvantages of the glucose effect were circumvented by the empirical development of the so-called fed-batch process before these regulatory relationships were known. To avoid a decrease in yield in the formation of ethanol, the sugar (molasses) is added batchwise according to the degree of growth in order to avoid the appearance of supercritical amounts of sugar and, consequently, to maintain derepressed growth. Since then, such a process has been used in all cases where glucose cannot easily be replaced by a nonrepressing sugar (e.g., lactose).

Product inhibition can be brought about by products that are formed in the course of the reaction. Their mode of action can be based on various mechanisms, whether by an impermissible change in the concentration of hydrogen ions (formation of acid) or by the "poisoning" of essential enzyme systems (e.g., by alcohol). In anabolic synthetic pathways (compare Figs. 7-1b, c and d), end-product regulation forms an important pathway for preventing the overproduction of individual structural units, which is effected by the mechanisms of the inhibition of enzymes or of the repression of transcription. In the biotechnical preparation of such substances as exert pronounced regulatory effects, such **feedback effects** are generally avoided by the use of suitable mutants. In principle, undesirable inhibitory effects can also be prevented by the removal of the product, by pH control (in the case of the formation of acids), or by immobilization methods. The nature of the inhibition of enzymes taking place (competitive or noncompetitive) can be deduced in batch and che-

Type 1: Candida sp.

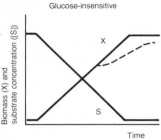

Glucose-insensitive

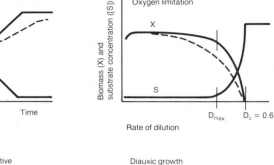

Monoauxic growth

Oxygen limitation

Type 2: Saccharomyces sp.

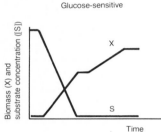

Glucose-sensitive

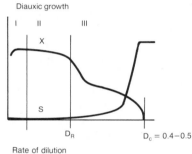

Diauxic growth

Type 3: Schizosaccharomyces sp.

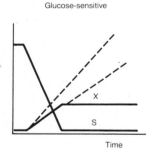

Glucose-sensitive

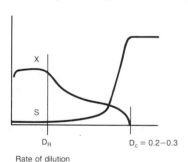

Secondary monoauxic growth

Fig. 7-3. Glucose effect in the growth of various types of yeasts.

Type 1: So called "respiration yeast"

Typical monoauxic growth. No formation of intermediate metabolites (D_{max} = dilution rate at maximum productivity, D_c = dilution rate at washout.)

Type 2: Glucose-sensitive yeats ("fermentation yeasts").

Diauxic growth. Formation of an intermediate metabolite (ethanol) during the first growth phase. After the consumption of glucose, ethanol acts as carbon substrate in the 2nd phase. (D_R = dilution rate).

Type 3: Secondary monoauxic growth.

Formally as type 2, but the substrate of the 2nd phase (ethanol) is consumed by respiration (no growth).

mostat charges so that suitable process formulations can be sought. Similar observations apply to the use of toxic substrates (ethanol, methanol) which bring about so-called substrate inhibition. The process can be formulated by the separate addition of these sources of carbon in such a way that high outputs can be achieved even in such cases. A typical example of this is the use of methanol as the sole source of carbon for the production of single cell protein (SCP) with bacteria where, in spite of extreme substrate inhibition, productivities of more than 10 g/L·h have been achieved (Puhar, 1980). The **localization** (intracellular or extracellular) and **identification** (inhibition or repression) of the regulatory effects observed are therefore of decisive importance for the optimum formulation of the process.

Catabolite Repression

Catabolite repression is of particular importance inasmuch as this regulatory mechanism is initiated by an **extracellular parameter** (glucose) (Pastan and Adhya, 1976). Although in the final account this is likewise a matter of transcription control, a decisive component is lacking in the operon model for it. In the induction of enzymes, in fact, the starting point is that the cyclic AMP (cAMP) necessary for the formation of the active activator/cAMP complex is actually available. The attachment of the complex to the promotor permits the initiation of the transcription of the structural proteins for enzyme formation. In the case of glucose repression, the formation of the cAMP itself is subject to a strict regulation which is associated with the glucose molecule not directly but through a mechanism coupled with its uptake. This has been substantially elucidated today for procaryotes (Peterkofsky's model) (Peterkofsky, 1977).

For eucaryotes this model does not possess definitive validity, but the phenomena of glucose repression are similar for a large number of microbes (Fiechter et al., 1981). In the case of glucose-sensitive cells, when supercritical amounts of these sources of carbon are present enzymes of the respiratory metabolic pathways are repressed, respiration falls off, and as a secondary result there is a complete change in the metabolism which, inter alia, is expressed in the secretion of intermediate products (such as ethanol). As a consequence of the formation of only small amounts of ATP, the efficiency of synthesis also falls of, which can be recognized from the drastic decrease in the cell yield, although not from the rate of growth. In addition to the enzymes of the citric acid cycle and of the glyoxylic acid shunt (anabolism), catabolic enzymes involved in the degradation of sugars (β-galactosidase) are also repressed. For this reason, in a suitable mixture of sugars, glucose is taken up until the supply is exhausted. The critical concentration for the repression effect is extraordinarily low and may be less than 50 mg/L.

Catabolite Inactivation

In the biological literature, the observed effects of free glucose are explained exclusively by **catabolite repression.** This would mean that the synthesis and – on the addition of the effector to derepressed cells – the degradation of the enzymes involved would be regulated. Consequently, only "slow" adaptation would be observed, but this is in contradiction with certain experimental results. Thus, extensive investigations on yeasts (Brändli, 1980; Hägele et al., 1978) have shown that the addition of glucose to derepressed cells leads to an immediate pulse response. The mechanism upon which this is based is termed **catabolite inactivation** (Holzer, 1976), and it has been established today that complex regulatory situations exist here which cannot be explained by catabolite repression alone (Entian, 1977).

This control principle is understood today as a mechanism that must be sought at the level of protein turnover. Proteolytic enzymes (proteases, proteinases) catalyze the degradation and the back-reaction (synthesis) of the proteins in question. This has in fact been shown by Isowa et al. (1977). In yeast, so far, endo-, exo-, and endoexoproteinases have been found. Their action spectra differ greatly in relation to specificity in that only one or else several peptide bonds may be cleaved. So far, seven different proteolytic enzymes with molecular masses of 32 000 to 640 000 dalton, including serine, thiol and carboxy proteinases and metalloproteinases have been found (Meussdoerfer, 1978). They are localized predominantly in the vacuoles (proteases A and B, carboxypeptidase Y, aminopeptidase). In addition, membrane-bound proteases with group-specific spectra have been found that act on transport processes. Some of them are capable of exerting signal functions for the transport of polypeptide chains through the membrane.

The regulation of the turnover of a given enzyme takes place very specifically. Proteolytic degradation can oppose stabilizing effects of corresponding coenzymes (Holzer et al., 1973). In addition, the energy regime appears to affect exergonic proteolysis.

The concept of catabolite inactivation was deduced from the fact that proteases can be inactivated by several systems. Five inhibitor proteins with low molecular masses have been described in detail and have been localized in the cytoplasm (Meussdoerfer, 1978). These inactivations offer possibilities of explanation for the rapid regulatory effects that can be observed. Particularly in the eucaryotic cell with its pronounced compartmentization, however, the situation is so complex that no definitve models are yet available.

Free glucose has an important regulatory action which, because of the complex molecular foundations, cannot always be directly distinguished from those of other extracellular effectors. However, a reliable identification of the relevant parameters is of decisive importance for the rational performance of the process.

7.2.4   Relevant Process Parameters

An effective performance of a process consists in the **optimization of expenditure and result (cost and benefit).** High process efficiencies must be achievable with acceptable means and the necessary reliability. Since the part of the cost for instrumentation in the construction of the apparatus is showing an increasing tendency, the **appropriate design** of the performance of the process is of decisive importance. It must start from the identification of the relevant process parameters, which, for complicated bioprocesses, frequently permits only an empirical procedure. The distinction between effects due to the apparatus and to biological factors frequently comes up against great difficulties, since biological regulation depends equally on the coded cell properties and on the freely selectable external process parameters. In spite of these difficulties, in the interest of a reduction in costs for process development a systematic procedure must be aimed at.

The controlling parameters of a bioprocess are, depending on its characteristics, of **physical, chemical, and biological** nature as is shown in Table 7-5.

7.3   Measurement Technique

7.3.1   Principles

Measuring Processes

In general, the magnitudes of interest in technology cannot be measured **directly** but their effects on

Table 7-5. Summary of the Classes of Parameters of Bioprocesses and Practical Aspects of Process Management.

Parameter	Measured magnitudes, practical aspects
Physical	Temperature, pressure, mass transport, viscosity, gas phase (oxygen, carbon dioxide), mixing (distribution/comminution, homogeneity), foam formation, phase separation, wall growth, maintenance of sterility, aeration, permissible function
Chemical	Substrate, metabolites, products, ions, redox state, dissolved gases (oxygen, carbon dioxide), composition and preparation of the medium, precipitates, open and concealed availability (limitations)
Biological	Specific growth rates, turnover rates, enzymes, DNA, RNA, $NAD^+/NADH_2$ ratio, total protein, ATP/ADP/AMP, regulatory effects, mutations, infections, growth coupling of product formation

other physical magnitudes are utilized in order to refer measurement to simple, controllable, processes.

Thus, previously, measurements were, quite generally, readily referred to measurements of length (clock, thermometer), since the measurement of length can be performed comparatively simply by comparison with a length unit and counting the units. Today, fundamental importance is attached to the measurement of electrical magnitudes which, at least as the last member of a possibly fairly long chain of different processes, by its electrical output signal creates the prerequisite of modern control technique and of automation in general. From a consideration of the energy appearing, therefore, the physical, chemical, or biological process is affected in such a way that part of the energy is converted into electrical energy. Together with this, a role is played by the transformation of chemical and mechanical energy into heat. In the determination of biomass by photometers, it is recognized that light, i.e., radiant energy, can also be used for measurement.

It can be said that practically all known physical and chemical effects are being utilized for measurement technique in biotechnology, but they cannot all be discussed here.

Measuring Setup

The usual measuring setup consists of a sensor at the position of measurement, a transducer, and an indicating or recording apparatus with the corresponding leads. All the above-mentioned units together are responsible for the accuracy of the measurement.

The **measurement sensor** must be placed in a representative measurement site, since reactors form profiles of the measurement magnitudes. For contact measurements in bioreactors a fouling of the measurement sensor is a very frequent cause of faulty measurements.

The **transducer** and **indicating apparatuses** are generally provided by the manufacturer with tolerance figures or information on their quality class.

The electrical leads and measurement cables in technical plants are particularly susceptible to interference by electric and magnetic fields. Some countermeasures are:

– adequate distance from conductors bearing large currents;

– measurement leads twisted together (scatters cancel one another in pairs);

– ferromagnetic sheathing of the cable (expensive);

– central grounding points (the mode of action of a so-called ground loop corresponds to a coil winding in which a voltage is induced);

– the use of coaxial cables (very expensive for long leads);

– filter technique (only when the interfering or useful frequency is known); and

– digital transmission of measurements with error code.

The **measured values** are basically subject to error unless it is a matter of a pure counting of events. Even here, errors creep in. Measurement is therefore carried out on the basis of a comparison of physical effects (e.g., the pressure in a conduit with the spring counterpressure of a Bourdon spring in a manometer). For this purpose, the system must be calibrated. The **calibration conditions** should, as far as possible, agree with those of the experimental conditions and those of the measurement.

If the measured value differs basically (due to the system) from the exact level, we have to deal with a **systematic error.** In the case where the measured value fluctuates statistically (accuracy of measurement, statistical fluctuations of other parameters), there is a **statistical error.**

The error Δx corresponds in its dimensions to the measured value x and is called the **absolute error.** In addition, the absolute error can be referred to the measured value ($\Delta x/x$) and can then be given as the **relative error.**

Methods of Measurement

The **continuous measurement** of all magnitudes would be ideal. Unfortunately, continuous measuring instruments are not available or economically applicable for all measured magnitudes. Chemical and biological compositions can often be determined only on samples that can be taken at relatively large time intervals. The results are available only after a rather long working time and cannot be used directly for controlling the process.

In some cases, however, it appears desirable and possible to develop devices for continuous sampling and automatic analysis which accelerate the availability of the measured figures. An example is the **autoanalyzer** described by Eppert (1976) and Vogelmann (1973), which can be used for determining cell densities and also for other analyses. Automatic sampling takes place at time intervals of between 15 minutes and several hours, so that it is possible to speak here of a semicontinuous measurement.

In the case of expensive measuring devices, it may become necessary to couple several processing units to a single measuring device and to sample the measured values of individual processes successively. If the time constants of the measuring devices are large (dead time, delay time), the use of such measuring arrangements likewise leads to **semicontinuous** measurement. As an example one may mention the multiplex process in waste-gas analysis (oxygen, carbon-dioxide) with which the waste air of various reactors can be investigated successively. Here, care should be taken that dead times due to transport pathways are kept as small as possible. The waste gas is sucked into the device even before the device is attached to the corresponding measuring channel. The time of the measurement is then determined essentially by the delay time of the measuring device. In the case of oxygen and carbon dioxide analysis, it is, for example, 2 minutes and therefore requires, depending on the evaluation, a measuring time of 2 to 2½ minutes. The measuring period is the product of the measuring time and the number of processes connected to ther device. The multiplex system makes data analysis difficult and requires particular care in automation.

In addition to the temporal sequence of measurements, attention must be devoted to the local arrangement of the measurement probes and sampling position, which depends fundamentally on the type of plant and of the process analysis. Here the mixing and residence times to be expected, and also local gradients, must be taken into account.

The **measuring site** permits a coarse but meaningful classification of measurement determinations: in the reactor, at the reactor, and outside the reactor.

Measurements **in the reactor** relate to determinations of the properties and compositions of the materials. Sterilizable measuring probes are necessary, which therefore cannot be taken over directly from the measuring devices supplied for related fields. Particular difficulties are to be expected in postcalibrations.

Parameters such as stirrer speed, torque, power, and rate of flow and temperature of coolant can be measured **at the reactor.** As a rule, they pose no special requirements that are due to biotechnology.

Sample analyses and investigations of the air fed and discharged – rates and compositions of the gas flow – can be performed **outside the reactor.** The measuring devices are largely taken over from chemical engineering. The oxygen and carbon dioxide analyses described are good examples of the many-sided utilization of physical effects in measurement technique. The use of mass spectrometers can take place in both the gas and the liquid phase and offers many-sided possibilities of application.

7.3.2 Exemplary Measurement Techniques

Temperature

The temperature is the most important parameter that is measured and controlled in most microbiological processes. The **methods of temperature control** are similar to those of the chemical and foodstuffs industries.

For large industrial plants, the solutions found are different from those for pilot or laboratory reactors. Depending on the dimensions of the reactor and the desired accuracy of regulation, expansion thermometers, metal resistance thermometers, semiconductor resistance thermometers (thermistors), or thermocouples may be considered.

Pressure

The measurement of the pressure is necessary in each case (sterilization). The measurement offers few difficulties, since pressure gauges with membrane connection can be built directly on to the vessel.

Flow rates of Liquid and Gaseous Media

The measurement of gas flows generally offers few difficulties, since the measuring devices can be arranged outside the sterile zone. Rotameters (if necessary, with remote indication) are generally used. If material balances are drawn up, the pressure and temperature figures must be determined simultaneously.

The control of the flow of liquid media (nutrient solutions) may be very troublesome because of the necessary maintenance of sterility. Depending on demands, measurement of the state of filling or determining the weight of the reservoirs may be adequate. In the case of very low rates of flow (< 100 mL/h) special measures must be taken. Here the automatic measurement of predetermined volumes with electronic control (Ruhm and Kuhn, 1980), for example, has proved satisfactory.

Measuring Sensors

Basically, potentiometric, amperometric (coulometric), and capacity- or conductivity-measuring electrodes are distinguished. **Potentiometric** are calomel, silver/silver chloride platinum/hydrogen, and glass pH electrodes, and many ion-sensitive electrodes. These electrodes develop a potential that depends on the concentration of the specific ion; more accurately: on the activity a (in mol/L) $= f C_S$ [f = activity coefficient; C_S = concentration (in mol/L) in solution]. The potential is determined in combination with a reference electrode.

The mathematical relationship between potential and concentration was derived by Nernst.

The potentiometric electrodes respond to activities (true concentrations). In dilute solutions ($< 10^{-2}$ mol/L), the difference between activity and analytical concentration is negligibly small.

During potential measurement, the system remains in equilibrium. A decisive factor is that there is no chemical transformation, since the potential is measured at zero current.

The effects of electrode geometry, rate of stirring, and viscosity of the solution being measured on the potential are slight. On the other hand, the temperature and ionic strength of the solution being measured are important. \

In the case of **amperometric** electrodes, e.g., the oxygen electrode, the determination of the concentration is based on the measurement of a current. The chemical equilibrium is changed by the substance to be analyzed (oxidation or reduction).

In contrast to potentiometry, in the case of amperometry, the electrode geometry, rate of stirring, and viscosity are of decisive importance.

Capacity and conductivity measurements are occasionally used for measuring states of filling or testing foam heights.

Partial Pressure of Oxygen, p_{O_2}

The **determination of dissolved oxygen** in the reaction solution gives an idea of the amount of oxygen available for the cell. Since this gas is comparatively poorly soluble in water, when there is a high demand, i.e., high rates of conversion (Q_{O_2} values) and/or high concentrations of biomass, the "reserve" in the solution is exhausted in a very short time. The limitation to the global reaction kinetics so caused can be prevented by an efficient further supply (gas flow rate, agitating device, increase in the partial pressure).

The following relationships apply.

Dissolved oxygen: oxygen molecules dissolved in the aqueous phase, C_S (in mg/L or in ppm)

Partial pressure of oxygen, p_{O_2}: according to Henry's law

$$p_{O_2} = C_S/H \qquad (H = \text{Henry's constant})$$

Oxygen activity ($\sim p_{O_2}$):

$$a = f C_S \qquad (f = \text{activity coefficient})$$

A membrane-sheathed electrode measures the oxygen activity ($\sim p_{O_2}$). The solubility or concentration is given by Henry's law.

A distinction must also be made between **oxygen demand** and **actual uptake of oxygen.** Since the latter depends not only on the biological activity (e.g., specific growth rate μ) but also on the availability, oxygen limitations cannot be detected directly. They must be determined in suitably designed experiments and be eliminated by appropriate measures. As experience has shown, the figures given in the literature for the critical (limiting) p_{O_2} values can be taken over to only a limited extent unless it has been proved that the observed kinetics is actually controlled by oxygen. In the correct procedure, however, the measurement of p_{O_2} provides an important signal, mainly for the monitoring of the process. Methods have also been described for the determination of Q_{O_2} and *OTR* (oxygen transfer rate) (outgassing or interruption of aeration) which, however, have as a prerequisite a disturbance of the process taking place. Consequently, these values are better determined by the analytical methods described above for the air flow rate and the waste air. On the other hand, the measurement of p_{O_2} can be used as the basis of a control circuit which acts through the mixing device (e.g., increase in the speed of the stirrer) or the aeration device on the control technique.

In principle, the dissolved oxygen can be measured polarographically or galvanically. For polarographic determination, an external source of current is necessary, while the **galvanic** electrode itself consumes oxygen, which in practical use can lead to erroneous indications (Lee and Tsao, 1979; Fatt, 1976). The sensors are therefore advantageously placed in the reactor at a position with intensive flow and new designs have, in addition, small cathode diameters. Measurements are usually carried out by the amperometric principle according to the processes

Cathode [platinum (Pt)]:
$$O_2 + 2\,H_2O + 4\,e^- \rightarrow 4\,OH^-$$

Anode [silver (Ag)]:
$$4\,Ag \rightarrow 4\,Ag^+ + 4\,e^-.$$

If gas diffusion electrodes are used, the partial pressure is measured. The oxygen diffuses into an electrode chamber closed by a membrane in which a platinum cathode and a silver anode produce the measurement signal. Interfering substances are excluded by the membrane. The electric current is produced by the chemical reaction, and the current is then amplified and, as a measure available as a voltage. The voltage is proportional to the partial pressure. The measurement is not ab-

solute, and the saturation of the liquid with oxygen is taken as the calibration value.

On sterilization, the liquid in the electrode can expand through overflow channels into the centering ring. This prevents an excessive stressing of the membrane and a change in the voltage that would alter the measurement signal.

Electrolytes that can be used are potassium chloride (KCl), potassium nitrate (KNO_3), and potassium phosphate (K_3PO_4). The phosphate has proved to be best in this electrode.

Today, mechanically robust designs that can be sterilized at 121°C and with easily changed membranes that exhibit the necessary long-term stability are available on the market. With special growth substrates, such as, for example, hydrocarbons, however, difficulties still arise (swelling of the membrane), and occasionally there are disturbances due to the settling of microbes on the surface of the membrane. Since a whole multiplicity of special electrodes has been developed for the various fields of application of biology, in the choice of apparatus the relevant documentation of the supplying firms and the literature must be consulted. A suitable review of this problem of measurement has been given by Lee and Tsao (1979).

In practice since the solubility of oxygen in the solutions used in biotechnology differs greatly from that in water, calibration can be performed only empirically. It must be carried out after sterilization and before inoculation. The zero point and saturation level are adjusted after outgassing with oxygen-free nitrogen and oxygen, respectively, and later postcalibrations during operations are possible at any time for the zero point. This process is quite sufficient in view of the long-term stability of modern designs.

Partial Pressure of Carbon Dioxide, p_{CO_2}

Dissolved carbon dioxide can affect the biological reaction. The mechanisms of its action have not been elucidated in all cases. One possibility consists in the fact that at pH > 6 carbonates (e.g., calcium or magnesium carbonates) precipitate, which leads to limitations in relation to alkaline-earth metal ions. However, in spite of the appropriate methods that are now available, the measurement of carbon dioxide in solution is usually omitted, since – as in the case of oxygen – its chemical determination in the waste gas leads to the same result without special effort.

In principle, with homogeneous mixing, the partial pressure of carbon dioxide in the liquid phase is in equilibrium with the gas phase. Recent electrode designs permit its determination in the liquid phase. In itself, the procedure has already been known for a relatively long time, but the types of electrode (according to Severinghaus) showed long response times and inadequate long-term stability and could not be sterilized. By improving the membrane material and filling the apparatus with carbonate buffer solution stability even after sterilization has been ensured. The carbon dioxide diffuses through a reinforced gas-permeable membrane and a small layer of bicarbonate electrolyte between the membrane and the pH electrode. This layer is kept constant by an incorporated nylon net.

The pH arises as a function of the concentration of carbon dioxide.

$$pH = pk - \log p_{CO_2}.$$

The potential of the internal electrode arises in accordance with the Nernst equation

$$E = E_0 - s\,pH \text{ (in mV)}$$
$$E = E_0 + s \log p_{CO_2} \text{ (in mV)}$$

(s = steepness)

Under normal conditions, values of about -120 mV are obtained with aeration, and about $+60$ mV for pure carbon dioxide.

Since the electrode shows the local p_{CO_2} level, similar problems arise for a representative determination to those of the oxygen electrode. Fouling prolongs the response time (Einsele and Puhar, 1980).

A special device is incorporated for calibration which makes it possible to carry out post-calibration subsequently and makes the procedure necessary in the case of the p_{O_2} electrode superfluous. Here, the bicarbonate solution between the membrane and the glass electrode is replaced by a special buffer solution, after the glass electrode has been somewhat withdrawn mechanically. The adjustment at the measuring amplifier is carried out with the glass electrode in this position, after which the special buffer is replaced and the electrode is reinserted. Since the manipulation is possible without dismantling the sensor, reliable signals can be obtained over very long times of operation.

pH

The monitoring of the optimum value of the **hydrogen ion concentration** is an indispensible requirement in any process, since pH changes occur in practically all cases. The hydrogen ion concentration can be measured potentiometrically. The pH can be calculated from the voltage in relation to a reference electrode. The measuring circuit therefore consists of a pH-active glass electrode and a reference electrode. At the glass electrode a potential arises which depends on the pH of the solution being measured. The takeoff system of the glass electrode consists of silver/silver chloride in a chloride-containing buffer. The takeoff system of the reference electrode likewise consists of silver/silver chloride, but in a concentrated potassium chloride (KCl) solution. A porous ceramic diaphragm forms the electrical contact between the glass and reference electrodes. Superimposition of a pressure on the reference electrode during sterilization prevents penetration of the solution being measured into the reference electrode.

Sterilizable impact-resistant measuring devices in which glass and reference electrodes have been combined into a single sensor have come into use. The current designs exhibit the necessary long-term stability and possess standardized mountings for incorporation into the reaction vessels. The signal produced is used almost solely for control purposes. The rates of formation of products changing the pH (acid formation) are better calculated from the consumption of a neutralizing agent.

The pH-control circuits are constructed in the usual manner (electrode-amplifier-controller-signal transducer for an electrical or a pneumatic signal). The controller signal activates a feed path for acid or alkali which works stepwise. Normally, to prevent overadjustment, timers are incorporated in the control circuit in flip-flop connection for pause/operation. The most frequent disturbances in practice arise through stray effects in the high-ohmic part of the measurement (sensor to amplifier). In the setting up of the arrangement, this part must be treated with particular care. With appropiate design, the result of control is better than ± 0.1 pH.

Redox Potential

The redox system consists of two components of which one is **oxidized** by the giving up of electrons and the other is **reduced** by the taking up of electrons. In a redox system, a potential can be measured with a bare noble-metal electrode which depends on the ratio of the amounts of the two components

$$E = E_0 + 2.303 \frac{RT}{hF} \log \frac{(Ox)}{(Red)}$$

E = redox potential relative to the reference electrode (in V)
E_0 = redox potential under standard conditions (in V)

h = number of electrons exchanged $(Ox \rightarrow Red)$
F = Faraday constant (in J/mol V)
R = gas constant (in J/K mol)
T = absolute temperature (in K)
$2.303 \dfrac{RT}{F}$ = Nernst voltage.

Since a multiplicity of redox systems occurs in bioprocesses, a clear definition of the measured magnitudes is impossible here. It has therefore been proposed to speak not of redox potential but of a **platinum electrode potential.**

With most redox pairs, the number of electrons exchanged depends on the presence of oxygen and on the pH, but in aerobic processes the measured value is determined decisively by the presence of oxygen. Since the participating redox pairs can hardly be defined in practice, the interpretation of the measured value is difficult. The use of redox measurement is therefore limited to strictly definable reaction systems. A review of theoretical and metrological aspects is given by Kjaergaard (1977).

Practical measurement is very simple, since a commercial sterilizable platinum electrode is adequate. It is used as a single-rod measuring circuit either together with a reference electrode [e.g., silver/silver chloride (Ag/AgCl)] or together with the reference electrode of a pH electrode. Obviously, combined sensors can also be obtained. The usual pH devices are suitable as amplifiers.

In accordance with what has been said above, the evaluation of redox values is mainly empirical. Individual values are of little significance. Under certain circumstances, complete redox curves over whole periods of time, particularly in combination with other figures, may enable the practical man to acquire important information. However, it must not be overlooked that in aerobic processes redox and oxygen monitorings often run in parallel. Simultaneous evaluation with pH and p_{O_2} curves is best. Their interpretation may give valuable information on regulation phenomena, technical disturbances, or effects of deliberate interventions.

Ion-sensitive Electrodes

Just like hydrogen ions, other ions also exert characteristic effects on the biological reaction. Under certain circumstances, they therefore represent important parameters for the performance of the process (Cheung, 1980). To determine the species in question, in addition to spectroscopic and colorimetric methods, more and more use is being made of ion-selective electrodes which form concentration-dependent potentials in accordance with Nernst's law:

$$E_a = E_0 \pm s \log a$$

E_a = the potential of the ion-selective electrode (in V)
E_0 = standard potential (in V)
s = $\dfrac{RT}{nF}$ (in V)
R = gas constant (in J/K mol)
T = absolute temperature (in K)
n = number of electrons liberated
F = Faraday constant (in J/mol V)
a = activity of the ions to be determined (in mol/L)
$(+)$ = for cation-selective electrodes
$(-)$ = for anion-selective electrodes.

The practical use of this measuring procedure must start from the fact that it is not the concentration but the activities of the ions that are determined, and for their part these are affected by other ions. The composition of the solution being measured must therefore be known. Consequently, definite conditions must be maintained for the measurement, which, together with the fact that the apparatus cannot be sterilized, in general makes an on-line measurement impossible. However, in samples pretreated appropriately, off-line de-

terminations can easily be performed by two procedures:

TISAB
(Total Ionic Strength Adjustment Buffer)

For maintaining pH constancy and ionic constancy and preventing undesired reactions of the solution being measured with the air or with the sensor. In practice, before the measurement the unknown solution is mixed with a TISAB adapted to the ion to be measured in a prescribed ratio.

Known Addition

In the known addition (calibration addition) method, the unknown concentration of the ion to be determined is raised by a definite, known, amount. The original concentration can be deduced from the measured change in potential.

By the addition of the calibration additive, with the volume kept the same as far as possible, the total concentration is raised by the amount c_a. A multiplication of the original concentration is achieved.

A review of the ion-sensitive electrons available today is given in Table 7-6 (Koryta, 1972).

For fast off-line measurements two electrodes are of particular interest:

Ammonium/Ammonia Electrode

The **ammonium electrode** consists of a glass electrode with a special glass membrane. The selectivity in relation to potassium and sodium is low. In addition, the pH must be between 6 and 9. Acid gases [carbon dioxide (CO_2), hydrogen sulfide (H_2S), and sulfur dioxide (SO_2)] interfere. This electrode is ster-

Table 7-6. Ion-Sensitive Electrodes and their Areas of Analytical Application.

Ion	Membrane	Measurement range (in mol/L)	pH range	Interfering ions: ions of
NH_3	gas	$1-10^{-6}$	10–12	volatile amines
NH_4	gas	$1-10^{-5}$	8–9	Ag, H, Na, K
NH_4	liquid	$1-10^{-6}$	2–8.5	Na, K, Ca
Br	solid	$1-5 \times 10^{-6}$	2–12	Hg, S, CN, I
Cd	solid	$1-10^{-7}$	3–7	Hg, Ag, S, Cu
Ca	liquid	$1-10^{-5}$	6–8	Zn, Fe, Pb
Cl	liquid	$10^{-1}-10^{-4}$	2–10	ClO_4, I, NO_3
Cl	solid	$1-10^{-5}$	2–11	Hg, S, CN, I, Br
Cu	solid	$1-10^{-7}$	2–7	Hg, Ag
CN	solid	$10^{-2}-10^{-6}$	10–12	Hg, S, I
F	solid	$1-10^{-6}$	4–8	OH
BF_4	liquid	$10^{-1}-10^{-5}$	3–10	I
I	solid	$1-10^{-7}$	3–12	Hg, S, CN
Pb	solid	$1-10^{-7}$	4–7	Hg, Ag, Cu
NO_3	liquid	$10^{-1}-10^{-5}$	3–10	I, Br, ClO_4, ClO_3
ClO_4	liquid	$10^{-1}-10^{-5}$	3–10	OH
K	glass	$1-10^{-6}$	9–12	Ag, H, Na, NH_4
K	liquid	$1-10^{-6}$	3–10	Rb, Cs
Ag	solid	$1-10^{-7}$	2–9	Hg
Na	glass	$1-10^{-6}$	9–12	Ag, H
S	solid	$1-10^{-7}$	13–14	Hg
SCN	solid	$1-5 \times 10^{-6}$	2–12	Hg, S, CN, I, Br

ilizable. The antibiotic membrane electrodes exhibit better selectivity. The ammonia electrode (Orion) is constructed in a similar manner to the carbon-dioxide electrode. Ammonia diffuses through the gas-permeable membrane and changes the pH of the internal solution (ammonium chloride).

Possibilities of an improvement are also conceivable with an arrangement such as is used for other volatile substances (see Volatile Substances, Ethanol) (flow of carrier gas through an immersed helical silicone tube).

ganic solvent which contains an organic calcium phosphate. Both are insoluble in water. Microporous filters, siliconized porous ceramic material, or poly(vinyl chloride) (PVC) is used as the support of the liquid membrane.

The main interfering ions are copper(II) ions (Cu^{2+}), lead(II) ions (Pb^{2+}), iron(II) ions (Fe^{2+}), zinc(II) ions (Zn^{2+}), and hydrogen ions (H^+). The lifetime of the liquid membrane electrodes is limited. The membrane and the internal solution must be changed frequently. The electrode is not sterilizable.

Calcium Electrode

The **calcium electrode** is a liquid membrane electrode. The membrane consists of an or-

Glucose

Chemical compounds such as glucose can be determined with the aid of immobilized sets of enzymes in electrode form in such a way that a measuring electrical signal arises (Rechnitz, 1975).

In a so-called **glucose electrode,** glucose is oxidized to gluconic acid on immobilized glucose oxidase. The hydrogen peroxide so produced is oxidized by a platinum electrode so that, with a suitable arrangement of the sensor, a current is formed which is proportional to the concentration of glucose.

At the present time, a multiplicity of designs have been described which cannot yet satisfy the demands of practice. The main disadvantages are inadequate long-term stability and temperature sensitivity, which exclude **in situ** sterilization. Frequently, also, the ranges of measurement that can be achieved are inadequate for use in an **in situ** measurement (too low sensitivity at high or very low glucose concentrations). On the other hand, for the manual injection of the solution to be measured good enzymatic measuring devices are available which provide reliable figures within seconds. Since, here also, the range of determination is still limited, the samples should be diluted to the appropriate degree before measurement. The adaptation of such apparatuses to on-line operation, whether in situ or in bypass operation, is therefore impossible without extra expense. However, it may be foreseen that solutions to the problem will be found in the next few years which do justice to the demands of an on-line measurement.

Volatile Substances
(Ethanol, Methanol).

Intermediate products of carbohydrate degradation are not easy to measure specifically. Older oxidation methods (permanganate, etc.) are laborious and cover several other components that occur in common process solutions (aldehydes, etc.). All **enzymatic processes** are, of course, highly specific. Thanks to the volatility of ethanol, methanol, etc., mass spectrometers or flame ionization devices can be used as detectors. Measurements can therefore be made directly in the waste gas of the aeration flow. Bach et al. (1978) have described a system, likewise for waste air measurement, which uses a gas semiconductor as sensor. This semiconductor changes its electrical conductivity when it comes into contact with combustible gases (hydrogen, carbon monoxide, methane, ether, propane) or organic vapors of alcohols, ketones, benzene, and others. The adsorption of a gas molecule on the surface of the semiconductor is based on the exchange of electrons between the semiconductor and the gas molecule. Sintered tin dioxide (SnO_2) is capable of adsorbing oxygen in this way. The occupancy of a semiconductor by oxygen leads to a rise in resistance of the semiconductor material. If this now comes into contact with a volatile substance such as ethanol, oxygen is desorbed, which raises the conductivity of the semiconductor. The change in conductivity is directly proportional to the gas concentration. Heating the surface of the sensor to 200°C accelerates the sorption/desorption processes. Selective measurement is possible, provided that the ranges of alteration of the resistance for individual substances do not overlap. It must also be borne in mind that the semiconductor reacts not only to the temperature but also, and sensitively, to water vapor. The direct introduction of the sensor into the waste-gas stream leads to measured values which depend on the speed of the stirrer, the rate of aeration, and the water vapor content of the waste air. If, however, it is possible to eliminate these effects by a suitable experimental arrangement, a very sensitive measurement can be realized in the ppm range.

Puhar et al. (1980) succeeded in making a silicone tube through which a carrier gas was flowing into a suitable form for its use as a sterilizable sensor in the reaction solution.

Yano et al. (1978) used this sensor system for the determination of methanol and analyzed the inert gas in a gas chromatograph (GC). In place of GC detection, however, a gas semiconductor can be used with advantage so that a comparatively cheap measurement is possible. It gives an electrical signal which can be processed further in any desired manner. The response time of the sensor is relatively short. In on-line use, stable end-values are reached after 6 to 8 min. The ranges of measurement can be adjusted by the choice of the sensor current and be adapted to practical requirements (10 g/L of ethanol at 0.5 mA).

Mass Spectrometry

Mass-spectrometric methods open up a wide analytical field. For biotechnology, it is particularly the partial pressures of the stream of gas and air at the outlet (oxygen, nitrogen, carbon dioxide, methane, hydrogen, ethanol, methanol etc.) that are of interest. Although at the present time it is exclusively the analytical possibility of the method that is being emphasized, its later use for process control is not excluded.

The samples must be transferred from the operating pressure to a high vacuum (10^{-6} bar). The molecules are ionized with an electron beam and the resulting ions are separated in a magnetic field or in the high-frequency alternating field of a quadrupole rod. The decisive characteristic for the sharpness of separation is the mass-charge ratio (m/z). The ions are trapped either on collector plates in Faraday cages or on secondary electron multipliers. Individual mass numbers or complete mass spectra can be determined by this method.

A continuous capillary inlet system is used for the determination of the components of a gas phase. Such apparatuses are available on the market today as complete units. These probes respond very rapidly: 95% of the end value is reached in about 200 ms. The measurement is characterized by an outstanding long-term stability.

For the measurement of dissolved substances, a sensor must be used which possesses a membrane as the closure member. Water should be retained as far as possible by the membrane; the various substances diffuse at different rates. In general, silicone or Teflon is used as the membrane material. In themselves, such sensors are sterilizable, so that on-line use in process control is quite conceivable. However, it must be borne in mind that a whole number of individual practical problems have so far prevented the routine use of mass spectrometry, in spite of the continuously falling prices for the measuring instruments. The first successful applications in biotechnology are to be found in reports by, for example, Reuss et al. (1975) and Heinzle (1978).

Waste-Gas Measurements

For **material balances,** the **composition of the waste gas** must be known in addition to that of the medium. Of nitrogen, oxygen, and carbon dioxide, at least two magnitudes (usually oxygen and carbon dioxide) must be measured. In addition, **volatile components** from the medium may be important. **Physical properties** that are utilized for gas analysis are: thermal conductivity, infrared absorption, and the paramagnetism of oxygen.

Thermal Conductivity

If a stream of gas is passed over an electrically heated wire, heat is taken up from the hot wire so that its resistance changes. The amount of heat taken up depends on the magnitude of the flow of gas and on the composition of the gas. If the composition of the gas is to be measured, the rate of flow of the gas must be kept constant. If the effect of the rate of flow of the mixture is to be utilized for measurement, the composition of the gas must be known. Carbon dioxide has a substantially lower thermal conductivity than nitrogen, oxygen, and carbon monoxide and can therefore be determined on the basis of its thermal conductivity. In order to reduce thermal effects, the resistances are arranged in the form of Wheatstone's bridges.

Infrared Absorption

Infrared rays produced by heated wires with a surface temperature of about 700 °C are absorbed particularly by carbon-containing gases. Each chemical compound has characteristic absorption wavelengths. By incorporating filters, therefore, devices can be used for measuring different gases (carbon dioxide, carbon monoxide, and C_2 and C_4 gases, etc.).

The gas takes up energy by absorption which is converted into heat. The amount of heat can then affect the electrical conductivity of a resistance and thereby produce a signal which is a measure of the concentration of the gas concerned.

Paramagnetism

In the determination of the concentration of oxygen use may be made of its paramagnetism, which sharply distinguishes oxygen from other gases. The magnetizability of the gas falls with the temperature. No dependence on other physical properties that play a part in process engineering can be detected. Consequently, magnetism is suitable for the determination of oxygen concentrations.

Oxygen Analyzer

As an example of a waste gas measuring instrument the oxygen analyzer will be described in more detail, since it gives a good insight into the many-sided application of physical effects in measurement tech-

nique. The measuring instrument is shown schematically in Fig. 7-4. The gas to be measured flows through an inhomogeneous magnetic field. A force acts on the oxygen molecules leading to the formation of a gradient of oxygen concentrations between points 1 and 2. If a comparison flow of gas divided into two parts is passed into the measuring gas tube at 1 and 2, the flow resistance of the comparison streams at the inlet points 1 and 2 will be different. This leads to the appearance of a pressure difference in the conduits of the comparison gas which can be measured at points 3 and 4.

In principle, the pressure gradient between 3 and 4 can be determined by the transverse flow, which affects the temperature and, therefore, the electrical resistance of a heater coil. In order to compensate the thermal dependence, the tube for the comparison gas can be widened and provided with a Wheatstone's bridge. In this case, the voltage is applied to the nodes 3/5 and 4/6, and the measuring signal is taken off between 7 and 8.

It can be seen that with this measuring device the following physical effects play a role: paramagnetism, flow resistance of gases, heat transfer, electrical conductivity, voltage division in interconnected resistances.

The range of greatest sensitivity of the measurements can be affected by the concentration of oxygen in the comparison gas. If the comparison gas contains no oxygen, the sensitivity will be high at low concentrations of the gas being measured. If a small percentage concentration of oxygen in the air is to be measured, it is recommended that dried air should be selected as the comparison gas and, by inserting a pneumatic resistance in conduit 2 of the comparison gas, the reading should be adjusted to zero when pure air is measured. In this way, the deviations from the concentration of oxygen in air are indicated sensitively.

The gas undergoing measurement and the comparison gas must be temperature-adjusted and dried. During use, the functional capacity of the drying unit, in particular, must be tested repeatedly.

Flame Ionization Detector (FID)

The FID is a very sensitive detector for the determination of organic carbon compounds in the waste

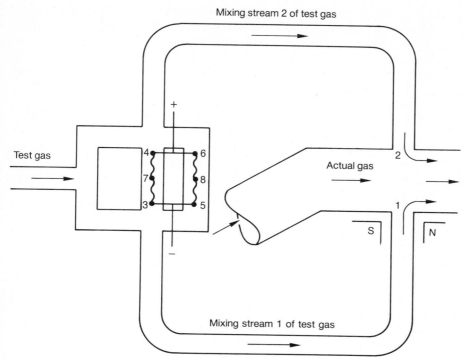

Mixing stream 2 of test gas

Test gas

Actual gas

Mixing stream 1 of test gas

Fig. 7-4. Principle of the oxygen analyzer.

gas from which, inter alia, concentrations of the compounds in the medium can be deduced. For example, when methanol is used as substrate its concentration in the medium can be calculated from measurements of the carbon compounds in the waste gas (Raoult's law).

The combustion of the organic substance gives rise to ions which are detected in an electric field. This physical principle is very simple: because of the flame that is present, safety regulations must be observed constructionally since highly combustible substances are frequently used at the points of application. Because of its sensitivity, the FID is highly favored in laboratories and pilot plants but it is often not desirable in production plants. The FID is independent of temperature and pressure and is insensitive to vibrations. The noise signal can be kept low if foreign organic compounds are excluded from the gas being measured. Trace impurities show up immediately. Consequently, the FID should be in operation for a relatively long time before the

measurement proper is started. During this time impurities that may be present in the FID and the feed conduits undergo combustion.

The FID yields a signal for the totality of the combustible carbon in the waste gas and therefore cannot be used for selective measurements. The measurement of individual components would be possible in special cases in combination with separating processes. Thus, chromatographic processes have been automated and used in biotechnology.

Photometry

Colorimetric and Enzymatic Analyses

Most components in a biological reaction solution can be determined by a **colorimetric** or **enzymatic analysis.** For **trace elements,** emission spectra are frequently measured. For this process the samples must be pretreated in a suitable manner, which requires much manual work. Consequently, for rationalization, multiform systems of analysis have been developed with which practically everything can be determined automatically and, with computer support, be evaluated. When the number of samples is very large but the number of different determinations is small, **automatic wet analysis** is extraordinarily advantageous (Mor et al., 1973; Weibel et al., 1974). The whole system is constructed of individual modules for the addition of reagents, for maintaining the reaction conditions, for photometry, and for issuing results and, by a suitable choice of the inserts in the modules, it can easily be adapted to the specific demands of an analytical operation.

The problem becomes more difficult to solve when smaller numbers of samples which, however, have to be subjected to many different analyses arise simultaneously and the values determined are to be used for on-line process control. The difficulties in automatic sampling and sample preparation as well as a completely automated operation lasting about an hour, have so far prevented the completely automatic monitoring of processes on the basis of this type of analysis.

Frequently, special devices give a great reduction in the amount of manual work for the analysis of individual substances. Glucose, nucleotides, ATP, and other substances can be analyzed relatively cheaply and rapidly today.

Fluorometry

In contrast to photometry in the visible region, in the case of fluorometry the analysis can be carried out directly in the reaction liquid without disturbance by air bubbles. Today, special designs of fluorometers are obtainable which can be built onto the vessel

(Einsele and Puhar, 1980). The signals from this measurement (excitation beam at 366 nm) can be used for the determination of the biomass and therefore of the growth rate (Zabriskie and Humphrey, 1978), of mixing times (Einsele et al., 1979), and of $k_L a$ values (Watteew et al., 1977). It can also be shown that an existing carbon limitation can be detected directly by fluorometry (Ristroph et al., 1977) and the redox state of growing cells can be followed on-line.

Determination of the Biomass (X)

The reliable on-line determination of the **number of cells** or the **weight of the cells** is still today the most important problem of measurement in biotechnology. A large number of calculable quantities that are of the greatest importance for evaluating the process depend on the quantification of the quantity X; for example:

- specific growth rate, μ
- productivity, μX or PX
- rates of conversion, Q_S, Q_{O_2}, Q_{CO_2}, etc.
- correlation between growth and product formation
- calculation of material balances.

Growth can be described by the increase in the amount of biomass (dry matter) or in the number of cells (N). The two quantities do not necessarily correlate in a constant manner. The choice of the method of determination must therefore be carried out in accordance with the purpose in view, and the principle upon which the measurement is based is decisive for its informatory value.

The **mass of the cells** forms the most important quantity that is used for material balances and rates of conversion. The most reliable method is to determine the **dry matter** (normally by drying overnight at 105°C). This method is very accurate and comparatively cheap. Disadvantages are the large time delay resulting from the long drying time and disturbances when foreign components that cannot be washed out, such as solid constituents of the medium or precipitates of insoluble salts, are present. When natural materials such as bran, soybean meal, etc., are used, therefore, this process cannot be employed. In such cases a switch is sometimes made to the determination of phosphorus, nitrogen, protein, or nucleotides, provided that a constant correlation with the formation of biomass can be demonstrated.

The **wet weight** can be determined rapidly by filtering the cells under standardized conditions, and with suitable procedures it can be correlated satisfactorily with the dry mass of the cells. However, all processes for the determination of mass require a relatively large amount of manual work and cannot be automated without considerable expenditure.

Numbers of cells

A distinction must be made between the total number of cells and the number of live cells. Because of the necessary dilution of the samples, the accurate counting of cells in cell chambers or electronic counting devices is very laborious. Counting devices which are based on the measurement of conductivity determine not only the number but also the volume of the cells.

The number of **live** cells can be determined by a culture experiment (plating out), and occasionally also by specific staining.

Photometry

Photometric measurements (turbidimetry, nephelometry) rapidly and simply yield results which can be correlated with growth (Pringle and Mor, 1975). A disadvantage is the rapidly falling accuracy with increasing cell density. Air bubbles and solid constituents of the nutrient solution interfere. For wet determination, therefore, the extinction value can be used only after careful standardization and calibration.

Because of the high numbers of cells and the air bubbles present, on-line measurement directly in the reaction solution presents great measuring difficulties. Today, sensors with integrated sources of light and photocells that can be built into the bioreactor are obtainable which give processable signals even when the absorption is intense. In special cases they provide good service but cannot avoid the interfering effects that have been mentioned. Development to automatic measurement is therefore taking place rather in the direction of adapting flow photometers in which the sample solution is continuously degassed and, if necessary, diluted.

Such a preparation of the samples in the bypass mode provides the possibility of combining other analyses with the determination of growth.

Other Biological Magnitudes

The comprehensive identification of a process includes a whole number of other magnitudes which can often be measured only by complicated methods. These include the determination of contaminations, mutations, inhibitors, and other magnitudes which are important for biological regulation, such as, for example, the energy loading [e.g., $EC = (ATP + 0.5\ ADP)/(ATP + ADP + AMP)$ or NADH]. Because of the unavoidable time delay in their determination, these magnitudes are not available for process control. Change in the course of the process that have biological causes must therefore be recognized directly from other measured magnitudes.

7.4 *Regulation Technique*

Regulation technique has the task of evening out disturbances or even undesired developments in the process. It is distinguished from control by the fact that the manipulated variable is changed as a function of the deviation of the actual value from the desired value of a process magnitude, i.e., the signal of the measured magnitude is compared with the desired value and fed back to the manipulated variable. A regulation can therefore be shown as a flow sheet, as in Fig. 7-5. The negative sign (−) indicates a negative feedback.

A simple form of regulation is **limiting value regulation** which responds only when a predetermined value is exceeded. An example is pH regulation such as is often carried out in biotechnology. If the pH measurement exceeds a value in the basic region, an acid is added and the pH is therefore shifted to lower values. The amounts added and the times for the examinations must be set on the regulator. The limiting value regulator can make only "yes or no" decisions. The regulating deviation plays no part here, and it can be taken into account only indirectly by adding the agent over several measurement intervals if the regulating deviation is too large and the value cannot be altered sufficiently rapidly.

Disadvantages of this type of regulation are undoubtedly this lack of consideration of the size of the control deviation and the resulting jumplike changes. For many tasks, however, limiting-value regulators are quite adequate.

An improvement in regulation can be achieved if the **control deviation,** i.e., the difference between the actual and the desired values, is taken into account. Thus, the adjustment of the manipulated variable may, for example, be made proportional to the deviation. But these **proportional regulators** also show considerable deviations in regulation, i.e., it is impossible to go below a minimum error.

A further improvement is achieved when the rate of change of the process magnitude is taken into account, e.g., with a slow change the manipulated variable is also changed slowly in order not to "overcontrol" the system.

Generally, a regulation can be made the more satisfactorily the greater the amount of information from the temporal behavior of the process, i. e., its dynamics, that is utilized.

Accordingly, in regulation technique one speaks of **proportional, differential,** and **integral regulators,** and the PID regulator, for example, is a proportional-integral-differential regulator. The regulated parameters are often determined empirically.

Simple examples are the evaluation of response functions to an impulse or jump in the input signal. When modern digital computers are used, an analysis of complicated disturbance signals is possible (Meiners and Rapmund, 1980; Isemann, 1974).

In addition to the representation of the dynamics in the **time field,** regulation engineers often use representation in the **frequency field,** the two representations being correlatable by mathematical formulations.

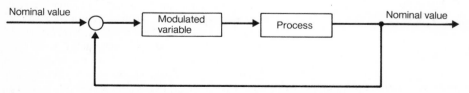

Fig. 7-5. Sketch of input magnitude regulation with negative feedback.

Often, however, the dynamic shows a pronounced time dependence, i.e., the coefficients are functions of the time. This applies to almost all fermentations, especially in batch processes. It is then appropriate to adjust the regulation parameters continuously. In this way we should have an **adaptive system of regulation.** According to Weber (1971), an adaptive system of regulation should be composed of three components:

- identification,
- decision process, and
- modification.

Identification is a more or less expensive system for the calculation or estimation of the differential equation, of the order of the system, and of the coefficients, and possibly for taking a dead time into account. In the **decision phase,** a distinction must be made between different models; statistical criteria can be used for this purpose. And finally, **modification** acts on the manipulated variable and therefore calculates the regulation parameters for the best model from the coefficients.

A representation of an adaptive system is shown in Fig. 7-6. Such solutions to the problem can be realized only with great difficulty in the analog mode, and therefore the digital computer is becoming more and more important for this task, as well.

Examples of Regulation Procedures in Practice

In biotechnology, regulation procedures for the pH and the temperature were introduced at a very early period. An important role was played here by the knowledge that the growth of microorganisms depends very greatly on the pH and the temperature, and therefore it was, in essence, a matter of keeping the magnitudes pH and temperature constant. As already mentioned, modern process performance requires variable process magnitudes (e.g., adaptive systems of regulation) and, in particular, the regulation of other process magnitudes. As examples, we shall mention here three simple systems of regulation, with the assumption in each case that a desired value is given beforehand at a definite point of time.

In general, no particularly high demands are made on the accuracy of regulation in bio-

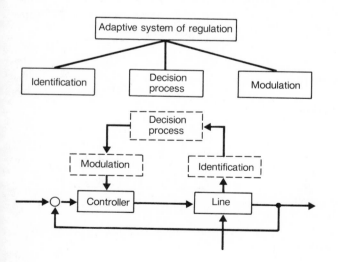

Fig. 7-6. Basic functions of an adaptive system of regulation (from Wolfgang Weber: "Adaptive Regelungssysteme").

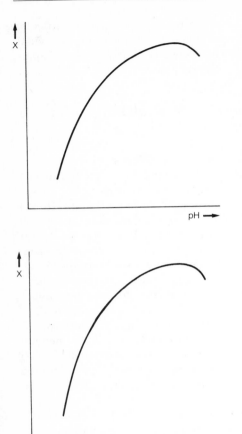

Fig. 7-7. Growth curves as functions of the pH and the temperature.

cies of regulation may be necessary from the aspect of measurement technique.

The **standard regulator for pH** is a two-point regulator. Small fluctuations are tolerated. The desired value is given beforehand and, in addition, an upper and/or a lower limiting value is defined. When the limiting values are transgressed, alkali or acid is added which bring the pH back into the specified working range.

The top part of Fig. 7-8 shows the specified desired value together with the upper and lower limits. In the example it is assumed that, because of the activity of the microorganisms, the pH has a tendency to assume high values, e.g., through the uptake of acids. When the upper limiting value is reached, a definite amount of acid is added which brings the pH back into the acid region. The bottom of the Figure shows the dosage. The amount injected can be adjusted on the metering device and must, of course, be chosen as a function of the amount of the culture and the size of the fer-

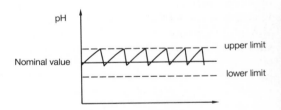

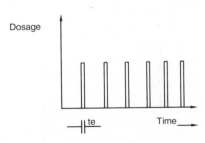

Fig. 7-8. pH metering and regulation during a fermentation.

technology, since, on the one hand, the microorganisms can cope well with slight variations and, on the other hand, growth curves as functions of pH and temperature show flat maxima so that the process can be carried out in a comparatively wide range. Figure 7-7 shows two examples of growth curves as a function of pH and temperature.

In laying down the accuracy of regulation, however, it should always be borne in mind that pH and temperature may very greatly affect other measurements and higher accura-

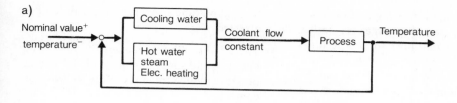

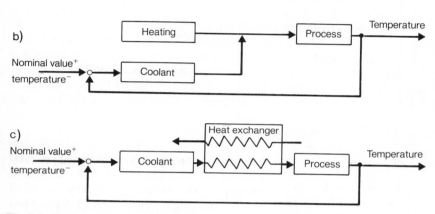

Fig. 7-9. Temperature regulation system.
a) Two-point regulator
b) Heated temperature-control system with equalization of the coolant flow
c) Closed cooling system with heat exchanger and coolant flow as direct manipulated variable.

menter but should also be adapted to the process. The amount injected is often determined by the injection time. In general, the comparison between the actual value and the limiting value is not carried out continuously but at predetermined time intervals so that the limiting values may be slightly exceeded.

Temperature regulation can also be realized by two-point regulators. When the temperature becomes too high, cold water is fed and when it becomes too low hot water or steam is applied or electric heating is switched on. For better regulation, in many cases heating is carried out continuously, e.g., with steam, and the temperature is adjusted by cold mains water. Naturally, such processes are not economic and permit rapid fouling of the cooling system. More appropiate, therefore, is a closed temperature system with the aid of heat exchangers which, in future, should also be used for pilot plants in research and development. The flow of coolant can then be selected as the actual manipulated variable for regulation. Figure 7-9 shows various possibilities for temperature regulation. In future, in the long term, regulation in a closed cooling circuit according to Fig. 7-9c should be used for fermenters larger than about 50 L.

As already mentioned, in future special metering devices will gain in importance. Technically, regulation through metering devices, even with small rates of flow, presents no problems. Basically, they can be constructed in the same way as for pH regulation.

As the last example of a regulation procedure we shall now describe **oxygen regulation,** which plays a large part both for the performance of the process and also for its economic efficiency, since, on the one hand, the transfer of oxygen often limits the fermentation and, on the other hand, aeration and stirring represent decisive operating costs.

The measurement signal is generally supplied by an oxygen electrode which measures the partial pressure of oxygen and is therefore pressure-dependent.

In accordance with the equation $Q_{O_2} = k_La(c^* - c)$ [k_La = volumetric mass transfer coefficient (in s^{-1} or h^{-1})], the transfer of oxygen can be affected by

- a change in the partial pressure of oxygen in the gas inlet, which alters c^*, the saturation concentration; and

- a change in the oxygen transfer coefficient, which alters the k_La value, c being the instantaneous concentration of oxygen in the liquid.

Again, for both methods there are various possibilities of realisation. c^* can be altered by the addition of pure oxygen to the air (or by the addition of nitrogen to the air if the total gas throughput is to be maintained at a low concentration of oxygen) but a change in the total pressure in the fermenter also acts on the partial pressure and the saturation. The k_La value can be altered by changing the speed of the stirrer system and the gas throughput, i.e., the rate of aeration. In the latter case, it should be borne in mind that the fermenter pressure likewise changes unless a pressure regulating system is installed. Figure 7-10 shows the most important possibilities of p_{O_2} regulation:

a) the speed of the stirrer is used as the manipulated variable i.e., regulation is carried out by a change in the k_La value. Air

throughput and fermenter pressure are not affected.

b) The air throughput changes the k_La value but also, and simultaneously, the fermenter pressure, which must therefore likewise be controlled.

c) A change in the concentration of oxygen in the feed gas regulates the p_{O_2} value in the liquid via a change in the partial pressure of oxygen in the feed gas. If the total gas throughput is to be kept constant, the variable addition of oxygen must be taken into account in the regulation of the rate of aeration. It can be lowered by the addition of nitrogen, but the process is not economically satisfactory.

In principle, the partial pressure of oxygen can likewise be affected by **changing the total pressure** but here the effects of the change in pressure, particularly the biological effects, as well as the process-engineering effects, must be borne in mind. Consequently, this principle cannot be recommended; however, it should be pointed out that it finds practical application in all p_{O_2} regulations by changing the gas throughput without regulating the total pressure, although, unfortunately, this has not been taken into account in many apparatuses on the market.

Table 7-7 and Fig. 7-11 give a comprehensive description of the mathematical magnitudes of a fermentation process that are to be determined by measurement, process regulation, and data acquisition, and the methodological procedures.

7.5 Process Computers

Proposals for the use of computers in biotechnology are numerous, and many problems

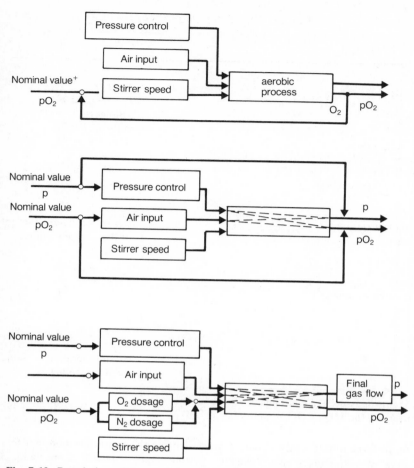

Fig. 7-10. Regulation of the partial pressure of oxygen in the fermenter.
a) Manipulated variable: stirrer speed
b) Manipulated variable: air throughput and therefore an effect on the pressure
c) Manipulated variable: additional feed of oxygen; the feed of nitrogen is uneconomic.

have already been discussed (Meiners, 1977; Blachère, 1973; Armiger et al., 1977). What tasks can be carried out by a process computer? Is the use of digital computers in biotechnological processes economically feasible? In answering these questions, a distinction must be made between the areas of research/development and of production.

In **research** the economic feasibility is always difficult to estimate. Research itself is so

greatly facilitated, or made possible for the first time, by the automatic processing of the ever-increasing amount of data that one can hardly renounce the process computer without falling behind.

The automatic acquisition of data can also be of great assistance in **production plants**, e.g., when cases of disturbance are to be analyzed. Data acquisition alone, however, would probably not be sufficiently economic to jus-

Table 7-7. Summary of the Required Process Data that can be Calculated.

Process data	Calculated from
a) **Material data**	
– Kinetics	
spec. growth rate, μ	Biomass, $[X]$, t
product formation, $P_{(t)}$	«Biomass, $\mu X \equiv DX$
(referred to X or V)	«other, $\mu P \equiv DP$
Coupling of growth and product	X, p, t, α, $\beta^{1)}$
and product formation	
Specific rates of conversion	$(S_0\text{-}S)_{(t)}$, O_2, CO_2, X, F_G
$S_{(t)}$, $O_{2(t)}$, $CO_{2(t)} \rightarrow Q_S$, Q_{O_2}, $Q_{CO_2}{}^{2)}$, $RQ_{(t)}$	Q_{O_2}, Q_{CO_2}
– Balance	
balancing of important substrates:	Results of the analysis
carbon, oxygen, nitrogen, phosphorus	of the medium and gas
b) **Technical data**	
– for managing the process	T, p, V, ...
temp. (T), pressure (p), pH, volume (V) ...	
– for organizing the process	
power input $(P/V)_{(t)}$	P, V, t
oxygen-uptake $O_{2(tot, t, V)}$	O_2, V, t
Product formation $= f(p)$	P, p
Energy balance	Mixing, aeration, heating, cooling.

[1] α and β: growth and nongrowth associated constants.
[2] $Q =$ specific rates of conversion for S, O_2, CO_2 (in mmol/L g h).

tify the use of computers in large plants. Only when computers can take over the tasks of process control with great certainty, leading to substantial reduction in the personnel costs and improving the performance of the process by:

– higher-quality products,
– lower operating costs, and
– shorter downtimes,

will their use pay.

    All the tasks of digital computers are covered by the term "computer control." Here it must be borne in mind that "control" is used both for the wide concept of "monitoring" and also for the narrower concept of "regulation, control,". Monitoring can indeed be carried out by data acquisition, but for computer-controlled and regulated fermentations the appropriate development work is still necessary.

7.5.1 Tasks of Process Computers

Data Acquisition

A prerequisite for all subsequent tasks is the acquisition of measured values (data). The figures are fed into the computer centrally and stored. Storage is carried out first in the computer (core memory) and is then transferred to external devices. Because of the importance of

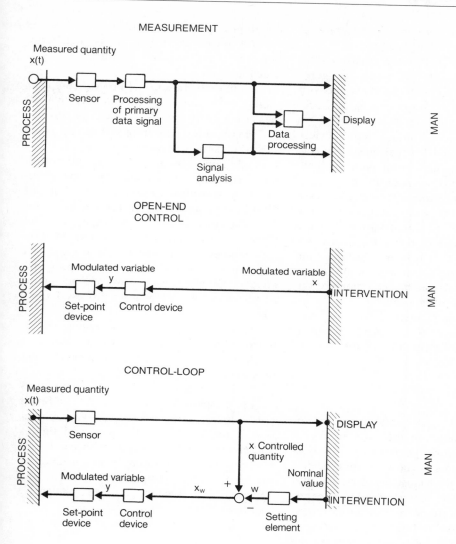

Fig. 7-11. Signal fluxes in measurement, control, and regulation. In biotechnology, the same basic laws as elsewhere apply for process monitoring. The reliable formation of the measuring signals is frequently made difficult by deficient specificity and long-term stability. For this reason, not every significant process parameter can be determined by an on-line measurement. In these cases, the samples taken must be analyzed separately and the variables controlled manually.

data acquisition the system for performing it will later be discussed in detail.

The **advantage of digital data acquisition** lies in the centralization of the measured figures and the subsequent possibility of storage with rapid access for further processing and presentation.

In **analog technique,** the individual devices are in the foreground but their measurements can be shown on the central panels which, nevertheless, are distinctly separated from one another and are therefore often difficult to see at a glance. The forms of presentation of the measurements are often predetermined by the apparatuses and are therefore frequently different. In process computer technique, the sensors are interrogated in series and the presentation of the data can be determined by the user and adapted to the problems.

Often, process computers are used only as data acquisition systems in order to facilitate the current and following operations.

Data Processing

The measurement signals obtained are available to the computer in the form of digital numbers which correspond to the electrical voltages or currents at the measuring device. For further use they must be converted into visible units. Such a transformation depends on the characteristic of the measuring instrument and, therefore, essentially on the measuring process. The relationship between the indication and the measured quantity must therefore be known.

This can be done, for example, by pointwise input. The measured value is then calculated by interpolation between two input points. The accuracy of the calculated measurement value depends on the density of the points. This type of transformation must always be recommended when approximately linear relationships exist and not too many stores for the input points are necessary. Another method consists in finding an analytical function (e.g., polynomial, logarithm, angular function).

The data structure in the process computer should be arranged in such a way that all measuring instruments can be treated alike.

Changes in the measuring system, e.g., drift effects, must be taken into account.

In addition to systematic errors, random errors frequently occur which must be eliminated by **statistical analyses.** One speaks of filtration or smoothing out. Basic work on **digital filtration** was carried out by Kalman (1960) and was introduced into fermentation technique by Svrcek et al. (1974). It requires a large amount of mathematical and programming effort which can, however, be diminished by the use of general process knowledge.

The simplest process is **averaging** which, however, is only permitted when a constant result is expected during the measurement time necessary for averaging.

Another comparatively simple method is the use of **spline functions** according to Späth (1973), these representing a piecewise adaptation of polynomials to the measured figures and giving smooth curves through conditions via continuous derivations. A minimization of the square error taking the dynamics of the apparatus into account has been shown by Meiners (1978).

Process Analysis

Advantages of the digital data acquisition and data processing that have been described, as compared with the analog technique, are the increase in accuracy and rapidity and also the clarity of presentation. Digital computer technique brings more significant advances for data analysis. It permits calculations to an extent that was not previously possible and with a rapidity which permits the results to be taken into account for the subsequent course of the process. One therefore speaks of on-line data analyses. Once the programs have been set up and tested, much work is saved and errors of calculation are avoided.

Data analysis is based on the use of balance equations such as material, energy and momentum balances, from which nonmeasurable parameters can be determined.

System Monitoring

The computer can monitor the technical plant, give alarm signals, and possibly also take countermeasures. However, this last task is difficult to realize and requires considerable development work.

If a failure of a part-system has occurred, an analysis of the measurements can give a rapid idea of what has happened. Thanks to its short access time and data processing, the rapid recognition of the situation becomes possible, which can lead to the cause of the error. Such **off-line analyses** are at the beginning of computer coupling. After a little experience with the computer on the process, one should be in a position by **on-line analyses** to recognize changes in the process that indicate possible errors.

A simple but useful method for the recognition of errors is **limiting value control.** The limits can be set before the beginning of the process or be calculated in correspondence with the work point.

When the limiting value of an important variable is exceeded, an alarm signal is given. The value of the process quantity concerned is shown on an indicating device. In addition, optical or acoustic signals may draw attention to the transgression of the limiting value.

With digital computers, it is also possible to monitor parameters that are not measurable

and that can be obtained only by extensive mathematical operations.

When limiting values are exceeded, a check must be made as to whether all the measuring instruments concerned are in order so that no false conclusions are drawn.

For a rapid review, the computer is capable of reducing the amount of data and producing the relevant magnitudes.

Data Storage

The representation of process magnitudes in time-dependent tables or diagrams presupposes a storage of the data. Data storage can be carried out to only a small extent with **core memories.** Consequently, the bulk of the data is stored on **peripheral equipment** such as disks, magnetic tapes, cassettes, perforated tapes, and cards. The advantage of digital storage lies in the accuracy of the representation and in a convenient and rapid access to the figures. The fastest access is achieved with the aid of disks, which must therefore always be recommended when earlier data are to be recovered for on-line analyses. Magnetic tapes are larger data stores and are appropriate for later off-line analyses. Cassettes are cheaper but contain only small storage capacities. Perforated cards and perforated tapes are now scarcely used for data but have been retained for the storage of programs.

Digital storage technique has the disadvantage that no gapfree storage is possible as is the case, for example, when a simple line recorder is used. The time intervals for storage operations must be selected in such a way that the essential characteristics of the process can be reconstructed while, on the other hand, no excessively large amounts of data have to be stored.

The **choice of time intervals** depends essentially on the aim of the analysis. If the dynamics of the process is to be determined, the interval is determined by the time constants of the process. In biotechnology, there are different types of constants for different process steps. The doubling time of a culture is in the order of magnitude of hours while, on the other hand, the substrate or oxygen in the medium may be consumed in seconds. Since fermentations may run for weeks, storage is not so simple as was often assumed at first. If the storage period were selected on the basis of the smallest time constants in the process, even with large-capacity storage peripheries the input capacity would be reached rapidly.

This applies particularly when a computer is coupled with several plants. Consequently, a reduction in the mass of data must be carried out. It is desirable to store measurements of process magnitudes with large time constants at wider intervals than those with small constants. Since the aim of the analysis may be different from process to process and from plant to plant, the **structure of the memory** should be variable.

It is appropriate to construct the **core memory** in such a way that from time to time parts of the core memory can be "displaced" to the external apparatus, e.g., as a submatrix of a core memory matrix.

An abnormal behavior of a process cannot always be determined by simple tests of limiting values. Consequently, more expensive methods must be used for the recognition of defects. In these, for example, tendencies of process variables may be analyzed, which presumes that the process is known to some extent and expected values from earlier experiments can be utilized.

If one is limited to individual measurement signals, these can be analyzed by statistical methods, without the use of any knowledge of the process, and changes in the signal behavior then lead to conclusions about the state of the plant. However, no applications of this type in biotechnology have so far been published.

Recording

For scientific work in the research area and also for the monitoring of the process in production, however, the acquisition of process data is only effective when these can be presented in manageable form. The digital computer with its possibility of storage offers various ways of representing the course of a process. It can give some summaries of the values of selected magnitudes at intervals of time and show clearly the instantaneous state of the process. If it is desired to follow changes of a number of process magnitudes, it is desirable to print out stored values or to show them graphically over the whole of the process time. In addition to time courses, two or three-dimensional representations of dependent process variables are often used.

Process Management

Digital computers are today capable of taking over not only control functions but also regulation functions and are comparable in price with the analog technique and superior to **analog regulators** in many points. Consequently, the management of the process in fermentations should include the use of digital regulation.

Several process variables change in the course of a fermentation. When the regulator parameters are fixed, therefore, the operation of a plant deviates from the optimum state. Systems of regulation which adapt themselves to the variable properties can be realized to only a limited extent by the analog technique.

Modeling and Parameter Identification

Models have substantially advanced the solution of scientific problems. Outstanding examples of this are shown, particularly, by physics and chemistry; e.g., the well-known Bohr model of the atom.

Models should simplify the individual steps in the complicated process and show them clearly in order that decisions can be taken about the design and performance of the plant. A criterion for the quality of a model is the possibility of predicting the process phenomena and adjusting the process in a favorable manner. Models always contain gaps and will not solve all problems.

The primary aim of the development of a model is to **improve our knowledge of the process** which then has repercussions on the planning, performance, and monitoring of the process.

If data are to be obtained for the design of plants, the steady state should be studied, while if the management of the process and the design of the control and regulating equipment is to be improved, the dynamic behavior of the plant must be investigated. In the first case, a **static model** is developed and in the second a **dynamic model.** However, these tasks cannot always be sharply delimited. In general, a dynamic model is more expensive and contains essential characteristics of the static model.

In addition to this distinction between static and dynamic models, we shall here go in somewhat more detail into the **method of modeling.** According to Fig. 7-12, we distinguish between theoretical and experimental analysis. The best-known and so far most successful is **theoretical analysis.** It is based on physical, chemical, and biological principles that are recognized as generally valid and known, e.g., heat transfer, mass transfer, reaction kinetics, etc. These principles have been confirmed experimentally and formulated mathematically.

The parameters may be generally known (e.g., heat transfer coefficients) or are determined by basic research. They do not necessarily need to be identified in the process if it is certain that the process conditions are adequately known. The mathematical aids are simple and the starting point is generally formed by the conservation laws.

The process computer has the task of performing the mathematical operations and comparing results with the measured process magnitudes. The process may be variable in time. As long as the basic equations apply, a solution may be expected. A disadvantageous feature is that the model is valid only for certain processes and cannot be used universally.

Experimental analysis always presupposes measurement directly on the process. A well-appointed process computer with an extensive software is necessary for the analysis.

The basis of the software consists of **mathematical equations,** e.g., differential equations. They are formulated in the most general possible manner, e.g., as a system of differential equations of order n, where $n = 1, 2, \ldots$ is variable. The coefficients of the differential equation are free and must be determined on the basis of the measurements: they have no physical, chemical, or biological significance. Models of various orders have been calculated and by adaptation to the measurements (method of least squares) the best estimated values of the coefficients and the probabilities of the individual model have been calculated and compared. The model with the highest probability is selected and can be used for the decision phase in the management of the process.

The model obtains its structure from the general mathematical formulas and not from the physical, chemical, or biological conditions. All information is obtained through measurements, and the model is therefore valid in only a small region around the working point. Consequently, continuous use of the process computer is necessary. The model is very suitable for regulation, since the differential equation found can be rapidly converted into equations for this purpose.

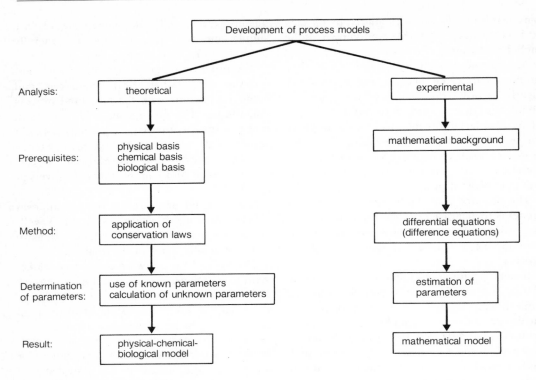

Fig. 7-12. Methods of modeling.

Models of this type have previously been used with success in other fields (Isemann, 1974). The first investigations in biotechnology have been reported by Stravs and Bourne (1976), Chen and Fan (1976), and Meiners and Rapmund (1980). If the experimental and theoretical analyses are compared, it is possible to find advantages and disadvantages for both. **Advantages of experimental analysis** are: no presuppositions concerning a knowledge of the process, universal applicability of the model, and simple transfer to regulation and therefore to process management. **Disadvantages** are: large amount of mathematical and programming effort in the development phase, and validity only within a narrow region of the working point, so that a continuous identification at the process is required

together with a high accuracy of measurement.

There is no doubt that the greater amount of information for biotechnology is obtained from theoretical analysis. However, it must be borne in mind that the theoretical analysis must also be confirmed by experiment, while, on the other hand, an experiment can only be performed correctly when the behavior of the plant is to some extent known. It is therefore important that it should be possible during a fermentation to keep as many process variables as possible constant in order to investigate the influence of one variable.

In multivariable systems, however, a change in one variable may affect many other parameters and complicate the interpretation of the analysis. If there were a model for a regulation magnitude obtained by the experimental method, favorable conditions could be created for measurements and theoretical analysis. Consequently, both methods, theoretical and experimental analysis, must be developed further and improved by mutual interaction in the hope that in this way adequate information and a better understanding of the process can be obtained.

7.5.2 Requirements for Process Computers

The requirements for process computers are determined substantially by the choice of computer tasks and the number and variety of the processes to be monitored. Several complicated tasks require an expensive computer system, which applies both to the hardware and to the software. Developments of the last few years in the computer market have lowered the importance of the hardware costs more and more as compared with the software, so that in the choice of systems the available software should be taken into account.

7.5.3 Hardware

General Hardware

The essential components of the hardware are the **central computer, core memory, external memory, signal acquisition, signal output,** and the **communication devices.** The measurement installation and the system of control and regulation may also be affected by the planned use of computers.

If only data acquisition tasks with storage and recording are to be carried out, compact systems are on the market which are easy to install and service and cost less than $ 20 000. Included in the cost is a basic software which can easily be expanded for the special requirements of the customers.

A data acquisition system contains a **central computer** with core memory, an external memory, a data-acquisition apparatus, and the communications periphery. In Fig. 7-13, a computer coupling is sketched, a minimum system being shown by full lines.

In the **memory periphery,** paper memories have become less important because of the fall in price of disk, magnetic tape, and cassette memories. In addition to disks, magnetic tapes, and cassettes, in the last few years a comparatively new disk system, called floppy disks, has come on to the market which for many purposes permits a favorable compromise in relation to access time, memory capacity, and economy.

If long lists of records are to be printed, **high-speed printers** are to be preferred above typewriters for the task, and for graphical representations with high demands a **plotter** can be used. For simple data acquisition systems the *console* **typewriter** is sufficient and simultaneously provides a record of the operating instructions. However, the provision of programs is substantially facilitated and accelerated by **visual display units.**

The data acquisition system is of fundamental importance for the use of computers. Analog signals of the process must be digitalized with the aid of **analog-digital converters** (ADCs). An ADC consists of the analog-digital conversion unit (AD) and a drive unit. Current ADCs work with voltages of up to 10 V, but are protected against higher voltages.

Typical **times** for data acquisition are a few μs and for conversion a few tens of μs and they are therefore substantially less than the time constants of the process.

Input rates of 200 channels per second and 20 measurements per channel per second are

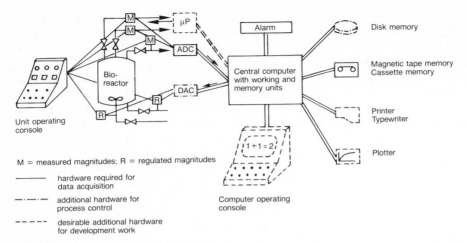

M = measured magnitudes; R = regulated magnitudes

——————   hardware required for
             data acquisition

—·——·—   additional hardware for
             process control

— — — —   desirable additional hardware
             for development work

Fig. 7-13. Computer coupled bioprocess.

sufficient for biotechnical processes and are not fully utilized in most cases.

The simplest possible **interference-free transfer** of the measurement to the process computer is important for a noise-free acquisition of data. For this purpose, high-frequency fields and alternating currents that may be produced by external apparatuses and machines must be screened out.

In linking the measuring instruments with the process computer by cables, it must be borne in mind that the AD converters contain capacitive and inductive elements and therefore form oscillating circuits which must not be brought into resonance with the measuring instruments. Resonance frequencies that occur can be changed by the incorporation of resistances.

Leads should be kept as short as possible. Not only is the distance between measuring instrument and computer important for an interference-free transmission but it may also have economic significance and therefore be decisive for the choice of the connecting principle.

Signal Output and Regulation

If the digital computer is to be used for process management tasks, a signal output is necessary which acts on the controlling and regulating system of the plant. There are various technical possibilities of realization of which we shall give two here that bring out the fundamental characteristics. In the first case an attempt will be made substantially to retain the analog technique and to allow the computer to act on the regulating system present. The digital computer therefore merely monitors the analog regulation, and the system is called "**supervisory computer control**" = SCC. On the other hand it is attractive to transfer all controlling and regulating functions to the computer and therefore to replace analog regulation by a digital regulation performed directly by the computer, which is called "**direct digital control**" = DDC.

Supervisory Computer Control

The preservation of essential elements of analog regulation is particularly advantageous in the initial phase of the incorporation of process computers, since:

a) the measuring, controlling, and regulating devices already present can be used;

b) in the case of failure of the computer, a return can be made directly to the conventional management of the process; and

c) it is possible to work first with the comparatively simple software which specifies only desired values.

Such a solution permits later more accurate investigations of the regulating sections with the aid of the computer and the provision of the software for the further assumption of regulation tasks by the computer.

It will now be assumed, therefore, that the computer has determined the desired value of a process quantity (in the simplest case, a predetermined standard figure) and the actual state is known. The actual and nominal values are stored in digital form but the regulating system expects an analog signal. A digital output module and a signal recognition module are necessary for this purpose.

The digital output can consist of a simple flip-flop relay which, for example, gives a signal to a motor which then changes a control member. The signal has a fixed value (e.g., 24 V) and the length of the Yes setting of the flip-flop determines the change in the control member. In order to be able to alter the control member in both directions, therefore two flip-flop relays are necessary. The time of the Yes setting can be predetermined by the difference between the desired and the actual values or, by continuous comparison, be broken off when the difference has fallen below a limit.

In addition to the signal output, signal interrogations are necessary. Interrupt signals, which start an action of the computer, and contact sensors, which are tested by the computer at regular intervals or before an envisaged activity of the computer, are important. The interrupt is started by a measuring device. The contact sensors can be activated by the

plant operator who can therefore choose between computer regulation and manual operation.

SCC regulation is comparatively slow but is adequate for many biotechnological processes. It can be realized without substantial program developments and can be improved in steps. It can at any time hark back to the analog regulation technique as a backup solution.

Such a system, which merely monitors the analog system of regulation, causes an additional financial load in the hardware configuration and for this reason is it probably not economic in production operation but must be regarded as a transitional solution in the technicum for the development of new systems of regulation.

Direct Digital Control

As the final aim, a solution is offered which substantially replaces the analog regulation technique and includes the digital computer in the regulation circuit. In the case of new plants, DDC does not mean an additional financial load through doubled hardware installations and offers the possibility of achieving optimum states of operation in the process with new strategies of regulation. However, a complete knowledge of the process and further developments in control and regulation systems of the plant are necessary for the realization of a DDC regulation in biotechnical processes.

DDC requires DA converters that possess variable outputs, i.e., output signals in a definite range of voltages which are digitally controlled. Because of the digital control, the outputs to the controlling devices are quantized, the number of steps depending on the resolution of the DA converter.

DDC requires new strategies and algorithms of regulation which is due essentially to the fact that the process takes place continuously while digital computers operate discretely, i.e., data acquisition and signal output take place only at discrete points of time. The control member is kept at a constant value in the meantime. In the analysis of regulation technique, this must be taken into account by a hold element. In contrast to continuous regulation, one speaks here of sampling regulation. Figure 7-14 shows the development of a process monitoring system with digital com-

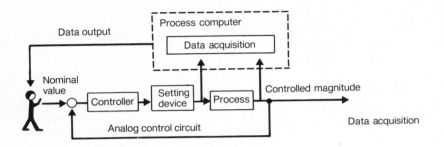

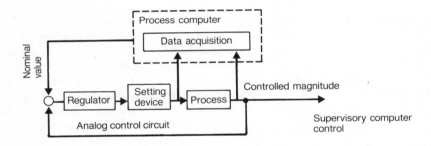

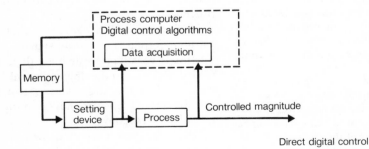

Fig. 7-14. The use of digital computers for process monitoring.

puters from the acquisition of data through the monitoring of the desired value to digital regulation. Sampling regulation requires new laws to be taken into account. Exhaustive descriptions are found in Tschannen (1960) and Ackermann (1972). Two time variables are involved in sampling regulations:

a) the **sampling time,** which is determined by the system of measurement, and

b) the **sampling period,** which is predetermined by the dynamics of the process and is therefore decisive for the regulation concept.

In the limiting case of infinitely small sampling periods, sampling regulation passes into continuous regulation. However, for the economic utilization of the computer it is necessary to select long sampling periods. The laws of sampling regulation should therefore be taken into account in the development of digital systems of regulation.

Regulation systems with large dead times can be treated particularly well by process computers. Another advantage of regulation by process computers is the interchangeability of regulation algorithms by means of the software.

The rapid developments in digital techniques are continually bringing further advantages of DDC. Today, even for DDC systems there are solutions which maintain operation in the case of computer failure so that a substantial disadvantage of DDC as compared with analog regulators can be eliminated.

New impulses are also expected from the further development of **microprocessors.** In this connection, reference must be made to the cost-benefit ratio of current pocket calculators. The decentralized use of microprocessors at individual centers or even at individual regulators could provide a convenient, economic, and safe solution. In any case, further devel-

opments should be observed. The programming of microprocessors still presents difficulties today.

7.5.4 *Software*

Efficient computers are available for the tasks mentioned. Nevertheless, comparatively few applications in biotechnology are known. Process computers have been used as data acquisition systems for laboratory and technical college plants. However, we are still far from an optimum process management of computer controlled production plants.

In the euphoric prognoses concerning computer couplings, the demands on the software have usually been underestimated. Process computers are not being developed for special tasks, e.g., process management on fermenters. Application to the process is carried out in the software used and therefore remains reserved to the experts of the application field, i.e., in our case, the biotechnological experts.

The software consists of two parts: the **basic software,** supplied by the computer firm, and the **application software,** provided by the user. The application software contains the special knowledge of the process. This includes the model, parameter identification, and the control and regulation algorithms.

The core of the basic software is the operating system. For process tasks, a **real-time operating system** must be present, i.e., the programs do not run according to fixed plans laid down beforehand but are determined by the course of the process. Storage disks must be reserved in the central computer for the operating system, and these are therefore no longer available for the application program and for data storage. Consequently, the size of the system must be taken into account in the design of the core memory.

In order to be able to use the core memory better, in many applications a disk system will be used for the external storage of the program and data, which can then be brought into the core memory at choice when necessary. In this case, the operating system is adjusted to the use of disks. Consequently, almost all manufacturers of process computers offer real-time disk operating systems.

The operating system supervises the course of the program. It does not need to be written or modified by the user. It is obtained (generated) at the beginning of the installation with the aid of programs supplied and requires only information concerning peripheral apparatuses, desired software structures on storage disks, etc. Also supervised by the operating system are the application programs that are set up by the user. Only to this extent must the operating system present be taken into account in programming. Also important in the choice of software are the available **programming languages.** Unfortunately, at the present time there is no uniform process language. By means of the project "Prozesslenkung mit DV-Anlagen (PDV)" (Process Control with Data-Processing Equipment), the Federal Republic of Germany has supported the development of a uniform process language PEARL (Process and Experiment Automation Realtime Language) and has attempted to introduce fundamental elements of this language into the international standardization. For smaller computers, programming languages are being developed which include parts of PEARL. However, PEARL has not yet achieved a true breakthrough as **the** process language.

Widely used is the language FORTRAN, known from large computer units and much used in research, which has been extended for process technique. ALGOL, PL1, BASIC, PASCAL, and others have been correspondingly extended and are in use.

An important factor is that the languages used contain the elements that are necessary for on-line processing:

– time-oriented instructions (starting instructions according to clock time, waiting instructions, etc.);

– instructions for the input of data, contacts, switch positions, and interrupt, and for output signals.

The available basic software is adequate. The success of a process computer depends on the development of user software for which, however, a number of experimental and theoretical investigations are necessary.

The software should be easily manageable. This can be achieved most simply by the introduction of data and program structures. Structured program languages are meanwhile available.

7.5.5   *Process Computers in Biotechnology*

The use of digital computers is being accelerated by the fall in price of the hardware and the rapid further development of electronics. It may be assumed that controlling and regulating systems will be substantially digitalized in future, as can already be observed in other fields and even in chemical technology. However, an increase in software costs can be recognized. It is calculated that the cost of the software is rising to as much as 90% of the total costs. Consequently, even today it is important in drawing up programs to take the modern techniques of information science into account in order to be able to incorporate the increasing tasks and growing programs into the existing software in the simplest possible way without substantial changes in the total concept, so that the probability of error should be decreased still further than has been the case hitherto. An important aid is the structuring both of the programs and of the data.

7.6   *Literature*

Ackermann, J.: *Abtastregelung*. Springer-Verlag, Berlin, Heidelberg 1972.

Armiger, W. B. and Humphrey, A. E.: "Computer applications in fermentation technology". In: *Microbial Technology*, Vol. II, 2nd Ed. Academic Press, New York 1979, p. 375.

Armiger, W. B., Humphrey, A. E. and Zabriskie, D. E., "Computer applications in fermentation technology", *Biotechnol. Bioeng. Symp.* **9** (1977).

Bach, H. P., Wöhrer, W. and Roehr, M., "Continuous determination of ethanol during aerobic cultivation of yeasts", *Biotechnol. Bioeng.* **20**, 799 (1978).

Blachère, H.: Proceeding of the First European Conference on Computer Process Control in Fermentation. INRA, Dijon, France, September 1973.

Brändli, E.: *Untersuchung zur Regulation und Funktion der Malat-Dehydrogenase in Schizosacch. pombe*. Dissertation, ETH Nr. 6549, Zürich 1980.

Chen, H. T. and Fan, L. T.: On-line dynamic forecasting in fermentation systems. *Int. Ferment. Symp. 5th,* **1976.**

Cheung, W. Y., "Calmodulin plays a pivotal role in cellular regulation", *Science* **207**, 19 (1980).

Cleland, W. W., "Substrate inhibition", *Methods Enzymol.* **63**, 500 (1979).

Demain, A. L., "Overproduction of microbial metabolites and enzymes due to alteration of regulation", *Adv. Biochem. Eng.* **1**, 113 (1971).

Einsele, A. et al., *Europ. J. Appl. Microbiol. Biotechnol.* **6**, 335 (1979).

Einsele, A. and Puhar, E., "On-line Erfassung von Fluoreszenz und Kohlendioxidpartialdruck in Bioreaktoren", *Acta Biotechnol.* **0**, 33 (1980).

Entian, K.-D., *Mol. Gen. Genet.* **158**, 201 (1977).

Eppert, K.: *Versuche zur Optimierung von Fermentationsprozessen mit Hilfe automatischer Stoffwechselanalysensysteme*. Dissertation, Technische Universität Braunschweig 1976.

Fatt, I.: *Polarographic Oxygen Sensors*. CRC Press, Cleveland (Ohio) 1976.

Fiechter, A.: "Batch and continuous culture of microbial, plant and animal cells". In: Rehm, H.-J. and Reed, G. (eds.): *Biotechnology*, Vol. 1. Verlag Chemie, Weinheim 1981.

Fiechter, A., Fuhrmann, F. G. and Käppeli, O., "Regulation of glucose metabolism in growing yeast cells", *Adv. Microb. Physiol.* **22**, 124 (1981).

Goldhammer, A. R. and Paradies, H. H., "Phosphofructokinase: Structure and function", *Curr. Top. Cell. Regul.* **15**, 109 (1979).

Hägele, E., Neff, J. and Mecke, D., *Eur. J. Biochem.* **83**, 67 (1978).

Heinzle, E.: *Wachstum und Synthese von Poly-β-Hydroxybuttersäure (PHB) in Alcaligenes eutrophus, Extraktion des Polymeren sowie deren mathematische Modellbildung*. Dissertation, Technische Universität Graz 1978.

Holzer, H., *Trends Biochem. Sci. Pers. Ed.* **1**, 178 (1976).

Holzer, H., Katsunama, T., Ferguson, E., Hasilik, A. and Betz, A., *Adv. Enzyme Regul.* **11**, 53 (1973).

Isemann, R.: *Prozeßidentifikation*. Springer-Verlag, Berlin 1974.

Isowa, Y., Ohmori, M., Ichikawa, T., Kurita, H., Sato, M. and Mori, K.: *Bull. Chem. Soc. Jpn.* **50**, 2762 and **50**, 2766 (1977).

Kalman, R. E., *J. Basic Eng.* **82**, 35 (1960).

Kjaergaard, L., "The redox potential: Its use and control in biotechnology", *Adv. Biochem. Eng.* **7**, 131 (1977).

Koryta, J., "Theory and application of ion-selective electrodes", *Anal. Chim. Acta* **61**, 329 (1972).

Kuhn, H.: *Einfluß der Temperatur auf das Wachstum von Bacillus caldotenax*. Dissertation, ETH Nr. 6435, Zürich 1979.

Lee, Y. H. and Tsao, G. T., "Dissolved oxygen electrodes", *Adv. Biochem. Eng.* **13**, 35 (1979).

Martin, J. F., "Control of antibiotic synthesis by phosphate", *Adv. Biochem. Eng.* **6**, 105 (1977).

Martin, J. F. and Demain, A. L., "Control of antibiotic biosynthesis", *Microbiol. Rev.* **44**, 230 (1980).

Meiners, M., "Application of simple algorithms for analysis of measurement data in fermentation and similar biotechnological processes", *Eur. Congr. Biotechnol. 1st* **1978.**

Meiners, M.: *Prozeßrechner*. DECHEMA-Grundkurs der Biotechnologie, Braunschweig (1977).

Meiners, M. and Rapmund, W., "Application of experimental methods to identify process dynamics of fermentation processes", *Adv. Biotechnol. Proc. Int. Ferment. Symp.* 6th **1980** (Publ. 1981).

Meussdoerfer, F.: *Untersuchungen über Inhibitoren*

der Proteinase A aus Hefe. Dissertation, Universität Freiburg/Br. 1978.

Mor, J.-R., Zimmerli, A. and Fiechter, A., "Automatic determination of glucose, ethanol, amino nitrogen and ammonia, cell counting and data processing", *Anal. Biochem.* **52,** 614–624 (1973).

Pastan, I. and Adhya, S., "Cyclic adenosine 5'-monophosphate in *Eschericchia coli*", *Bacteriol.* **40,** 527 (1976).

Peterkofsky, A., "Regulation of *Escherichia coli* adenylate cyclase by phosphorylation-dephosphorylation", *Trends Biochem. Sci. Pers. Ed.* **2** (1977).

Pringle, J. R. and Mor, J.-R., "Methods for monitoring the growth of yeast cultures and for dealing with the clumping problem", *Methods Cell Biol.* **11,** 131 (1975).

Puhar, E., Guerra, L. H., Lorences, I. and Fiechter, A., "A combination of methods for the on-line determination of anabols in microbial cultures", *Eur. J. Appl. Microbiol. Biotechnol.* **9,** 227 (1980).

Puhar, E., Einsele, A., Bühler, H. and Ingold, W., "A steam-sterilizable pCO_2 electrode", *Biotechnol. Bioeng.* **22,** 2411 (1980).

Rechnitz, G. A., "Membrane electrode probes for biological systems", *Science* **190,** 234 (1975).

Reuss, M., Piehl, H. and Wagner, F., "Application of mass spectrometry to the measurement of dissolved gases and volatile substances in fermentation", *Eur. J. Appl. Microbiol.* **1,** 323 (1975).

Ristroph, D. L., Watteeuw, C. M., Armiger, W. B. and Humphrey, A. E., *J. Ferment. Technol.* **1977,** 599–608.

Ruhm, K. and Kuhn, H. J., "Measurement of small volumetric flow rates in small-scale chemostats", *Biotechnol. Bioeng.* **22,** 655 (1980).

Späth, H.: *Spline-Algorithmen zur Konstruktion glatter Kurven und Flächen*. R. Oldenbourg-Verlag, 1973.

Stravs, A. and Bourne, J. R., "A description of biological system dynamics", *Adv. Biotechnol. Proc. Int. Ferment. Symp. 5th* **1976.**

Svrcek, W. Y., Elliott, R. F. and Zagic, Y. E., "The extended Kalman filter applied to a continuous culture model", *Biotechnol. Bioeng.* **16,** 27 (1974).

Tschannen, J.: *Einführung in die Theorie des Abtastsystems*. R. Oldenbourg-Verlag, 1960.

Vogelmann, H., 3. Symposium für technische Mikrobiologie, Berlin 1973.

Watteew, C. M., Ristroph, D. L. and Humphrey, A. E., ACS Meeting, Chicago 1977.

Weber, W.: *Adaptive Regelsysteme*. R. Oldenbourg-Verlag, 1971.

Weibel, K. E., Mor, J.-R. and Fiechter, A., "Rapid sampling of yeast cells and automated assay of AMP, ADP, ATP, citrate, pyruvate and glucose-6-phosphate pools", *Anal. Biochem.* **58,** 208 (1974).

Yano, T., Kobayashi, T. and Shimuzu, S.: *J. Ferment. Technol.* **1968,** 421.

Zabriskie, D. W. and Humphrey, A. E., *Appl. Environ. Microbiol.* **35,** 337 (1978).

Chapter 8

Product Recovery in Biotechnology

Günter Schmidt-Kastner and Christian Gölker

8.1   Introduction

Bioproducts are produced by living cells or are localized in cells from which they must be isolated. This means that the majority of substances are **sensitive compounds** the structure and biological activity of which can be maintained only within sharply defined conditions of the medium. Accordingly, methods for their recovery and processing must be used that are adapted to their labile structures and range within narrow limits in relation to temperature, salt concentration, or pH. In addition, the recovery of enzymes ist frequently restricted to the use of aqueous solutions, since in most cases organic solvents bring about a denaturation of proteins.

While the methods for the recovery of bioproducts were originally taken over from the repertoire of chemical process engineering, recently special methods have been developed to an increasing degree. Furthermore, recovery methods that can be carried out under sterile conditions are gaining importance, particularly in the pharmaceutical industry.

8.2   Separation

The size of an individual bacterial cell ranges from about 0.2 to 5 μm in its largest dimension. The specific gravity of bacterial cells is in the order of 1.03, i.e., the difference in density between the particles to be separated and the suspending medium is very small, which makes separation extraordinarily difficult. The separation of bacteria therefore, as a rule, requires a pretreatment of the suspension to be separated. This situation is more favorable in the separation of, for example, yeast cells with sizes in the order of 15 to 20 μm, which

can be concentrated by the use of separators up to a very high solid-matter content in the separated deposit. The operations shown in Table 8-1 may be considered both for the mechanical separation of cells and for the concentration of products for the subsequent purification steps.

8.2.1   Flocculation and Flotation

It can be deduced from the Stokes law for the settling velocity of a particle that an increase in this velocity can be achieved by increasing the diameter of the particle, i.e., the separation of cells from culture solutions can be facilitated by the agglomeration of individual cells to larger flocs. **Reversible flocculation** can be achieved by the neutralization of the charges present on the cell surface by polyvalent ions of opposite charge, the cells then coming into close contact with their neighbors. On the other hand, the use of polymeric compounds leads to an **irreversible** agglomeration into flocs because of the formation of bridges between individual cells. Flocculating agents that can be considered include inorganic salts, mineral hydrocolloids, and organic polyelectrolytes. However, compounds

Table 8-1. Methods for the Separation of Cells and the Concentration of Products.

Operation	Separation according to	Particle size [nm]
Filtration	particle size	$\approx 10^5$
Ultrafiltration	molecular size	$> 10^2$ to $< 10^5$
Reverse osmosis	molecular size/ solubility	$< 10^2$
Centrifugation	specific gravity	$< 10^4$
Flotation	electric charge/ surface forces	$< 10^4$
Ion exchangers	electric charge	$< 10^3$

such as proteins, polysaccharides, and nucleic acids which bring about an agglomeration of individual cells may also be liberated by partial autolysis. The flocculation of cells depends on various factors, such as temperature, ionic environment, physiological age of the cells, surface forces, and the nature of the organisms, as has been shown by investigations with various organisms (*Pseudomonas fluorescens, Escherichia coli,* and *Lactobacillus delbrückii;* McGregor et al., 1969). Polyelectrolytes have been used extensively for the treatment of sewage. The action of 50 different flocculants under various conditions on fermentation liquors of *Candida intermedia* has been studied by Gasner and Wang (1970). The most effective agents are mineral colloids and polyelectrolytes. Their activity as flocculants depends substantially on the state of the cell surface and of the flow situation during the flocculation process. The cell surface is normally negatively charged but can on balance exhibit positive total charge through the absorption of ions from the fermenter liquor, which explains the good effect of negatively charged polyelectrolytes.

The fact that the state of the cell surface represents a main factor in the mechanism of the flocculation reaction is confirmed by the observation that cells grown on glucose behave differently towards surface-active agents as flocculants compared to cells that have grown on hydrocarbons. In the latter case, the cell surface is coated with a hydrophobic layer, which increases the effect of surface-active agents. Also important is the method of stirring during the flocculation reaction, since a certain shear force is necessary for the formation of flocs while excessively high shear forces can result in the breakdown of already formed flocs.

An exhaustive account of the theoretical principles of the flocculation reactions has been given by Atkinson and Daoud (1976).

In those cases where flocculation reactions lead only to the formation of unstable agglomerates of cells, **flotation** can be used for the enrichment of microorganisms. In flotation, particles are adsorbed on gas bubbles which are either blown into the suspension or are generated in the suspension. The separated particles collect in a foam layer and can be taken off. The formation of a stable foam layer is supported by the use of insoluble **"collector substances"**, such as longchain fatty acids or amines. Microflotation processes have been developed in experiments with bacteria and algae by Rubin et al. (1966) and Rubin (1968). The separation effect in flotation is highly dependent on the size of the gas bubbles. With electrolytically produced nascent hydrogen/oxygen, very small (ca. 30 μm) gas bubbles can be produced in the suspension to be separated, while in normal flotation processes sufficiently small gas bubbles (ca. 40 μm) can be obtained only at pressures of at least ca. 5 bar. By electroflotation from a preflocculated suspension of bacteria with a cell concentration of 16 g/L Seipenbusch et al. (1977) succeeded in achieving a solid-matter concentration in the flotate of about 100 g/L with a good sharpness of separation. Gnieser (1977) has given the enrichment factors collected in Table 8-2. The disadvantage of electroflotation consists in the possibility of damage to the biomass through oxidation processes that may take place.

8.2.2 Filtration

In filtration, a distinction is made according to the mechanism of separating the particles between

- surface filtration (cake filtration),
- depth filtration, and
- sieving filtration.

Information on the general principles of filtration has been given by, for example, Alt

Table 8-2. Separation of Activated Sludge by Electroflotation (after Gnieser, 1977).

Residence time in electroflotation [h]	Current density [A/dm³]	Biomass in the raw water [g/L]	Residual content in the flotate [g/L]	Biomass of the flotation sludge [g/L]	Enrichment factor
0.75	1.8	2.5	0.09	39.2	15.7
1	1.8	1.9	0.06	39.3	20.7
2.5	1.8	2.5	0.017	38.6	15.4

(1972). Reviews on the construction and use of the most diverse types of filter have been given by Alt (1972) and by Trawinski (1976a), among others.

filtration is widely used for the clarification of liquids and for obtaining a great number of different active substances.

The economic performance of a cake filtration requires a relatively high solid-matter content (ca. 3 to 5%) and also good permea-

Surface (Cake) Filtration

In **cake filtration,** the particles are retained on the filter medium (Fig. 8-1) and form a filter cake, while the liquid flows through the filter medium. The flow through the filter layer depends, *inter alia* on the effective **pressure difference, the area of the filter,** and on the **filtration flow resistance,** α, of the filter medium and the filter cake. On the assumption that the particles do not penetrate into the filter medium, the filtration flow resistance of the filter medium can be regarded as constant, while the flow resistance of the filter cake increases through the continuous growth of the thickness of the cake. In the separation of biomass, in many cases, compressible filter cakes are obtained so that the filtration resistance also depends on the effective pressure difference. For the filtration of yeast cells, Rushton et al. (1977) found the relation $\alpha = 1.25 \cdot 10^{11} \cdot \Delta p^{0.9}$ in the range of pressures from 100 to 250 kN/m². On the basis of these properties, and because of lower costs, vacuum filters are used more frequently than pressure filters for the filtration of biomass. On the other hand, pressure

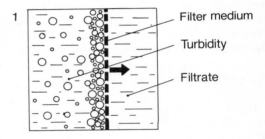

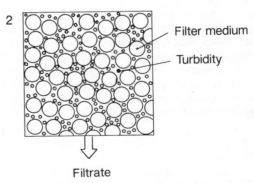

Fig. 8-1. Schematic drawing of cake filtration (1) in comparison with depth filtration (2).

bility of the filter cake. In order to ensure such permeability even in the filtration of suspensions with a tendency to agglutinate the filter layer, filter aids may be added or devices may be used which permit a "renewal" of the filter layer in each filtration cycle.

Plate filters (Fig. 8-2) are suitable for the filtration of small amounts of suspensions, since their uptake capacity for solids is limited. However, they are used widely for the clarification of solutions with a low residual solid matter content.

Typical data for the filtration of various suspensions with the aid of plate filters have been given by Wyllie (1971).

Rotary drum vacuum filters are used most frequently for the separation of microorganisms. The mode of action of this type of filter is shown schematically in Fig. 8-3. The filter cake can be taken off by means of cloths, strings, or a knife. In the last case, the knife is moved towards the drum at a given speed. With each rotation of the drum, in addition to the solid matter that has separated on it part

of the filter aid applied as a precoat is taken off, so that a clean layer is available for the following filtration cycle, and this prevents a continuous increase in the flow resistance. The influence of various factors (nature of the filter aid, speed of rotation of the drum, depth of immersion of the drum, speed of approach of the knife, quality of the vacuum, temperature of the suspension) on the efficiency of the filtration process has been investigated in detail by Bell and Hutto (1958). Gray et al. (1973) studied the filtration of yeast cells with a rotary vacuum filter after their disruption in a homogenizer. Because of the high filtration resistance of the disrupted yeast cells the rate of filtration was independent of the thickness of the layer of precoat. The clarification of the filtrate is better than the separation of cell constituents achieved in the overflow from centrifuges of comparable capacity. The yield of protein in the filtrate measured with a 20% suspension of yeast was 91%. The corresponding figures for the yields of various enzymes are:

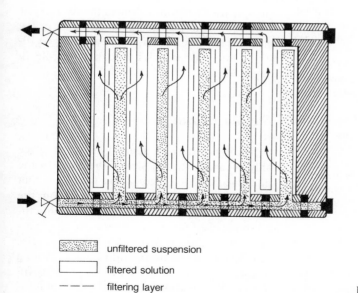

▨ unfiltered suspension

▢ filtered solution

--- filtering layer

Fig. 8-2. Plate filter.

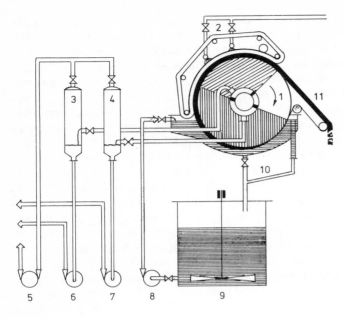

Fig. 8-3. Schematic representation of the mode of action of a rotary drum vacuum filter.

1 Drum filter
2 Cake-washing device
3 Separator for the wash filtrate
4 Separator for the filtrate
5 Vacuum pump
6 Pump for the wash filtrate
7 Pump for the filtrate
8 Pump for suspension
9 Tank for suspension with stirrer
10 Emptying and overflow conduit
11 Filter cake

Fumarase	84%
Alcohol dehydrogenase	67%
Glucose 6-phosphate dehydrogenase	90%
6-Phospho-D-gluconate oxidoreductase	92%

The **Roto-Shear pressure filter** contains filter plates with channels in them. Rotating disks are arranged between the filter plates so that the suspension is kept in motion and a deposition of solids on the filter medium is substantially prevented. The solid matter remains in suspension and is concentrated on its passage through the series-connected chambers.

Rotary pressure filters permit a continuous separation of solids. The filter cake can be washed and blown dry on the filter. Cake removal is carried out automatically.

Belt filters are particularly suitable for the continuous filtration of crystalline precipitates which have subsequently to be washed (Prinssen, 1979).

Depth Filtration

In depth filtration, the separation of the particles takes place through **adsorption** on the skeleton of the filter medium around which the turbid matter is flowing, after penetration of the particles into the filter medium. Depth filtration is a method for clarification of solutions with a low degree of turbidity. It is less suitable for filtrations in which the recovery of the cake is the primary goal. In many cases, electrostatic interactions between charged filter layers and particles also play a role in depth filtration.

Sieving Filtration

In sieving filtration, separation takes place only according to the **size of the pores** of the filter medium. A precondition for this is that the deposited particles are removed from the surface of the filter immediately. If sieving filtration is used for the separation of large particles, the removal of the separated particles can be facilitated by operating with slanting or shaking sieves. A special case of sieving filtration is represented by cross-flow microfiltration and by ultrafiltration. These methods are described in more detail in section 8.4.3.

8.2.3 Centrifugation

The following expression applies to the acceleration u_c of a particle in a centrifugal field:

$$u_c = \frac{d_p^2(\rho_p - \rho_L)}{18\,\eta} \cdot b$$

$$b = r \cdot \omega^2 = \frac{1}{2}(d_a + d_i)\frac{\pi^2 \cdot n^2}{1800}$$

d_p = diameter of the particle
ρ_p = density of the particle
ρ_L = density of the liquid
η = viscosity of the medium
b = centrifugal acceleration
r = radius of the drum
ω = angular velocity
d_a = outer diameter of the drum
d_i = inner diameter of the drum
n = number of revolutions

The ratio of the acceleration in the centrifugal field to the acceleration due to gravity is called the acceleration factor or centrifugal effect Z:

$$Z = \frac{b}{g} = \frac{d \cdot n^2}{1800}$$

g gravitation
d diameter of the drum

A measure of the capacity of a centrifuge is the clarification area Σ as product of the surface of the rotor F and the centrifugal effect:

$$\Sigma = F \cdot Z$$

Since the product includes, via F, the length of the centrifuge drum and, via Z, the number of revolutions n and the diameter of the drum d, it is obvious that the capacity of a centrifuge can be increased both by increasing its length and by raising its speed or increasing the drum diameter. The dependence of F on the length L has led to the construction of

long tubular bowl centrifuges. Another method for intensifying the clarification effect consists in reducing the sedimentation pathway, which is achieved in separators by the installation of stacks of plates. A detailed discussion of the theoretical principles and a description of the most diverse types of centrifuge have been given by Trawinski (1972, 1976).

Filter Centrifuges and Sieve-type Centrifuges

Filter centrifuges and sieve-type centrifuges are used in great numbers for the separation of bioproducts. As in filtration, the throughput depends on the properties of the filter cake that forms in them. Various types of centrifuges based on this principle are shown in Fig. 8-4.

Basket centrifuges are used for the batchwise separation of enzymes and active agents. They provide moderate centrifugal forces (up to 3000 g) and require relatively large particles in order to achieve adequate separation. It is impossible to separate bacterial cells with these centrifuges.

Peeler centrifuges and **pusher centrifuges** can also be used for continuous processes because of devices which permit an automatic removal of the cake.

Sieve-type centrifuges: by a suitable choice of the pore size of the sieve these centrifuges permit not only the dewatering of the product but simultaneously a classification according to particle size.

Decanter and Sedimenting Centrifuges

In **bowl centrifuges,** the constituents of the suspension are separated according to their specific gravities and collected at the wall of the drum. The bowl centrifuges, of which typical representatives are shown in Fig. 8-5 operate on the overflow principle. The untreated mixture is added continuously during the centrifugation process, and the light phase, after

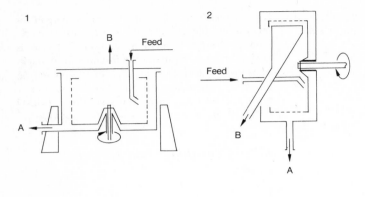

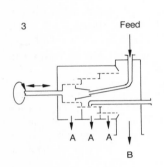

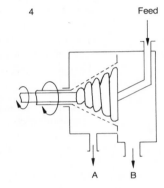

Fig. 8-4. Schematic representation of filter centrifuges.
1 Centrifuge with perforated basket
2 Knife discharge centrifuge
3 Pusher centrifuge
4 Sieve scroll centrifuge
A Liquid discharge
B Solid discharge

separation, keeps flowing over the inner weir of the drum. The discharge of the dense phase may take place continuously (liquid-liquid separations in the solid bowl separator; solids in the nozzle separator) or discontinuously. In the latter case the batchwise removal of the solid is achieved without stopping the drum by a particular design of the discharge device. In the case of tubular bowl super centrifuges, however, the discharge of the solid can only be carried out manually after the drum has stopped.

Separators are used traditionally in the yeast industry for the production of bakers' yeast and in the fermentation industry for the clarification of the most diverse fermentation liquors. A **nozzle separator** is best used for the separation of bacteria; the solids content may

amount to 30% but in general the concentration ratio is somewhat lower than for the intermittently discharging separators. Very high throughputs (referred to the equivalent clarification surface) are reached, since the continuous discharge of the concentrated phase simultaneously ensures uniform flow conditions in the drum. In intermittently discharging separators the solids content of the feed may, in general, be about 2% and in exceptional cases it may amount to as much as 8%. Recent developments are also permitting a complete emptying of the drum and therefore a CIP (cleaning in place) cleansing operation even with nozzle separators, as in the case of the intermittently discharging separators (Hemfort, 1979). **Chamber separators** are suitable particularly for the clarification of liquids

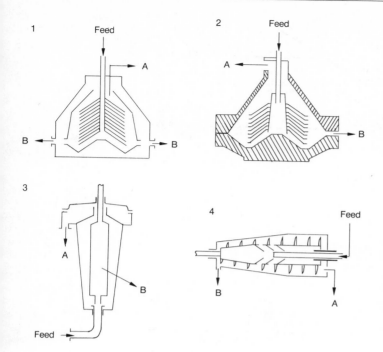

Fig. 8-5. Schematic representation of solid-bowl centrifuges.
1 Nozzle separator
2 Intermittently-discharging separator
3 Tubular bowl centrifuge
4 Decanter
A Light phase discharge
B Heavy phase discharge

with a low solids content. They are used, for example, in the processing of blood and plasma fractions. They can be cooled very satisfactorily and have a larger uptake capacity for solids than tubular bowl centrifuges. In the separations of bacterial mass in separators, an improvement in the separation can be achieved by the addition of flocculants, as the results shown in Fig. 8-6 demonstrate (Seipenbusch et al., 1977).

According to these investigations, an increase in the throughput up to a value of log (throughput/amount of concentrate) of about 0.7 is possible. A separation without pretreatment is successful only if very high centrifugal effects are reached, since in these separation processes the equivalent clarification area Σ is not sufficient for judging the separation capacity of the machine. The separation of particles with sizes down to 0.5 μm is possible with newly developed separators in which the double-conical solids space is emptied through several axial

channels. These channels are sealed by a ring piston which is hydraulically controlled and is capable of axial displacement (Hemford, 1979).

Decanter centrifuges: in decanter (scroll type) centrifuges, sedimentation of the solid particles takes place on the rotating drum wall. The deposited solid is removed by means of a helical screw rotating at a differential speed. Decanter centrifuges are used, for example, for the further dewatering of yeasts obtained in separators and, especially, in the production of single-cell protein.

Tubular bowl centrifuges have a comparatively very simple construction and permit very high g-forces (averaging about 15 000 g and rising in special cases to 60 000 g). They therefore permit the separation of even very small particles.

Their disadvantage is the discontinuous mode of operation and a relatively low sludge

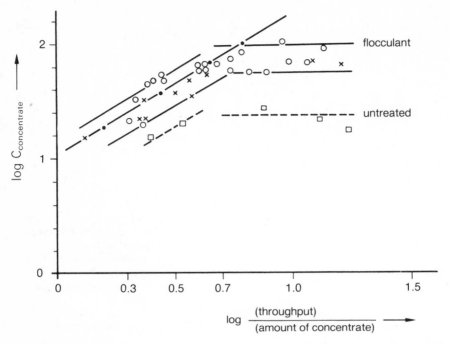

Fig. 8-6. Separation of bacteria in a separator after pretreatment with flocculants (Seipenbusch, 1977).

holdup capacity. Apart from the separation of bacteria and microorganisms, this type of centrifuge is particularly suitable for the separation of protein precipitates.

8.3   Disintegration

Many of the substances to be isolated are present within cells or bound to certain cell structures. As the first step in recovery, therefore, the intact cell structure must be destroyed in order to liberate the desired products. Hence methods must be available which disrupt the cell but simultaneously act in a gentle enough manner to prevent an inactiva-

tion of the biological substances to be isolated. This applies particularly in the isolation of high-molecular-weight compounds with secondary and tertiary structures.

8.3.1   Disintegration of Animal and Plant Tissue

Because of their nonrigid structure, cells from animal organs or plant material can normally be comminuted satisfactorily by **mechanical methods.** A series of various **mills** and **breakers** such as are used elsewhere in the chemical industry are available for this purpose. A review has been given by, for example, Samans (1973). Mechanical comminution can be assisted by the milling of the products in the deep-frozen state, which leads to additional shear forces through the breakdown of ice crystals. The disintegration of organs by the actions of enzymes has been described by Schutt (1976) for the case of the recovery of kallikrein-trypsin inhibitor from cattle lungs. Enzymes are often localized in special organs. In addition to the tissue actually to be disintegrated, therefore, considerable amounts of fatty tissue must be removed, since fat often interferes with the subsequent purification operations.

8.3.2 Disintegration of Microorganisms

Great difficulties arise here, since the cells of microorganisms are very stable and an osmotic pressure of up to 30 bar may exist in the interior of the cell. In addition to the cell membrane, therefore, the rigid cell wall must also be broken down. Besides, these are sub-

stantially smaller particles than are normally ground in mills and, consequently, larger forces must be applied. The methods used for the disintegration of microorganisms can be classified according to the scheme shown in Fig. 8-7 (Wimpenny, 1967; Hughes et al., 1971).

Mechanical Methods

Those methods in which the disintegration of the cells is brought about by **shear forces** applied to the solution possess particular importance: milling in agitator ball mills or colloid mills, the application of pressure and its subsequent release (homogenizers), and the disintegration of the cells by the action of ultrasound. The breakdown of cells in agitator ball mills (Rehaćek et al., 1977) takes place through the effect of shear forces and deformation stresses even during the primary compression when dry matter is to be disinte-

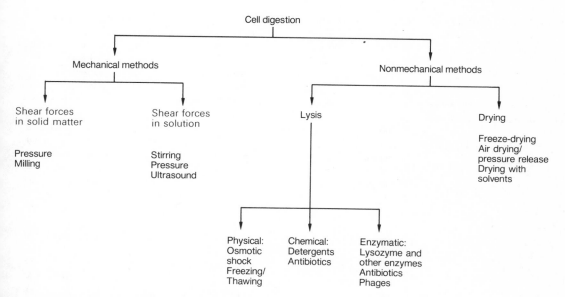

Fig. 8-7. Methods for the disintegration of cells.

grated, while by milling in suspension hydraulic shear forces are responsible for the destruction of the cells. The shear forces that occur at the ends of rapidly rotating knives are usually not sufficient to break down solid cell walls. The mill is therefore filled with the microorganisms together with small **glass beads** (ballotini). The efficiency of this method has been shown by Zetelaki (1969) in comparison with other methods of disintegration by means of measurements of the glucose oxidase activity liberated from *Aspergillus niger* (Table 8-3).

Curie et al. (1972) investigated the release of proteins from bakers' yeast in an industrial mill with the addition of glass beads. This release follows a first-order reaction the rate constant of which depends on several factors: stirrer speed, temperature, amount of glass beads serving as the grinding elements, the size of the beads used, the flow rate, and the concentration of yeast. When all the parameters were optimized, a cell breakdown of 90% could be achieved.

A widely used method for the disintegration of microorganisms uses high pressure followed by immediate pressure release as the cell suspension passes through a nozzle (Fig. 8-8).

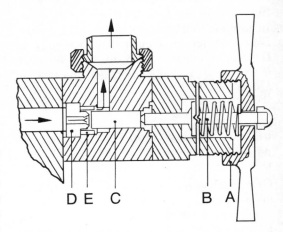

Fig. 8-8. Pressure-quenching valve of a high-pressure homogenizer.

Table 8-3. Comparison of Various Methods for the Liberation of Enzymes from Mycelium *(Aspergillus niger)*.

Method	Moist mycelium/ water ratio	Temperature after disintegration [°C]	Time [min]	Glucose oxidase activity [U]	Yield [%]
Manual trituration with quartz sand	500 mg + 1500 mg quartz	–	15	86	100
Vibration disintegrator	500 mg/10 mL	12	60	51	59
Ultrasound	500 mg/10 mL	55	25	44	52
X-Press	15 g/30 mL	–	–	110	128
Laboratory homogenizer	100 g/2 L	19	–	42	49

Ball mill rpm kg of beads					
800 3	800 g/2.4 L	26	40	66	76
800 3	400 g/2.4 L	25	40	76	88
800 3	800 g/2.4 L	26	40	67	77
800 6	800 g/2.4 L	29	40	93	108
1200 6	800 g/2.4 L	31	40	115	133

In a valve the handwheel A presses the plug C by means of the shaft B against the valve seat D. During discharge, the material to be disintegrated is forced through the gap between the plug and the seat and impinges on the deflecting ring E.

Here the disintegration of the cells takes place through hydrodynamic shear forces and cavitation (Follows et al., 1971). The following facts have been found for the release of various enzymes from yeast: acid phosphatase and invertase are set free faster than the bulk of total protein while alcohol dehydrogenase, glucose-6-phosphate dehydrogenase, and 6-phosphogluconate dehydrogenase are released at a rate comparable with that of the total protein and alkaline phosphatase and fumarase more slowly. This finding is in agreement with the localization of the enzymes within the cell.

Ultrasonic action is used for the disintegration of cells mainly in the laboratory field. The effect is ascribed mainly to cavitation in the solution. Attempts have also been made to perform the method continuously (James et al., 1972).

Nonmechanical (Thermal, Chemical, Enzymatic) Methods

Drying as a method of disintegration: various drying methods have been used for the disintegration of microorganisms (Gunsalus, 1955; Hugo, 1954). The mode of action is based on a **change in the structure of the cell wall** during the drying process so that it is subsequently possible to extract the constituents of the cell, for example, by buffer solutions. Microorganisms can be dried by air, whereupon partial autolysis occurs, or by freeze-drying. The elimination of water can also be carried out by the introduction into at least a tenfold volume of an organic solvent, such as acetone, at low temperatures.

The lysis of cells can be achieved by physical, chemical, or enzymatic procedures (Wiseman, 1969). In particular, animal cells, the cell membrane of which is very sensitive, can be disintegrated by **osmotic shock.** In the case of microorganisms, additional measures must often be taken because of the rigid cell wall. Through osmotic shock, Gram-negative bacteria release a group of "binding" proteins which play a part in active transport (Heppel, 1969, 1967). **Chemical autolysis** in combination with enzymatic cell disintegration is used in the production of invertase from yeast: the yeast is liquefied by incubation with toluene and the invertase is then set free by digestion with papain. **Salt-induced autolysis** is used in the production of toxins from Clostridium. Cholesterol oxidase can be liberated very specifically by the action of surface-active agents, such as Triton X-100, with a yield of 70%, only 2% of the total protein being dissolved (Buckland et al., 1974). The **enzymatic lysis** of bacteria can be achieved by inhibiting cell wall synthesis during the growth phase or by the action of enzymes on the cell wall. Gram-positive bacteria are very sensitive to an attack of lysozyme. Gram-negative bacteria are likewise lysed by lysozyme in the presence of ethylenediaminetetraacetic acid and tris buffer.

In addition to lysozyme, other enzymes bring about bacteriolysis, e.g., enzymes from various soil bacteria, enzymes of various species of Streptomyces, and snail enzymes. Treatment with lysozyme has proved to be the most effective method for the liberation of penicillin V-acylase from *Erwinia aroidea,* as Fig. 8-9 shows (Vandamme et al., 1975).

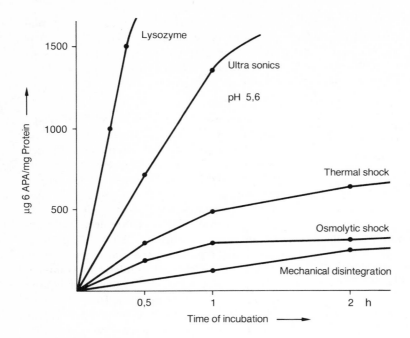

Fig. 8-9. Disintegration of cells of *Erwinia aroidea* by various methods.

8.4   Enrichment

8.4.1   Concentration by Thermal Processes

Because of the thermolability of bioproducts, only equipment with short residence times can be considered for an economic process of concentration. In the case of distillation in rotary vacuum evaporators or stills, which is still frequently used for small volumes, only relatively low temperatures can be employed, since the residence time is relatively long and, because of the hydrostatic pressure of liquid, the risk of an overheating of the liquid is high. For concentration with short residence times there exist thin-layer apparatuses, a selection of which is shown in Fig. 8-10. For the theory of evaporation, reference may be made to the literature (Rant, 1977; Billet, 1965; Schaefer,

1972). Economic aspects for the choice of evaporators have been treated by Walter et al. (1975).

Plug flow evaporator: this apparatus permits the concentration of solutions in a single passage with a reduced residence time as compared with conventional recycling evaporators.

Falling film evaporators: the vapors flowing in the same direction as the material to be concentrated lead to an additional movement of the downward-flowing thin layer in the tubes and thereby improve the heat transfer. The residence time of the product is reduced further as compared with so-called plug flow evaporators (ca. 1 min.). Because of the long design, a large heat-exchange surface is available for the evaporation of a given amount of product, so that this type of evaporator can be operated economically with very small temperature differences between the solution and the heating medium (ca. 4°C). A disadvantage is the risk of liquid film rupture, which may lead to an overheating of the wall and cause damage to the product. Falling film evaporators can be used for solutions with vis-

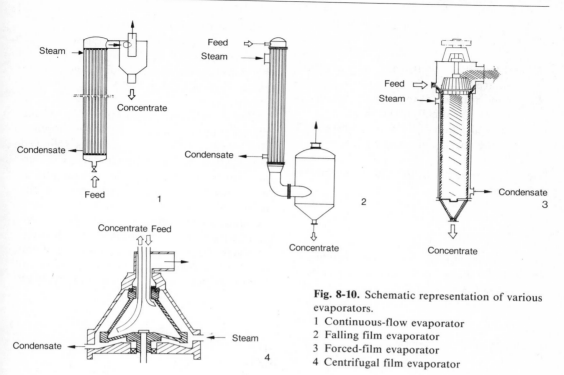

Fig. 8-10. Schematic representation of various evaporators.
1 Continuous-flow evaporator
2 Falling film evaporator
3 Forced-film evaporator
4 Centrifugal film evaporator

cosities of up to about 1.5 Pa s. They are widely used in the foodstuffs industry (Wiegand, 1971).

Forced-film evaporators with liquid films produced mechanically, are also suitable for the concentration of sulutions with high viscosities and, in certain cases, even for concentration as far as to the dry product (Widmer, 1971). In the forced-film evaporator, the film of liquid is set by rotating wiper blades to a predetermined layer thickness. High turbulence is achieved in the liquid layer so that a good heat transfer is produced. The residence times of the product range from a few seconds to a few minutes.

Centrifugal forced-film evaporators permit a further reduction of the residence time of the product (in the seconds range), so that even temperature-sensitive substances can be concentrated under very gentle conditions. Evaporation proceeds on heated conical surfaces or plates over which the transport of the liquid takes place through the centrifugal force produced by the rotating drum (Billet, 1974).

8.4.2 Extraction

Extraction is used to separate active substances mainly after the removal of cell constituents. It is primarily an enrichment process and is used in most cases as the first step in the **manufacture of antibiotics.** Further purification can be carried out by reextraction although in most cases this is done after the elimination of the solvent by purification processes that are treated in the next chapter.

The carrier phase loaded with the extractable material is mixed with the solvent. After phase segregation has taken place, the extract and a raffinate which, in the ideal case, contains no more extractable material, are obtained. The distribution of the active substance between the carrier phase and the extractant is determined by the Nernst distribution law:

$$_AK_v = \frac{_AC_O}{_AC_U} = \text{const.}$$

$_AK_v$ = distribution coefficient of active substance A

$_AC_O$ = concentration of the active substance A in the specifically light phase

$_AC_U$ = concentration of the active substance A in the specifically heavy phase

The extraction factor of the active substance is defined as

$$_AE = {_AK_v} \cdot \frac{\% \text{ Vol } O}{\% \text{ Vol } U}$$

$_AE$ = extraction factor of active substance A

$_AK_v$ = distribution coefficient of active substance A

% Vol O = vol.-% of the light phase
% Vol U = vol.-% of the heavy phase

The most common types of extractors are shown schematically in Fig. 8-11 according to Schreiner (1969).

Mixer-separators: the arrangement of the greatest simplicity and of the widest applicability consists of a mixing chamber followed by a settling device. Distinct density differences must exist between the various phases since otherwise the time of separation in the settling device becomes too long.

Countercurrent columns: in sieve-plate columns with an efficiency of 0.3 to 0.5 theoretical plates per step, and plate distances of 150 to 400 mm, efficiencies of about 2 to 3 theoretical plates per meter of column are obtained.

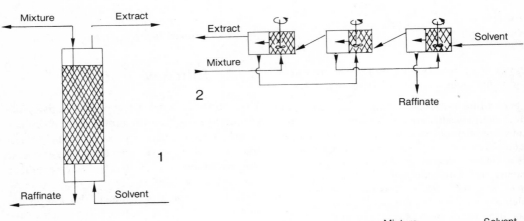

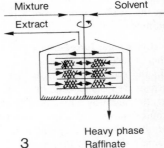

Fig. 8-11. Schematic representation of the most common types extractors (Schreiner, 1969).
1 Extraction column
2 Mixer followed by settling vessel
3 Extraction centrifuge

In order to improve the efficiency, the droplets in the column are dispersed by pulsation or by rotating internals in order to give a better mass transfer between the phases.

Extraction centrifuges: since many active agents are damaged by the action of solvents or by the extraction conditions, endeavors must be made to achieve the shortest possible residence time in extraction and also rapid reextraction, e.g., into buffer solutions.

This condition is satisfied by extraction centrifuges, e.g., of the type of the Podbielniak or the Luwa extractor. Here extraction takes place in a centrifugal field in order to achieve a sufficiently large velocity of flow of the phases at a small difference in density. The residence times are in the order of one minute. These apparatuses are also used with advantage in those cases in which the two phases tend to form emulsions.

In extraction with centrifuges, several machines frequently have to be connected in series, since the number of theoretical plates is relatively small with 3 to 4. In the case of the extraction of penicillin, for example, the maximum possible volume flow of such machines amounts to 30 m^3/h.

6-Aminopenicillanic acid can be isolated from aqueous solutions by extraction with a small volume of a water-immiscible organic solvent in which 0.5 to 10 wt.-% of an amine has been dissolved (Batchelor et al., 1963; Christmann et al., 1969).

An interesting method of enzyme extraction has been developed by Kula et al. (1978a, 1978b). Depending on the concentrations of the two polymers, aqueous mixtures of polyethyleneglycol and dextran form two phases which can be separated in a separator. After liberation from the cells, enzymes can be separated from cell constituents and be extracted in this system.

In this way, it was possible to isolate pullulanase from *Klebsiella pneumoniae* in a single step with a yield of 88%. α-Glucosidase has been isolated in the same way from *Saccharomyces carlsbergensis* and various aminoacyl-tRNA synthetases from *Escherichia coli*.

Active substances from animal organs can be extracted by mixtures of organic solvents and salt solutions (Schultz, 1961).

Fundamentals of the calculation of liquid-liquid extraction processes and descriptions of various types of apparatus together with uses in the pharmaceutical industry have been given by Schreiner (1967, 1969) and by Todd et al. (1973). For theoretical background of extraction, reference may be made to the literature, e.g., Müller (1972).

Fig. 8-12 shows possible arrangements of two different extraction processes.

8.4.3 Membrane Filtration

The basic process in membrane filtration consists in the **convective transport of dissolved particles** to the surface of a membrane. Under the influence of a hydrostatic pressure, certain particles pass through the membrane while other particles are retained at the membrane. The decisive magnitude in membrane processes is represented by the **osmotic pressure**. The situation is shown in Fig. 8-13:

When two solutions are separated by a semipermeable membrane, an equilibrium prevails if the concentration ratios on the two sides of the membrane are identical (a). If a concentrated solution is present on one side of the membrane and a dilute solution or pure solvent on the other, solvent passes through the membrane into the concentrated solution, which has a higher osmotic pressure (b). The solution becomes more dilute until the hydrostatic pressure built up corresponds to the osmotic pressure. The transport of solvent can be brought to a halt by the application of an external pressure (c). If this external pressure is increased above the osmotic pressure the flow of solvent reverses and pure sol-a)

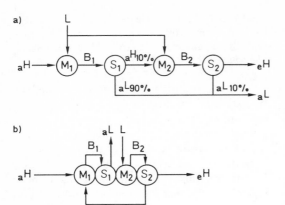

b)

Fig. 8-12. Representation of extraction methods.
a) 2-stage extraction
b) 2-stage countercurrent extraction in the Lu-
    westa extractor

L   Solvent (light phase)
$_aL$ Solvent with active substance (light phase
        with active substance)
$_aL_{10\%}$ Solvent with 10% of active substance
$_aH$ Carrier phase (heavy phase) with active
        substance
$_eH$ Carrier phase (heavy phase) extracted
B   Mixture of light and heavy phases
M   Mixer
S   Separator
M S   Separator-mixer

vent flows from the concentrated solution to the dilute solution (d).

   In principle, these considerations apply to
all membrane filtration processes. The fact
that with increasing particle size the osmotic
pressure falls sharply, however, permits a
quantitative distinction between ultrafiltration
and reverse osmosis. By **ultrafiltration,** molecules of different molecular sizes and molecular weights greater than 1000 are separated
from one another or from solvent molecules.
Here the membrane can be regarded as a sieve
with very small pores (porous membrane).
The separation of the materials is based on a
geometric sieve action in which the theoretical
separating effect depends only on the operating pressure. Material transport takes place by
convection, and the amount passing through
the cross-section of the membrane depends on
the pressure applied. In **reverse osmosis,** on
the other hand, molecules with comparable
molecular weights are separated and here the
concept of a porous membrane fails. Separation based on interactions between the molecules to be separated takes place at the membrane as the result of different solubilities in
the homogeneous polymer membrane (solubility membrane). The permeation of a solute
through a solubility membrane is determined

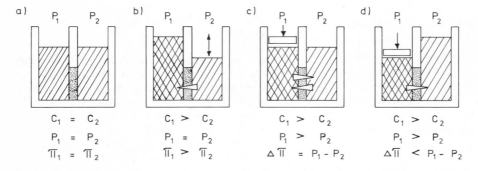

Fig. 8-13. Representation of the processes taking place during ultrafiltration.

by the concentration gradient and the coefficients of diffusion in the membrane. It is practically independent of the passage of the solvent. The separating capacity is therefore hardly influenced by the operating pressure. It holds for both types of membrane that the mass transport is inversely proportional to the thickness of the membrane. In order to achieve adequate flow rates, the membrane should be only 0.1 to 0.2 μm thick. To achieve this, so-called "asymmetric membranes" consisting of a supporting layer of 0.2 to 0.4 mm and the membrane with a thickness of 0.2 to 0.5 μm are used.

Criteria for distinguishing between ultrafiltration and reverse osmosis are summarized in Table 8-4.

In all membrane filtration systems, the flow of liquid in the direction of the membrane and the retention of molecules at the surface of the membrane result in an increase in the concentration of these molecules at the surface of the membrane, an effect which is known as concentration polarization. The concentration of a substance increases with approach to the membrane and then, behind the membrane, falls suddenly. With rising concentration at the surface of the membrane, a concentration-dependent back-diffusion of molecules into the solution begins. An equilibrium is set up which results in a layer of raised concentration at the surface of the membrane of certain thickness. Consequently, in this area the osmotic pressure rises and the filtration capacity of the membrane falls. In addition to the decrease in capacity, the separation characteristics may change because of the "secondary membrane" located in front of the membrane. In a membrane filtration, the concentration polarization and the back-diffusion must be limited. Technically, this is ensured by stirring the solution or by the use of so-called "cross-flow systems", i.e., by the enforcement of turbulent flow in the case of relatively large cross-sections or laminar flow in thin channels or "hollow fiber" systems.

The principles of the processes occuring in membrane filtration, the preparation of membranes, and the description of apparatus can be found, for example, in Matsuura (1978), Marquardt (1973), Strathmann (1978), Saier and Strathmann (1975), Porter (1972), and Madsen and Olsen (1974).

The range of application for ultrafiltration and reverse osmosis is summarized in Table 8-5.

Table 8-4. Criteria for Distinguishing between Ultrafiltration and Reverse Osmosis.

Criterion	Reverse osmosis	Ultrafiltration
Size of the dissolved particles retained	MW < 500–1000	MW > 1000
Osmotic pressure	considerable, may rise to 800–1000 N/cm^2	negligible
Working pressure	greater than 100 N/cm^2 and up to 1500 N/cm^2	up to 100 N/cm^2
Principal processes	transport by diffusion; the material of the membrane may affect transport properties	separation according to molecular size; sieve effect; the material of the membrane has no influence, the important characteristic being the pore size

It is evident from these data that mainly ultrafiltration processes are used in the biotechnological field. Preferred areas of application in the **foodstuffs industry** are the concentration and processing of fruit juices and also, to an increasing extent, the processing of whey for the recovery of proteins and lactose (Fig. 8-14). The retention rate for protein amounts to as much as 99%. The protein concentrate formed has a solids content of 12 to 15% and can be processed directly in a spray-dryer.

Products of low molecular weight after enzymatic reactions, e.g., in the liquefaction of starch or the proteolytic degradation of proteins from whey, can advantageously be isolated by ultrafiltration (Porter, 1972). In the enzymatic cleavage of penicillins, the resulting 6-aminopenicillanic acid can be isolated by ultrafiltration (Cawthorne, 1974).

A process for the manufacture of protein-containing foodstuffs and fodder materials in which microorganisms are propagated in whey likewise makes use of ultrafiltration for the isolation of the protein formed, the solution being concentrated in the presence of the microorganisms (Müller, 1974).

In the purification of enzymes, ultrafiltration can be used advantageously for the demi-

Table 8-5. Examples of the Application of Ultrafiltration and Reverse Osmosis.

Type of membrane	Type of filtration Application	Molecular-weight cut-off
"Desalination membrane"	treatment of effluents, desalination of brackish water	MW > 150
"Hyperfiltration membrane"	concentration of active pharmaceutical compounds; concentration of dyestuffs; recovery of lactose; partial desalination	MW > 220 **organic compounds**
"Ultrafiltration membrane"	fractionation; dialysis; processing of whey; recovery of protein; manufacture of enzymes	MW > 10 000 **high-molecular-weight compounds, e.g., albumins, globulins**

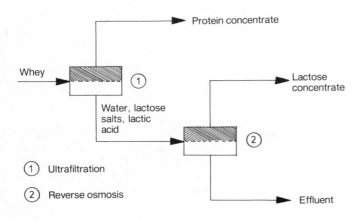

① Ultrafiltration

② Reverse osmosis

Fig. 8-14. Schematic representation of a membrane filtration plant for the processing of whey.

neralization and concentration of protein solutions.

It has been possible to concentrate penicillin acylase 20-fold. The total yield in terms of enzymatic activity averaged 92.7% (Table 8-6). With a rate of flow of 1200 L/h through a membrane area of 7 m²,

Table 8-6. Demineralization and Concentration of Penicillin Acylase from *Escherichia coli*.

Concentration ratio	Yield % activity
1:4	80.2
1:5 to 1:7	94.9
1:7 to 1:10	93.8
>1:10	98.0
>1:20	107.2

permeate outputs of between 200 L/h and 50 L/h for the original solution and the solution after concentration, respectively, were obtained. Melling and Westmacott (1972) showed that the retention rate for penicillin acylase from *Escherichia coli* (MW 22 000) with a membrane having a cut-off of 30 000 varies between 1.6% and 55% as a function of the pH and the ionic strength of the solution. A hollow fiber ultrafiltration apparatus has been used successfully by Weiss (1980) for the concentration of a virus.

8.4.4   Freeze-concentration

This method permits a very gentle concentration by freezing out pure water from solutions of active substances. It is used mainly in the foodstuffs industry. A schematic representation of the process is shown in Fig. 8-15 (Hüper and Schmidt-Kastner, 1973). A new process (vacuum countercurrent freeze concentration) has been described by Steinbach (1974).

8.4.5   Ion-exchange Processes and Adsorption with Adsorber Resins

Ion-exchange or adsorption with special polymer resins may be considered for the isolation of hydrophilic metabolites that cannot be extracted with organic solvents. In addition to the use of ion-exchange resins for the enrichment of active materials, they can also be used for the separation of undesired by-products and for pH adjustment in cases where foreign ions are undesirable. The fine purification of active substances by ion-exchange chromatography is considered in more detail in section 8.5.2.

Solid Ion-exchangers

Solid ion-exchangers can be described by the following parameters:

Functional groups:

- carbonyl
- sulfonic acid
- primary, secondary, and tertiary amines
- quaternary amines

Basic matrix:

- styrene-divinylbenzene
- acrylate
- methacrylate
- polyamine
- cellulose
- dextran

Microscopic form:

- gel
- macroporous

Macroscopic form:

- granulate
- beads.

An extensive literature exists on ion-exchangers although most of it deals with the use of ion-exchangers for water treatment. A general review on ion-exchangers has been given by Dorfner (1963).

Active substances from fermentation liquors can be isolated from the culture broth either after filtration or directly by adsorption on ion-exchangers. The isolation of sisomicin is carried out by the first method (Weinstein et al., 1974), while streptomycin, for example, is isolated from the culture broth without prefiltration (Bartels et al., 1958). The separation of

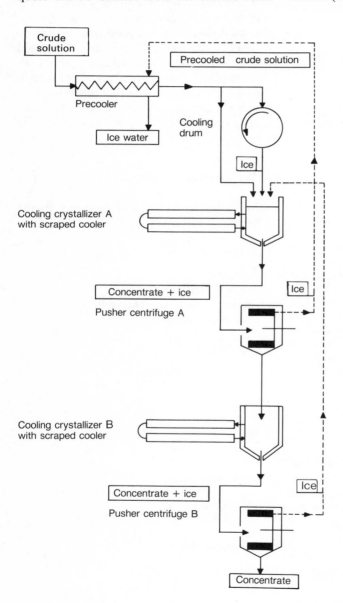

Fig. 8-15. Schematic representation of a two-stage continuous plant for freeze-concentration.

an antibiotic directly from the culture solution has also been described by Belter et al. (1973): for the isolation of novobiocin, the total culture liquor is treated with an anion-exchanger in stirred columns connected in series. The columns are equipped with sieve-plates which permit a passage of the cells of the culture broth but retain the resin within the columns. For the adsorption, a mathematical model has been developed which permits process optimization to be carried out when the production conditions change. The use of ion-exchangers for the separation of bacterial mixtures has been described by Daniels et al. (1966), and also by Rotman (1960).

Liquid Ion-exchangers

The choice of liquid ion-exchangers is limited. However, they have some advantages over solid ion-exchangers. While in the case of solid ion-exchangers the particles must have a **definite minimum size** to permit an adequate rate of flow in columns, which may have an adverse influence on the properties of the exchangers, these hydraulic and kinetic problems are negligible in the case of liquid ion-exchangers. With the liquid exchangers there is a **selective transfer** of a solute from an aqueous phase into an organic phase that contains the liquid exchanger. For technical application, the following properties are desirable: low solubility in water, high selectivity, good miscibility with organic solvents, good stability, easy regenerability, and low costs.

The technical processes for the application of liquid ion-exchangers have already been described, in section 8.4.2.

Typical liquid ion-exchangers are amines and organic acids with molecular weights of 250 to 500 having one functional group in the molecule. Liquid ion-exchangers can be characterized in the following way:

Functional groups:

- primary, secondary, tertiary amines
- phosphoric acid monoesters
- phosphoric acid diesters

Structure:

- unbranched carbon chain
- branched carbon chain
- aromatic compounds.

As an example of the use of a liquid ion-exchanger, the recovery of cephalosporin is shown in Fig. 8-16 (Voser, 1977). A good review of the properties and use of liquid ion-exchangers has been given by Kunin and Winger (1962).

In Table 8-7, solid and liquid ion-exchangers are compared with respect to their properties and possible applications.

Adsorber Resins

Various manufacturers have developed resins without functional groups, so-called macroporous or macroreticular adsorber resins. The binding of substances to these resins takes place nonstoichiometrically by adsorption. Important characteristics of these resins are, therefore, **pore volume, specific surface,** mean **pore diameter,** and **pore distribution.** Summarizing, these resins can be described in the following manner:

Chemical nature:

- nonpolar: styrene-divinylbenzene
- semipolar: acrylic esters
- polar: sulfoxides, amides, polar N-O groups

Physical properties:

- internal surface 20 to 800 m^2/g (bone charcoal ca. 60 m^2/g)

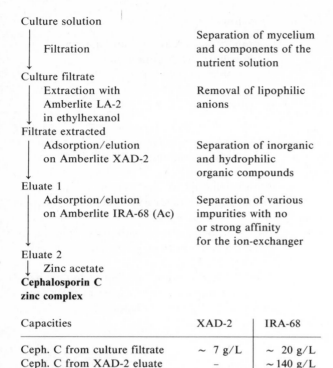

Culture solution	
Filtration	Separation of mycelium and components of the nutrient solution
Culture filtrate	
Extraction with Amberlite LA-2 in ethylhexanol	Removal of lipophilic anions
Filtrate extracted	
Adsorption/elution on Amberlite XAD-2	Separation of inorganic and hydrophilic organic compounds
Eluate 1	
Adsorption/elution on Amberlite IRA-68 (Ac)	Separation of various impurities with no or strong affinity for the ion-exchanger
Eluate 2	
Zinc acetate	
Cephalosporin C zinc complex	

Capacities	XAD-2	IRA-68
Ceph. C from culture filtrate	~ 7 g/L	~ 20 g/L
Ceph. C from XAD-2 eluate	–	~ 140 g/L
Pure cephalosporin C	~ 20 g/L	~ 200 g/L

Fig. 8-16. Recovery of cephalosporin with ion-exchange.

– pore volume 0.5 to 1.2 mL/g
– mean pore diameter 5 to 130 nm (bone charcoal ca. 13 nm).

In the last few years, the adsorber resins have proved satisfactory in many cases for the isolation of active substances from fermentation solutions. According to Fiedler (1977), any substance that can be extracted from aqueous solution with an organic solvent can also bind to adsorber resins. In many cases, elution can be carried out with organic solvents. In contrast to ion-exchangers, in many cases the capacity of adsorber resins increases in the presence of salts. Descriptions of adsorber resins and of their use and manufacture have been given by Kennedy (1973) and by Corte and Meyer (1970).

8.4.6 Precipitation Reactions

The precipitation of active substances by the addition of salts or organic solvents is used mainly for the enrichment of macromolecular compounds. Organic solvents lower the dielectric constant of the medium and therefore increase the Coulomb forces of attraction between differently charged molecules, so that the solubility decreases. In addition to this, the solvation of the molecules is altered by organic solvents. In concentrated salt solutions,

Table 8-7. Comparison between Solid and Liquid Ion-exchangers.

Characteristic	Solid ion-exchangers	Liquid ion-exchangers
Function	practically all types obtainable	limited predominantly to amines and alkyl phosphates
Matrix	rigid cross-linked polymer units	diluent acts as carrier of the active group
Exchange	comparatively slow (diffusion-controlled)	extremely fast
Selectivity	dependent on the functional groups, the degree of cross-linking, the substituents, and the matrix	dependent on the functional and substituted groups and the diluent
Mechanism	ion exchange in a hydrated resin particle	ion exchange in the boundary layer of the two liquid phases (in a water-free droplet)
Process technology	mainly flow through a column filled with resin	same apparatus as for liquid-liquid extraction

the decrease in the solubility of proteins is a function of the ionic strength of the solution which is expressed by the equation

$$\log S = \beta - K_O \cdot \Gamma$$

where S = solubility of the protein, Γ = ionic strength, and β and K_O are constants. Proven precipitants for the enrichment of proteins from crude solutions are ammonium sulfate and sodium sulfate. The recovery of enzymes from *Bacillus subtilis* by precipitation with sodium sulfate has been described by Pelluet (1970), and a process for the precipitation of penicillin acylase from *Escherichia coli* with tannin has been reported by Delin et al. (1972). As an example of the precipitation of proteins with solvents, reference may be made to plasma fractionation (Fig. 8-17; Cohn et al., 1950; Green and Hughes, 1955).

Proteins and viruses can be enriched and purified by precipitation with polyethylenglycols (PEGs) of different molecular weights. In the concentration of viruses by PEGs, the mechanism appears to consist in a phase separation of PEG-salt solutions, although macroscopically only one phase can be recognized (Yamamoto et al., 1970). As well as by concentration, viruses can be separated on the basis of symmetry and size differences (Yamamoto et al., 1970). In the purification of L-asparaginase, likewise, an enrichment step involving precipitation by polyethyleneglycol has been used (Wagner et al., 1968). In the field of low-molecular-weight compounds, organic acids are enriched mainly by precipitation in the form of salts; for example, in the technical isolation of citric acid this is precipitated as the calcium salt (Schulz and Rauch, 1972).

8.5 *Purification*

A number of different processes is available for further purification of bioproducts:

– crystallization
– chromatography
– countercurrent distribution
– electrophoresis
– electrodialysis.

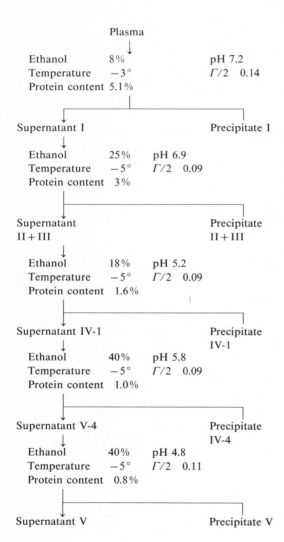

Fig. 8-17. Scheme of fractionation for human plasma with alcohol (Γ: ionic strength of the solution).

Electrophoretic processes have so far been used for purification mainly on the preparative laboratory scale. A very effective method is **countercurrent distribution.** It is also used technically, e.g., for the isolation of citric acid from citrus juice (Zang et al., 1966).

The main processes for the purification of bioproducts are crystallization and chromatography.

8.5.1 Crystallization

The crystallization of **citric acid** is carried out on the large scale. The solution coming from the concentration step is fed continuously to a cooled vacuum crystallization process. The steep solubility curve requires an accurate control of the amounts of water to be added and removed. In order to obtain citric acid monohydrate, crystallization must be carried out below 36.5 °C (Schmitz, 1977).

In the pharmaceutical industry, various **antibiotics** are purified by crystallization and recrystallization from organic solvents. Crystallization can also be used for the **purification of enzymes** and often takes place from solutions saturated with ammonium sulfate. For the theoretical principles of crystallization, reference may be made to, for example, Matz (1972) and Mullin (1972).

8.5.2 Chromatography

The purification of substances by chromatography is based on the high selectivity of this procedure. The components are distributed between a stationary and a mobile phase as the result of different binding forces. The separating apparatus most commonly used is a column filled with the particular support material. The mixture of components to be separated is passed through the column. A separation of the components is achieved by the subsequent elution procedure, in which their binding forces are compensated to different extents. Various types of chromatography are distinguished according to the nature of the binding forces and the principle of separation (Table 8-8).

Apart from the high selectivity in separation, another advantage of chromatography consists in the mild **reaction conditions.** In general, it takes place at room temperature in buffered solutions. No shear forces arise which result in damage of the product. The separation of a mixture of similar compounds on a chromatographic column is affected by two contrary factors:

– The degree of separation depends on the different levels of retention of the various components on a given stationary phase using a given eluent.

– The separation is affected by "zone broadening". This broadening of the zones migrating through the chromatographic column is affected by three factors:
In the column, a diffusion takes place in the longitudinal direction which cannot be prevented. Its adverse effect can be limited by a high linear velocity of flow.
Because of the finite velocity of flow, only an incomplete establishment of equilibrium between the stationary and the mobile phase takes place, which has the consequence of a displacement of the concentration between the leading and trailing edges of the migrating zones. This adverse influence can be reduced only by the smallest possible linear velocity of flow.

Irregularities in the packing material and different qualities of the packing of the column lead to the formation of solvent channels and therefore to different flow situations over the cross-section of the column.

It can be seen from what has been said so far that an **optimum velocity of flow** exists for any chromatographic column, which is generally very small. In order to be able to perform a chromatographic process economically, it is preferred to work outside the optimum range. This is possible, because the **separation quality** of a chromatographic column changes appreciably only at large deviations from the optimum. From this it follows that for scaling up of chromatographic processes the following factors must be kept constant:

– the length of the column (the increase in volume must be achieved by choosing a larger diameter and not by increasing the height of the column)

– the linear velocity of flow

– the ratio of the volume of the sample to the volume of the chromatographic matrix.

Table 8-8. Distinguishing Characteristics for Chromatographic Processes.

Name	Action principle	Separation according to
Adsorption chromatography	surface binding	surface affinity
Ion-exchange chromatography	ion binding	charge
Molecular sieve chromatography	pore diffusion	molecular size, molecular shape
Affinity chromatography	biospecific adsorption/desorption	molecular structure
Hydrophobic chromatography	hydrophobic complex-formation	molecular structure
Partition chromatography	partition equilibrium	polarity
Covalent chromatography	covalent binding	functional groups

In the case of affinity chromatography, the following additional factors must be kept constant for scaling up:

– the degree of substitution of the adsorbent

– the adsorption and elution kinetics.

A detailed treatment of the parameters important for scaling up in chromatography is given by Janson and Dunnill (1974).

Adsorption Chromatography

In adsorption chromatography, the components are separated on the basis of different valence forces between them and the surface of the solid. The **method of manufacture** and the **pretreatment of the support** play a large role for the separating behavior. Support materials that can be used are inorganic substances such as silicates, hydroxylapatite, and alumina, and also organic materials such as activated carbon or synthetic polymers with surfaces of between 100 and 1000 m^2/g. Vogelmann and Wagner (1977) have reported the separation of natural materials with synthetic polymer resins. Adsorber resins can also be used for the purification of proteins. The kallikrein-trypsin inhibitor from cattle organs, for example, has been purified in this way (Rauenbusch and Gölker, 1972).

Ion-exchange Chromatography

In ion-exchange chromatography, substances are separated by reversible ionic binding on the basis of charges of opposite sign or of the same sign but different magnitudes to a matrix which contains charged groups. The carriers used for ion-exchange chromatography may be either solid or liquid, in contrast to all other chromatographic methods in which only

solid supports are used. A large number of ion-exchangers has been developed on the basis of synthetic polymers. Today, ion-exchangers are also used on the technical scale for the purification of, for example antibiotics and enzymes, and also for demineralization or decoloration in the downstream processing of bioproducts. When ion-exchangers based on polystyrene are used, the hydrophobic nature of the polymer chain may have adverse effects on the native structure of enzymes and proteins. For such separations ion-exchangers based on **dextran** or **cellulose** have proved very satisfactory in the laboratory. For a long time, the compressibility of these ion-exchangers and the poor rates of flow were against their use in large columns in the technical field. In the last few years, however, special columns have been developed which permit outstanding separations with these materials even on the technical scale (Janson, 1971). Figure 8-18 shows a prototype of a production column with a volume of 300 L.

In the purification of albumin, in addition to other methods, two chromatographic steps are carried out with the ion-exchangers DEAE-Sepharose and SP-Sephadex (Fig. 8-19).

Molecular Sieve Chromatography

In molecular sieve or gel chromatography, the separation of mixtures of substances takes place on a matrix with a defined "sieve structure". Here, the small molecules can penetrate into the pores and are therefore retarded in comparison with larger molecules. The separation depends not only on the size but also on the shape of the molecules. A definite degree of swelling must be maintained for the gel, since the pore structure of the gel depends on this factor. Enzymes, nucleic acids, carbohydrates, and peptides can be separated by gel chromatography. In addition, sensitive bio-

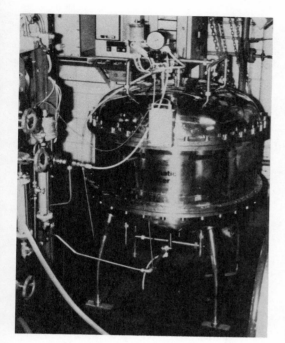

Fig. 8-18. Chromatographic column with a volume of 300 L (Pharmacia).

products can be desalted by "gel filters". An exhaustive description of the theory and application of gel chromatography has been given by Determann (1967).

Affinity Chromatography

Affinity chromatography uses a biospecific effector to isolate and/or purify a complementary molecule by highly selective adsorption and desorption. The biospecific effector and the biospecific complementary molecule act as lock and key. The effector is usually covalently bound to a support and can be filled into a column for selective adsorption/desorption. High-molecular-weight compounds such as enzyme inhibitors and low-molecular-weight

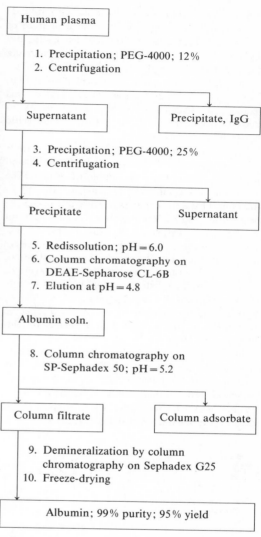

Fig. 8-19. Purification of albumin from human plasma.

compounds such as substrate analogs can be used as effectors.

The following example shows schematically an affinity chromatographic process in three steps (Fig. 8-20). The biospecific effector, e.g., an enzyme inhibitor I_1, attached to a water-insoluble support binds the complementary enzyme E_1 from a mixture of enzymes E_1, E_2, E_3, and E_4. The enzymes E_2, E_3, and E_4 are not bound and are washed off. By changing the pH, for example, the binding of the enzyme inhibitor I_1 to the enzyme E_1 is loosened and the enzyme is released from the effector and eluted. This example shows schematically the separation of enzyme E_1 from enzymes E_2 + E_3 + E_4 by biospecific adsorption.

However, affinity chromatography also permits the dual utilization of biospecificity. In the second example, a bivalent enzyme inhibitor I_b is used. The biospecifically complementary enzymes E_1 and E_2 are bound from the complex mixture of enzymes E_1 and E_2, E_3, and E_4. The enzymes E_3 and E_4 are not bound and are washed off. By using a substrate analog A_1 to enzyme E_1, the latter can be eluted selectively from the bivalent enzyme inhibitor and be isolated in pure form. In a second step, the enzyme E_2 is eluted with the substrate analog A_2. This example shows schematically the separation of enzyme E_1 from E_2 and from enzyme E_3 and E_4 by biospecific adsorption in combination with a biospecific elution (Fig. 8-21).

An example of the use of a high-molecular-weight effector is the isolation of the Kunitz inhibitor with trypsin (Werle and Fritz, 1972). A low-molecular-weight effector, in this case N^6-(6-aminohexyl)adenosine, bound to Sepharose 4B as support (I), is used for the separation of dehydrogenases.

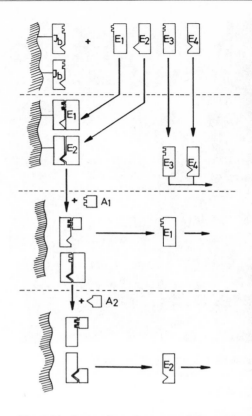

Fig. 8-21. Separation of enzymes from a mixture of enzymes by the use of a bivalent inhibitor.

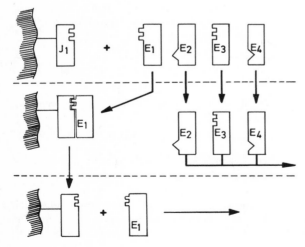

Fig. 8-20. Separation of an enzyme by biospecific adsorption.

Fig. 8-22 shows the separation of albumin from four dehydrogenases by biospecific adsorption and the separation of the four dehydrogenases by pH-gradient elution (Mosbach et al., 1974).

Fig. 8-23 shows the separation of the five lactate-dehydrogenase-isoenzymes by affinity chromatography on I and selective desorption by the use of a NADH gradient (Brodelius and Mosbach, 1973).

An example of a high specifity of a bioeffector is the isolation of the vitamin B_{12}-binding protein transcobalamin II from the Cohn-III fraction of human plasma with an enrichment factor of 24000. The effector used was vitamin B_{12} bound to Sepharose 4B through 3,3'-diaminodipropylamine as spacer. The starting material was 1400 L of human plasma. 6.3 mg of vitamin B_{12}-binding protein was obtained, which corresponds to a total yield referred to the Cohn-III fraction of 31% (Allen et al., 1972). The individual purification steps are summarized in Table 8-9.

Sepharose 4B ---NH—CH_2 CH_2 CH_2 CH_2 CH_2 CH_2 —NH CH_2-O-PO_3H_2 OH OH

I

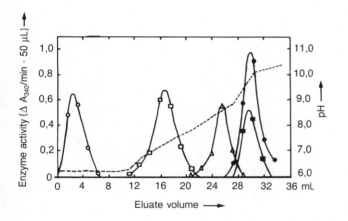

Fig. 8-22. Separation of glucose phosphate dehydrogenase, alcohol dehydrogenase, malate dehydrogenase, and lactate dehydrogenase from albumin by biospecific adsorption.

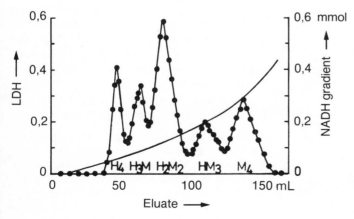

Fig. 8-23. Separation of the lactate dehydrogenase isoenzymes by affinity chromatography.

Table 8-9. Purification of Transcobalamin II from Human Plasma (Cohn-III fraction).

Process step	Yield of the step[a]	% yield of the step	Purity[b]	Enrichment factor
Cohn-III fraction (372 g from 1400 L of human serum)	573	100%	0.11	–
CM-Sephadex eluate	447	78%	0.59	5.4
Affinity chromatography on (vit. B_{12})-Sepharose	353	80%	14000	24000
DEAE-Cellulose and diaminodipropylamino-Sephadex chromatography	258	73%	25400	1.8
Sephadex G150 chromatography	179	69%	28600	1.1
		(31% overall yield)		

[a]   (Vitamin B_{12}) binding in mg
[b]   ng of (Vitamin B_{12}) binding/mg of protein

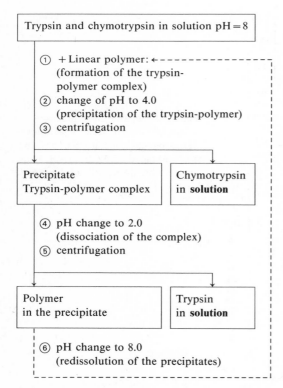

Fig. 8-24. Separation of trypsin and chymotrypsin by affinity precipitation.

The surface specifity of the cell membrane also permits the separation of cells by affinity chromatography. Thus, for example, antigen-specific cells can be selected with lectin-biospecific effectors (Schlossmann and Hudson, 1973; Chess et al., 1974).

A special case of affinity chromatography is represented by **affinity precipitation.** An example of this method is the separation and purification of trypsin and chymotrypsin (Schneider, 1975). The effector in this case is an aminobenzamidine derivative which together with N-acryloyl-p-amino-benzoic acid as precipitate and with acrylamide becomes a water soluble bifunctional linear copolymer.

By changing the pH into the acid range, the dissociation of the p-aminobenzoic acid derivative is suppressed and the soluble polymer is precipitated.

The separation of trypsin and chymotrypsin by this scheme is summarized in Fig. 8-24.

For more detailed information on the problems and chances of affinity chromatography, the following literature is recommended: Dunlap (1974), Jakoby et al. (1974), Lowe et al. (1974), Turkova (1978), Hoffmann-Ostenhoff et al. (1978), and a Pharmacia brochure (1979).

Hydrophobic Chromatography

Hydrophobic chromatography is based primarily on an interaction between a hydrophobic or hydrophobic-substituted support and hydrophobic regions in biopolymers, especially in proteins and polypeptides. A simplifying idea of the hydrophobic interaction between hydrophobic matrix and corresponding regions in the protein assumes the intercalation of an alkyl or aryl residue into hydrophobic pockets of the protein or the addition of alkyl or aryl residues to the surface of a hydrophobic region. In both cases, a **multipoint attachment** is possible. Biospecific interactions are excluded. Other binding mechanisms that influence the situation to a greater or smaller extent may be superposed on the hydrophobic interaction.

In aqueous solutions, proteins bind to hydrophobically substituted agarose (Er-el et al., 1972; Hofstee, 1973). Shaltiel and Er-el (1973) have shown that the separation of enzymes depends on the **length of the alkyl chain** of the substituted agarose. Alkyl-substituted agaroses (I) are obtained from (cyanogen bromide)-activated agarose by treatment with primary amines with different chain lengths. A hydrophobic carrier prepared in this manner also contains in the neighborhood of the carrier surface a basic function which may affect the separation. The proteins to be separated in this way are adsorbed at a low ionic strength and are desorbed selectively with an eluent having increasing ionic strength. Hydrophobic carriers without an additional basic function

(II) have been developed by Hjerten (1973), among others. The proteins to be separated are bound more strongly at a high than at a low ionic strength.

A decisive factor for the application of hydrophobic chromatography in biotechnology is the **separating power** of the hydrophobic carrier, its **mechanical stability**, its **permanent capacity**, and, finally, its price, which contribute to the economics of a bioproduct. The separating power depends on the **tertiary structure of the proteins** in the mixture of proteins. For each given protein mixture, therefore, a special hydrophobic carrier must be developed or a known carrier must be optimized. For each system the adaptation of the hydrophobic carrier to the mixture to be separated requires a high expenditure on development. A scaling up of hydrophobic chromatography to the large technical scale is ensured by the development of modern equipment.

At the present time, hydrophobic chromatography is mainly used for the separation of proteins, especially enzymes. However, its application is not limited to this class of substances but, in principle, covers all bioproducts that exhibit a hydrophobic interaction. It likewise comprises the reversible adsorption of cells (erythrocytes). The combination of hydrophobic chromatography with other chromatographic methods permits the manufacture of high-purity bioproducts for pharmaceuticals or diagnostics. The demand for a high quality of bioproducts will decisively affect the further development of modern separating processes in biotechnology and, therefore, also the further development of hydrophobic chromatography.

Partition Chromatography

Here, substances are distributed between two immiscible or only partially miscible phases on the basis of different solubilities of the components. In **column chromatography**, a hydrophilic stationary phase is usually used which is capable of retaining the aqueous phase. The mobile phase consists of an

I $\quad \}-O-\overset{\overset{NH}{\|}}{C}-NH-(CH_2)_n-CH_3$

II $\quad \}-O-CH_2-CHOH-CH_2-O-(CH_2)_n-CH_3$

organic solvent. The mixture of substances to be separated migrates through the column and is distributed between the phases. The separation depends on the **partition coefficient** K_D, i.e., on the ratio of the equilibrium concentration of a component in the stationary phase to that in the mobile phase. The results of the separation are frequently affected by **temperature** and the concentration of the components. Since an equilibrium must be established, only very low rates of flow are achieved. **"Reversed phase chromatography"** uses a matrix coated with a hydrophobic material that is saturated with an organic solvent. The aqueous phase forms the mobile phase. Partition chromatography in columns has so far played no part in technical processes.

Covalent Chromatography

Covalent chromatography makes use of the interaction of specific groups. The active principle will be explained in connection with the purification of the enzyme **urease** (Carlsson et al., 1976). The purification is based on the reciprocal thiol-disulfide exchange on an agarose pyridin-2-yl disulfide as water-insoluble effector. The enzyme urease is bound to a support present in a column through a covalent bond in the form of a disulfide bridge. Elution is carried out with low-molecular-weight SH compounds such as dithiothreitol (Fig. 8-25). The enrichment factors obtained can be seen from Table 8-10. The yield in one step amounts to 86%.

Another example of the efficacy of the method is the purification of mercaptalbumin. By covalent chromatography on a Sepharose-(glutathione pyridin-2-yl disulfide) conjugate it was possible to achieve a separation of albumin into mercaptalbumin with a thiol group content of 1.00 to 1.02/mol and non-mercaptalbumin with a thiol group content of < 0.02/mol (Carlsson et al., 1974). A separation of SH-group-containing proteins from proteins without SH groups is also possible by covalent chromatography on agarose-(5,5'-dithiobis(2-nitrobenzoate)) (Lin et al., 1975).

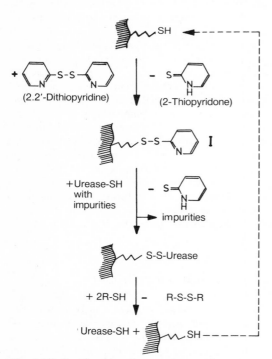

Fig. 8-25. Purification of urease by covalent chromatography.

8.6 Drying

For the bioproducts treated within this review, only very gentle methods of drying can be considered because of their heat-sensitive structure. To eliminate water or solvent from a moist product, heat must be supplied to the material to be dried. Depending on the method of heat transfer, a distinction can be made between:

– contact dryers
– convection dryers
– radiation dryers.

Table 8-10. Enrichment Factors and Yields in the Purification of Urease.

Process step	Yield of the step in units	% yield of the step	Purity in units/mg of dry matter	Enrichment factor
Ethanol extract	56 100	100%	9	–
Covalent chromatography	48 000	86%	1500	167
Molecular sieve chromatography	40 200	72% (62% overall yield)	2515	1.7

Table 8-11. Principles of the Action of Frequently Used Drying Apparatuses.

Type of dryer	Heat transfer through	Movement of the product
Chamber dryer	convection and contact	none
Tumbler dryer	contact	moderate mechanical
Drum dryer	contact	slight mechanical
Thin-layer dryer	contact	intensive mechanical
Belt dryer	convection	slight mechanical
Pneumatic conveying dryer	convection	intensive due to gas flow
Fluidized bed dryer	convection	intensive due to gas flow
Spray-dryer	convection	intensive due to gas flow
Freeze-dryer	contact and radiation	none or mechanical

For the principles and the general review of drying procedures and dryers reference may be made to the literature, e.g., Vogelpohl and Schlünder (1972).

Some common dryers are listed in Table 8-11.

8.6.1 Contact Dryers

Batchwise drying is carried out in many contact dryers with mechanically moved layers in which the movement of the material is carried out by rotating internals. The advantage of these dryers as compared with a simple chamber dryer is the uniform thermal stressing of the material being dried, higher throughputs, and the possibility of the automatic feed and discharge of the apparatus. To some extent, these dryers can also be used for the subsequent mixing of different components with one another, which is very important in pharmaceutical chemistry, for example (Juergens and Knetsch, 1977). Stein (1976, 1977) has performed investigations on the economic aspect of the choice of contact dryers. When drying is carried out in **double-conical dryers** and **disk dryers,** the material to be dried must be flowable even in the moist state in order to prevent the formation of cakes and lumps in the dryer. The drying process may therefore be preceded by a granulation step. The mode of operation in the disk dryer is continuous. For special cases, **thin-layer dryers** with extremely short residence times of the product are available (Widmer, 1971).

8.6.2 *Convection Dryers*

In many convection dryers, the movement of the material to be dried is effected by the flow of a gas. They permit the drying of large streams of product in a relatively short time. The most important convection dryer for bioproducts is the **spray dryer.** The material to be dried is fed to the dryer in the form of a concentrated sulution, a suspension, or a moist but still flowable solid. Extremely fine particles are generated by nozzles or rotating atomizing disks and these immediately come into contact with a stream of hot air. Here, even in the case of sensitive bioproducts, the temperatures may be in the region of 150 to 200°C. Because the heat of evaporation is removed at stroke, the temperature of the particles is kept so low that the bioproducts suffer no thermal damage.

Spray dryers are used in the recovery of antiotics as pure substance, in the manufacture of antibiotics for animal husbandry in the form of dried mycelium, in the manufacture of single-cell protein (Bennoit el al., 1975), and in the recovery of residues (manufacture of foodstuffs, fermentation) (Masters and Vestergaard, 1978).

For discontinuous processes in which small amounts of product arise, **chamber dryers** (vacuum drying cabinets, shelf dryers) are still in use today. The product is charged onto shelves and the transfer of heat takes place partly by contact but mainly by convection. The material to be dried undergoes practically no mechanical stress but the distribution of thermal stress is very nonuniform and therefore only relatively low drying temperatures can be used.

8.6.3 *Freeze-dryers*

The freeze-drying (sublimation drying) process has continuously gained importance in the last few years both for the drying of pharmaceutical and biological products and also in foodstuffs technology. In the pharmaceutical industry, the following bioproducts, *inter alia,* are manufactured by freeze-drying: viruses, bacteria (live vaccines, cultivation of strains), serum fractions for the purposes of concentration, preserved plasma and sera for blood transfusion, hormones, enzymes, and vitamin preparations.

If one considers the phase diagram of water, it can be seen that the sublimation process can take place only below the triple point since only here does water exist exclusively in solid form as ice. In most of the products coming into consideration for freeze-drying, the phase diagrams are more complex than for pure water. An essential factor for freeze-drying is the temperature at which only a solid phase still exists (eutectic point or eutectic range). In the case of products of complex composition, this temperature is generally much lower than for water, and the partial pressure of water vapor at the sublimation surface is therefore low. The temperature of the material to be dried must not be higher during the drying process in order to avoid thawing.

Sublimation requires an energy of about 2800 kJ/kg of water. During the freeze-drying process, this energy must be transported from the exterior to the sublimation zone. The transport of heat takes place through contact, radiation, and, to a varying extent, depending on the vacuum in the drying chamber, by convection. Since practically no heat transfer by convection is possible below 10^{-2} mbar, the vacuum must always be kept as poor as is just tolerable for the total process. Consequently the regulation of the pressure in the equipment must be very accurate. As drying proceeds, the sublimation zone is covered by a layer of dried material. Acting as a very good insulator, this layer, on the one hand, impedes the transfer of heat by radiation and, on the other hand, it also hinders the removal of the water vapor. Fig. 8-26 tries to clarify the situa-

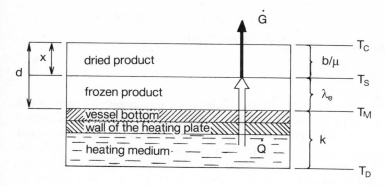

Fig. 8-26. Heat and mass transport in freeze-drying.
T_D temperature of the heating medium
T_M maximum product temperature (wall surface temperature)
T_S sublimation temperature
T_C condenser temperature
$\dot{Q}$ heat flux
$\dot{G}$ mass flux
k heat-transfer coefficient
λ_e coefficient of conductivity in the frozen product
b/μ mass transfer coefficient.

tion relating to the transport of heat and water vapor.

In order to prevent thawing of the product, the amount of heat supplied must be in equilibrium with the amount of heat required for sublimation. Following Strasser et al. (1966), the transport of heat and mass can be deduced from the shape of the temperature curves (Fig. 8-27). Curve TG 1 shows that more heat is supplied than necessary. In the case of curve TG 2, the transport of heat and mass are in equilibrium, while at TG 3 the transport of heat to the sublimation surface is smaller than the permitted maximum.

The water sublimed can be removed by various methods:

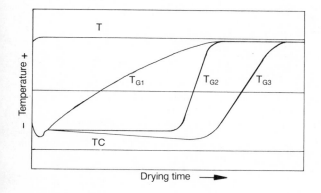

Fig. 8-27. Curves of the change in temperature during freeze-drying
T heating temperature
T_C condenser temperature

– suction with pumps
– deposition on cooled surfaces
– absorption by chemical compounds.

When it is realized that at a pressure of, for example, $1.3 \cdot 10^{-3}$ mbar 100 g of water vapor occupies a volume of 100 m^3, it is not difficult to see that in the case of large units suction with pumps alone is inadequate. A schematic representation of a freeze-drying unit for batch operation is shown in Fig. 8-28. Continuous units are used in the **foodstuffs industry.** In the future, this technology will certainly be used in the area of the production of **active pharmaceutical** agents, as well.

For the principles and applications of freeze-drying refer to the following literature: Rowe (1971), Goldblith et al. (1975), Liapis and Litchfield (1979), and Morgan and Spotts (1979).

8.7 Evaluation of Separation Processes

Each process for the isolation and purification of a bioproduct from microorganisms, animal organs, or plant cells consists of a sequence of individual process steps. The choice of the individual process steps is governed by the properties of the bioproduct to be isolated, and also by the properties of the accompanying substances that are to be removed. Important evaluation parameters of a process step are:

The yield of the step: The yield of the step, given in amounts (e.g., g or kg), or in units (or in mega units = millions of units), documents the scale of the

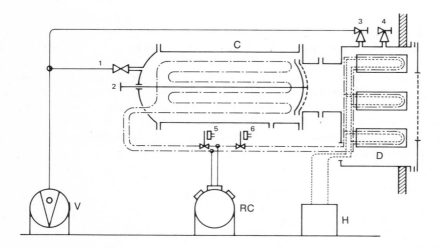

1	vacuum valve	
2	condenser-chamber connecting valve	
3	vacuum valve	
4	air inlet valve	
5	valve between cooling system and condenser	
6	valve between cooling system and drying chamber	

D   drying chamber
C   condenser
V   vacuum pump
RC refrigerating compressor
H   heating

Fig. 8-28. Schematic representation of a freeze-drying unit.

process step and the batch size and permits conclusions concerning the equipment used.

The percentage yield of a step:

$$100 \cdot \frac{\text{units (or amount) after purification}}{\text{units (or amount) before purification}}$$

indirectly evaluates the loss of bioproduct in the process step.

The purity of the bioproduct after enrichment or purification is given as amount of bioproduct/total amount, units/total amount, or, for example, units/mg of protein.

The enrichment factor is defined as:

$$\frac{\text{purity of the bioproduct after purification}}{\text{purity of the bioproduct before purification}}$$

The common evaluation of enrichment factor and percentage yield of the step permits a statement concerning the efficiency of the technology used in the process step. The product of purification factor times percentage yield of the step is termed the **efficiency.**

Technical and scientific parameters alone are not sufficient for the evaluation of a process step. Economic aspects must also be included, especially the **manufacturing costs** of the bioproduct. For calculating these, all types of costs, such as

- material costs
- personnel costs
- energy costs
- costs of repair
- depreciations
- costs for waste treatment, and
- overheads

must be added and the result is divided by the yield of the step. The manufacturing costs are given in

$$\frac{\text{total costs}}{\text{kg of bioproduct}} \quad \text{or} \quad \frac{\text{total costs}}{\text{mega units of bioproduct}}$$

and they integrate the economic and technical parameters of the process step. The purity of the bioproduct that has been achieved in the step is brought into relationship with the manufacturing costs.

The evaluation of the total process results from the evaluation of the individual process steps. Thus, the **percentage total yield** may be obtained by multiplying all the percentage step yields, and the **manufacturing costs of the end product** by adding all types of costs of all process steps and dividing by the **overall yield** in

$$\frac{\text{total costs}}{\text{kg of bioproduct}} \quad \text{or} \quad \frac{\text{total costs}}{\text{mega units of bioproduct}}$$

The technical and economic classification of a process into process steps does not only permit an **optimization of the process** but also an immediate adaptation to necessary **changes in the process** even when they are independent of the process itself.

8.8 Literature

Allen, R. H. and Majerus, W. P., "Isolation of vitamin B_{12}-binding proteins using affinity chromatography. III. Purification and properties of human plasma transcobalamin II", *J. Biol. Chem.* **247,** 7709–7717 (1972).

Alt, G.: "Filtration". In: *Ullmanns Encyklopädie der Technischen Chemie,* Vol. **2,** 4th Ed. Verlag Chemie, Weinheim 1972, pp. 154–198.

Atkinson, B. and Daoud, I. S., "Microbial flocs and flocculation in fermentation process engineering", *Adv. Biochem. Eng.* **4,** 41–124 (1976).

Bartels, C. R., Kleinmann, G., Korzun, J. N. and Irish, D. B., "A novel ion-exchange method for the isolation of streptomycin", *Chem. Eng. Prog.* **54** (8), 49–51 (1958).

Batchelor, F. R., Rolinson, G. N. and Stove, E. R.: Verfahren zur Anreicherung von 6-Aminopenicillansäure. D.O.S. 1,152,418 (1963).

Bell, G. R. and Hutto jr., F. B., "Analysis of rotary precoat filter operation – New concepts, Part I", *Chem. Eng. Prog.* **54,** 69–76 (1958).

Belter, P. A., Cunningham, F. L. and Chen, J. W., "Development of a recovery process for novobiocin", *Biotechnol. Bioeng.* **15,** 533–549 (1973).

Bennoit, H., Schütz, J. and Sittig, W.: "Abstimmung von mechanischer Flüssigkeitsabtrennung und thermischer Trocknung bei der mikrobiellen Proteingewinnung aus Kohlenwasserstoffen". Lecture to the GVC Expert Committee on Drying Technology, Erlangen (April 10, 1975).

Billet, R.: *Verdampfertechnik.* Bibliographisches Institut, Mannheim 1965.

Billet, R., "Trennwirkung im Dünnschichtverdampfer mit extrem kurzer Produktverweilzeit", *CZ-Chem. Tech.* 3 (1), 9-12 (1974).

Brodelius, P. and Mosbach, K., "Separation of the isoenzymes of lactate dehydrogenase by affinity chromatography using an immobilized AMP-analogue", *FEBS Lett.* 35, 223-226 (1973).

Buckland, B. C., Richmond, W., Dunnill, P. and Lilly, M. D., "The large-scale isolation of intracellular microbial enzymes: Cholesterol oxidase from Nocardia", *Ind. Aspects Biochem.* 30 (Part I), 65-79 (1974).

Carlsson, J., Olsson, I., Axén, R. and Drevin, H., "A new method for the preparation of jack-bean urease involving covalent chromatography", *Acta Chem. Scand.* B 30, 180-182 (1976).

Carlsson, J. and Svenson, A., "Preparation of bovine mercaptalbumin by means of covalent chromatography", *FEBS Lett.* 42, 183-186 (1974).

Cawthorne, A. M.: Verfahren zur Erzeugung von 6-Aminopenicillansäure. D.O.S. 2,356,630 (1974).

Chess, L., MacDermott, R. P. and Schlossmann, St. F., "Immunologic functions of isolated human lymphocyte subpopulations", *J. Immunol.* 113, 1113-1121 (1974).

Christman, C. C. and Robinson, A. C.: Verfahren zur Herstellung einer ein Derivat der 6-Aminopenicillansäure enthaltenden Lösung und deren Verwendung zur Herstellung von Penicillinen. D.O.S. 1,814,085 (1969).

Cohn, E. J., Gurd, F. R. N., Surgenor, D. M., Barnes, B. A., Brown, R. K., Derounaux, G., Gillespie, J. M., Kahnt, F. W., Lever, W. F., Liu, C. H., Mittelman, D., Mouton, R. F., Schmid, K. and Uroma, E., "A system for the separation of the components of human blood: Quantitative procedures for the separation of the protein components of human plasma", *J. Am. Chem. Soc.* 72, 465-474 (1950).

Corte, H. and Meyer, A.: Verfahren zur Herstellung von vernetzten Mischpolymerisaten mit Schwammstruktur. D.O.S. 1,745,717 (1970).

Curie, J. A., Dunnill, P. and Lilly, M. D., "Release of protein from baker's yeast *(Saccharomyces cerevisiae)* by disruption in an industrial agitator mill", *Biotechnol. Bioeng.* 14, 725-736 (1972).

Daniels, S. L. and Kempe, L. L., "The separation of bacteria by adsorption onto ion exchange resins", *Chem. Eng. Prog. Symp. Ser.* 62, (69), 142-148 (1966).

Delin, P. S., Ekström, B. A., Sjöberg, B. O. H., Thelin, K. H. and Nathorst-Westfelt, L. S.: Verfahren zur Herstellung von 6-Aminopenicillansäure. D.O.S. 1, 966, 427 (1972).

Determann, H.: *Gelchromatographie.* Springer-Verlag, Heidelberg 1967.

Dorfner, K.: *Ionenaustauscher.* Verlag Walter de Gruyter und Co., Berlin 1963.

Dunlap, R. B., "Immobilized biochemicals and affinity chromatography", *Adv. Exp. Med. Biol.* 42 (1974).

Er-el, Z., Zaidenzaig, Y. and Shaltiel, S., "Hydrocarbon-coated sepharose. Use in the purification of glycogen phosphorylase", *Biochem. Biophys. Res. Commun.* 49, 383-390 (1972).

Fiedler, H.-P.: "Isolierung von mikrobiellen Stoffwechselprodukten mit Hilfe von Adsorberharzen". Working meeting: Aufarbeitung in der Biotechnologie. ETH Zürich (May 6, 1977).

Follows, M., Hertherington, P. J., Dunnill, P. and Lilly, M. D., "Release of enzymes from baker's yeast by disruption in an industrial homogenizer", *Biotechnol. Bioeng.* 13, 549-560 (1971).

Gasner, L. L. and Wang, D. C. I., "Microbial cell recovery enhancement through flocculation", *Biotechnol. Bioeng.* 12, 873-887 (1970).

Gerstenberg, H., Sittig, W. and Zepf, K.-H., "Aufarbeitung von Fermentationsprodukten", *Chem. Ing. Tech.* 52, 19-31 (1980).

McGregor, W. C. and Finn, K. R., "Factors affecting the flocculation of bacteria by chemical additives", *Biotechnol. Bioeng.* 11, 127-138 (1969).

Gnieser, J.: "Separierung von Biomasse durch Elektroflotation". Working meeting: Aufarbeitung in der Biotechnologie, ETH Zürich (May 6, 1977).

Goldblith, S. A., Rey, L. and Rothmayer, W. W. (Eds.): *Freeze-drying and Advanced Food Technology.* Academic Press, New York 1975.

Gray, P. P., Dunnill, P. and Lilly, M. D., "The clarification of mechanically disrupted yeast suspensions by rotary vacuum precoat filtration", *Biotechnol. Bioeng.* 15, 309-320 (1973).

Green, A. A. and Hughes, W. L., "Protein fractionation on the basis of solubility in aqueous solutions of salts and organic solvents", *Methods Enzymol.* **I,** 67–90 (1955).

Gunsalus, I. C., "Extraction of enzymes from microorganisms (bacteria and yeast)", *Methods Enzymol.* **1,** 51–63 (1955).

Hemfort, H., "Diversifikation von Separatoren mit Düsen-, selbstreinigenden und Vollmantel-Trommeln", *Chem. Ing. Tech.* **51,** 479–484 (1979).

Heppel, L. A., "The effect of osmotic shock on release of bacterial proteins and on active transport", *J. Gen. Physiol.* **14,** 95–113 (1969).

Heppel, L. A., "Selective release of enzymes from bacteria", *Science* **156,** 1451–1455 (1967).

Hjerten, S., "Some general aspects of hydrophobic interaction chromatography", *J. Chromatogr.* **87,** 325–331 (1973).

Hoffmann-Ostenhoff, O., Breitenbach, M., Koller, F., Kraft, D. and Schreiner, O.: *Affinity Chromatography.* Pergamon Press, New York 1978.

Hofstee, B. H. J., "Hydrophobic affinity chromatography of proteins", *Anal. Biochem.* **52,** 430–448 (1973).

Hüper, F. and Schmidt-Kastner, G.: Anwendung eines Verfahrens zur Gefrierkonzentrierung von wäßrigen Lösungen von Arzneimitteln. D.O.S. 2,204,598 (1973).

Hughes, D. E., Wimpenny, J. W. T. and Lloyd, D., "The disintegration of microorganisms", *Methods Microbiol.* **5** B, 1–54 (1971).

Hugo, W. B., "The preparation of cell-free enzymes from microorganisms", *Bacteriol. Rev.* **18,** 87–105 (1965).

Jakoby, W. B. and Wilchek, M., "Affinity techniques", *Methods Enzymol.* **34** (1974).

James, C. J., Coakley, W. T. and Hughes, D. E., "Kinetics of protein release from yeast sonicated in batch and flow systems at 20 kHz", *Biotechnol. Bioeng.* **14,** 33–42 (1972).

Janson, J. C., "Columns of large-scale gel filtration on porous gels. Fractionation of rape seed proteins and insulin", *J. Agric. Food Chem.* **19,** 581–588 (1971).

Janson, J.-C. and Dunnill, P., "Factors affecting scale-up of chromatography", *Ind. Aspects Biochem.* **30** (Part I), 81–105 (1974).

Juergens, H.-H. and Knetsch, D., "Trocknung phar-mazeutischer Zwischenprodukte", *CZ-Chem. Tech.* **6** (7), 273–276 (1977).

Kennedy, D. C., "Macroreticular polymeric adsorbents", *Ind. Eng. Chem. Prod. Res. Dev.* **12** (1), 56–61 (1973).

Kula, M.-R., Kroner, K. H., Hustedt, H., Granda, S. and Stach, W.: Verfahren zur Abtrennung von Enzymen. D.O.S. 2,639,129 (1978a).

Kula, M.-R., Buckmann, A., Hustedt, H., Kroner, K. H. and Morr, M., "Aqueous two-phase systems for the large scale purification of enzymes", *Enzyme Eng.* **4,** 47–53 (1978b).

Kunin, R. and Winger, A. G., "Technologie der flüssigen Ionenaustauscher", *Chem. Ing. Tech.* **34** (7), 461–467 (1962).

Lowe, C. R. and Dean, P. D. G.: *Affinity Chromatography.* Wiley, London 1974.

Lin, L. J. and Foster, J. F., "Agarose-DTNB column for binding sulfhydryl-containing proteins and peptides", *Anal. Biochem.* **63,** 485–490 (1975).

Liapis, A. I. and Litchfield, R. J., "Optimal control of a freeze dryer – I. Theoretical development and quasi steady state analysis", *Chem. Eng. Sci.* **34,** 975–981 (1979).

Madsen, R. F. and Olsen, O. J., "Anwendung von Ultrafiltration und Hyperfiltration als Vorkonzentrierungs- und Reinigungsstufen in der pharmazeutischen Industrie und Nahrungsmittelindustrie", *CZ-Chem. Tech.* **3** (3), 81–84 (1974).

Marquardt, K., "Umgekehrte Osmose und Ultrafiltration – Anwendungsmöglichkeiten und Beschränkungen des Verfahrens sowie der gegenwärtige Trend im Anlagenbau", *CZ Chem. Tech.* **2** (6), 245–253 (1973).

Masters, K. and Vestergaard, I., "Spray drying techniques for by-product recovery", *Process Biochem.* **13,** (1), 3–26 (1978).

Matsuura, T., "Transportvorgänge in Membranen zur umgekehrten Osmose", *Chem. Ing. Tech.* **50** (8), 565–573 (1978).

Matz, G.: "Kristallisation". In: *Ullmanns Encyklopädie der Technischen Chemie*, Vol. **2,** 4th Ed. Verlag Chemie, Weinheim 1972, pp. 672–681.

Melling, J. and Westmacott, D., "The influence of pH value and ionic strength on the ultrafiltration characteristics of a penicillinase produced by *Escherichia coli* Strain W 3310", *J. Appl. Chem. Biotechnol.* **22,** 951–958 (1972).

Morgan, S. L. and Spotts, M. R., "How to select a

pharmaceutical freeze-drying system", *Pharm. Technol.* **3,** 95–101/114 (1979).

Mosbách, K., Larson, P. O., Brodelius, P., Guilford, H. and Lindberg, M., "Synthesis and application of matrix bound AMP, NAD$^+$ and other adenine nucleotides", *Enzyme Eng.* **2,** 237–242 (1974).

Müller, E.: "Flüssig-Flüssig-Extraktion". In: *Ullmanns Encyklopädie der Technischen Chemie* Vol. **2,** 4th Ed. Verlag Chemie, Weinheim 1972, pp. 546–574.

Müller, H.: Verfahren zur Herstellung hoch eiweißhaltiger Nahrungs- und Futtermittel. D.O.S. 2,344,317 (1974).

Mullin, J. W.: *Crystallization.* 2nd Ed. Butterworths, London 1972.

Pharmacia brochure: *Affinity Chromatography. Principles and Methods.* Pharmacia Fine Chemicals. Uppsala, Schweden 1979.

Pelluet, J.: Verfahren zur Extraktion von Enzymen. D.O.S. 2,046,596 (1970).

Porter, M. C., "Applications of membranes to enzyme isolation and purification", *Biotechnol. Bioeng. Symp.* **3,** 115–144 (1972).

Prinssen, A. A. J. A., "Vacuum belt filters", *Filtr. Sep.* **16,** 176–180 (1979).

Rant, Z.: *Verdampfer in Theorie und Praxis,* 2nd Ed. Verlag Sauerländer, Aarau, Frankfurt/M. 1977.

Rauenbusch, E. and Gölker, Ch.: Verfahren zur Gewinnung des Kallikrein-Trypsin-Inhibitors aus Rinderorganen. D.A.S. 2,116,377 (1972).

Reháček, J. and Schaefer, J., "Disintegration of microorganisms in an industrial horizontal mill of novel design", *Biotechnol. Bioeng.* **19,** 1523–1534 (1977).

Rotman, B., "Uses of ion exchange resins in microbiology", *Bacteriol. Rev.* **24,** 251–260 (1960).

Rowe, T. W. G., "Machinery and methods in freeze-drying", *Cryobiology* **8,** 153–172 (1971).

Rubin, A. J., Cassel, E. A., Henderson, O., Johnson, J. D. and Lamb, J. C., III, "Microflotation – new low gasflow rate foam separation technique for bacteria and algae", *Biotechnol. Bioeng.* **8,** 135–151 (1966).

Rubin, A. J., "Microflotation: Coagulation and foam separation of *Aerobacter aerogenes*", *Biotechnol. Bioeng.* **10,** 89–98 (1968).

Rushton, A. and Khoo, H. E., "The filtration characteristics of yeast", *J. Appl. Chem. Biotechnol.* **27,** 99–109 (1977).

Saier, H.-D. and Strathmann, H., "Asymmetric membranes: preparation and application", *Angew. Chem. Int. Ed. Engl.* **14,** 452–459 (1975).

Samans, H., "Zerkleinerungstechnik im Bereich der chemischen und pharmazeutischen Industrie. Einführung in die Technologie des Zerkleinerns weicher bis mittelharter Stoffe", *CZ Chem. Tech.* **2** (9), 345–350 (1973).

Schaefer, F.: "Verdampfer". In: *Ullmanns Encyklopädie der Technischen Chemie,* Vol. **2,** 4th Ed. Verlag Chemie, Weinheim 1972, pp. 650–663.

Schmitz, R., "Problemlösungen bei der Aufarbeitung von Fermentationslösungen zu reiner Citronensäure", *CZ Chem. Tech.* **6** (7), 255–259 (1977).

Schneider, M.: Verfahren zur Extraktion eines Polypeptids, insbesondere eines Enzyms, aus einer wäßrigen Lösung. D.O.S. 2,611,258 (1975).

Schlossmann, St. F. and Hudson, L., "Specific purification of lymphocyte populations on a digestible immunoabsorbent", *J. Immunol.* **110,** 313–315 (1973).

Schreiner, H., "Flüssig-Flüssig-Extraktion – Teil I: Berechnungsgrundlagen", *Chem. Ztg.* **91,** 667–676 (1967).

Schreiner, H., "Flüssig-Flüssig-Extraktion – Teil II: Extraktionsapparate", *Chem. Ztg.* **93,** 971–982 (1969).

Schultz, F.: Verfahren zur Herstellung von reinen Lösungen des Kallikrein-Inaktivators. D.B.P. 1,084,433 (1961).

Schulz, G. und Rauch, J.: "Citronensäure". In: *Ullmanns Encyklopädie der Technischen Chemie.* Vol. **9,** 4th Ed. Verlag Chemie, Weinheim 1972, pp. 624–636.

Schutt, H.: Verfahren zur Herstellung des Kallikrein-Trypsin-Inhibitors aus Rinderlunge. D.O.S. 2,509,482 (1976).

Shaltiel, S. and Er-el, Z., "Hydrophobic chromatography: Use for purification of glycogen synthetase", *Proc. Nat. Acad. Sci. USA* **70,** 778–781 (1973).

Seipenbusch, R., Birckenstaedt, J. W. and Grosse, A.: "Ökonomische Überlegungen zur Aufarbeitung von Einzellerprotein". Working meeting: Aufarbeitung in der Biotechnologie, ETH Zürich (May 6, 1977).

Stein, W. A., "Chargenweise Trocknung mit unterschiedlichen Vakuumkontakttrocknern (Teil 1)", *Verfahrenstechnik* **10** (12), 769–774 (1976).

Stein, W. A., "Chargenweise Trocknung mit unterschiedlichen Vakuumkontakttrocknern (Teil 2)", *Verfahrenstechnik* **11** (2), 108–111 (1977).

Steinbach, G., "Vakuum-Gegenstrom-Gefrierkonzentrieren – Vorschlag für ein neues, leistungsfähiges Verfahren", *CZ Chem. Tech.* **3** (10), 363–366 (1974).

Strasser, J., Heiss, R. and Görling, P., "Der Wasserdampf- und Wärmetransport bei der Vakuum-Sublimationstrocknung im Hinblick auf einen technisch günstigen Ablauf des Prozesses", *Kältetech. Klim.* **18**, 286–293 (1966).

Strathmann, H., "Anwendung von Membranprozessen zur Trennung molekularer Gemische", *CZ Chem. Tech.* **7** (8), 333–347 (1978).

Todd, D. B. and Davies, G. R., "Centrifugal pharmaceutical extractions", *Filtr. Sep.* **10**, 663–666 (1973).

Trawinski, H., "Filter-Apparate", *Chem. Ing. Tech.* **48**, 1124–1132 (1976).

Trawinski, H.: "Zentrifugen und Hydrozyklone". In: *Ullmanns Encyklopädie der Technischen Chemie,* Vol. **2**, 4th Ed. Verlag Chemie, Weinheim 1972, pp. 204–224.

Trawinski, H., "Zentrifugen", *Chem. Ing. Tech.* **48**, 1112–1124 (1976).

Turkova, J.: *Affinity Chromatography.* Elsevier, Amsterdam 1978.

Vandamme, E. J. and Voets, J. P., "Properties of the purified penicillin V-acylase of *Erwinia aroidea*", *Experientia* **31**, 140–143 (1975).

Vogelmann, H. and Wagner, F.: "Trennung von Naturstoffen an Amberlite XAD-2", Working meeting: Aufarbeitung in der Biotechnologie, ETH Zürich (May 6, 1977).

Vogelpohl, A. and Schlünder, E. U.: "Trocknung fester Stoffe". In: *Ullmanns Encyklopädie der Technischen Chemie,* Vol. **2**, 4th Ed. Verlag Chemie, Weinheim 1972, pp. 698–721.

Voser, W.: "Aufarbeitung hydrophiler Metabolite". Working meeting: Aufarbeitung in der Biotechnologie. ETH Zürich (May 6, 1977).

Wagner, O., Bauer, K., Kaufmann, W., Rauenbusch, E., Arens, A. and Irion, E.: Verfahren zur Anreicherung von L-Asparaginase. D.O.S. 1,767,158 (1968).

Walter, R. O. and Kondorosy, P., "Wirtschaftliche Entscheidungsgrundlagen für die Systemwahl bei Verdampfungsprozessen", *CZ Chem. Tech.* **4** (3), 87–92 (1975).

Weinstein, J. M., Wagman, G. H. and Luedemann, G. M.: Antibiotikum 66-40 (Sisomicin) und seine pharmazeutisch annehmbaren funktionellen Derivate, Verfahren zu ihrer Herstellung und diese enthaltende pharmazeutische Mittel. D.O.S. 1,932,309 (1974).

Weiss, S. A., "Concentration of baboon endogenous virus in large-scale production by use of hollow-fiber ultrafiltration technology", *Biotechnol. Bioeng.* **22**, 19–31 (1980).

Werle, E. and Fritz, H.: Verfahren zur Anreicherung von Polypeptiden, vorzugsweise von Enzymen und Enzym-Inhibitoren. D.O.S. 1,768,934 (1972).

Widmer, F., "Zum Einsatz von Dünnschichtapparaten bei hochviskosen Medien und bei der Erzeugung von Trockenprodukten", *Chem. Ztg.* **95**, 772–780 (1971).

Wiegand, J., "Falling-film evaporators and their applications in the food industry", *J. Appl. Chem. Biotechnol.* **21**, 351–358 (1971).

Wimpenny, J. W. T., "Breakage of microorganisms", *Process Biochem.* **2** (7), 41–44 (1967).

Wiseman, A., "Enzymes for breakage of microorganisms", *Process Biochem.* **4** (5), 63–65 (1969).

Wyllie, D. M., "Sheet filters", *Process Biochem.* **6** (9), 53–54 (1971).

Yamamoto, K. R., Alberts, B. M., Benzinger, R., Lawhorne, L. and Treiber, G., "Rapid bacteriophage sedimentation in the presence of polyethylene glycol and its application to large-scale virus purification", *Virology* **40**, 734–744 (1970).

Zang, J. A., Moshy, R. J., and Smith, R. N., "Electrodialysis in food processing", *Chem. Eng. Prog. Symp. Ser.* **62** (69), 105–110 (1966).

Zetelaki, K., "Disruption of mycelia for enzymes", *Process Biochem.* **4** (12), 19–27 (1969).

Part III: Processes and Products

Chapter 9

Biotechnological Processes for the Manufacture of Foodstuffs and Fodders

Michael Teuber, Arnold Geis, Uli Krusch, Jürgen Lembke, and Otto Moebus

9.1   Introduction

The biotechnological processes in the food industry are severely challenged in several respects by a variety of quality requirements. The articles produced must not only satisfy criteria that can be measured chemically and physically but must also be tested with the most sensitive analytical tools of man – by the tongue, nose, eyes, and hands of the consumer. With many foodstuffs, in addition, details such as the nature of the raw material, the manufacturing and ripening procedure, chemical composition, keepability, and hygienic status are laid down by legal provisions. Difficulties may arise through seasonal fluctuations in the composition of the plant and animal raw materials and through the effects of climate and the natural degree of contamination (cereals, vegetables) or the nature of the feeding and health of animals (milk, meat).

The microflora involved in the fermentations have to cope with the characteristics of the complex substrate and also with the selected technological conditions. Their mastery requires long practical experience and a close cooperation and harmonization between the microbiologist and the food technologist.

The technological spectrum in the production of foods and fodders ranges from simple technologies taking place spontaneously (fermentation of tea, coffee, and chocolate and the preparation of silage) to the completely automatically controlled industrial manufacture and packaging of baked products and fermented milk products.

Table 9-1 shows the economic importance of fodders and foodstuffs produced biotechnologically in the Federal Republic of Germany. In 1978, the value of the foodstuffs concerned amounted to more than 20 thousand million DM. The value of the silage is difficult to determine, since it is a so-called domestic fodder which is only occasionally sold from farm to farm. In the case of sausages, the proportion that is manufactured with starter cultures is unknown.

9.2   Foodstuffs and Fodders of Plant Origin

9.2.1   Silage

Silages are **plant fodder materials** preserved by **natural lactic acid fermentation.** To make silage, fodder plants are subjected to fermentation with the exclusion of air. The lactic acid so formed leads to a preservation of the fermented material. In this process, smaller losses of nutrient material take place (10 to 40%) than is the case in the preparation of hay (25 to 55%).

Fermentability		
Ready	Less good	Difficult
Silo corn	horse beans, silo-ripe	red clover
Moist cereals	meadow grass, 1st cut	horse beans, beginning of flowering
Sunflowers	hay pasture grass, 1st cut	rape, turnips, oil radish
Turnip leaves	meadow grass, 2nd + 3rd cuts	alfalfa (lucerne)
Jerusalem artichoke	grass-clover mixture, 1st cut	common vetch
Marrowstem kale	hay pasture grass, 2nd + 4th cuts	

Table 9-1. Extent of Production and Value of Important Types of Foodstuffs and Fodders with a Biotechnological Basis in the Federal Republic of Germany and in the EEC.

Product	Federal Republic of Germany[1] in 1982		EEC (9) in 1981[2]
	Production (in 1000 tons)	Value (in millions of DM)	Production (in 1000 tons)
Silage	50 000.0[5]		
Sauerkraut	164.0[4]	315.0	
Pickles	146.5[4]	300.5	
Baked goods	1 897.7[4]	8152.5	
Bakers' yeast	89.8[4]	112.0	
Aroma substances	15.5[4]	207.4	
Butter	463.4[4]	4086.6	1902
Hard cheese	131.4[4]	934.6	727
Semihard cheese	199.4[4]	1306.3	799
Soft cheese	73.7[4]	596.7	716
Fresh cheese	361.3[4]	1006.7	810
Sour milk curds and cheese	19.2[4]	83.4 ⎫	
Yoghurt	463.1[4]	416.2 ⎬	1568
Raw, cooked, and scalded sausages	660.5[4]	5825.9	
Coffee	283.6[4]	3564.6	
Tea	12.4	333.7	
Chocolate	113.8	1367.4[2]	
Tobacco, raw		1542.5[3]	

[1] Statistisches Jahrbuch über Ernährung, Landwirtschaft und Forsten [Statistical Yearbook on Nutrition, Agriculture, and Forestry]. Landwirtschaftsverlag, Münster-Hiltrup 1983, pp. 239 ff.
[2] Statistik der bayerischen Milchwirtschaft 1982 [Statistics of the Bavarian Dairy Industry]. Bayerisches Staatsministerium für Ernährung, Landwirtschaft und Forsten, pp. 69 ff.
[3] Import
[4] Produced in factories and enterprises with more than 20 employees.
[5] 1978

Raw Materials: All types of green fodders can be ensilaged. The list at the bottom of p. 326 gives a classification of the types of fodder according to their fermentability (Gross and Rabe, 1974).

Important factors for fermentability are the amount of fermentable carbohydrates and also the amounts of water and protein in the fodder plants. Ensilability is the better the larger the amount of readily fermentable carbohydrates and the lower the proportion of crude protein and of water.

Silo ripeness, i.e., the degree of suitability according to the state of vegetation of the plants, is another important criterion for the fermentability of fodder plants.

Technology of Ensilage

Forms of Silo

A large number of different forms of silo are available for ensilage. Economic, local, and climatic conditions and also the type of fodder to be ensilaged are the main criteria in the choice of the silo system. In addition to systems constructed on the massive scale as tower, low, and pit silos, a whole series of different sheeting silos are in use. Suitable materials for the construction of massive silos are wood, concrete (including prefabricated parts), glass-fiber reinforced plastics, metals, and other materials. For most materials, acid-resistant internal coatings are necessary for protection against the corrosive action of the lactic acid. Foil silos usually consist of PVC and polyethylene foils (Orth, 1961; Gross and Rabe, 1974).

Preparation of Silage

For ensiling, the plant material to be fermented must be packed as tightly as possible into the silo. If freshly cut fodder is used for this purpose, one speaks of **fresh silage.** In the case of **withered and semihay silages** (haylage) the starting material is withered or dried out plant material. This can be fermented more satisfactorily than fresh plants of a high moisture content. As a rule, the silos are charged with material cut into small pieces. In addition to the optimum utilization of space, this also achieves the densest possible storage and therefore early anaerobic conditions, which promote fermentation. The following measures must be taken into account in the preparation of the fodder and the charging of the silo (Orth, 1961):

– as far as possible, the fodder should be dried out beforehand;
– any contamination must be avoided;
– the silo must be filled rapidly (1–2 days);
– the fodder must be comminuted;
– the fodder must be packed as tightly as possible.

After the silo has been filled, the fodder should be compressed and the silo be made airtight.

Ensilaging Additives: To control the course of fermentation and to avoid fermentation losses through incorrect fermentation, ensilaging additives must frequently be used with the fodder. The ensilaging salts commercially available generally contain a mixture of germination inhibitors (hexamethylenetetramine, etc.), together with various salts of organic and inorganic acids (e.g., formic or propionic acid) and sugars.

Microbiology of the Production of Silage

The lactic acid fermentation that takes place spontaneously during the ensiling of fodder plants is performed by lactic acid bacteria, essentially Lactobacillus species. These microorganisms pass into the silo with the plant material together with many other species of bacteria. The proportion of lactic acid bacteria in the epiphytic microflora of fodder plants is very low, often amounting to less than 100 organisms per gram (Beck, 1966; McDonald, 1976).

At the beginning of fermentation there is a rapid growth of aerobic and coliform bacteria, the number of which rapidly decreases once anaerobic conditions and increasing acidification have been achieved. The increasing anaerobiosis and the rising concentration of acids promote the multiplication of the lactic acid bacteria, the bulk of which is formed by the homofermentative Lactobacilli together with streptococci and Leuconostoc species (Beck, 1966; Gross and Rabe 1974). After the main fermentation has taken place, the pH of the silage has fallen to levels of about pH 4.

When insufficient lactic acid is formed, the appearance of butyric acid bacteria *(Clostridium butyricum, Clostridium tyrobutyricum)* is possible. These microorganisms ferment the lactic acid to butyric acid, carbon dioxide, and hydrogen. The resulting rise in the pH leads to the development of putrefactive organisms. Their metabolic products can lead to the complete spoilage of the fodder.

The milk of cows fed with silage is not suitable for the manufacture of Emmental cheese (see page 364) since it hardly permits a contamination with *Clostridium tyrobutyricum* to be avoided. This contamination leads to the dreaded defect of "late blowing". Such a blown cheese is unsuitable for human consumption.

In addition to butyric acid bacteria, another main cause of faulty fermentations is the pronounced growth of yeasts, usually caused by the entry of air during the removal of silage, which leads to a high loss of nutrient material and therefore to a fall in the quality of the fermented fodder.

9.2.2 Fermented Vegetables

Sauerkraut

Definition of the Product

Sauerkraut is a product made from white cabbage preserved by natural lactic acid fermentation with the addition of common salt, with a characteristic acidic taste.

The German Food Law prescribes the following quality standards for: sauerkraut or pickled cabbage, delicatessen sauerkraut or delicatessen pickled cabbage:

Properties: ripened solid white cabbage, cut into long uniform pieces, pickled by natural lactic acid fermentation with the addition of common salt, acidic taste, pH 4.1 or below, pure spicy smell, light color, unobjectionable consistency, not more than 10% natural brine after draining for 5 minutes (no tolerance).

Permissible: addition of natural spices, herbs, and sugars, and also burst white cabbage heads if they satisfy the other requirements.

Impermissible: addition of vinegar and lactic acid, chemical preservatives, chemical bleaching agents, artificial sweeterners, and other foreign materials.

Raw material: Slowly growing varieties of cabbage with firm heads and thin leaf ribs are mainly used for the manufacture of sauerkraut. (Klein, Rabe, and Weiss, 1978).

The vitamin C content (30 to 70 mg/100 g of cabbage) is largely retained in the sauerkraut, if its processing has been satisfactory, and explains the particularly nutritional and physiological value of this product (Müller, 1974).

Technology of the Manufacture of Sauerkraut

Heads of white cabbage dried for 1 to 2 days are freed mechanically from stalks and the outer leaves and are then cut into strips 1 to 3 mm wide. The cut cabbage is charged into the fermentation vessel together with common salt. The optimum amount of salt is 2 to 2.5 per cent by weight. The **amount of salt** and also the most **homogeneous distribution** possible are important factors for a satisfactory course of the fermentation the nonobservance of which frequently leads to faulty fermentations (Pederson and Albury, 1954). The wooden vats previously used as fermentation vessels have today been replaced by concrete troughs with an acid-resistant inner layer or by fiber-glass tanks with capacities of up to 100 tons. After filling, the fermentation vessels are made airtight with plastic foils and loaded in such a way that the dense-packed cabbage is completely covered with brine. Fermentation is regarded as completed when the lactic acid concentration has reached 1.5%. In the conventional methods of fermentation at 18 to 20°C, the process lasts four or more weeks.

A further developed process with external recycling of the brine permits the fermentation to be monitored and is said to improve the quality of the product and also to accelerate the pickling process (Noel, 1979).

A pronounced **shortening of the time of fermentation** can be achieved by the addition of starter cultures. In this process, very differing results in relation to the quality of the product are achieved. Consequently, and also because of the additional expense, the use of starter cultures has not been taken up widely in the manufacture of sauerkraut.

Today, sauerkraut is marketed mainly in small packages, in cans or plastic bags. To prolong its keepability, the sauerkraut is frequently pasteurized. Unsterilized sauerkraut must be stored under cool conditions with the exclusion of air.

A problem in the manufacture of sauerkraut is the production of large amounts of highly loaded effluents in the order of magnitude of 1000 to 1500 L per ton of cut white cabbage. The BOD amounts to 5.2 kg and the concentration of NaCl to 8 kg per ton of cut raw material (Hang et al., 1972).

Microbiology of Sauerkraut Fermentation

The fermentation of sauerkraut is a multistage biological process. During it, various microorganisms, separated from one another in time,

develop and bring about certain chemical transformations (Fig. 9-1). The cell juice issuing from the cabbage is a good nutrient medium for the microorganisms introduced into the fermentation vessel with the raw material. At the beginning, aerobic organisms, mainly Gram-negative bacteria, yeasts, and fungi, develop. The aerobic microorganisms die with increasing deficit of oxygen. The high salt content and also the anaerobic conditions promote the growth of the lactic acid bacteria which originally made up only a small proportion of the total bacterial population. The lactic acid fermentation is initiated by *Leuconostoc mesenteroides*. This heterofermentative lactic acid bacterium degrades the sugars in the cell juice to lactic acid, acetic acid, alcohol, and carbon dioxide.

With increasing acid content, the growth of *L. mesenteroides* is inhibited. Fermentation is carried further by *Lactobacillus brevis* and *Pediococcus cerevisiae* and, finally, by *Lactobacillus plantarum* (Pederson, 1969, 1979). The lactic acid content rises at this stage to 1.5 to 2%. At this high concentration of acid, the growth of even the acid-insensitive lactic acid bacteria is inhibited.

Inadequate technological and hygienic conditions, and also unsuitable raw material frequently lead to faulty fermentations which can result in the complete spoilage of the end product.

Pickled Gherkins (Sour Pickles, Dill Pickles)

Definition of the Product

Pickled gherkins are green gherkins preserved by natural lactic acid fermentation.

The German Food Law lays down the following quality standards for 1st-quality pickled gherkins:

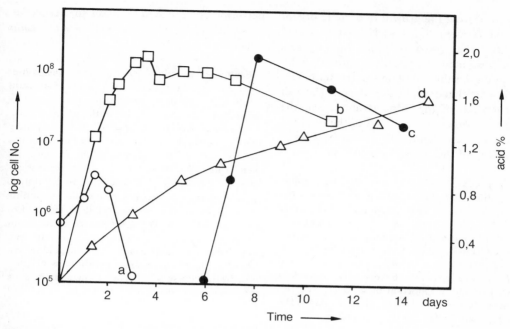

Fig. 9-1. Development of the bacterial population during the fermentation process and the production of acid,

a aerobic germs

b heterofermentative lactic acid bacteria

c homofermentative lactic acid bacteria

d production of acid

(drawn up from figures due to Noel et al., 1979).

Properties: green, firm, spot-free, well-formed undamaged gherkins preserved by natural lactic acid fermentation with the addition of salt, spices, and herbs.

Impermissible: deformed gherkins, hollow and half gherkins, addition of vinegar, lactic acid, and preservatives.

The manufacture of products not conforming to the standards is not prohibited. However, such products must not be designated 1st quality (Klein, Rabe and Weiss, 1978). Gherkins preserved by fermentation, together with sauerkraut, are among the most widely used vegetable lactic acid products. In 1972 in the USA 511 000 tons of gherkins with a value of approximately $ 500 millions were processed into fermented products (Etchells, Fleming, and Bell, 1975).

Technology

Carefully cleaned gherkins are placed in layers in suitable fermentation vessels and completely covered with 4 to 8% salt brine. Spices and herbs, especially dill, are frequently added to the fermentation charge. In order to prevent the growth of aerobic organisms, the fermentation vessels must be sealed airtightly. The growth of film-forming yeasts can be prevented by irradiation with UV light. Depending on the temperature, the fermentation is completed in 3 to 6 weeks. The salt concentration of the brine is about 3%, the lactic acid content 0.7 to 1%, and the final pH value 3.5. These conditions guarantee a good keepability of the product on cold storage.

Etchells et al. (1975) have described a controlled fermentation with the use of starter cultures. The washed gherkins are disinfected in a chlorine solution and placed in brine. This is acidified with acetic acid and buffered with sodium acetate. The fermentation is initiated by the addition of starter cultures of *Lactobacillus plantarum* or *L. plantarum* and *Pediococcus cerevisiae*. Excess carbon dioxide is removed by the introduction of nitrogen. The fermentation is completed after 10 to 12 days. The product is said to be of very good quality.

Microbiology

The fermentation of gherkins is a very complex multistage microbiological process which differs only inessentially from the fermentation of sauerkraut. *Leuconostoc mesenteroides, Pediococcus cerevisiae,* and *Lactobacillus plantarum* are the most important microorganisms involved. They are introduced into the fermentation charge with the raw material, to which they adhere. The natural microflora of gherkins is very variable and contains bacteria, yeasts, and fungi. The lactic acid bacteria form only a quite small proportion of the bacterial population which consists mainly of aerobic and coliform microorganisms (Etchells, 1975).

Increasing anaerobiosis, the high salt content, and the acids formed by the lactic acid bacteria rapidly inhibit the growth of the undesirable species of microorganisms.

The lactic acid fermentation is initiated by *L. mesenteroides*. The main fermentation is performed by the acid-resistant species *Pediococcus cerevisiae* and, especially, *Lactobacillus plantarum*.

Faulty fermentations are frequently the consequence of the growth of acid- and salt-tolerant yeasts. The lactic acid decomposition performed by these organisms causes a rise in the pH and therefore permits the growth of acid-sensitive spoiling agents. The rise in the pH caused by the yeasts frequently leads to the softening of the product and even to its complete unusability. Today this is ascribed to the action of pectinolytic and cellulolytic enzymes. These enzymes break down the supporting tissue of the gherkins or the cellulose included in the plant cell wall. The main source of these enzymes is formed by fungi which enter the fermentation charge on the gherkins. Pectin-degrading enzymes are, moreover, natural constituents of gherkins. In the course of a correct fermentation, these enzymes are inactive because of the low pH value of the brine.

Olives

For preservation, olives are subjected to a lactic acid fermentation in brine in a similar manner to gherkins. Ripe (black) or unripe (green) fruit are used for this purpose. Olives contain a bitter-tasting glycoside, oleuropein. To remove this bitter constituent, the fruit is subjected to treatment with 1.25 to 2% caustic soda before fermentation.

The olives are then washed with fresh water. In order to keep the loss of water-soluble materials such as sugars, amino acids, and mineral salts as low as possible an excess of water is avoided. After one to four washings, the still alkaline fruit is placed in the brine. As a rule, this contains about 10% of common salt and 3% of lactic acid to neutralize the residual caustic soda. Because of the liberation of water from the fruit, the concentration of salt in the brine falls considerably. In order to achieve the salt content of 7 to 8% that is necessary for an optimum fermentation, further salt is added after a few days.

The fermentation vessels – wooden barrels or wooden or plastic tanks; bottle-shaped polyethylene vessels with a capacity of about 1550 L are also often used – are sealed airtightly. To accelerate the fermentation, brines from batches already undergoing fermentation, pure starter cultures of *Lactobacillus plantarum,* and also fermentable sugars such as glucose and sucrose, may be added. Depending on the variety of olives, the salt content, the pH, and the temperature, the fermentation process lasts between two weeks and several months. In order to obtain a keepable and well-tasting product, the concentration of acid must be at least 0.6 to 0.7%. The microbiological course of fermentation resembles that of the sauerkraut and gherkin fermentations.

Other Fermentable Vegetables

Various types of turnips, cauliflower, asparagus, green tomatoes, green beans, fresh peas, radishes, pepper pods, and many other vegetables are preserved by natural lactic acid fermentation in salt brines. In spite of numerous regional features, the fermentation of these vegetables takes place in a similar manner to the fermentations described above.

9.2.3 Asian Fermentation Products

In the Far East (Japan, China, Korea, and adjacent regions) a number of fermented plant products in the manufacture of which definite fungi are employed are used for human nutrition. For these products the protein-rich soybean (35%) is the most important raw material. The role of the fungi resides in the provision of amylases and proteases for the enzymatic digestion of the polymeric constituents

for the alcoholic fermentation and lactic acid fermentation that then take place. This centuries-old experience with traditional fungal fermentations has contributed substantially to the leading position of Japan in the biotechnology of enzymes, antibiotics, amino acids, and other products of microbial metabolism. The two most important products are soy sauce (shoyu) and soybean paste (miso).

Soy Sauce (Shoyu)

Definition

Soy sauce is a dark brown liquid with a salty taste and a typical pleasant aroma. It is manufactured by the fermentation of **soybeans** or defatted soybean meal and **wheat** in the presence of NaCl with fungi, yeasts, and bacteria. In 1974 the Japanese production was more than 10^9 L with a consumption per head per year of 10.2 L.

Manufacture (Flow sheet 9-1)

The beans are softened at room temperature with frequent changes of water for 10 to 12 h and finally steamed at 120°C for 1 h. Defatted soybean meal is sprayed with water and steamed in the autoclave for 45 min.

The wheat is first parched and is then coarsely ground. This additive has the aim of better growth of the fungi. More enzymes are formed in mixtures of soybean and wheat than in the individual constituents separately. Wheat affects the taste and color. It is a source of sugars, alcohols, organic acids, and aroma components.

The salt acts as a preservative and a component of the taste. The first step in fermentation consists in the treatment of the mixed substrate, consisting of wheat and soybeans in a ratio of 1:1 with fungal starter cultures of *Aspergillus oryzae* or *A. soyae* (0.1 to 0.2%). These consist of dried spores (about $2.5 \cdot 10^7$/g) obtained from steamed rice with the addition of 2% of wood ash. The inoculation takes place at 30°C in flat wooden chests covered with moist cloths. The substrate must be regularly stirred in order to achieve a uniform temperature (27 to 37°C), aeration, and humidity. The inoculation is complete after 72 h. The resulting product (in Japanese, **koji**) has a dark green color, a pleasant aroma, and a sweet but at the same time bitter taste, together with high protease and amylase activities. The koji is transferred to deep concrete or wooden vessels and is mixed with the same volume of common salt brine so as to give a salt concentration of 17 to 19% on the mash. In order to inhibit the causative agents of spoilage, the NaCl content must not be below 16%. This mash is called **moromi** in Japanese. During the following 8- to 10-month fermentation, yeasts and pediococci develop, so that the pH falls from its original value of 6.5-7 to 4.6-4.8. The optimum for the yeast is 5.5. Frequent stirring prevents the growth of anaerobic bacteria and ensures a uniform temperature and the elimination of the carbon dioxide formed. The time of fermentation can be shortened to six months by controlled management of the temperature (one month at 15°C, 4 months at 28°C, and one month at 15°C).

The finished fermented product is separated by pressing into a liquid phase (crude soy sauce) and a press-cake (fodder). After pasteurization (70 to 80°C) and filtration the sauce is bottled. In Japan, benzoic acid and butyl p-hydroxybenzoate can be added for preservation.

Each 1 ton of soybeans, wheat, and common salt gives 5000 L of soy sauce containing an average of 18% of salt, 1.2 to 1.3% of glutamic acid, 1.5 to 1.6% of total nitrogen, 0.7 to 0.9% of amino nitrogen, 1.9 to 4.4% of reducing sugars, and 1.5 to 2.1% of alcohol.

Soybean Paste (Miso)

Definition

Soybean paste (miso) is manufactured in a similar manner to soy sauce from **soybeans, rice** and **salt** by fermentation with fungi, yeasts, and bacteria. The consistency resem-

bles that of peanut butter. The color may be light yellow to red-brown. The aroma resembles that of soy sauce. Just as in the case of cheese in Europe, there are many different types depending on composition and manufacturing conditions. In Japan, up to 80% of the pastes are made from rice and soybeans (rice miso) and the remainder from barley and soybeans or from soybeans alone. The annual production of commercial miso amounts to about 600000 tons and of that made in the home about 150000 tons. The consumption per head per year is 6.7 kg.

Manufacture (Flow sheet 9-2)

Hulled rice is washed, swollen at 15°C for 20 h to a water content of 35%, and steamed for 40 min. After cooling to 50°C it is inoculated with koji starter as in the case of soy sauce and is incubated in a rotary fermenter at suitable atmospheric humidity until a pervading formation of mycelium has been achieved but before there is any formation of spores **(white koji)**. This koji has a pleasant smell which is in no case musty or earthy. It tastes relatively sweet. It is mixed with salt in order to stop the further development of the fungus to spores. It is mixed with soybeans which, as in the manufacture of soy sauce, have been washed, swollen, steamed, and coarsely ground. The mixture is inoculated with starter cultures of pediococci, streptococci, and yeasts. Water is added to a moisture content of 48%. It is packed firmly into containers where the fermentation takes place at 25 to 50°C (2 to 3 months). During fermentation, the product must be transferred into other tanks at least twice. At the end of fermentation, miso is allowed to stand at room temperature for two weeks in order to finish ripening. The ripened product is comminuted, pasteurized, and packed in wooden boxes, polyethylene bags, or tubes. Sorbic acid (1‰) is used as preservative. Freeze-dried miso powders are also on the market. The product may contain 44 to 45% of moisture, 8 to 19% of protein, 2 to 33% of reducing sugars, 2 to 10% of fat, and 5 to 13% of sodium chloride.

Flow sheet 9-1. Manufacture of soy sauce.

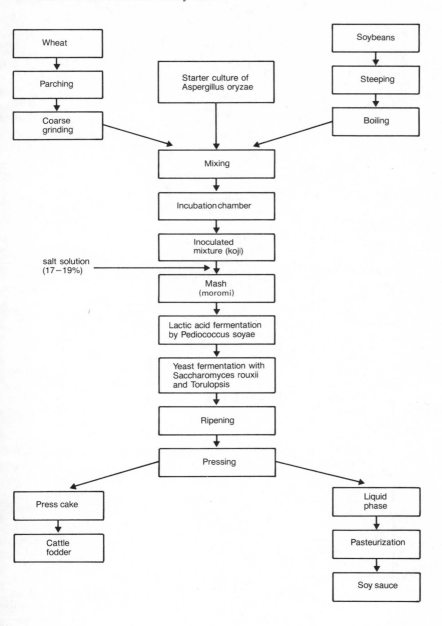

Flow sheet 9-2. Manufacture of miso (Wang and Hesseltine, 1979).

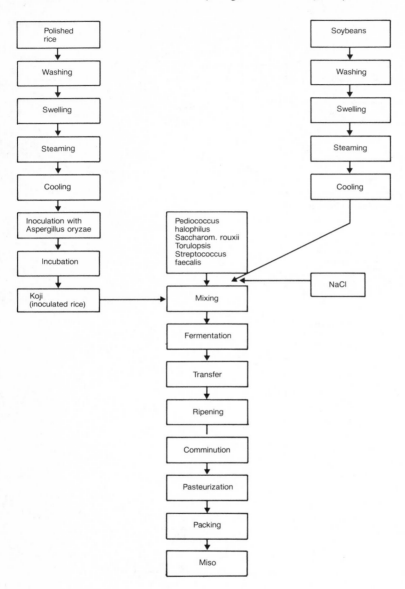

Other Asian Products

a) **Hamanatto** (black beans): whole soybeans that have been fermented with *Aspergillus oryzae,* streptococci, and pediococci.

b) **Sufu:** a Chinese product resembling "fresh cheese" made from acid-coagulated soybean protein salted and fermented with various mucor species.

c) **Tempeh:** Rhizopus-fermented soybeans from Indonesia.

d) **Ang-khak:** rice that has been fermented with *Monascus purpureus* from China, which is used for coloring foodstuffs.

Note: the formation of mycotoxins, such as aflatoxin in fungus-fermented products is practically excluded today by the use of defined starter cultures.

9.2.4 Raising Agents for Baked Products

Bakers' Yeast

Definition of the Product

A raising agent is necessary for the manufacture of bread and baked products from wheat flour. Compressed or dried bakers' yeast is used for this purpose, causing a loosening of the structure of the dough through the formation of carbon dioxide by fermentation. Yeast is also sometimes added to rye dough to simplify the handling of the dough and thus takes over the function of the sourdough yeast present in sourdough. The loosening of the dough is achieved by carbon dioxide stemming from fermentation of the maltose (as generated from starch by α-amylase or from malt containing compounds) or perhaps from added sucrose.

According to Schulz (1962) by **compressed yeast** is understood a top-fermenting yeast manufactured from sugar-containing raw materials which may not be marketed in mixtures with brewers' bottom yeast or with starch flour. *Saccharomyces cerevisiae* is used almost exclusively for the manufacture of bakers' yeast. These strains are also used in the manufacture of alcohol (Kretzschmar, 1955). The yeast must possess good raising power in the dough, the color must be white or slightly yellowish, and good keepability is required. The proportion of film-forming yeasts in the compressed yeasts must be only low, since otherwise its suitability for the bakery is adversely affected. Just like the sourdough yeast present in sourdough, compressed yeast must exhibit a high resistance to acids.

The compressed yeast contains 27% (w/w) of dry matter. By gentle drying, e.g., in a fluidized bed, bakers' yeast can be processed into **dried bakers' yeast.** The dried bakers' yeast has about 3 to 4 times the raising power of compressed yeast, corresponding to its higher dry-matter content of 90 to 93% and is resistant to relatively high temperatures and bacterial actions and undergoes no autolysis. The dried bakers' yeast retains its raising power on vacuum packing and storage without cooling for more than a year. An agent for rehydration is added to the dried bakers' yeast.

Processes for the Manufacture of Bakers' Yeast

Today, **molasses** from the manufacture of sugar is used almost exclusively for the manufacture of bakers' yeast. The supply of nutrients in the molasses must be supplemented by a source of additional nitrogen such as ammonia or ammonium salts, by a source of additional phosphates, for example, in the form

Flow sheet 9-3. Manufacture of bakers' yeast.

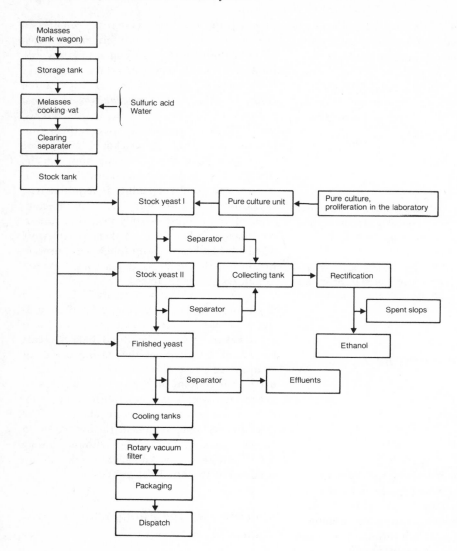

of an ammonium phosphate or as superphosphate, and possibly also by vitamins. A process common in yeast factories for the manufacture of bakers' yeast from molasses is shown in Flow-sheet 9-3. Details of the manufacture of bakers' yeast can be obtained from the account by Butschek and Kautzmann (1962), and possibilities for the arrangement of the apparatus in the individual process steps have been treated by Kretzschmar (1968).

Below, Flow sheet 9-3 for the production of yeast from molasses will be explained in more detail. The molasses is weighed out and diluted in a molasses cooking vat with hot water, acidified with sulfuric acid, and boiled. The treated molasses is separated from lime and protein sludge and is kept in a storage tank until it is used for the manufacture of yeast.

The cultivation of the bakers' yeast starts from a factory yeast culture which is kept as **permanent culture.** A regeneration of the yeast, for example, by passage of the culture through malt wort, is necessary at intervals of 4 to 6 months. The factory strain can be produced from a pure strain of yeast in the form of a single-spore culture, a single-cell culture, or a multicell culture. The **single-spore cultures** have the advantage that they are genetically very stable. According to Butschek and Kautzmann it is not advantageous to use a mixture of different strains of yeast as a factory culture, since the overwhelming multiplication of one strain of yeast or another cannot be adequately controlled, which gives rise to an uncertainty factor in the process.

The propagation of the initial yeast is carried out in the laboratory of the yeast factory under sterile conditions in glass vessels. An amount of yeast is made in this way which is then multiplied further in a technical apparatus, a **yeast pure culture unit,** under sterile conditions. The pure culture unit consists of two or three (steel) tanks of increasing size with possibilities for aeration with sterile air and for the addition of sterile wort.

The yeast so made is multiplied by at least two further stock yeast stages in order to prepare the amount of inoculum for the last step, the manufacture of the **finished yeast.** During the multiplication

of the stock yeast part of the molasses is added immediately but only a little aeration is used. Under these conditions the yeast forms a large amount of alcohol since with oxygen deficiency the respiratory metabolism is switched to fermentation metabolism. This switch of the metabolism is known as the **Pasteur effect.**

The residual solutions arising after the separation of the yeast by means of the separator are collected and are worked up by the yeast factories with a distilling license to give alcohol. Yeast factories without a distilling license add the alcohol-containing residual solutions to the following more highly aerated finished-yeast stage in order to utilize the alcohol for an intensified formation of cell substance.

The centrifuged stock yeast of the last stage is used as **inoculation yeast** for the manufacture of the **finished yeast.** During cultivation in the stock yeast stages, the metabolism of the yeast is directed to fermentation, so that it can be used as a powerful raising yeast. During the cultivation of the finished yeast, there is a pronounced multiplication of the yeast during which the raising power of the yeast must not decrease. In order to prevent a more pronounced formation of alcohol as a consequence of the Crabtree effect (Hartmeier, 1972), the molasses is introduced in a continuous-addition ("fed batch") process in such a way that the yeast can just take up the sugar and a limiting concentration of the sugar is not exceeded. In addition, the yeast must be aerated in the optimum manner in order to avoid the formation of alcohol. The addition of the molasses wort and the nutrient salts can be carried out with programmed control. Another possibility is control via the analysis of the waste air by measuring the concentration of alcohol or carbon dioxide. During the yeast-forming process, the pH is kept at 4.5. This can be done through the addition of the sources of nitrogen by adding, as required, ammonia to raise the pH or ammonium sulfate for acidification. In the case of ammonium sulfate, the yeast takes up only the ammonia of the salt, so that the free sulfuric acid remains in the solution. During the production of yeast, the temperature of the batch rises from about 26°C to 33°C. The batch is cooled by spraying the wall of the tank or by built-in cooling coils. An excessive development of foam is prevented by the addition of an antifoaming agent. Various aeration systems are used which differ in efficiency. An air consumption of 8 to 13 m³ has been given for the consumption of 1 kg of compressed yeast (27% of dry matter) when a nozzle-type aeration system is used, and 1 to 8 m³ of air in the case of a rotary aerator. Technical aeration systems have been described by Kretzschmar (1968).

The time of multiplication of yeast in the final yeast stage amounts to 9 to 12 hours. After the ending of the yeast-forming process, the yeast is separated from the residual solution by means of a centrifuge (nozzle separator), washed with fresh water, and centrifuged again. The yeast is immediately pumped into cooled reservoirs and can be stored at temperatures below 10 °C.

The cooled yeast cream is dewatered by means of a rotary vacuum filter. The yeast scraped off the rotary vacuum filter, with a dry-matter content of 26 to 28%, is compressed in one operation, and is then packed.

A characteristic of new yeast factories is the system for discharging effluents. The process water, particularly the water arising after the separation of the finished yeast with the components of the molasses that have not been utilized by the yeast, is concentrated by evaporation and used as cattle fodder.

Economic Importance of the Bakers' Yeast Industry

The growth of the bakers' yeast industry follows primarily the increase in world population. Peppler (1978) gives an annual world production of yeast of 187 700 tons (referred to dry matter). In additon to increasing the capacity of existing plants, new bakers' yeast factories have been brought into operation in the last few years (in Denmark, Czechoslovakia, Zaire, California (USA), Brazil, and Iran). New yeast products with special functional properties will in future achieve ever-increasing importance in the foodstuffs industry and face biotechnology with new problems. Possible developments are indicated in Johnson's (1977) review of US patent specifications.

Sourdough and Yeast Dough

Definition

Sourdough and yeast dough are **microbiological raising agents** that are necessary for the manufacture of baked goods such as bread, rolls, and cakes. They serve primarily for the adjustment of the desired loose consistency of these products by means of the carbon dioxide formed during the preliminary proof (in the ripening of the dough) and the final proof (during the baking process). Other by-products of the fermentation of dough such as ethanol, acetic acid, and acetoin, biacetyl, and fusel oils make decisive contributions to the aroma and taste, particularly, of bread. In the Federal Republic of Germany alone there are about 280 different varieties of bread (Spicher, 1974).

The microorganisms responsible for the sourdough fermentation are homo- and heterofermentative lactic acid bacteria and various acid-tolerant yeasts (see Table 9-2).

For yeast dough, pure cultures of top-fermenting yeasts of the species *Saccharomyces cerevisiae*, which are also called bakers' yeast, are used (see Section 9.5.1). The source of carbohydrate for the fermentation taking place are the free sugars such as glucose, fructose, and sucrose present in the flour or added separately and the maltose and glucose formed from starch during the preparation of dough and the baking process by the cereal amylases of the flour. The addition of microbial amylase has been described.

Manufacture of Sourdough

Sourdough is necessary for the processing of rye flour which exhibits the necessary optimum swelling of its constituents only at pH 4.3. This is a precondition for the formation of an elastic and wholesome crust of mixed, rye,

Table 9-2. Lactic Acid Bacteria and Yeasts in Commercial Starter Cultures for Sourdough (Spicher and Schröder, 1978).

Commercial starter culture	Bacteria	Yeasts
Product A	*Lactobacillus fructivorans*	*Saccharomyces cerevisiae*
	L. fermentum	*Torulopsis holmii*
Product B	predominantly *L. brevis* and	*Candida krusei*
	L. brevis var. *lindneri*	*Pichia saitoi*
Product C	*L. brevis*	n.d.*
	L. plantarum	
	L. alimentarius	

* not described

and fine- and coarse-grained wholemeal breads (Spicher, 1974).

The acetic and lactic acids formed (in a ratio of about 2:8) in the lactic acid homo- and heterofermentation are responsible for the strong and characteristic taste and also the pH of 4.2 to 4.3 in rye bread, 4.4 in rye mixed bread, and 4.7 to 4.8 in wheat mixed bread. The yeasts of sourdough that are important for the formation of gas have their optimum between pH 4.0 and 5.6 (Spicher and Schröder, 1980).

Essentially, two processes are in use for the production of sourdough.

a) Multistage process (Flow sheet 9-4)
   This is the classical and conventional method of preparing sourdough. Since lactic acid bacteria and yeasts have different growth requirements, multistage processes are more suitable for satisfying these requirements [the lactic acid bacteria require higher temperatures during fermentation (> 30°C), and the yeasts somewhat lower temperatures (< 30°C)]. On the other hand, they require a great expenditure of time and labor, so that they are used preferentially in large factories

(Spicher, 1974). Referred to the mass of flour the fermentation losses may amount to 2.0 to 2.5%.

b) Single-stage process
   Simplified processes for producing sourdough are achieved by performing only the lactic acid fermentation with sourdough. The raising power of the dough must then be ensured by the addition of bakers' yeast. With large additions (20% of the flour to be soured) of sourdough and high fermentation temperatures of 35 to 36°C, the required acidification can be achieved within three hours in the "Berlin short-souring process". The amount of yeast that must be added then comes to 1 to 1.5%. Continuous processes for the preparation of sourdough have also been described. However, on prolonged operation a segregation of the complex microflora is observed which may lead to undesired changes in the aroma of the bread.

Manufacture of Yeast Dough

In the industrial area, two processes are dominant for the manufacture of white bread:

Flow sheet 9-4. Manufacture of sourdough from 85% of R 1150 rye flour and 15% of W 812 wheat flour – four-stage process (Müller, 1974).

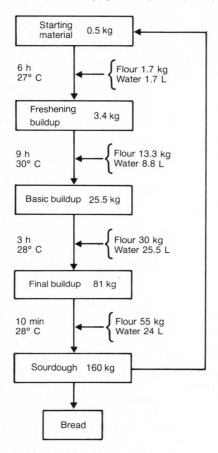

a) Classical, indirect process

In this process, yeast is made into a dough with flour and water and is left for a few hours at 25°C or overnight at 20°C. The ripened dough is worked up with more flour and water to give the finished dough. The fermentation losses are between 1 and 3%. This process needs less yeast but is not so microbiologically safe as the direct process.

b) Direct process

The necessary amount of yeast is distributed uniformly in the dough right at the beginning. Re-ferred to the amount of flour, 2 to 3% is needed for white bread, 3 to 4% for rolls, 3 to 5% for cakes, 7 to 9% for cookies, and 8 to 10% for stollen (fruit loaves). The dough is first fermented at 20 to 30°C for 10 to 60 minutes. The main fermentation ("proof") which causes the desired raising of the product takes place after kneading and shaping. The fermentation temperatures are between 28 and 32°C.

9.2.5   Fermentation of Semiluxury Consumer Goods

Coffee

Coffee beans are the fermented and roasted seeds from the berries of the coffee tree *(Coffea arabica)*. Each berry contains two seeds which are surrounded by a husk or "parchment."

The purpose of the fermentation of the coffee is the **breakdown of this husk.** It is carried out by either a dry or a wet process. In the **dry process,** the berries are dried in the sun, which brings about the desired fermentation. In the **wet process,** the beans freed mechanically from the berry husks are fermented in a tank. The fermentation of the coffee takes place **spontaneously.** During it there is a pronounced increase in the number of Gram-negative microorganisms and an almost complete degradation of the pectin-containing flesh of the berries. The predominating microflora of the coffee beans consists of bacteria from the genera Erwinia, Escherichia, and Paracolobactrum. The species *Erwinia dissolvens* is of particular importance, since it is the only one of the species concerned that forms pectinolytic enzymes (Franck, 1965). The significance of the lactic acid bacteria that occur in the later stages of fermentation is not clear. By the formation of lactic acid they possibly prevent the growth of agents causing spoilage. In addition to microorganisms, the enzymes of the plant itself are involved in the fermentation of coffee.

Chocolate

Chocolate is prepared fromt the seeds of the cacao tree *(Theobroma cacao)*. The cacao beans, removed mechanically from the fruit, are subjected to a fermentation in which the residues of the flesh of the fruit is removed and the seedlings are killed. In addition to this the desired changes in the aroma, the taste and the color of the cacao beans take place. Fermentation is carried out in wooden fermentation boxes or in pits. In order to prevent the temperature rising above 46 to 50°C, the fermentation batch is occasionally aerated. At the beginning of fermentation, yeasts of the genera Saccharomyces, Hansenula, Pichia, etc., predominate. The ethanol which they form is subsequently oxidized to acetic acid by acetic acid bacteria *(Acetobacter oxydans, A. rancens, A. aceti,* and *A. melanogenus)*. During fermentation, the content of tannin, caffeine, and reducing sugars falls. Fermentation is complete in 2 to 9 days (Forsyth and Quesnel, 1963).

Tea

Tea is the name given to the processed leaves of the tea plant (*Camellia sinensis* or *Thea sinensis*). A distinction is made between fermented black and unfermented green teas.

In the case of unfermented tea, after harvesting the leaves are briefly heated. This inactivates the enzymes of the plant. No further transformations take place. For fermentation, the tea leaves are withered for 18 to 20 hours. In the following rolling process, the plant cells are broken and the cell sap becomes distributed over the surface of the leaves. The subsequent fermentation changes the color of the tea leaves and the characteris-

tic taste and smell develop. The concluding drying process gives the tea its final black color.

Fermentation is based on the activities of oxidizing enzymes native to the plant. In addition to these, however, the microflora of the leaves (bacteria and yeasts) have an influence on the quality and taste of black tea (Pederson, 1979).

Tobacco

Tobacco is the name given to the dried and fermented leaves of the tobacco plant *(Nicotiana tabacum, Nicotiana rustica)*.

For fermentation, the tobacco leaves are moistened and arranged in layers in large stacks. Under these conditions the temperature rises through the biological heat of the microflora of the leaves to a maximum of 70°C. The fermentation then taking place, in which bacteria, as well as the plant enzymes, play a part (Jensen and Parmele, 1950) brings about an improvement in structure, a degradation of proteinaceous materials, starches, and sugars, and the formation of aroma substances. The exact processes taking place during fermentation are unknown.

9.2.6   Cultivation of Edible Fungi

The demand for edible fungi has risen greatly in the last three years and has greatly exceeded the supply of wild-growing fungi. Increased demand has been answered by an expansion and improvement of the production of cultivatible fungi. In 1978, the world production was more than 700 000 tons.

In Europe and North America it is mainly the cultivated mushroom *Agaricus bisporus,* the asphalt mushroom *Agaricus bitorquis,* and the oyster mushroom or oyster pleurotus *Pleurotus ostreatus* that are cultivated. In Asia, in addition, the shiitake, *Lentinus edoides* and the rice straw fungus *Volvariella volvacea* are produced in comparable amounts.

The production of the shiitake is a tradition going back almost 2000 years in Japan. The substrate for this consists of logs of the shii tree *(Pasania cuspidata)*. After they have been pervaded by mycelium, small cylinders of wood inoculated with spores are hammered into holes in the logs. After storage for a year, the logs are thoroughly watered. In the autumn and spring, the formation of fruiting bodies takes place at between 12 and 20°C. The wood is exhausted and rotten after about six years.

The padi straw mushroom, a tropical fungus, is traditionally cultivated on slightly composted rice straw. Banana leaves, sugar cane and cotton wastes are also used as substrates. Recently, the modern techniques of mushroom cultivation have been applied to the cultivation of this fungus.

Today, the cultivation of the oyster pleurotus is frequently carried out on the large technical scale. The substrate used is straw. Before inoculation with the fungal spores, it is chopped, treated with water, pasteurized at 80°C, and compressed into balls. The yield of fruiting bodies amounts to 40 to 50% of the dry substrate used.

However, in the Western world it is the cultivation of the common mushroom that is of true economic importance. In the last few decades, biotechnological methods have been developed that permit a mass cultivation of this fungus on the large scale.

Flow sheet 9-5 shows mushroom cultivation as it is carried out by a large American firm. The biotechnology of the modern cultivation of mushrooms includes two process steps: 1) the preparation of suitable composts, and 2) growth of the mycelium and fructification.

The preparation of the compost is carried out in two phases. As a first step, a mixture of horse manure and various additives (urea, gypsum, etc.) is subjected to hot rotting. In the preparation of com-

Flow sheet 9-5. Cultivation of mushrooms (after Hatch and Finger, 1979). The figures in parentheses give the daily amounts used per day in tons.

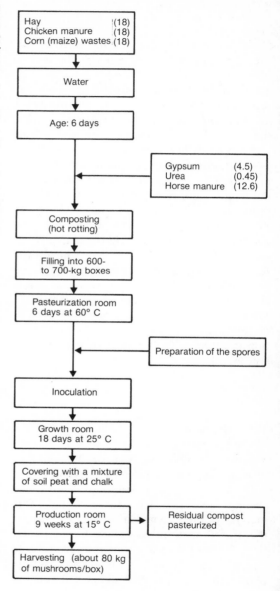

Table 9-3. Natural and Pretreated Wastes from Agriculture and Industry as Starting Materials for Substrates for the Cultivation of Mushrooms (Grabbe and Zadrazil, 1979).

Function	Material	Constituents valuable for mushroom cultivation	% C	% N
Basic substrate (alone or combined)	horse manure	litter: cellulose, lignin, excrements		
	straw	cellulose		~1
	sawdust	lignin		
	garbage compost			
Additives from agricultural production processes	liquid manure from animal stocks	undigested constituents of fodder: cellulose, lignin, protein, mineral substances		3–5
	drainage juice from silage	sugars, acids, proteins	>40	~1–2
	whey	sugars, acids, proteins		~1
Additives from industrial production processes	sulfite waste liquor	lignin		~<1
	extraction residues (formation of aroma)	cellulose, lignin		
	fungal mycelium (production of metabolites)	cell wall constituents: glucosamine; cell contents		~3–5
	marc and draff (manufacture of wine and beer)	cellulose, lignin, protein		~<1
	molasses	sugars		

post, today a whole series of wastes from agriculture and industry is processed. Table 9-3 gives a review of the materials used. In the hot rotting process, the temperature within the heap soon reaches 60 to 70 °C. Composting is accelerated by the repeated turning over of the layers in the heap. After 8 to 9 days the compost is packed into boxes and subjected to pasteurization at 60 °C. This kills animal pests (e.g., nematodes, mites), and also harmful microorganisms. The free ammonia present in the compost, which is toxic for fungi, is eliminated by thermophilic microorganisms (phase II).

The compost treated in this way is now cooled to 25 °C and is inoculated with fungal spores in amounts of 0.5 to 1% of the mass of the substrate and is placed in an incubation chamber with a controlled air temperature (17 °C). After some lag phase of a few weeks, rapid mycelial growth sets in. At a compost temperature of about 25 °C, the mycelium has pervaded the compost completely in about 3

weeks. The compost is now covered with a mixture of soil, peat, and chalk. The formation of fruiting bodies is induced by lowering the temperature of the compost (14 to 17 °C) and by a copious supply of oxygen. The first mushrooms can be harvested after about 3 weeks. During the whole harvesting period of 6 weeks, yields of 0.5 to 1 kg of mushrooms per kg of compost dry matter or 15 to 30 kg per m² of cultivation area can be obtained. The residual compost, which has now been about 50% degraded, is pasteurized and used as a fertilizer.

The fundamental problems in the cultivation of mushrooms are, on the one hand, the preparation of uniformly good compost and, on the other hand, the attack of the cultures by harmful organisms. Infections with viruses, bacteria, and fungi and attacks by worms and insects can greatly affect the yield of mushrooms.

9.3 Foodstuffs and Fodders of Animal Origin

9.3.1 Milk and Dairy Products

Milk

Introduction

The milk of domestic animals – in our region that of domestic cattle – is one of the most valuable nutrients from the aspect of nutritional physiology (for its composition, see Table 9-4). Because of its ready digestibility, a large proportion of the production of milk is marketed in the form of keepable fermented products such as sour milk, sour cream, cheese, and sour-cream butter. For 1978, the world output of these products can be taken as about $2 \cdot 10^{10}$ kg. In the Federal Republic of Germany, fermented milk products cover about 8% of the supply of energy, about 25% of the supply of animal fats, about 8% of the supply of protein, about 20% of the calcium, and about 15% of the supply of vitamin A to the population (Ernährungsbericht [Nutritional Report], 1976).

Table 9-4. Composition of Cows' Milk (Mean values in 100 g of edible component). According to Souci et al. (1979).

Component	Content	
Water	87.5	g
Protein (N × 6.38)	3.33	g
Casein	2.66	g
Albumin + globulin	0.51	g
Fat	3.78	g
Carbohydrates (lactose)	4.65	g
Crude fiber	–	
Minerals	0.74	g
Potassium	157	mg
Calcium	120	mg
Iron	0.046	mg
Phosphorus	92	mg
Vitamin A	30	µg
Carotene	18	µg
Vitamin D_2	0.063	µg
Vitamin E	88	µg
Vitamin K	17	µg
Vitamin B_1	37	µg
Vitamin B_2	0.18	µg
Nicotinamide	90	µg
Pantothenic acid	0.35	µg
Vitamin B_6	46	µg
Biotin	3.5	µg
Folic acid	–	
Vitamin B_{12}	0.42	µg
Vitamin C	1.7	mg

Quality of the Raw Milk

In the manufacture of dairy products of all types, the quality of the initial substrate, raw milk, is decisive for the quality of the product made from it (Frank, 1969). The composition and taste of the milk and the suitability for processing are affected by the genetic constitution, the state of health, and the state of lactation of the milk-yielding animal, and also by the climate, the geological subsoil of the fodder-producing meadows, and the type of the fodder plants and additives. In this respect, by collecting and mixing the milk from a large number of animals from various producers a certain equalization is achieved.

The greatest influence on the suitability of the milk for further processing has the **treatment** to which the milk is exposed between the milking process and its further use. Apart from the high sensitivity of the taste to the action of external factors such as light, mechanical stress, or contamination, the first point that must be mentioned is the **multiplication of microorganisms** in the milk that has taken place up to the moment of its processing. The metabolism of bacteria of many species, the numbers of which rapidly increase in the excellent nutrient medium that milk provides, leads to continuing biochemical changes of all constituents which have an adverse effect on the taste and suitability for further use of the milk and may lead to complete spoilage.

Dairy products must be manufactured from milk which, if possible, should contain not more than 10^5 to 10^6 microorganisms per mL. The widespread collection of the milk from the producer in a two-day rhythm and the cold storage of the raw milk before processing for up to three days associated with this system must be regarded critically. Under these conditions, psychrotrophic components of the original milk flora acquire growth advantages, since the components of the lactic acid bacteria of the flora that have a regulating effect are switched off at these temperatures. These psychrotrophic microorganisms, especially those which decompose protein and fat, and which grow with generation times of 8 to 14 hour even at 4 to 8 °C, liberate into the milk heat-resistant proteolytic and lipolytic enzymes which withstand pasteurization and to some extent ultra-high-temperature treatment without substantial losses in activity. Although the microorganisms are killed by these processes, nevertheless undesirable changes in the substrate may still continue in the treated product and lead to deteriorations in quality (Angevine, 1976).

Pretreatment of the Milk

The delivered raw milk is stored in vats with a capacity of up to 200 000 L. Samples for quality control are taken on receipt from the delivering vehicle. As a rule, the smell and taste, the pH, the numbers of microorganisms and somatic cells present, and also the amounts of protein, fat, calcium, etc., and possible inhibitors are analyzed. From the reservoir, the milk is freed by purifying centrifuge from coarse impurities such as hairs and the like. The milk may then be subjected to intermediate storage or be passed immediately to the cream separator (cream centrifuge) and the skim milk (fat content below 0.3%) and cream (fat content about 30%) be separated from one another.

The skim milk is further processed directly into the products of the skim-milk stage, or it is standardized to the desired fat content by the addition of cream and/or to the dry-matter content desirable for the particular product by the addition of dried milk or edible casein.

The milk is then heated to 70 °C in a heat exchanger and is homogenized at a pressure of 35 to 200 bar depending on the type of machine and the purpose for which it is to be used. This treatment leads to a substantial decrease in the size of the droplets of fat ($\sim 1\ \mu m$) and thus greatly reduces the tendency to creaming. The milk is then pasteurized at 71 to 74 °C for 30 seconds or at 86 °C for 15 seconds. In several cases, other temperatures and times of heating may be necessary for the manufacture of dairy products. The heat treatment substantially kills the vegetative germs, including any pathogenic ones. Some thermoresistant bacteria such as *Streptococcus faecalis* and *S. thermophilus* and also the spores of spore-forming bacteria survive pasteurization.

Following the thermal treatment, the milk is cooled in a heat exchanger to the temperature of storage or to the particular production temperature.

Clotting (Curdling, Coagulation) of Milk

The curdling of milk necessary for the manufacture of sour milk products and cheese is the consequent of a destabilization of the colloidally dissolved casein micelles which can be achieved biophysically by lowering the pH or biochemically-biophysically by means of the proteolytic enzyme preparation rennet or by a combination of the two processes.

About 75 to 80% of the milk protein consists of casein ("cheese substance") and 15 to 25% of whey protein (lactoglobulin, lactalbumin, serum and immune globulins). The casein fraction is heat-resistant and acid-labile, and the whey proteins are denatured by heating but remain in a solution in the critical lactic acid pH range of about 4.

The caseins are organized into casein micelles the size of which is between 50 and 300 mm. There are about $70 \cdot 10^{13}$ of these porous particulate colloids per mL of milk. In their turn, the casein micelles consist of submicelles (see Fig. 9-2). The micelles contain 42% of α-casein (MW 23 615), 28% of β-casein (MW 23 983), and 14% of κ-casein (MW 19 023, see Fig. 9-3), together with 10% of other casein components, 2.9% of calcium, 0.5% of magnesium, 0.8% of organically bound phosphorus, 1.4% of non-bound phosphorus, 0.5% of citric acid, 0.3% of N-acetylneuraminic acid, 0.2% of galactose, and 0.2% of galactosamine (Schmidt and Payens, 1976). The isoelectric point of the casein micelle is at pH 4.6.

The amino acid sequences of α-, β-, and κ-caseins are known (Mercier et al., 1973). α_{s1}-casein is characterized by eight and β-casein by five phosphoric acid residues esterified with serine hydroxy groups. κ-Casein contains only one serine phosphate residue but it contains a glycosyl residue at threonine-131 (N-acetylneuraminyl-(2→3 (6))-galactosyl-(1→3(6))-N-acetylgalactosaminyl→Thr). The

casein micelle is probably stabilized by hydrophobic interactions and salt bridges. Referred to 1 mole of casein, the micelle contains 24 moles of calcium, 8 moles of organically bound phosphoric acid, 11 moles of inorganic phosphate, and one mole of citric acid. On the basis of this composition, the casein micelle is often called a caseinate-calcium-phosphate complex. An experimentally substantiated and descriptive model of the casein micelle has recently been developed by Schmidt (1980). Figure 9-2 shows this idea in comparison with electron micrographs (Fig. 9-3) which demonstrate, on the one hand, the calcium-phosphate-containing regions of the micelle and, on the other hand, the construction of the micelles from submicelles.

a) The curdling of milk by lactic acid fermentation.

With decreasing pH, the casein micelles lose calcium. Phosphoric acid is also dissociated. From a pH of 5.2 to 5.3, i.e., even before the isoelectric point of 4.6 is reached, the calcium- and phosphorus-impoverished micelles begin to precipitate. In this pH region, the jelly formed occupies the whole of the original volume of the

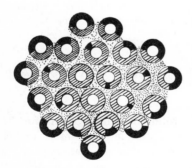

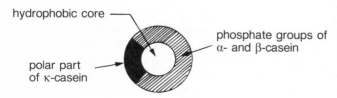

hydrophobic core

polar part
of κ-casein

phosphate groups of
α- and β-casein

Fig. 9-2. Model of casein micelle (Schmidt, 1980). The micelle is constructed of submicelles which, for their part, consist of caseins α_{s1}, β, and κ. The intramicellar colloidal calcium phosphate (dotted regions) is the lute that binds the submicelles into micelles. The splitting out of the polar region of the κ-casein by rennet leads to the denaturation of the micelle and thereby to the clotting or curdling of the milk.

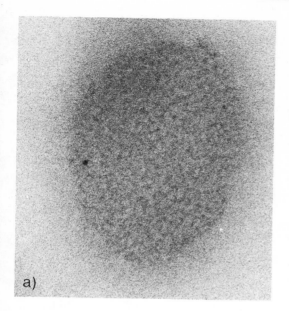

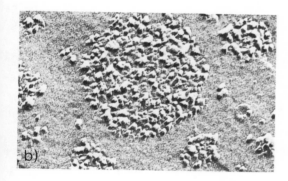

Fig. 9-3. Electron microscopy of a casein micelle from milk.
a) Uncontrasted section through a casein micelle which shows only the colloidal calcium phosphate (compare the casein model in Fig. 9-2). Magnification 200 000 × (taken by Dr. A. M. Knoop, Bundesanstalt für Milchforschung [(German) Federal Institute for Dairy Research], Kiel).
b) Freeze-fractured preparation of casein micelles that clearly shows the submicelles. Magnification 100 000 × (taken by Dr. W. Buchheim, Kiel).

milk. Only by mechanical agitation (cutting and stirring) and raising the temperature (heating) does a further aggregation of the casein (syneresis) take place with a consequent liberation of whey.

b) Curdling of the milk with rennet.
Rennet is an aqueous extract from the fourth stomach of unweaned calves which is marketed in aqueous form or as rennet powder. As an important constituent it contains the proteolytic enzyme chymosin (rennin, E.C. 3.4.4.3). Chymosin cleaves the κ-casein molecules very specifically between phenylalanine-105 and methionine-106 (Mercier et al., 1973):

$$\kappa\text{-casein} \xrightarrow{\text{rennet}}$$

$$\underset{\text{(insoluble)}}{\text{p-}\kappa\text{-casein}} + \underset{\text{(soluble in whey)}}{\text{glycosylmacropeptide}}$$

However, in milk, rennet-induced curdling is a two-phase process which takes place only when sufficient calcium is available. In the absence of calcium, κ-casein is in fact cleaved, but there is no coagulation. In a third phase, during the ripening of the cheese over long periods, other caseins are also hydrolyzed slowly. Pepsin and chymotrypsin act quite similarly, so that today calf rennin is very often mixed with these enzymes from other sources (cattle, pigs, hens); however, such addition is limited for reasons of taste (risk of formation of bitter peptides). Microbial enzymes (rennet substitutes) from *Mucor miehei* and *Mucor pusillus* are also permitted and are marketed as such or mixed with rennin.

Sour Milk Products

General Observations

Sour milk has probably been used for more than 5000 years for human nutrition. Its preparation was first carried out empirically by spontaneous lactic acid fermentation.

Under suitable conditions (22 to 45°C), the **lactic acid bacteria** from the very complex mixture of microflora present in milk fresh from the cow can multiply selectively at a high rate and thereby ferment part of the lactose present in the milk to lactic acid. The resulting decrease of the pH and the redox potential suppress many of the other species of microorganisms of the original milk flora and, in particular, the causative agents of spoilage and disease, such as staphylococci. This lactic acid fermentation produces from milk a keepable well-tasting and highly nutritious product.

In various regions of the world different practices for milk treatment have developed on the basis of the existing climatic effects. Depending on the type of milk used, products arise such as curdled (sour) milk in Europe, **yogurt** in the Balkans, **kefir** in the Caucasus, **koumiss** (see p. 355) in Central Asia, **dahi** in India, and **leben** in Egypt (Klupsch, 1968; Kosikowski, 1977).

The mild acidification in the sour milk product (pH 4.0 to 4.5) brings about a precipitation of the casein in the form of fine flocs and therefore produces a better digestibility.

The lactic acid formed promotes the acidification of the medium in the stomach and the retention of the important mineral calcium by the formation of the readily resorbable calcium lactate. The decrease in the lactose content of the milk caused by lactic acid fermentation also permits people with lowered lactose tolerances to enjoy these milk products. The pleasant fresh taste of sour milk products induces children, the sick, and the old to accept them more readily than milk.

Definition

Sour milk products are products which have been obtained by the use of lactic acid bacteria (lactic acid streptococci and lactobacilli). Special products are also manufactured by the addition of microorganisms not belonging to the typical lactic acid bacteria or by the exclusive use of only certain of them. The initial substrate is pasteurized or heat-treated homogenized milk such as whole milk, partially defatted milk, skim milk, milk the fat content of which has been adjusted by the addition of cream, and cream. The amount of dry matter in the milk can be raised by evaporation or by the addition of dry skim-milk powder or of edible casein.

Corresponding to their fat contents, the following groups of sour milk products exist:

- cream stage with a fat content of 10.0%
- whole-milk stage with a fat content of 3.5%
- fat-poor stage with a fat content of 1.5% to 1.8%
- skim-milk stage with a fat content < 0.3%.

The sour milk products include:

a) fermented milk soured with mesophilic cultures of lactic acid bacteria:
   sour milk, curdled milk, sour cream, buttermilk.

b) Fermented milk soured with special thermophilic lactic acid bacteria:
   yogurt

c) fermented milk manufactured with special mesophilic or thermophilic cultures which contain, in addition to typical lactic acid bacteria, other bacteria or yeasts, or which are manufactured only with other bacteria:
   acidophilus milk, BIO-ghurt, Sanoghurt, kefir, koumiss, etc.

Flow sheet 9-6. Manufacture of curdled milk, sour cream, etc.

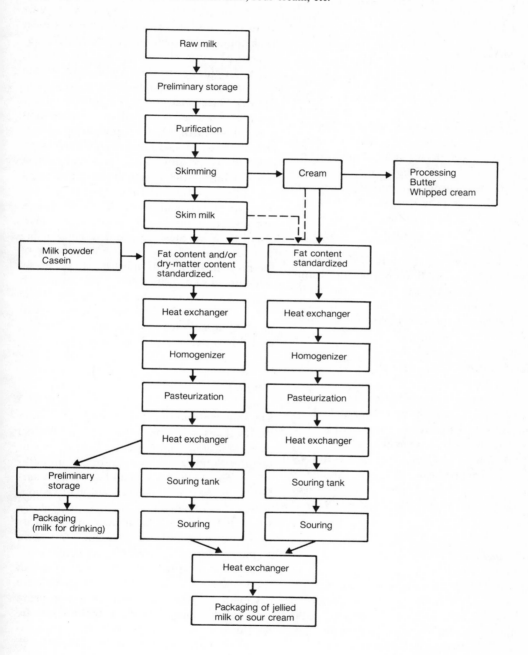

Curdled milk (Sour Milk, Defatted Sour Milk)

(Flow sheet 9-6)

For the preparation of curdled milk, the adjusted and pasteurized milk is cooled in the heat exchanger to 22°C or 30°C, depending on the process, and is inoculated with 2 to 5% or 0.1 to 1% of culture. It is mainly cream-souring cultures or dairy cultures consisting of *Streptococcus cremoris, S. lactis* subsp. *diacetylactis* and/or *Leuconostoc cremoris* that are used. Souring (to about pH 4.6) and coagulation take place in the souring tank in about 16 hours. The sour milk is then cooled to 7 to 10°C and packed.

In another process, the milk is packed immediately after the addition of the culture and it is soured and curdled in the package. Souring at low temperatures promotes the development of aroma (Klupsch, 1968).

Sour Cream (Sour-cream Milk)

For the manufacture of sour cream, cream is adjusted to a fat content of 10% or 20 to 25%, homogenized, and incubated at 18 to 20°C with 2 to 4% of a creamery culture. After about 9 hours, a pH of between 5.1 and 4.9 has been reached. After this, the product is cooled to 4°C, packed, and stored cold (see flow sheet 9-6) (Mann, 1980; Spreer, 1978).

Buttermilk

Buttermilk is a high-value sour milk product. It arises as a by-product in the manufacture of sour-cream butter. It is also obtained by the subsequent souring of the sweet-cream whey that remains after preparation of sweet-cream butter.

Buttermilk may contain up to 10% of water added for reasons of creamery technology or up to 15% of skim milk. **Pure** buttermilk must be manufactured without additives. The fat content of buttermilk is less than 1%.

The origin of the buttermilk and of the sweet-cream whey are described in the section "Butter" (see page 368). The souring of the sweet-cream whey is carried out as in the preparation of curds. In the manufacture of buttermilk, a pH of 4.65 must be achieved as accurately as possible and then maintained, since at higher pH values the casein precipitates as coarse flocs and at lower pH values it does so in granular form. In the drainage, pumping, and filling of the product, the incorporation of air must be avoided, since rising bubbles of air bring about a sedimentation of the protein. Buttermilk must be stored in the well-cooled state, since the production path offers possibilities of recontamination. If its keepability is to be increased by heat treatment, hydrocolloids such as alginates must be added in order to stabilize the protein.

Yogurt

The sour milk product yogurt originated from the Balkans and the Middle East. Goats', ewes', and cows' milk are used for its manufacture. Solid yogurt is a product of milk-white color with a porcelain-like smooth surface. It possesses a creamy solid gel-like consistency, can be cut, and does not release whey. It has a fresh lactic-acid smell and its taste is characteristic, pleasant, full, and slightly to intensely sour. Yogurt is manufactured from heat-treated milk of various fat grades or from cream, and also from milk the dry matter of which has been increased, using cultures of lactic acid bacteria that are **specific** for this purpose. As a product ready for consumption, it usually contains large numbers of living yogurt bacteria.

Flow sheet 9-7. Manufacture of yogurt.

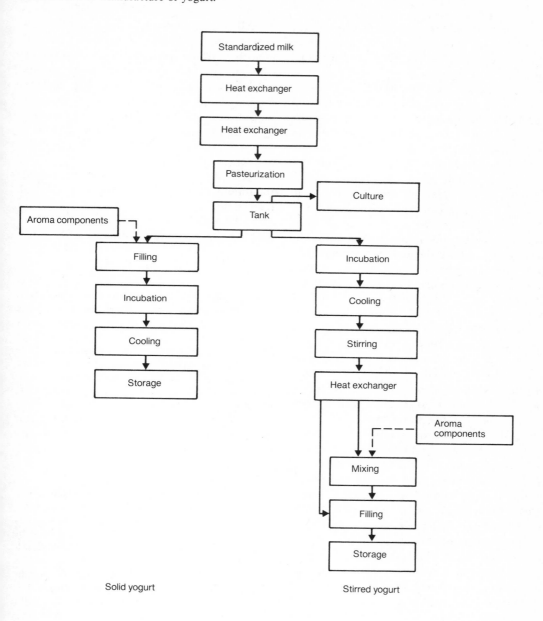

Solid yogurt   Stirred yogurt

The specific yogurt culture used for the manufacture of yogurt consists of thermophilic lactic acid bacteria from the species *Streptococcus thermophilus* and *Lactobacillus bulgaricus,* which live together in symbiosis. In place of *L. bulgaricus,* it is possible occasionally to use *L. jugurti,* a biotype of *L. helveticus.* The yogurt organisms are found in milk curdled in hot countries but can otherwise be isolated from calf stomachs. The two species of bacteria activate one another. *S. thermophilus* rapidly lowers the redox potential and produces the formic acid that promotes the growth of *L. bulgaricus* and some carbon dioxide. *L. bulgaricus* is a more powerful proteolyte. It produces the amino acids and peptides required by *S. thermophilus.* Thus, the two species of bacteria grow in a common culture better, sour faster, and give the product more aroma components than either of the strains alone could do (Moon and Reufold, 1976; Shankar and Davies, 1977; Veringa et al., 1968). In a good yogurt culture the two species are present in a numerical ratio of about 1:1. This composition can always be readjusted by the choice of incubation temperature. Since *S. thermophilus* has its temperature optimum at 40 to 45°C and *L. bulgaricus* at 45 to 50°C, cultivation temperatures under about 45°C permit the number of *S. thermophilus* to rise faster and temperatures above about 45°C lead to the faster multiplication of *L. bulgaricus* (Puhan and Banhegyi, 1974).

In the manufacture of yogurt, *S. thermophilus* multiplies faster at the beginning of fermentation and first brings about souring. At an acid content of about 0.6%, its activity falls off, to die out at about 0.8% of lactic acid. *L. bulgaricus* then takes over the souring process to a maximum of 1.5 to 2% of lactic acid. A mild yogurt ready for consumption contains 0.8 to 0.9% of lactic acid, and a very sour yogurt 1.0 to 1.3%.

Fermentation products are, mainly, lactic acid [D($-$) and L($+$)] and small amounts of volatile fatty acids, carbonyl compounds, and alcohols. The characteristic taste of yogurt is evoked by a bouquet of aroma materials the synthesis of which sets in at a pH of 5, falls off then to a pH range or 4.4 to 4.3, and diminishes greatly at about pH 4. Prolonged storage at low values leads to the loss of the most important aroma components. The characterizing substance of the yogurt aroma is acetaldehyde, and others are acetone, ethanol, butan-2-one, biacetyl, and ethyl acetate (Gesheva and Rusev, 1979).

According to Rasić and Kurmann (1978), the total acid in yogurt is made up of 59% of lactic acid, 28% of citric acid, 5.3% of acetic acid, 2.4% of formic acid, 2.3% of succinic acid, and small amounts of other acids.

Manufacture of yogurt (flow sheet 9-7)

Because of the extreme sensitivity of the yogurt bacteria, the milk must be completely free of antibiotics and other inhibitors. It is adjusted to the desired fat content and the necessary dry-matter content. After this it is heated to 60°C and, to improve the taste and also to increase the firmness of the gel it is homogenized at a pressure of about 200 bar and is finally heat-treated in the pasteurizer at 75 to 95°C for 5 to 40 minutes. After cooling to the ripening temperature of 42 to 45°C, 1.5 to 3% of yogurt starter culture is added to the milk.

Solid yogurt

A rapid decrease of the pH and the incipient coagulation of the milk leads to steep rise in viscosity. Since a uniformly solid structure not releasing whey is required, after the inoculation the milk must be filled into beakers within 20 minutes. Incubation is carried out at 42 to 45°C for 2.5 to 3 hours. When a pH of 4.6 has been reached, the product must be cooled as rapidly as possible to temperatures below about 5°C. This substantially reduces the metabolic activities of the yogurt flora in order to avoid oversouring. Slight postsouring takes place even at these temperatures. From the sealing of the yogurt containers until cooling, shaking must be avoided at all costs in order to prevent the appearance of fissures in the gel that is forming, with an associated release of whey.

At the moment of filling, flavoring components of the most diverse types – for example, in the form of fruit – can be added to the yogurt, so that a broad spectrum of yogurt products can be obtained.

Stirred yogurt

In the manufacture of stirred yogurt, incubation is carried out in the ripening tank. Shortly before a pH of 4.7 had been reached, the tank is cooled so that the yogurt can be stirred at pH values of 4.7 to 4.6 at about 20°C. After this, the substrate is cooled in a heat exchanger to 5°C and is either filled directly or is first mixed with flavoring components and then filled. Because of the tendency to postsouring, storage must take place at 5°C.

Kefir

Kefir originated from the Caucasus. It was obtained there from cows', goats', or ewes' milk. Today, kefir is produced in large amounts, particularly in Russia (in 1971, about 1 116 000 L of whole-milk kefir). In many countries, the popularity of kefir is only slightly less than that of yogurt.

Kefir is a thick-flowing creamy, slightly effervescent or foaming beverage of milk-white color. It contains 0.8 to 1% of lactic acid, 0.3 to 0.8% of ethanol, and carbon dioxide. The alcohol and carbon dioxide, together with small amounts of biacetyl, acetaldehyde, and acetone, contribute greatly to its characteristic refreshing taste.

Today, kefir is manufactured from pasteurized milk or cream, the fat content or dry-matter content of which has been adjusted, by the use of cultures specific for this purpose.

The **kefir cultures** or **kefir grains** (also known by Mohammedans as millet of the Prophet) are whitish-yellow clumps of pea to walnut size with cauliflower-like shape. These agglomerates, the structure of which consists of the sparingly water-soluble but highly swellable polysaccharide kefiran and acid-coagulated casein, contain a **symbiotic microflora.** In addition to lactose-fermenting yeasts, such as *Saccharomyces kefir* and *Candida kefir* (5 to 10% of the culture), it also contains homofermentative and heterofermentative lactobacilli (e.g., *L. kefir*), mesophilic lactic acid streptococci, flavor-forming Leuconostoc, and occasionally acetic acid bacteria (Mann, 1979). The composition of the mixed kefir culture is variable, according to the process, the climate, or the milk used without, however, this giving rise to fundamental changes.

Manufacture of kefir (Flow sheet 9-8)

The prepared milk is heated in the heat exchanger to 70°C and is then homogenized and is heat-treated in the pasteurizer at 85°C for 30 min. Pasteurized milk is cooled to the fermentation temperature of 18 to 28°C, usually 22°C. In the ripening vessel 3 to 5% of kefir culture is added to the milk and, depending on the amount of innoculum, it is incubated for 10 to 20 hours. When a pH of 4.6 to 4.4 has been reached, the soft coagulate is stirred. The kefir grains are then separated off. These may, after being washed well with cold germ-free water, be added to a new production batch. The kefir is cooled to 7 to 12°C and is then filled either into glass bottles or plastic beakers and sealed. It can be issued directly for consumption or it can be left to postripen at 7°C for 24 to 48 hours, depending on the taste. When an airtight seal is opened kefir tends to foam. If kefir is stored in bottles the closure of which permits carbon dioxide to escape, alcohol is also lost from the product. Kefir filled into plastic containers tends to blow, to cause the containers to swell. This is a normal behavior for a living fermented product and does not mean that the product is spoiled (Spreer, 1978).

Koumiss

Koumiss comes from Central Asia. It was originally prepared from **mares' milk.** The prod-

Flow sheet 9-8. Manufacture of kefir.

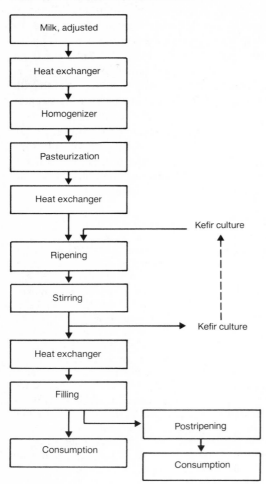

uct is recommended today, particularly in Russia, for dietetic treatment in the case of intestinal diseases because of its wholesomeness, ready digestibility, and its vitamin content.

Koumiss is a homogeneous, slightly foaming, sour milk drink. Its taste is due to a simultaneous lactic acid and alcohol fermentation, and the taste-affecting metabolic products of the organisms of the koumiss culture. Koumiss contains 0.7 to 1.8% of lactic acid, 0.5 to

2.5% of ethanol, and carbon dioxide. According to Saigin (1978), in the year 1980 in Bashkir 200000 mares were to be available for the production of milk, and in the near future 5620000 L were to be fermented. In addition to this, **modified cows' milk** is being used in increasing amounts. Cows' and mares' milks have substantially differing chemical compositions. In particular, the lower protein content in mares' milk and the ratio of casein to whey proteins of approximately 1:1 lead to the situation that a soured mares' milk coagulates only quite feebly, which is characteristic for koumiss.

Consequently, the composition of **skimmed cows' milk** intended for the manufacture of koumiss is brought close to that of mares' milk by the addition of whey proteins and it is then fermented (Gallmann and Puhan, 1978; Schamgin, 1977).

The cultures used are mixed cultures of yeasts (Torula, Kluyveromyces, Candida, and Brettanomyces), lactobacilli (*L. bulgaricus, L. acidophilus*), streptococci (*S. lactis, S. thermophilus*). Yeasts and mixtures of bacteria are preincubated separately and are then added to the milk in ratios of 1:1 to 1:10.

In principle, the manufacture is similar to that of kefir.

Types of Acidophilus Milk

After Metchnikoff's publication "Prolongation of Life" the opinion was held for a long time that the bacteria populating the human gut which were said to affect health and lifespan by the liberation of toxic products, are inhibited or suppressed by lactic acid bacteria colonizing the gut, especially *Lactobacillus acidophilus*. Therefore large numbers of *L. acidophilus*, which is capable of surviving all obstacles to a passage through the gastrointestinal tract, should be added through foodstuffs. Because of taxonomic difficulties, at first *L. bulgaricus,* belonging to the yogurt flora, which is itself incapable of existing in the gut, was taken for *L. acidophilus.* Yogurt therefore gained great popularity as a promotor of health.

At the present time, in many countries of the world sour milk products containing typical inhabitants of the human gut (*L. acidophilus, Bifidobacterium bifidum* or *L. casei*) are on sale.

As an effect of these products during long-term consumption in many subjects slight changes in the composition of the intestinal flora have been observed. In cases with diarrhoeas and disturbances of the intestinal equilibrium due to treatment with antibiotics, operations, or old age, alleviations and improvements have been described. However, a medical-therapeutic action due to *L. acidophilus* has not yet been satisfactorily proved.

Attempts have been made to obtain products with a fresh lactic acid smell, a pleasant aromatic sour taste, and a high number of *L. acidophilus* germs by combining *L. acidophilus* with normal sour milk or yogurt starters.

L. acidophilus has its temperature optimum at 35 to 38 °C, the organisms of the cream-souring culture have theirs at 25 to 27 °C, and those of yogurt at 40 to 48 °C. It is therefore understandable that when *L. acidophilus* germs are added to normal starters and these mixed cultures are used under the conditions normal for the particular products, materials with inadequate numbers of *L. acidophilus* germs arise.

Consequently, other ways have been found for the manufacture of *L. acidophilus*-containing milk products.

Bioghurt in Germany: sour milk manufactured with the use of *L.acidophilus* and *Streptococcus lactis* var. *taette.*

Aco-Joghurt in Switzerland: a concentrate of *L. acidophilus* containing up to $5 \cdot 10^7$ microorganisms in 200 mL is added to normal yogurt.

Produkt A-38 in Denmark: nine parts of normal yogurt are mixed with one part of *L. acidophilus* sour milk.

Yakult in Japan: sweetened and flavored milk is soured with *L. casei.*

Acidophilus sour milk in Czechoslovakia: nine parts of curdled milk are mixed with one part of acidophilus milk.

"Di-gest", sweet acidophilus milk in the USA: to homogenized, pasteurized, semicream milk are added a *L. acidophilus* concentrate with $8 \cdot 10^6$ germs/mL and vitamins A and D. After filling, the milk is well cooled, and is stored at 4 to 6 °C until consumed. In this way, in spite of the high number of living germs, the milk undergoes no change in its organoleptic quality (Speck, 1978; Spreer, 1978).

Keepability of Sour Milk Products
(Flow sheet 9-9)

In the manufacture of sour milk products, increasing popularity, the concentration and expansion of production units, and limitation of the factories to individual products are leading to an increasing supply of products to superregional and distant markets. This leads to a demand for an improvement in the keepability of these products. The elimination of contaminants (coliform germs, yeasts, and fungi) and the inactivation of the souring cultures used with the consequence of an inhibition of postsouring can be achieved most simply by hot or aseptic filling. Unlimited keepability resulting from a possible technologically safe sterilization process is not necessary here since it is always fresh products that are involved which would lose their desirable or organoleptic properties during excessive periods of storage even under sterile conditions.

Cheese

Definition

Cheeses are fresh products or products with various degrees of maturation which have

Flow sheet 9-9. Manufacture of keepable sour milk products (Puhan, 1979).

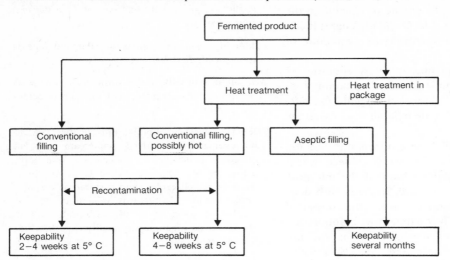

been manufactured from curdled cheese milk.

In contrast to sour milk products, the curdling of the milk need not take place only through microbially induced lactic acid fermentation (as in the case of the sour-milk cheeses) but also, and in particular, by means of **proteolytic enzymes** such as calf rennet, pepsin, or microbial rennet (on the mechanism, see the general introduction to this chapter). A further difference from sour milk products is that in the case of cheese a larger or smaller part of the aqueous phase of the milk is eliminated as whey by the processing of the product. The larger the amount of whey removed, the harder is the consistency of the cheese or the higher is its dry-matter content.

The degree of **elimination of whey** is determined essentially by the syneresis (separation of hydrophobic colloids) of the coagulum or curd (coagulated casein). The degree of syneresis and therefore the release of whey during cheese manufacture is increased by mechanical stirring and, in particular, by heating the coagulum. Systematically, the manufacturing

process for a cheese can be subdivided into the following steps:

– Preripening of the cheese milk (kettle milk)
  Raw milk or pasteurized milk is inoculated with a small amount (0.1%) of a culture of lactic acid bacteria and is incubated overnight at 12 °C. This preripening step acts essentially as a process of conditioning the milk for the manufacture of cheese. The exact biochemical processes that occur are not yet known. Undoubtedly, an important factor is the resulting fall in the redox potential of the kettle milk.

– Renneting of the milk and curdling
  The preripened milk treated with starter culture is coagulated by the addition of rennet (rennet preparation). Curdling may also take place by souring alone.

– Cutting of the curdled milk
  This process is necessary in order to permit the release of the whey and to make the cheese curd formed capable of being processed.

– Heating the cheese curd
Heating has the aim of promoting syneresis (see above) and, consequently, an increased release of whey. The larger the amount of whey that is to be removed, the longer and the hotter must the heating process be.

– Elimination of the whey and formation of the cheese mass
In the case of soft and hard cheeses, the whey is removed by mechanical sieves, and in the case of fresh cheeses so-called curd separators are used for this purpose.

– Pressing the cheese
This process has the aim of eliminating more whey, after the final shaping of the cheese. During pressing, lactic acid fermentation also proceeds further.

– Salting the cheese
If the curd has not been dry-salted before the formation of the cheese, the shaped and molded cheeses are immersed for a few days in a salt bath. With certain types of cheese, the cheeses can also be dry-salted (see Roquefort).

– Ripening of the cheese
The ripening of the cheese has the aim of imparting to the final product the desired consistency, taste, and aroma. The microbiology and biochemistry of cheese ripening is not yet known in all its details.

Mair-Waldburg (1974) lists some hundreds of varieties of cheese. Below, the manufacture of some characteristic varieties of cheese will be described in more detail (Mair-Waldburg, 1974).

Fresh Cheeses

Fresh cheeses are natural, unripened, products. They are manufactured from pasteurized or tempered milk of adjusted fat content by the use of **souring cultures** and **rennet** or rennet substitutes or with souring cultures alone by the precipitation of the casein and the separation of whey, and are marketed in the fresh state. Keepability can be improved by heat treatment (Puhan, 1979; Kielwein and Melling, 1978).

Fresh cheese preparations are obtained by incorporating flavoring additives in the cheese mass. The fresh cheeses include quark and granular fresh cheese (cottage cheese).

Quark (fresh cheese, fresh cream cheese, white cheese, fresh double-cream cheese, layer cheese).

Quark forms the main fresh-cheese product in large parts of Europe. It is manufactured only from pasteurized skim milk the fat content of which has been adjusted or, for the higher-fat grades, from milk with the later incorporation of cream. Quark possesses a white to cream-yellow uniformly soft, smooth to paste-like dough without any skin or rind whatever, without the release of whey, and without granular or gritty structures and a clean slightly lactic acid taste (Loos and Nebe, 1980). Quark is prepared with souring cultures and small amounts of rennet (sour-rennet quark) or souring cultures alone (sour-milk quark). In the low-temperature souring process at 20 to 30°C (time of souring 15 to 22 hours), mesophilic cultures, creamery cultures (see under that heading), or single-strain cultures of *S. cremoris* are used. In the warm souring process at 38 to 40°C (souring time 3 to 5 hours), thermophilic lactic acid bacteria (*S. thermophilus* and *L. bulgaricus*) are used.

Manufacture of quark (Flow sheet 9-10)

– Preparation of the milk
Milk of adjusted fat content from the primary stock tank is heated to approximately the temper-

Flow sheet 9-10. Manufacture of edible quark.

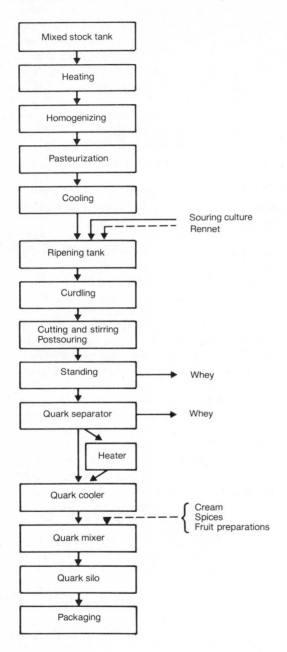

ature of pasteurization, homogenized, and then pasteurized in the pasteurizer at 72°C for 15 seconds or at 85 to 95°C for a few seconds, cooled in the cooler to 20 to 27°C or 38 to 42°C, according to the process being used, and pumped into ripening tanks with a capacity of 15000 to 50000 L.

– Souring and curdling
  In the souring tank, 0.5 to 2% of the souring culture in the low-temperature process and 3 to 4% in the warm souring process is added, with, if required, the rennet preparation, and the mixture is thoroughly stirred for about 2 minutes. Then the milk is left to rest until it has curdled. Small amounts of rennet are said to accelerate the coagulation through slight proteolysis and therefore also to have a favorable effect on the stability of the consistency of the casein gel. In no case may the rennet in the quark bring about a far-reaching decomposition of the casein through proteolytic cleavages going beyond this.

– Cutting and stirring
  After 8 to 12 or 2 to 3 hours, when a pH of 4.8 has been reached, the coagulum is cut by an integrated cutting and stirring device in the souring tank into sections with an edge length of about 10 to 20 cm and is slowly stirred. In another 6 to 8 or 1 to 2 hours, with souring proceeding further, whey slowly separates out and the coagulum sinks in the whey.

– Separation
  As soon as the pH has fallen to 4.65 to 4.6, the stirring is stopped and the supernatant whey is run off. After this, the quark and the residual whey are removed from the tank. The quark can now be heat-treated at 60°C to stop the activity of the rennet and to kill recontaminants and souring bacteria, i.e., to prolong keepability. Then, at a temperature of 30°C, the substrate passes through the quark separator for the elimination of more whey and for the adjustment of the desired dry-matter content of the product. After this the quark is cooled to 4 to 8°C.

– Mixing
  The quark is processed to a uniform consistency in a kneading and mixing machine. Pasteurized

cream, spices, fruit preparations may be incorporated at the same time. The finished product is first stored in a quark silo and is then fed into packaging devices where filling is carried out with the greatest possible efforts to avoide recontamination. Quark pumps, piping, separators, and mixing devices of the unit must be so designed that the acid-coagulated casein micelles are not damaged by shearing forces, which would lead to a continuing release of whey (Dolle, 1977; Spreer, 1978; Kessler, 1976).

Granular Fresh Cheese (Cottage Cheese)

Cottage cheese is a fresh-cheese speciality. In the USA, it forms the main fresh cheese product. Edible quark is largely unknown there.

Cottage cheese is obtained from pasteurized skim milk with the addition of souring cultures, and also with the addition of rennet, by the acid coagulation of casein, and by special further treatment as a granular product and to improve its taste it is mixed with cream and with the addition of common salt, and filled into containers.

Manufacture of cottage cheese
(Flow sheet 9-11)

– Preparation of the milk
Selected skim milk is homogenized and subjected to gentle pasteurization (72 to 75 °C for 15 seconds).

– Souring
The souring cultures used are mesophilic mixed cultures and also creamery cultures. These populations consist overwhelmingly of organisms of *S. cremoris,* a small proportion of *S. lactis,* and from 1% to a maximum of 3% of aroma-forming agents (*S. lactis* subsp. *diacetylactis* and/or *Leuconostoc cremoris*). Larger proportions of aroma-forming agents in the culture adversely affect the product by the pronounced formation of gas. These cultures are added to the milk. To facilitate

curdling and the release of whey and to improve the granular texture by proteolysis, small amounts of rennet may be added to the milk.

The amount of starter culture and the temperature determine the time until the milk curdles.

Milk, starter culture, and any rennet are mixed directly in the cheese vat and the mixture is left unstirred until it curdles.

However, the milk may also be preripened in a preripening tank by the souring culture until a pH of 5.7 is reached. It is then pumped into the cheese vat with the addition of the desired amount of rennet. The vats contain 5000 to 12000 L of milk. They are provided with cutting and stirring devices and also with heatable jackets. In the pretreatment of milk up to the stage of the coagulation of the casein, any introduction of gas bubbles whether by entrainment during pumping or stirring or through gas-forming microorganisms must be avoided, since the production of curds containing bubbles of gas make processing difficult and cause losses of yield.

– Cutting and stirring
The solid curd with a pH of 4.7, corresponding to 0.4 to 0.5% of lactic acid, is cut into pieces with an edge length of 1 to 2 cm. Slow stirring prevents the pieces of curd from coalescing again and promotes the release of whey. Pronounced turbulence in the vat which leads to the abrasion of cheese dust from the pieces of curd is avoided because of the loss of yield.

– Scalding
About 30 minutes after cutting, the contents of the vat are heated quite slowly to temperatures of 42 to 60 °C by blowing hot water or steam into the jacket of the vat with simultaneous stirring and are left under these conditions for some time. This promotes the uniform release of whey from the grains of curd, so that a firm elastic curd arises with no formation of skin. This process lasts 1 to 3 hours.

– Washing
After this, part of the whey is run off and, with stirring, the grain is washed with cold germ-free water and finally with ice water, which cools it to 8 °C, and the water is run off.

Flow sheet 9-11. Manufacture of cottage cheese (Niederauer, 1978).

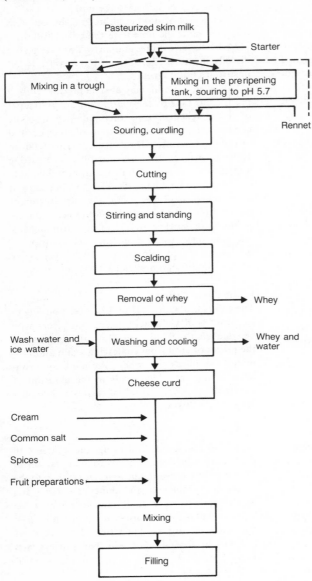

Flow sheet 9-12. Manufacture of Harzer cheese.

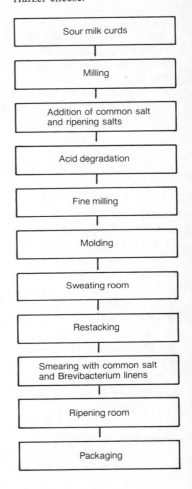

- Mixing

The curd is mixed with cream, if desired with the addition of common salt. Spices or fruit preparations may also be added. After this, the granular fresh cheese is filled into packages.

Composition of cottage cheese according to Niederauer (1978):

Water	78.5%
Protein	12.3%
Fat	4.3%
Lactose	3.3%
Lactic acid	0.4%

Granular fresh cheese, especially when it contains flavoring additives, should be stored at 5°C in order to retain its organoleptic quality (Dolle, 1977; Diessel, 1976; Klein et al., 1980; Niederauer, 1980).

Harzer cheese

Manufacture (Flow sheet 9-12).

This was originally manufactured from pure sour-milk quark, but today it is also made from quark that has been obtained by a mixed rennet-lactic acid coagulation process. The lactic acid fermentation can be carried out with mesophilic cultures (*Streptococcus lactis* and *S. cremoris*) or with thermophilic cultures (*Lactobacillus helveticus*, etc.). The dry-matter content should amount to at least 32%.

Quark from various productions and manufacturers is milled to walnut size and mixed with 3 to 4% of common salt and 0.5 to 1.5% of ripening salts (NaHCO$_3$, CaCO$_3$). This is intended to neutralize part of the lactic acid in order to give a pH of 4.8 to 4.9. A further decomposition of the acids by yeasts is achieved by storage at room temperature for several hours to one day. After fine comminution, the curd is shaped in special machines. The freshly formed cheeses are incubated on boards in the "sweating room" at 20 to 25°C in 95% atmospheric humidity for 2 to 3 days. During this process, the surface of the cheese is deacidified by film-forming yeasts. After the formation of a light yellow smooth skin the cheeses are coated on all sides with a solution of 50 to 75 g of common salt and 50 to 100 mL of a culture of *Brevibacterium linens* in a liter of water. After drying overnight, the cheeses are transferred to the ripening room where, at 12 to 18°C and a relative humidity of 90 to 95%, the typical red streak is formed. The cheeses can then be packaged and marketed.

Emmental (Swiss) Cheese

Manufacture (Flow sheet 9-13)

Emmental cheese is produced from raw milk mainly in Switzerland, Germany, Finland, France, and Austria. There is a classical procedure of manufacture in the cheese vat in which 1000 L of milk gives one cheese. In addition, however, there are already many large-scale manufactures in which up to 12 000 L of milk are processed in each cheese vat. The evening milk preripened overnight (12°C) is mixed with the fresh morning milk. The added starter culture consists of 1 to 2% of a culture of thermophilic streptococci (*S. thermophilus*) and lactobacilli (e.g., *L. helveticus*) in whey. In addition, a few drops of a culture of propionic acid bacteria must be added. The curdling time with rennet is about 30 minutes. The cutting of the curd and preliminary cheese formation require 45 min. The mixture of curd and whey is heated with stirring to 53°C within 30 to 40 min and is stirred for another 30 to 60 min. After the treatment, the grains of curd are about 2 to 3 mm in size. After the settling of the curd, it is taken up with a cloth and placed in molds. At first it is compressed under a load of 500 kg for 20 min, and then under 1000 kg for 60 min and finally under 1200 kg. During this procedure it must be turned several times. After overnight pressing, by the next morning the lactose should have been fermented quantitatively to lactic acid. The pH of the cheese is then about 5.25. After this, the cheeses are placed in a salt bath for 2 to 3 days at 15°C. After drying in the salting room, which requires about 10 to 14 days, the cheeses are stored in the warm room for 6 to 8 weeks. At temperatures of 22 to 24°C, the lactic acid formed is fermented by the propionic acid bacteria to carbon dioxide and acetic and propionic acids, which gives rise to the characteristic formation of "eyes" and to the development of the taste of the Swiss cheese. After the conclusion of gas formation, the cheeses are ripened in the storage cellar at 12 to 14°C. During this time,

Flow sheet 9-13. Manufacture of Emmental cheese.

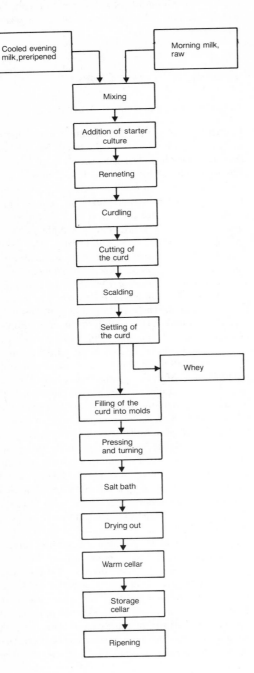

the surface of the cheeses must be freed from the fungal coating that forms by washing. The optimum time of ripening is six months and the maximum time of storage another 12 months at 15°C.

The dreaded **late blowing** (see section 9.2, p. 329) is caused by spore-forming bacteria which ferment the lactic acid not to propionic acid but to butyric acid and hydrogen (e.g., *Clostridium tyrobutyricum*). These bacteria cannot be avoided in the milk when the cows are fed with fermented fodder (silage). For this reason, in the German and Swiss production are- as the feeding of silage is forbidden if the milk is to be supplied for the preparation of Emmental cheese. Another fermentation failure is the so-called **Nachgärung** [postfermentation] in which, after the "eyes" have been formed, the production of carbon dioxide does not stop. This leads to fissures in the cheese and therefore to a lowering of it commercial value, although not always to an effect on the taste of the cheese. The microbiological reasons for this occurrence are so far unknown.

Cheddar Cheese

Manufacture (Flow sheet 9-14)

Cheddar cheese is the preferred cheese product of the Anglo-Saxon countries (United Kingdom, USA, New Zealand).

The milk for its manufacture is heated at 72.2°C for 15 sec and cooled to 31°C and is then treated with 1.5% of a single- or multistrain starter. 21.8 mL of rennet per 100 kg of milk is stirred in mechanically in the vat. The curdling time amounts to 30 to 35 min. After this, the curd is cut into cubes with a size of about 1 cm³. Five minutes after the end of this process and within less than 30 minutes the material is heated (scalded) to 38 to 39°C. The mixture is stirred at this temperature to an acidity in the whey of 0.15% of lactic acid (about 6.7 °SH*) (about 2.5 h). The curd is allowed to settle and the

---

* °SH is the result of the Soxhlet-Henkel method for determining the titrable acidity of dairy products. °SH = mL of NaOH (c = 0.25 mol/L) per 100 mL of product.

Flow sheet 9-14. Manufacture of Cheddar cheese.

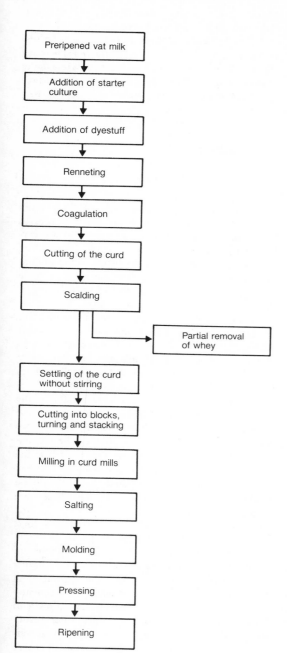

whey is run off through filters. A rake-type stirrer is then drawn through the mass of curd several times during a period of 20 min in order to achieve the desired grain size. During this process the acidity rises to about 0.23 to 0.24% of lactic acid. The mass of curd is now heaped up in order to achieve its coalescence ("cheddaring"). After this heaping procedure, pieces weighing 8 to 12 kg are cut out from this mass of curd and are placed in layers above one another. During this period of storage of about 2 to 2.5 h, the lactic acid content rises to 0.5 to 0.6% with a simultaneous drainage of whey. The cheddared blocks are then milled to form shreds of curd and are salted (about 3 kg of salt/100 kg of cheese mass). The salted mass is filled into molds and pressed. After this, the cheeses are taken from the molds and coated with plastic foil or hot wax. In this form they are placed in the ripening cellar. They remain there at 7 to 10°C under a relative humidity of 55% for 1 to 12 months. Cheddar cheese can be colored by the addition of dyestuffs (usually carotenoids).

Limburg Cheese

Manufacture (Flow sheet 9-15)

The pasteurized kettle milk is treated with 0.2 to 0.5% of mesophilic starter. Then 15 to 20 mL of liquid rennet (1:10000) is added per 100 L of kettle milk. The temperature at adding the rennet is between 29 and 35°C, depending on the fat content. The whole curdling time amounts to 40 to 45 minutes. The curd is cut into 1.5- to 2-cm pieces. After 10 min, it is cut again and after 15 min some whey is taken off and the coagulum is agitated for 5 to 10 min in order to make it somewhat firmer. The coagulum is charged into molds, and after about 1 hour it is turned in the molds. Limburg cheese is then kept for 24 h in the salt bath (16 to 18% NaCl between 16 and 18°C). After the salt bath, the cheese is allowed to drain and dry out. It is dried for another 2 to 3 days in the ripening cellar. Then it is greased, i.e., coated with a red smear culture (*Brevibacterium linens*). Greasing must be repeated three to eight times, depending on the size of the cheese, in order to obtain a thick surface growth, particu-

Flow sheet 9-15. Manufacture of Limburg cheese.

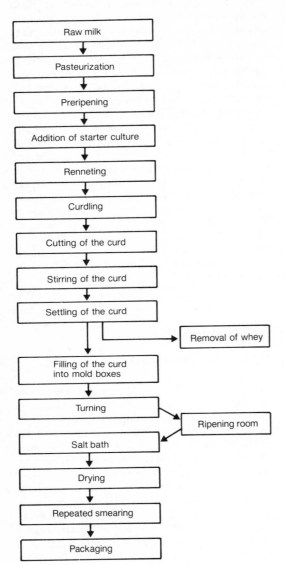

larly when the cellars are relatively dry and have somewhat high temperatures, since otherwise the growth of moulds takes place. Good ripening conditions are 14°C and a relative humidity of 90 to 95°C. After 3 to 4 weeks or, in the smaller cheeses, after only 2 to 3 weeks, as soon as the red smear has developed well, the cheeses are packed. While in the classical cheese dairy the greasing of the surface was carried out by hand, today this task is performed mechanically.

Camembert Cheese

Manufacture (Flow sheet 9-16)

Pasteurized milk is inoculated with 1 to 2% of starter. Today, the addition of suspension of spores of *Penicillium caseicolum* or *P. camemberti* is also carried out before the addition of rennet, as a rule. The renneting temperature is 35 to 36°C and the amount of rennet 20 to 25 mL (1:10000) per 100 L of kettle milk. The curdling time is 15 to 20 min. This may be followed by a thickening time of 40 to 50 min. The curd is carefully cut into cubes with a size of 1.5 to 2 cm. From cutting to the removal of the curd takes about 25 min. The curd is filled into suitable molds. After having stood for 10 minutes, the cheeses are turned, and the process repeated two or three times in the course of a day. In order to permit souring to take place during this period, the temperature of the room should be about 20 to 24°C. Before the cheese is immersed in the salt bath, the pH should have fallen to about 4.8 to 5. Depending on the fat content and the size of the cheeses, they are left in the salt bath (18 to 20% NaCl, 16 to 20°C) for between 40 and 220 min. The salt bath itself should be slightly acidic (about 20 to 40 °SH). The cheeses are transferred from the salt bath racks to the ripening racks. They are first stored in the drying room for 2 to 3 days (19°C, then falling to 17°C). In the ripening room a temperature of 16°C then falling to 14°C is possible. The relative humidity in the drying room should be 70 to 80%, and in the ripening room 85 to 95%. The cheeses are turned fairly frequently in the ripening and drying rooms. The growth of mold appears after about 3 to 4 days. After 9 to 11 days, the cheese can be packed in foil and marketed. Camembert is one of the varieties of cheese

Flow sheet 9-16. Manufacture of Camembert.

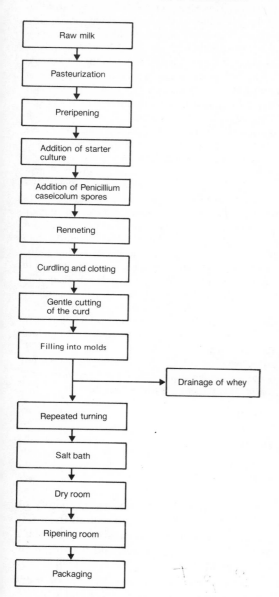

which, because of the growth of molds rapidly ripens or changes its consistency at a suitable storage temperature after the customer has acquired it. The proteolytic enzymes of the Camembert mould then lead to a softening of the cheese mass, coupled with a liberation of aroma products and, finally, ammonia through the action of deaminating enzymes. This has the consequence that contaminating microorganisms such as coliform bacteria that may have passed into the cheese during its production can develop well in the Camembert.

Roquefort Cheese

Manufacture (Flow sheet 9-17)

Roquefort cheese is produced from fresh raw ewes' milk. The average protein content is 6.5% and the average fat content 8%. As a rule, whey from the cheese production of the previous day, which contains a mixed culture of lactic acid streptococci and lactic acid bacilli, is used as the starter culture. The temperature for the growth of this culture is 35°C. *Penicillium roqueforti* is added to the kettle milk in the form of a suspension of spores. The fungus can also be cultivated on bread and then be dusted on to the cheese curd with the dry spores during the shaping process. The renneting temperature is 30°C and the curdling time 120 to 150 min with 25 mL of rennet (1:10 000) to 100 L of kettle milk. The curd is cut into 1- to 3-cm cubes. During the next few hours, the curd is stirred a few times. Then it is allowed to settle and the whey is drawn off. The coagulum is filled into suitable stoneware or tinplate molds (diameter 20 cm, height 10 cm). The drainage of the whey in the molds lasts about four days. They are turned once a day. During this phase a slight heterofermentation of the lactic acid type takes place in the coagulum which serves to create cavities for the development of the fungus. These still soft cheeses are transported (from as far away as Corsica and the Pyrenees) to Roquefort. They are salted by hand with coarse sea salt in salting rooms (temperature 9 to 10°C) (several times in the course of 3 to 5 days). The salt-tolerant microorganisms that develop are removed from the surface by brushes. Then the cheeses are manually or mechanically pierced with needles in order to create access to the mass of

Flow sheet 9-17. Manufacture of Roquefort.

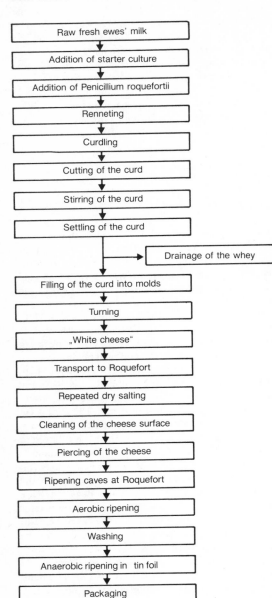

```
┌──────────────────────────────────┐
│     Raw fresh ewes' milk          │
└──────────────────────────────────┘
              ↓
┌──────────────────────────────────┐
│   Addition of starter culture     │
└──────────────────────────────────┘
              ↓
┌──────────────────────────────────┐
│ Addition of Penicillium roquefortii│
└──────────────────────────────────┘
              ↓
┌──────────────────────────────────┐
│           Renneting               │
└──────────────────────────────────┘
              ↓
┌──────────────────────────────────┐
│           Curdling                │
└──────────────────────────────────┘
              ↓
┌──────────────────────────────────┐
│      Cutting of the curd          │
└──────────────────────────────────┘
              ↓
┌──────────────────────────────────┐
│      Stirring of the curd         │
└──────────────────────────────────┘
              ↓
┌──────────────────────────────────┐
│      Settling of the curd         │
└──────────────────────────────────┘
              ↓   ────────→  ┌──────────────────────────┐
              │             │   Drainage of the whey    │
              ↓             └──────────────────────────┘
┌──────────────────────────────────┐
│   Filling of the curd into molds  │
└──────────────────────────────────┘
              ↓
┌──────────────────────────────────┐
│            Turning                │
└──────────────────────────────────┘
              ↓
┌──────────────────────────────────┐
│         „White cheese"            │
└──────────────────────────────────┘
              ↓
┌──────────────────────────────────┐
│     Transport to Roquefort        │
└──────────────────────────────────┘
              ↓
┌──────────────────────────────────┐
│      Repeated dry salting         │
└──────────────────────────────────┘
              ↓
┌──────────────────────────────────┐
│  Cleaning of the cheese surface   │
└──────────────────────────────────┘
              ↓
┌──────────────────────────────────┐
│     Piercing of the cheese        │
└──────────────────────────────────┘
              ↓
┌──────────────────────────────────┐
│   Ripening caves at Roquefort     │
└──────────────────────────────────┘
              ↓
┌──────────────────────────────────┐
│       Aerobic ripening            │
└──────────────────────────────────┘
              ↓
┌──────────────────────────────────┐
│            Washing                │
└──────────────────────────────────┘
              ↓
┌──────────────────────────────────┐
│ Anaerobic ripening in tin foil    │
└──────────────────────────────────┘
              ↓
┌──────────────────────────────────┐
│           Packaging               │
└──────────────────────────────────┘
```

cheese for the oxygen necessary for the growth of the fungus. Ripening must take place exclusively in the natural cellars at Roquefort which run for several kilometers through the mountain. The temperature in these cellars is constant at 7 to 10 °C and the atmospheric humidity is between 90 and 100%. At first, the cheeses are stored in layers on edge at 8 to 10 °C and a relative humidity of 96% for 18 to 23 days. Yeasts and bacteria that develop on the surface of the cheeses are scraped off. After the end of this **aerobic ripening,** to induce the **anaerobic phase** the cheeses are packed into tinfoil and are stored at 7 to 8 °C, again on edge. Because of the lack of oxygen the growth of the fungus slows down. Ripening, proteolysis, and lipolysis proceed further under the action of the proteolytic and lipolytic enzymes that have already been secreted in the cheese dough. This anaerobic phase lasts at least three months. A ripened cheese can be stored at 1 °C for another 5 to 10 months. After the conclusion of ripening, the cheeses are taken from the tin foil and are packed in aluminium foils or plastic bags. The high quality blue cheeses known in other European countries, such as Danish Blue, Bavaria Blu, and Bresse Bleu, are cheeses made from cows' milk which, however, is otherwise treated as in the manner of Roquefort. The speciality "Bavaria Blu" is a cheese in the interior of which the Roquefort fungus has grown but which has on the surface the white *Penicillium caseicolum.* It is therefore a true white-blue cheese.

Butter

Introduction

Butter is a plastic mass consisting mainly of milkfat that has been manufactured from fat-enriched milk (cream). It consists of 82 to 84% of fat, 14 to 16% of water, and 0.8 to 2% of nonfat solids.

Butter is marketed as sweet-cream or sour-cream butter. In the case of **sweet-cream butter** the cream is made into butter without the addition of the aroma- and acid-forming lactic acid bacteria that are used in the case of **sour-cream butter.** 86% of the butter manufactured in the Federal Republic of Germany is sour-cream butter. In a process recently developed in Holland (NIZO process), aroma-forming lactic acid bacteria are incorporated in an already prepared sweet-cream butter (van den Berg, 1976). This "soured" butter resembles conventional sour-cream butter in taste and keepability.

Salted butter, where it contains more than 0.1% of salt, must be labeled accordingly.

Manufacture (Flow sheet 9-18)

Treatment of the cream

The fat content of the cream is adjusted to 25 to 35% in the churn in the case of discontinuous buttermaking and to 35 to 50% in the buttermaking machine for the continuous process. Then the cream is subjected to a heat treatment (102 to 110°C). This serves to kill microorganisms and to inactivate proteolytic and lipolytic enzymes. After heating, the cream is cooled into the setting region of the fat, during which process the fat should crystallize out only partially.

The **cooling** and **ripening** of the **cream** form important phases in the technological course of buttermaking. They create the physical requisites for the crystallization of fat that is necessary for the formation of butter.

In the case of the production of sour-cream butter, the taste and aroma components that are typical for this product are formed by the lactic acid bacteria added to the cream. After being heated, the cream intended for **sweet-cream butter** is cooled to 6 to 8°C and is generally left to ripen to the following morning but in any case for at least two hours. During the cooling and storage of the cream crystallization processes take place in the butterfat.

The cream intended for **sour-cream butter,** after cooling, is inoculated in the cream ripener with 2 to 5% lactic acid bacteria. These microorganisms, known in practice as starter cultures are usually mixtures of the acid-forming *Streptococcus lactis* and *Streptococcus cremoris* with the predomonantly aroma-forming strains of *S. lactis* subsp. *diacetylactis* and of *Leuconostoc cremoris*. They convert the

Flow sheet 9-18. Technology of butter manufacture.

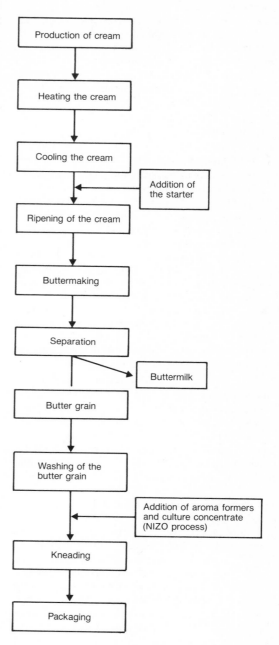

lactose present into lactic acid and the citric acid into biacetyl (butter aroma) and acetoin.

The ripening of the sour cream is completed at the desired pH (pH 4.8 to 5.0). The physical properties (e.g., spreadability) of the finished sour-cream butter are favorably affected by appropriate temperature control (cold-warm souring of winter cream and warm-cold souring of summer cream) during the course of the ripening of the cream.

Buttermaking

a) Batch process in the churn
Here buttermaking is carried out by the mechanical treatment of the cream which, because of the unsymmetrical construction of the churn in relation to the axis of rotation and its partial filling, is powerfully shaken and beaten as the churn is rotated (Mohr and Koenen, 1958). After agglomeration of the globules of fat into grains of butter (time: 40 to 60 min) and the drainage of the buttermilk, the butter grain is washed with cold water to eliminate adhering particles of buttermilk. The elimination of the protein- and sugar-rich particles of buttermilk leads to an improved protection of the butter against premature microbial spoilage. After washing, the butter grains are kneaded in the churn into a homogeneous mass of butter.

In kneading, salt, bubbles of air, and drops of buttermilk are worked into the mass. The distribution and size of the droplets of buttermilk have a decisive influence on the keepability of the butter. Droplets with diameters of less than 7 μm in the finished butter offer microorganisms no possibility for multiplication, which ensures good protection against microbial spoilage.

b) Continuous process in buttermaking machines
The first usable continuous machine for the manufacture of sweet-cream butter (Fritz, 1946) consisted essentially of a buttermaking cylinder and an extruder. In it, the cream was fed to the cylinder and was subjected there to the action of a high-speed rotating beater. After this intensive treatment of the cream, the butter grains formed in 3 to 35 seconds and they were then separated from the buttermilk on sieves. Then they were washed and were fed to the extruder for kneading. The homogenized butter mass left the machine as a continuous slab.

The modern **continuous buttermaking processes** have substantially driven batch buttermaking processes from the market.

The ripening of the cream with the addition of starters is time-consuming and requires a careful control of the course of the process. A direct addition of the starter to preprepared sweet-cream butter gives not only a saving of time but also advantages in relation to an optimization of the treatment of the cream (better crystallization of the fat) and of the cultivation of the starter (better aroma formation). In buttermaking by the NIZO process (p. 369), aroma-forming starters and the acid-forming filtrate from lactic acid bacteria, separately, are added in metered amounts to the sweet-cream butter. The aroma cultures added to the mixture are strains of *Streptococcus lactis* subsp. *diacetylactis* and of *Leuconostoc cremoris* grown in skim-milk. The last-mentioned strain is capable of transforming acetaldehyde (bad flavor) formed by the the the *S. lactis* subsp. *diacetylactis*. The bacterial filtrate is obtained from pasteurized whey after inoculation with *Lactobacillus helveticus,* and after the removal of the cell substance it is concentrated by evaporation. When 1 to 2% of the aroma-forming starter and 0.5 to 0.7% of the acid-forming concentrates are added, the biacetyl content of the finished butter is 1.5 to 2.0 mg/kg and the pH is 4.9 to 5.2. After storage for seven days, the biacetyl content rises to 2.2 to 2.5 mg/kg of butter and is then equal to that of sour-cream butter (Kessler, 1976).

Bacteriophage Problems in the Manufacture of Fermented Milk Products

Fermented milk products are manufactured with the use of lactic acid bacteria (lactic acid streptococci, lactobacilli). These microorganisms cause a rapid souring of the inoculated milk which inhibits the growth of undesirable microorganisms. Other metabolic actions (proteolysis, lipolysis, aroma, gas) affect the organoleptic properties of the finished products.

Disturbances to fermentation – souring, abnormal formation of aroma or gas – affect the quality of the product and may have serious economic consequences. Causes of disturbances in fermentation are: 1) genetic changes in the starter culture, 2) inhibitors in the milk (e.g., antibiotics, disinfectant residues), and, above all, 3) infections of the starter with bacteriophages. In the opinion of experts, today more than 80% of disturbances to fermentation are caused by **phages,** and the tendency is rising.

The phages of the lactic acid streptococci are very resistant to physical and chemical attacks. Pasteurization and spray-drying are incapable of inactivating them. They survive drying out in whey without harm. These phages are also extraordinarily resistant to many disinfectants.

Little is known about the nature of the phages of streptococci and their interactions with the host bacteria in the complex biotope "dairy." In the case of mesophilic – and recently also thermophilic – lactic acid streptococci, so far more than 25 types of phages capable of morphological differentiation have been isolated of which three are particularly important from the economic aspect (Lembke et al., 1980).

The dairy is a permanent **reservoir of phages,** and the fight against them is correspondingly difficult. Measures for combating phages include:

a) a use of mixedstrain starters in temporal alternation (rotation process),

b) a direct inoculation of the cheese vats with deep-frozen ($-196\,^{\circ}$C) starter concentrates,

c) a separation of cultivation and production units within the dairy, and, above all,

d) careful and regular cleansing and disinfection measures on all articles coming into contact with whey.

When these points are carefully observed, disturbances of fermentation due to phages can be kept within economically tolerable limits.

9.3.7 Meat and Sausage Products

Various types of fresh sausage, such as salami, cervelat (saveloy), and Mettwurst and also cured meat products such as hams, are **microbially ripened** meat products. The fermentation processes taking place during ripening have the aim not only of preservation but also of forming the aroma, taste, and color of the product.

Manufacture of Fresh Sausages

Fresh sausages are reddened sausage products which can be stored in the uncooled state (above $10\,^{\circ}$C) and are usually marketed in the uncooked form and which are spreadable or have become firm after a ripening process associated with drying out (Klein, Rabe and Weiss, 1980).

In the manufacture of fresh sausages, microbial starter cultures have been widely used for a long time. The composition of these cultures differs from region to region. Species of Penicillium, in particular, are used for the manufacture of raw sausages. They are applied only externally. The white, dry, uniform, and well-adhering coating of mold that forms on ripening imparts its characteristic aroma and appearance to the product (e.g., Hungarian or Italian salami). Only tested mycotoxin-free strains should be used for the inoculation of raw sausages with fungal cultures (Coretti, 1977).

The use of starter cultures increases production safety, shortens production time, and leads to an improvement of the quality of the end product. The bacteria added to the raw sausage mass rapidly multiply in it. The lactic acid arising from the enzymatic degradation of the muscle glycogen and added sugar lowers the pH to about 5 and below. This low pH value inhibits the growth of acid-sensitive spoilage organisms. In addition to this preservative action, the lowering of the pH also leads to changes in the consistency of the sausage mass. The isoelectric point of meat protein is at pH 5.3, and at this value the protein passes into a gel-like state. The solidity so arising is partially responsible for the firmness of the raw sausage.

The **nitrite** added to the raw mass with the curing salt is of decisive importance for the formation of the color. In the presence of reducing substances nitrite can be reduced chemically, and it can also be reduced by nitrite-reducing bacteria. The nitric oxide so produced binds with the myoglobin of the meat to form nitrosomyoglobin. This stable pigment complex imparts to the raw sausage the red color that is so prized by the consumer. In addition to the formation of the desired red coloration, the addition of nitrite also improves the keepability of the products in relation to bacterial spoilage. The addition of nitrite to meat products inhibits the development of pathogenic germs. Thus, the germination of *Clostridium botulinum* is prevented. Since nitrites can form carcinogenic nitrosamines with secondary and tertiary amines, their use in food technology is not uncontested (Lück, 1977). The degradation and transformation products formed from the carbohydrates, the fats, and the nitrogen-containing compounds of the meat during fermentation have a substantial effect on the aroma and taste of the product.

Cured Raw Meat Products

For the manufacture of raw cured products it is preferred to use parts of meat from the hindquarters. In essence, the following three methods of curing are used in practice (Liepe and Scheffold, 1978):

– Dry salting: in this process, the mixture of curing salts, containing mainly common salt, nitrate and/or nitrite, is thoroughly rubbed into the meat.

– Dry- and wet-curing: after dry salting, the pieces of meat are cured further in a brine.

– Injection curing: brine is injected into the pieces of meat by means of an automatic syringe, and the meat is subsequently also rubbed with curing salt mixture.

The curing phase proper is followed by a second phase of **postripening** and **drying** (scalding and hanging), sometimes with an additional **smoking** step.

The processes that take place in the meat during curing are the same in principle in all the three operations mentioned. Curing is a complex process in which changes take place in the meat that have physical, biochemical, and microbiological causes. Through the activity of the enzymes of the meat itself and the cooperation of curing bacteria, far-reaching changes take place in the color, aroma, taste, structure, and chemical state of the meat.

In contrast to the manufacture of dry sausages, in the curing of raw meat products the use of starter cultures has not come into general practice. This is due for the most part to our still inadequate knowledge of which microflora is to be regarded as typical and decisive for the result of curing. Micrococci of various species, vibrios, lactobacilli, and related species probably have a substantial effect on the course of a curing process. In addition to these species a number of other bacterial species have been found in the brine and on cured meat, but their influence in curing is obscure (Coretti, 1975).

Recently, an account has been given of experiments on the manufacture of cured products with the aid of starter cultures from *Staphylococcus simulans* (Liepe and Scheffold, 1978).

9.4 Starter and Ripening Cultures

9.4.1 Definition

By starter and ripening cultures are understood pure and mixed cultures of various microorganisms that are used for the manufacture of foodstuffs, semiluxury consumer articles, and fodders. They must be optimized for the desired purpose (see Table 9-5). Particular care must be taken that these cultures are not contaminated with spoilage-producing and pathogenic germs, since a multiplication of such germs in the manufacture of foodstuffs must be avoided under all circumstances.

9.4.2 Manufacture

Starter cultures are supplied as liquid cultures, in freeze-dried form, or deep frozen in liquid nitrogen by the culture manufacturer to the food industry and, in particular, to the milk-processing industry. While hitherto these cultures were used in the factories as mother cultures for the factories' own starters, the trend now is to **deep-frozen culture concentrates** or lyophilizates which permit a direct inocula-

Table 9-5. Examples of Starter and Ripening Cultures in Industry.

Product	Culture (conventional name)	Main functions of the culture
Fodders		
Silage (fermented fodder)	autochthonous lactic acid bacterial flora	preservation by spontaneous souring
	pure culture of *Lactobacillus plantarum*	promotion of spontaneous souring in order to avoid faulty fermentations
FACW (fermented ammoniated concentrated whey)	*Lactobacillus bulgaricus* (Stieber et al., 1977)	quantitative formation of ammonium lactate from the lactose of cheese whey for ruminant nutrition
Foodstuffs		
Sauerkraut, pickled gherkins	autochthonous lactic acid bacterial flora	preservation and the formation of flavor by spontaneous souring
Soy sauce, soybean paste	*Aspergillus oryzae*	formation of amylases for the hydrolysis of starch and proteases
	Pediococcus soyae, P. halophilus, S. faecalis, Saccharomyces rouxii and Torulopsis	lactic acid fermentation and alcoholic fermentation
White bread	bakers' yeast *(Saccharomyces cerevisiae)*	dough raising by the CO_2 from alcoholic fermentation

Table 9-5. Examples of Starter and Ripening Cultures in Industry.

Product	Culture (conventional name)	Main functions of the culture
Rye bread	pure culture sour (mixture of lactobacilli such as *L. brevis, L. fermentum, L. plantarum* with yeasts such as *S. cerevisiae, Candida krusei, Torulopsis holmii,* or *Pichia saitoi*)	lowering of the pH to 4.3 by lactic acid fermentation (optimum swelling of the rye constituents) taste formation by the products of hetero- and homolactic acid fermentation (e.g., acetic and lactic acids) raising of the dough by fermentation CO_2
Sour milk (curdled milk)	starter culture (homofermentative lactobacilli and lactic acid streptococci)	souring and preservation separation of the casein (curdling) formation of taste and aroma components
Yogurt	yogurt culture (*Streptococcus thermophilus* and *Lactobacillus bulgaricus* in a ratio of 1:1)	souring curdling aroma formation (acetaldehyde)
Quark (fresh cheese)	*Streptococcus lactis, S. cremoris*	curdling and souring aroma formation
Edam and Gouda cheeses	starter consisting of *S. lactis, S. cremoris, S. lactis* subsp. *diacetylactis, Leuconostoc cremoris*	souring aroma formation (biacetyl) and the formation of eyes by the CO_2 from citrate proteolysis (ripening)
Swiss cheese	spontaneous whey culture from previous production of commercial starter culture consisting of thermophilic lactobacilli such as *L. helveticus* and *Streptococcus thermophilus* propionic acid bacteria *(P. shermanii)*	souring (consumption of the lactose) proteolysis (ripening) formation of propionic acid as a flavor component and eye formation (CO_2 from lactate)

Table 9-5. Examples of Starter and Ripening Cultures in Industry.

Product	Culture (conventional name)	Main functions of the culture
Tilsit Harzer cheese Romadur Appenzeller	starter as for Edam cheese; additional red smear, yellow smear (*Brevibacterium linens*)	surface ripening: mature taste due to the action of lipases (free butyric acid from milkfat)
Camembert Brie	starter as for Edam cheese; in addition, fungal culture (spores of *Penicillium camemberti, P. caseicolum*)	ripening of the cheese from outside mainly by proteolysis (softening)
Roquefort Danish blue Edelpilzkäse Gorgonzola	starter as for Edam cheese; in addition, fungal culture (spores of *P. roqueforti*)	ripening and formation of a mature taste by lipolytic and proteolytic enzymes
Sour cream Sour-cream butter	creamery culture (starter) consisting of *S. cremoris, S. lactis, S. lactis* subsp. *diacetylactis*, and *Leuconostoc cremoris*	formation of acid production of aroma (biacetyl from citrate)
Raw ham Raw sausages Bologna	*Micrococcus aurantiacus* *Staphylococcus simulans* *Pediococcus cerevisiae* *Lactobacillus plantarum* *Lactobacillus brevis* *Streptomyces griseus*	formation of lactic acid, suppression of the causative agents of spoilage reduction of nitrate to nitrite (reddening) aroma formation mold coating, aroma, reduction of nitrate
Salami	*Penicillium nalgiovensis*	typical appearance of salami (fungal coating) and aroma

tion of the milk without an intermediate culture. In this way it is possible substantially to improve the microbiological safety of these milk industry fermentations, which take place under nonsterile conditions.

Manufacture of a freeze-dried yogurt culture (Tamine and Robinson 1976)

Step 1: Multiplication of the starter culture consisting of *Streptococcus thermophilus* and *Lactobacillus bulgaricus* in autoclaved reconstituted skim milk (16% dry matter); amount of inoculum: 2%, incubation at 42°C for 4 h.

Step 2: Storage of the culture at 5°C for 18 h, filling of 2 to 3 mL into sterile glass tubes, freezing at −40°C for 2 to 3 h.

Step 3: Freeze-drying (for up to 36 h).

Step 4: Sealing the tubes under vacuum.

Step 5: Dispatch and storage (5°C) until use.

Step 6: Reactivation
a) The contents of one tube are mixed with 250 mL of autoclaved reconstituted skim milk (9% dry matter) and are incubated at 42°C for 12 to 15 h.
b) In order to achieve full activity, subcultivation is carried out once or twice in the same medium with an inoculum of 2% and an incubation time of 4 h at 42°C. The ratio of *S. thermophilus* to *L. bulgaricus* should be 1:1.

Manufacture of concentrated deep-frozen starter cultures exemplified by lactic acid streptococci (Stanley, 1977)

The medium used is skim milk which has been digested by proteolytic enzymes such as papain to give a clear solution. The sterilized medium is inoculated with the desired culture, and incubated at 22°C for 16 to 18 h. For a high yield of cells the necessary pH in the weakly acid region must be maintained by an appropriate addition of alkali. The number of cells can also be increased by the addition of catalase, which destroys the hydrogen peroxide formed by the streptococci. At the end of the growth phase, the culture is rapidly cooled. The bacterial cells are separated from the medium in a self-cleansing separator and are filled semiautomatically into suitable disposable syringes which are frozen in liquid nitrogen and dispatched. In this way it is possible to manufacture culture concentrates which contain up to 10^{11} viable germs per mL. Similarly high germ numbers can be achieved when the lactate formed during cultivation is removed continuously by dialysis (Osborne, 1977).

Manufacture of *Penicillium roqueforti* spores (Moskowitz, 1979)

For the manufacture of the spores necessary for the inoculation of the cheese, *P. roqueforti* is cultivated on sterilized bread or on a nutrient agar containing casein and glucose. After 16 to 22 days the conidia are washed off and are freeze-dried ($5 \cdot 10^8$ spores/g) or are marketed as a liquid suspension. The manufacturing process must be carried out with great

care in order to prevent contamination with foreign fungi. *P. roqueforti* can be separated selectively from other fungi by growth on nutrient substrates containing 0.5% of acetic acid (Engel and Teuber, 1978).

Manufacture of spores of the Camembert fungus (Schulz, 1965)

Penicillium camemberti or *Penicillium caseicolum* is cultivated on wort agar or sterilized malt grains in the dark at 18 to 20°C. After the optimum formation of the conidia, they are washed off with common salt solution or mains water. These cultures should contain 1 to $5 \cdot 10^6$ or, even better, 2 to $5 \cdot 10^7$ spores capable of germination. In the case of good cultures, at least 20% of the spores should germinate on wort agar at 20 to 22°C within 8 to 10 hours. At refrigerator temperatures, good cultures can be kept for a maximum of 2 to 3 months.

9.5   Literature

Angevine, N. C., "Cures for some cottage cheese problems", *Cult. Dairy Prod. J.* **11** (14), 16–17 (1976).

Beck, Th., "Die Mikrobiologie der Gärfutterbereitung", *Wirtschaftseigenes Futter* **12**, 227–263 (1966).

van den Berg, G., "Eine alternative Methode für die Herstellung von Sauerrahmbutter", *Molk. Ztg. Welt der Milch* **30** (42), 1275 (1976).

Butscheck, G. and Kautzmann, R.: "Backhefefabrikation. In: *Die Hefen,* Vol. II. Verlag Hans Carl, Nürnberg 1962, pp. 501–504.

Coretti, K., "Rohwurst und Rohfleischwaren. II. Teil. Rohfleischwaren: Pökelprozeß und Pökelbakterien", *Fleischwirtschaft* **10**, 1365–1376 (1975).

Coretti, K., "Starterkulturen in der Fleischwirtschaft", *Fleischwirtschaft* **3**, 386–394 (1977).

Deutsche Gesellschaft für Ernährung e. V.: *Ernährungsbericht 1976.*

Diessel, W.: Vorrichtung zur Herstellung von Sauermilchquark. D.B.P. 1,942,488 (1976).

Dolle, E., "Technik des Thermoquark-Verfahrens", *Dtsch. Milchwirtsch. Gelsenkirchen Fed. Rep. Ger.* **28**, 709–712 (1977).

Eisenreich, L.: "Butter. Allgemeines und Herstellung". In: *Handbuch der Lebensmittelchemie,* Vol. III/Part 1: Tierische Lebensmittel. Springer-Verlag, Berlin, Heidelberg, New York 1968, pp. 447–476.

Engel, G. and Teuber, M., "Simple aid for the identification of *P. roqueforti* Thom", *Eur. J. Appl. Microbiol. Biotechnol.* **6**, 107–111 (1978).

Etchells, J. L., Fleming, H. P. and Bell, T. A.: "Factors influenzing the growth of lactic acid bacteria during fermentation of brined cucumbers". In: Carr, J. G., Cutting, C. V. and Whiting, G. G. (eds.): *Lactic Acid Bacteria in Beverages and Food.* Academic Press, London 1975, pp. 281–305.

Food and Agriculture Organisation: *FAO Production Yearbook* (1979).

Food and Agriculture Organisation: *FAO/WHO Report of the Joint Expert Committee on the code of principles concerning milk and milk products* (1977).

Forsyth, W. G. C. and Quesnel, W. C., "The mechanism of cacao curing", *Adv. Enzymol. Relat. Subj. Biochem.* **25**, 457–491 (1963).

Fritz, W., "Butterungsprozesse, neue Wege und Anschauungen", *Milchwissenschaft* **1/2**, 2–6 (1946).

Frank, H. A., Lum, N. A. and La Cruz, A. S., "Bacteria responsible for mucilage-layer decomposition in kana coffee cherries", *Appl. Microbiol.* **13**, 201–207 (1965).

Frank, H. K., "Milcheigene Faktoren, die das Wachstum von Joghurt-Bakterien beeinflussen können", *Milchwissenschaft* **24**, 269–276 (1969).

Gallmann, P. and Puhan, Z., "Anwendung der Ultrafiltration zur Herstellung von Kumys aus Kuhmilch", *Dtsch. Molk. Ztg.* **99** (36), 1244–1253 (1978).

Gesheva, B. and Rusev, P., "Gas chromatography and spectral method application for the study of the Bulgarian yoghurt flavour", *Nahrung* **23**, 385–392 (1979).

Grabbe, K. and Zadrazil, F., "Verwendung von Reststoffen pflanzlichen und tierischen Ursprungs im Pilzanbau", *Forum Mikrobiol.* **1**, 13–18 (1979).

Gross, F. and Riebe, K.: *Gärfutter.* Verlag Eugen Ulmer, Stuttgart 1974.

Hamdan, I. Y., Kunsmann, J. E. and Deane, D. D., "Acetaldehyde production by combined yoghurt cultures", *J. Dairy Sci.* **54**, 1080–1082 (1971).

Hang, Y. D., Downing, D. L., Stamer, J. R. and Splittstoesser, D. F., "Wastes generated in the manufacture of sauerkraut", *J. Milk Food Technol.* **35**, 432–435 (1972).

Hartmeier, W.: *Untersuchungen über die Kinetik der mikrobiellen Sauerstoff-Aufnahme und den Einfluß des Sauerstoff-Partialdruckes auf den Stoffwechsel von Saccharomyces cerevisiae.* Dissertation, TU Berlin 1972.

Hatch, R. T. and Finger, S. M.: "Mushroom fermentation". In: Peppler, H. J. and Perlman, D. (eds.): *Microbial Technology – Fermentation Technology,* Vol. II. Academic Press, Inc., New York 1979, pp. 179–199.

Jensen, C. O. and Pannele, H. P., "Fermenting of cigar-type tobacco", *Ind. Eng. Chem.* **42**, 519–522 (1950).

Johnson, J. C.: *Yeasts for food and other purposes.* Food Technology Review No. 45. Noyes Data Corporation, New Jersey, USA 1977.

Jones, J. D., Etchells, J. L., Veldhuis, M. K. and Voerhoft, O., "Pasteurization of genuine dill pickles", *Fruit Prod. J. Am. Vinegar Ind.* **20**, 304–307 (1941).

Kessler, H. G.: *Lebensmittel-Verfahrenstechnik – Schwerpunkt Molkereitechnologie.* A. Kessler-Verlag, Freising 1976.

Kielwein, G. and Melling, H., "Ein Beitrag zur Haltbarkeit von Sauermilch, Joghurt und Sauermilchquark", *Dtsch. Molk. Ztg.* **99**, 1023–1024 (1978).

Kiermeier, F. and Lechner, E.: *Milch und Milcherzeugnisse.* Verlag Paul Parey, Berlin, Hamburg 1973.

Klein, G., Rabe, H.-J. and Weiss, H.: *Lebensmittelrecht.* B. Behr's Verlag, Hamburg (State at January 1980).

Klupsch, H. J.: *Sauermilcherzeugnisse.* Verlag Th. Mann GmbH, Hildesheim 1968.

Kretzschmar, H.: *Hefe und Alkohol.* Springer-Verlag, Berlin, Göttingen, Heidelberg 1955.

Kretzschmar, H.: *Technische Mikrobiologie.* Verlag Paul Parey, Berlin, Hamburg (1968).

Lawrence, R. C., Thomas, T. D. and Terzaghi, B. E.,

"Reviews on the progress of dairy science: cheese starters", *J. Dairy Res.* **43,** 141–193 (1976).

Lembke, J., Krusch, U., Lompe, A. and Teuber, M., "Isolation and ultrastructure of bacteriophages of group N (lactic) streptococci", *Zentralblatt Bakteriol. Abt. 1 Orig. C* **1,** 79–91 (1980).

Liepe, H.-U. and Scheffold, A., "Probleme und Methoden der Pökelwarenherstellung", *Fleischwirtschaft* **8,** 1294–1297 (1978).

Loos, H. and Nebe, Th.: *Das Recht der Milchwirtschaft in der EWG und BRD,* Vol. III A 3 Milcherzeugnisse; A 5 Käseverordnung (State at 20. 3. 1980).

Lück, E.: *Chemische Lebensmittelkonservierung.* Springer-Verlag, Berlin 1977.

McDonald, P., "Trends in silage making", *Soc. Appl. Bacteriol. Symp. Ser.* **4,** 109–123 (1976).

Mair-Waldburg, H.: *Handbuch der Käse.* Volkswirtschaftlicher Verlag, Kempten 1974.

Mann, E. J., "Cottage cheese", *Dairy Ind. Int.* **41,** 372–353 (1976).

Mann, E. J., "Kefir", *Dairy Ind. Int.* **44,** 39, 41, 47 (1979).

Mann, E. J., „Cultured cream", *Dairy Ind. Int.* **45,** 29, 39, 59 (1980).

Mercier, J. E. et al., "Primary structure of bovine κ-casein", *Eur. J. Biochem.* **35** (2), 222–235 (1973).

Mohr, W. and Koenen, K.: *Die Butter.* Milchwirtschaftlicher Verlag Th. Mann, Hildesheim 1958.

Moon, N. J. and Reufold, G. W., "Commensalism and competition in mixed cultures of *Lactobacillus bulgaricus* and *Streptococcus thermophilus*", *J. Milk Food Technol.* **39,** 337–341 (1976).

Moskowitz, G. J.: "Inocula for blue-veined cheeses and blue cheese flavour". In: Peppler, H. J. and Perlman, D. (eds.): *Microbial Technology – Fermentation Technology,* Vol. **II.** Academic Press, New York, San Francisco, London 1979, pp. 201–210.

Müller, G.: *Mikrobiologie pflanzlicher Lebensmittel.* Dietrich Steinkopf-Verlag, Darmstadt 1974, pp. 151–154.

Niederauer, Th., "Cottage cheese: Herstellung und Eigenschaften", *Ernähr. Umsch.* **27,** 243–246 (1978).

Niederauer, Th., "Frischkäse: Herstellung und Eigenschaften", *Ernähr. Umsch.* **27,** 119–126 (1980).

Noel, C., Deschamps, A. M. and Lebeault, J. M., "Sauerkraut-fermentation: new fermentation vat", *Biotechnol. Lett.* **1,** 321–326 (1979).

Orth, A.: *Silage und ihre Verfütterung.* DLG-Verlag, Frankfurt/M. 1961.

Osborne, R. J. W., "Production of frozen concentrated cheese starters by diffusion culture", *J. Soc. Dairy Technol.* **30,** 40–44 (1977).

Pederson, C. S., "Sauerkraut", *Adv. Food Res.* **10,** 233–291 (1960).

Pederson, C. S.: *Microbiology of food fermentation,* 2nd Ed. AVI-Publishing Co, Inc., Westport, Conn. 1979.

Pederson, C. S. and Albury, M. N., "The influence of salt and temperature on the microflora of sauerkraut fermentation", *Food Technol. Chicago* **8,** 1–5 (1954).

Pederson, C. S. and Albury, M. N., "The sauerkraut fermentation", *Bull. N. J. Agric. Exp. Stn.* **824** (1969).

Peppler, H. J., "Yeasts", *Annu. Rep. Ferment. Processes* **2,** 191–202 (1978).

Perlman, O. (ed.): *Microbial Technology Fermentation Technology,* Vol. II. Academic Press, New York, San Francisco, London 1979, pp. 95–129.

Puhan, Z. and Banhegyi, M., "Beeinflussung des Verhältnisses *Lactobacillus bulgarius : Streptococcus thermophilus* in Joghurt durch die Bebrütungstemperatur", *Schweiz. Milchwirtsch. Forsch.* **3,** 9–13 (1974).

Puhan, Z., "Heat treatment of cultured dairy products", *J. Food Prot.* **42,** 890–894 (1979).

Rasić, J. Lj. and Kurmann, J. A.: *Yoghurt. Scientific grounds, technology, manufacture and preparations.* Stämpfli und Cie. AG, Bern 1978.

Robinson, R. K., Tamine, A. Y. and Chubb, L. W., "Acetaldehyde as an indicator of flavour intensity in yoghurt", *Milk Ind.* **79,** 4–6 (1977).

Saigin, I., "Bashkir horse", *Dairy Sci. Abstr.* **40,** 312 (1978).

Schamgin, V. K., Salaschko, L. S., Motschalova, K. Vj. and Pastuchova, S. M.: Verfahren zur Herstellung von Kumyß aus Kuhmilch. D.O.S. 2,555,146 A 1 (1977).

Schmidt, D. G., "Colloidal aspects of casein", *Neth. Milk Dairy J.* **34,** 42–64 (1980).

Schmidt, D. G. and Payens, T. A. J., Surf. Colloid Sci. **9,** 165–229 (1976).

Schulz, A.: "Backhefe und Bäckerei". In: *Die Hefe,*

Vol. II. Verlag Hans Carl, Nürnberg 1962, pp. 695–728.

Schulz, M. E., "Die Technologie der kontinuierlichen Sauerrahmbutter nach dem Separierverfahren", *Milchwissenschaft* **17**, 235–245 (1962).

Schulz, M. E. and Voss, E.: *Das große Molkerei-Lexikon*. Volkswirtschaftlicher Verlag, Kempten 1965.

Shankar, P. A. and Davies, F. L., "Associative bacterial growth in yoghurt starters; initial observations on stimulatory factors", *J. Soc. Dairy Technol.* **30**, 31–32 (1977).

Sharpe, M. E., "Lactic acid bacteria in the dairy industry", *J. Soc. Dairy Technol.* **32**, 9–18 (1979).

Souci, S. W., Fachmann, W. and Kraut, H.: *Die Zusammensetzung der Lebensmittel. Nährwert-Tabellen*. Wissenschaftliche Verlagsgemeinschaft mbH, Stuttgart (updated to 1979).

Speck, M. L., "Acidophilus food products", *Dev. Ind. Microbiol.* **19**, 95–101 (1978).

Spicher, G.: "Brot und andere Backwaren". In: *Ullmanns Encyclopädie der Technischen Chemie*. Vol. **8**. Verlag Chemie, Weinheim 1974, pp. 702–730.

Spicher, G. and Schröder, R., "Die Mikroflora des Sauerteiges. IV. Untersuchungen über die Art der in „Reinzuchtsauern" anzutreffenden stäbchenförmigen Milchsäurebakterien (genus *Lactobacillus Beijerinck*)", *Z. Lebensm. Unters. Forsch.* **167**, 342–354 (1978).

Spicher, G. and Schröder, R., „Die Mikroflora des Sauerteiges. VII. Untersuchungen über die Art der in „Reinzuchtsauer" auftretenden Hefen", *Z. Lebensm. Unters. Forsch.* **169**, 77–81 (1979).

Spicher, G. and Schröder, R., "Die Mikroflora des Sauerteiges. VIII. Die Faktoren des Wachstums der im „Reinzuchtsauer" auftretenden Hefen", *Z. Lebensm. Unters. Forsch.* **170**, 119–123 (1980).

Spreer, E.: *Technologie der Milchverarbeitung*. VEB Fachbuchverlag, Leipzig 1978.

Stamer, J. R., Dikinson, M. H., Brouke, J. B. and Stoyla, B. O., "Fermentation patterns of poorly fermenting cabbage hybrids", *Appl. Microbiol.* **18**, 323–327.

Stamer, J. R.: "Recent developments in the fermentations of sauerkraut". In: Carr, J. G., Cutting, C. V. and Whiting, G. C. (eds.): *Lactic Acid Bacteria in Beverages and Food*. Academic Press, New York 1973, pp. 267–280.

Stanley, G., "The manufacture of starters by batch fermentation and centrifugation to produce concentrates", *J. Soc. Dairy Technol.* **30**, 36–39 (1977).

Stieber, R. W., Coulman, G. A. and Gerhardt, P., "Dialysis continuous process for ammonium-lactate fermentation of whey: experimental tests", *J. Appl. Environm. Microbiol.* **34**, 733–739 (1977).

Tamine, A. Y. and Greig, R. I. W.: Some aspects of yoghurt technology. Dairy Industry Intern. **44** (9), 8–27 (1979).

Tamine, A. Y. and Robinson, R. K., "Recent developments in the production and preservation of starter cultures for yoghurt", *Dairy Ind. Int.* **41**, 408–411 (1976).

Veringa, H. A., Galesloot, T. E. and DaVelaar, H., "Symbiosis in yoghurt (II). Isolation and identification of a growth factor for *Lactobacillus bulgaricus* produced by *Streptococcus thermophilus*", *Neth. Milk Dairy J.* **22**, 114–120 (1968).

Wang, H. L. and Hesseltine, C. W.: "Mold-modified foods". In: Peppler, H. J. and Perlman, O. (eds.): *Microbial Technology – Fermentation Technology*, Vol II. Academic Press, New York, San Francisco, London 1979, pp. 95–129.

Weigmann, H.: "Das Reinzuchtsystem in der Butterbereitung und in der Käserei". In: Lafar, F. (ed.): *Handbuch der Technischen Mykologie*. Vol. 2. Mykologie der Nahrungsmittelgewerbe. Gustav Fischer Verlag, Jena 1905–1908, pp. 293–309.

Chapter 10

Fermentation Processes – Ethanol, Wine, Beer

Friedrich Drawert, Werner Klisch, and Gert Sommer

10.1 Ethanol

Friedrich Drawert and Werner Klisch

10.1.1 General Observations

The economic production of alcohol for nutritional and technical purposes is the business of the fermentation industry (alcohol industry). In wide areas, the process technique available for this purpose does not correspond to the state of modern technology of comparable sectors. Just as in other biotechnological processes, so also in the manufacture of alcohol is the creation of the optimum conditions (nutrient medium, temperature, pH, mass transfer, etc.) for suitable microorganisms of importance. The **nutrient substrate** necessary can be obtained from various starting materials (carbohydrates) which, for their part, determine the manufacturing process. In their choice, the costs of the raw material and of the processes involved (including energy costs) are in the foreground.

At the present time, the **fermentation process** (formation of alcohol) is overwhelmingly carried out discontinuously (batch process), but in principle it can also be performed continuously. The microorganisms used **(yeasts)** which bring about the formation of alcohol biochemically (enzymatically) are cultivated directly in the fermentation substrate, or as an external process step, in a suitable nutrient medium. At the present time, the alcohol of the fermented substrate is obtained exclusively by thermal separating processes **(distillation)**.

10.1.2 Importance of Alcohol

Ethanol (ethyl alcohol, C_2H_5OH) arises as the main product in the fermentation of sugar. The synthesis of alcohol from ethylene is losing importance because of its high costs. Ethyl alcohol is a colorless liquid with a burning taste and spirituous smell that is miscible with water in all proportions. Mixtures of ethanol and water are known as spirits. Absolute alcohol is spirit with less than 0.2% of water. Pure alcohol (A) exhibits a boiling point of 78.4°C (at 1013.25 hPa) and a density of 789.35 kg/m^3. It is combustible; its calorific value (H_u) is about 27 MJ/kg (or 6440 kcal/kg). Ethanol forms a stimulant with a definite physiological action and is a constituent of alcoholic beverages in the most various concentrations (Pieper et al., 1977; Wüstenfeld and Haeseler, 1964).

In the technical field, its use as a raw material (e.g., the basic material for chemosyntheses) and as an auxiliary material (e.g., as a solvent) in the chemical and cosmetic industry and in pharmacy and medicine is many-sided. Its use as a liquid energy carrier is gaining importance because of the cost and increasing shortage of petroleum; e.g., as a fuel for automobiles with alcohol engines or as an additive to gasoline for the purpose of reducing additions of lead (improvement in knock resistance), so that the pollution of the environment associated with this is decreased (Bernhardt et al., 1979; Bernhardt and Menrad, 1979; Pieper, 1981).

Brazil produced about 5 million m^3/year of ethanol for this purpose in 1983 (Schreier, 1980; Anderle, 1982). In the USA, the production of fermentation ethanol for fuel use amounted to 0.7 million m^3 in 1981 (PERP-Report 81-5).

10.1.3 Raw Materials

Basically, all raw materials can be used for the production of alcohol that contain either fermentable sugars or constituents (starch, cellulose) which can be converted into sugars by suitable treatment.

10.1.3.1 Alcohol-containing Raw Materials

To manufacture concentrated alcohol it is also possible to use raw materials in which alcohol has been formed previously by fermentation, e.g., wine, wine yeast, and wastes from the production of beer and yeast. Other raw materials and constituents have been given by Kreipe (1972, 1981) and Rehm (1980).

10.1.4 Auxiliary Materials

The addition of chemicals (acids, bases) or biochemical auxiliaries **(enzymes)** is necessary for the conversion (hydrolysis) of starch or cellulose into sugars. While the hydrolysis of starch is mostly performed enzymatically, at the present time the saccharification of cellulose is carried out overwhelmingly by chemical auxiliaries. Green and kiln-dried malt have lost importance as bearers of enzymes. Technical (microbial) enzymes (Gutcho, 1974; Aunstrup, 1978; Schreiber, 1980) are offered on the market in liquid and powder form for single use. The employment of suitable microorganisms and their culture broths that can provide the enzymes is conceivable. The use of **immobilized enzymes** is the aim of current research.

Because pure starch, cellulose, molasses, and fruit materials are deficient in nutrient materials for yeasts, they are upgraded by the addition of nitrogen compounds (ammonium salts) and growth, mineral, and buffer substances.

10.1.5 Fermenting Organisms (Yeasts)

Yests are single-celled fungi (eucaryotes) with a specific morphological structure and characteristic growth form (mean size about 7 to 9 μm). Their multiplication takes place by budding, in which cell division is subjected to mitosis (identical reproduction of the genetic material); under special conditions, spores are formed. In nature a multiplicity of species and variations exists with different physiological and physical properties. Yeasts are distinguished as cultivated yeasts *(Saccharomyces cerevi-*

siae), such are used in the brewery and distillery and elsewhere, and wild yeasts (mold yeasts, Candida species etc.). Cultivated yeasts are obtained as pure-culture yeasts from a single cell (Reiff et al., 1961, 1962).

The special metabolic and physiological properties of yeasts consist in their rapid conversion of sugars into alcohol. Almost all yeasts can ferment the monosaccharides glucose, fructose, and many can also ferment galactose. Of the disaccharides, sucrose and maltose are fermented by the majority of yeasts. Some yeasts can also ferment lactose, melibiose, and trehalose – although only after relatively long adaptation – and also the trisaccharide raffinose.

Depending on the supply of oxygen, yeast cells are capable of performing respiration under aerobic conditions (metabolism for cell formation) and a fermentation metabolism (production of energy) under anaerobic conditions (Pasteur effect). The cells can still multiply at concentrations of alcohol of up to about 10 vol %. In the fermentation metabolism, up to 18 vol % of alcohol is tolerated. However, the specific growth rate or specific rate of fermentation falls off with increasing concentration of alcohol. The special physical properties of yeasts include their capacity for **agglomeration** (flocculation), as occurs in the so-called **flocculating yeasts,** and therefore for sedimentation.

On the other hand, other yeasts exist as single cells and therefore possess a certain capacity for remaining suspended in the nutrient substrate **("powdery yeasts").** Of prime interest for the production of alcohol are highly fermenting races of yeast (so-called **fermentation yeasts, distillery yeasts**), which produce a large amount of alcohol in a very short time (high rate of fermentation) with a high alcohol tolerance. The **fermentation capacity** of the various yeasts is mainly determined by their enzyme content ("zymase complex"). Also of importance for multiplication and fermentation are the temperature (20 to 35 °C) and the pH (3.5 to 6) of the extracellular medium. The demand for nutrients and growth substances of yeast is largely known (Reiff et al., 1961, 1962). Under aerobic conditions they possess the capacity of synthesizing certain substrates "essential" for an anaerobic medium. The **metabolism of the formation of alcohol** as a special form of the dissimilatory metabolism and also as part of the intermediate total metabolism of the yeast cell has been described in some detail by Karlson (1977). In simplified representation, the disproportionation of sugar (hexoses) to ethanol and carbon dioxide (CO_2) is an exothermic reaction:

$$C_6H_{12}O_6 \rightarrow 2C_2H_5OH + 2CO_2 \quad \Delta H = -84 \text{ kJ.}$$

It takes place in a total of 12 enzymatically catalyzed reaction steps. Some of the heat of the reaction is converted into biochemically utilizable energy (ATP). In the yeast cell, the ATP (adenosine triphosphate) acts as a source of energy for a number of reactions which, using the most diverse substrates, lead to new cell substances.

10.1.6 Preparation of the Fermentation Substrate

The fermentation process proper is preceded by the **production of a suitable fermentation substrate** (sugar solution, wort, mash). The total liquefaction of all plant cell structures (e.g., crude fibers) by their conversion into small fragments in dissolved form by an exclusively biochemical pathway has not so far been possible because of the long reaction times. A more or less satisfactory liquefaction is achieved by mechanical and/or thermal means with a combined or subsequent chemical and biological treatment depending on the initial raw material. For many raw materials a pretreatment (e.g., purification) is necessary.

10.1.6.1 Sugar-containing Raw Materials

Sugar-containing raw materials in liquid form, e.g., molasses, are adjusted to a sugar concentration (g of sugar/L) that is favorable for an optimum fermentation and, if necessary, they are improved by the addition of nutrients and growth substances. If the pH is unfavorable, this is corrected. Solid sugar-containing raw materials are disintegrated by mechanical comminution (milling), e.g., fruit materials (by fruit cutters) or sugar cane (by cane mills) so as to make the sugars accessible to the yeast. In the case of sugar cane and sugar beet, the juice may also be obtained in extraction units. In the case of sugar beet, the consumption of energy amounts to about 1 MJ/L A (A = alcohol; Misselhorn, 1980).

10.1.6.2 Starch-containing Raw Materials

Starch-containing raw materials require different pretreatments for processing into a fermentable mash according to the particular raw material used. While grains can be processed without pretreatment, tubers or roots must be freed from adherent soil by a washing process. The subsequent disintegration of cell structures of the raw material is carried out mechanically (milling, e.g. by hammer mills), thermally (boiling, steaming), or as a combined process. The combined **milling and cooking process** is encountered predominantly in the USA in the processing of cereals (Scheller, 1977; Prescott and Dunn, 1949).

The **hydrolysis of starch** (saccharification) is carried out mainly by an enzymatic method. Karlson (1977) has given information on the chemical structure of starch (amylum) and the mode of action of amylases. Native starch is hardly soluble, and in this form it cannot be hydrolyzed enzymatically. Enzymatic hydrolysis must be preceded by the gelatinization (hydration) of the starch (at about 65 to 80°C). If the raw material is milled, gelatinization must take place during milling or as a subsequent process step.

The preparation of mashes by the classical process is carried out discontinuously in a Henze steam cooker (disintegration of the raw material, and gelatinization of the starch) and in a mash tun. In the mash tun the starch is hydrolyzed enzymatically to fermentable sugars at temperatures between 55 °C (saccharification with glucoamylase) and 85 °C (liquefaction with α-amylase) (Fig. 10-1).

However, **high-pressure steaming** (4 to 6 bar = 150 to 165 °C) promotes Maillard reactions which lead, on the one hand, to losses of sugar (lower yields of alcohol) and on the other hand to undesired reaction products (3-phenylfuran) (Misselhorn and Brückner, 1979), which can have a toxic action on fermentation organisms. The discontinuous mode of operation is associated with a high input of energy (6 to 8 MJ/L A). Only a small part of the thermal energy supplied can be recovered. The recovery of heat can be realized only in continuous processes. The development of usable processes has very recently been pursued with great intensity. In such processes, the gelatinization and saccharification of the starch must be preceded by mechanical comminution (milling) of the raw material. Kreipe (1980) has reported on a discontinuous process for the disintegration (grinding) and digestion of cereals into mashes ("cold mash process"). Borud (1971) has described a continuous steaming and mashing process which works according to well-known principles and can be used for the production of mash from starch production wastes.

The **basic principle for a continuous process** for the treatment of starch-containing raw materials, which can be regarded as the state of the art, has been described by Misselhorn (1980). In this process, the complete recovery of heat is not yet realized, and part of it is removed via cooling water. The temperature difference of the material flows between the raw material inlet and the mash outlet is about 40 °C. The energy consumption has been given as about 2 MJ/L A. A pure countercurrent process in the gelatinization region is aimed at (Fig. 10-2).

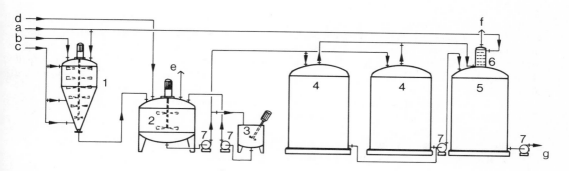

Fig. 10-1. Raw material disintegration, starch saccharification, and fermentation by the classical process (after Misselhorn, K. and Starcosa GmbH, 1980).

1 = steam cooker (Henze)
2 = mash tun
3 = pure culture container
4 = fermentation tank
5 = intermediate container
6 = carbon dioxide washer
7 = pump

a = process water
b = starch-containing raw materials
c = steam
d = enzymes
e = exhaust steam
f = carbon dioxide
g = fermented mash to distillation

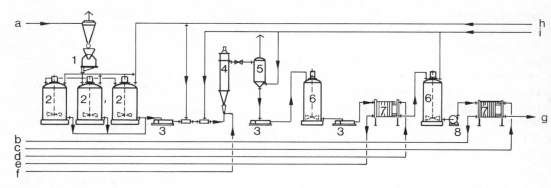

Fig. 10-2. Scheme of a plant for the continuous digestion of starch-containing raw materials into fermentable mashes (after Misselhorn, K. and Starcosa GmbH, 1980).

1 = scales	a = raw material, cleaned and comminuted
2 = mashing tank	b = deep-cooling water outlet
3 = special pump	c = deep-cooling water inlet
4 = converter	d = cooling water inlet
5 = cyclone separator	e = cooling water outlet
6 = mash container	f = steam
7 = cooler	g = saccharified mash (sweet mash)
8 = pump	h = caustic soda
	i = enzymes

A process (Supramyl process) for the gelatinization and saccharification of suspensions with up to 40% of starch dry matter has been described briefly by Stegemann (1980) and Misselhorn (1981). The marked rise in viscosity which usually occurs during the gelatinization of starch is avoided by thermomechanical gelatinization in the Supraton machine. The energy demand for this continuous process is about 0.7 MJ/L A.

The continuous preparation of mash with a unit characterized by extremely fine comminution of the raw material has been carried out successfully on the semitechnical (Drawert, 1979) and, in modified form, on the technical scale (Klisch and Drawert, 1982). The coarse, preliminary, comminution of the raw material is followed by extremely fine milling (particle size less than 100 μm) and the gelatinization of the starch by indirect (Thermalizer-heat exchanger) or direct (injection of steam) heat exchange. The feed of enzymes for saccharification is carried out continuously. Heat can be recovered by countercurrent heat exchange. The consumption of energy, without the recovery of heat is about 2 MJ/L A.

In the **enzymatic hydrolysis of starch,** in a very short time (15 to 30 min) a degree of saccharification (glucose, maltose, maltotriose) of from only about 40% (technical enzymes) to about 80% (malt enzymes) is achieved, the residue remaining as oligosaccharides. The saccharification enzyme is competitively inhibited by the low-molecular-weight products (product inhibition). When the sugars are removed (by dialysis or fermentation) there is an immediate secondary saccharification.

10.1.6.3 Cellulose-containing Raw Materials

At the present time, **acid hydrolysis** is the usual method by which simple sugars (especially glucose) can be prepared from cellulose and hemicellulose on the large technical scale. However, acid hydrolysis exhibits several disadvantages (Dellweg, 1978), such as high capital costs (operating costs), the destruction by a high concentration of acid of glucose already formed, undesirable side reactions, and the environment-polluting conversion products (e.g., gypsum). About 200 processes for the saccharification of wood are known but differ by their choice of acid and their technology. For economic reasons and process-engineering considerations (recovery of acid), only a few processes have acquired importance on the large technical scale.

In the **Bergius process** (Rheinau process), the cellulose hydrolysis of the precomminuted material (timber wastes) is preceded by a prehydrolysis (hemicellulose hydrolysis) in a countercurrent diffusion battery with a high concentration of acid. As the acid flows through the material its concentration in the hydrolysate falls and the sugar content rises to a maximum of 30%. The hydrolysate is evaporated in vacuum to a sugar syrup (recovery of the hydrochloric acid) and is subjected to a secondary hydrolysis. Purification follows demineralization (ion-exchange), evaporation, and crystallization (Fig. 10-3). The yield from 100 kg of dry matter of coniferous wood is about 55 kg of wood sugar, of which about 70% is glucose (Kretzschmar, 1955).

The **Scholler-Tornesch process** works by the percolation principle (pressure percolation). The cellulose of wood chips is hydrolyzed at a low concentration of acid (H_2SO_4) under the pressure-pulse-like action of steam (about 8 bar) at temperatures of 170 to 180°C. The hydrolysate obtained contains about 5 to 6% of fermentable sugars. The solution is neutralized with lime and can be concentrated to form a wood-sugar molasses. The lignin arising is burnt to obtain operating energy (Kretzschmar, 1955).

At Madison in the USA the Scholler process has been modified and improved with the aim of achieving higher yields.

The firm Projektierung Chemische Verfahrenstechnik has made known a **digestion process** for the production of sugars from plant residues and wastes (broad-leaved and coniferous trees, straw, bagasse). The raw materials are comminuted by conventional processes and are digested in a special cooking process (saturated steam, about 160 to 230°C). In the following refiner, the still hot material is disintegrated and in various washing steps is leached successively with water (recovery of xylan) and with an aqueous solution of alkali (0.6% NaOH). The fi-

brous residue can be hydrolyzed enzymatically in spite of its high lignin content.

Very recently, because of the disadvantages in acid hydrolysis, processes have been discussed and realized on the laboratory and technical scale in which **the cellulose is hydrolyzed enzymatically.** So far no processes on the large technical scale have become known. In contrast to the acid digestion processes, cellulolytic enzymes act specifically; there are no side reactions and, moreover, they do not require extreme conditions of temperature and pH. It is preferred to use **cellulase-forming microorganisms,** in order to avoid the use of expensive cellulase preparations (two to three times more expensive than, for example, amylases). In general, thermophilic (temperature > 55°C) microorganisms (e.g., actinomycetes, clostridia, sporocytophages) have advantages over mesophilic organisms (e.g., *Trichoderma reesii*), since they are characterized by faster growth, greater enzymatic activity, and more stable enzyme systems (Bellamy, 1978).

In the present state of the process, the conversion of about 50% of the cellulose (waste cellulose) into low-molecular-weight sugars, mainly glucose, has been mastered. In plants, lignin, as a protective sheathing of the cellulose, prevents enzymatic hydrolysis. The lignocellulose material must therefore be comminuted to form particles smaller than 100 μm ("pulverization", creation of a surface for the adsorption of enzymes) in order to liberate at least a large part of the cellulose [or it may be subjected to other pretreatments: steam (about 180°C) or NaOH]. The fact that total hydrolysis takes place *in vitro* only slowly must be ascribed to the predominantly crystalline structure of native cellulose (β-1,4-glucan chains), which opposes the penetration of water and enzyme molecules, and to inhibitory mechanisms (competitive inhibition and assumed substrate inhibition).

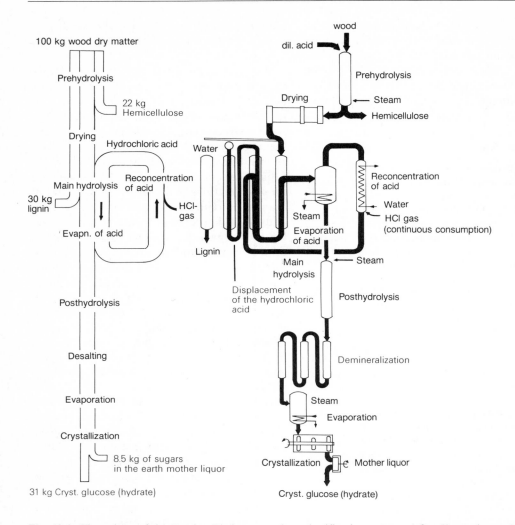

Fig. 10-3. Flow sheet of the Bergius-Rheinau wood saccharification process (after Kretzschmar, 1955).

The results of some groups of workers (e.g., Bruchmann or Dellweg) show the difficulty that must be reckoned with in a technological utilization. In the case of the enzymatic degradation of cellulose by fungal cellulases it may be assumed today that an endoglucanase attacks the native cellulose, an exoglucanase degrades this to cellobiose, and the cellobiose is finally cleaved by a β-glucosidase to form glucose. A distinction must also be made between fungal cellulases and bacterial cellulases; Bruchmann (1973, 1979) and Schmid (1977) have dealt in very great detail with the inhibition of cellulolysis and also with the optimization of the bacterial fermentation of cellulose, for example, by the addition of manganese(II) salts. Linko (1978) has recently come to the conclusion that *Trichoderma reesii* – earlier known as *Trichoderma viride* – is the most suitable microorganism for the production of a stable cellulase complex that catalytically accelerates the hydrolysis of native cellulose. As a rule, the formation of cellulases can be observed only when the organisms grow in the presence of cellulose or of cellobiose, sophorose, gentiobiose, or lactose, which all contain a β-glucosidic bond. According to Pathak and Ghose (1973), sophorose induces the formation of cellulases about 200 times more strongly than cellobiose. The total reaction is highly inhibited by the product. However, Yamane et al. (1970) have established that with a low concentration of sugars in the culture medium the addition of a source of carbon such as glucose, mannose, or cellobiose stimulates the production of cellulases. This finding was later confirmed by Nagai et al. (1976), who found that a controlled addition of a source of carbon to *Trichoderma reesii* cultures intensifies the formation of hydrolases. The extracellular formation of cellulases by fungi can be intensified by the addition of surface-active agents to the culture medium, as is also known in other cases.

Processes are being sought that will eliminate unfavorable inhibition mechanisms. In a two-stage process, the glucose formed is eliminated with a dialysate, e.g., by membrane filtration, while unconverted cellulose and the enzyme are returned to the saccharification reactor (residence time about 48 h; degree of saccharification about 60%). The conversion of the sugar into ethanol is carried out in a separate reactor (Ghose and Kostick, 1970). Single-stage processes work with mixed cultures. Gauss (1979) has described a one-stage process in which *Trichoderma reesii* (fermentation of cellulose) and *Saccharomyces cerevisiae* (formation of ethanol) are active simultaneously. Inhibition by cellobiose or glucose is avoided by the fact that the sugars formed are fermented immediately. It has not been possible to detect the mycolytic action of the cellulases in relation to yeast cells that was originally assumed.

In mixed cultures of thermophilic organisms, the hydrolysis of cellulose is carried out, for example, with sporocytophages and the formation of ethanol by a suitable bacillus at 50 to 65°C and pH 7 to 8 (Bellamy, 1978).

In order to avoid inhibitions of the bacillus and of the cellulases by alcohol, the alcohol formed can be drawn off during fermentation by means of a partial vacuum (130 to 530 hPa).

The **production of enzymes** proves to be the **main cost factor** in the enzymatic degradation of cellulose. As compared with batch processes, it has been possible to achieve a greater production with cell recycling systems in cell cultivation (multiplication). In place of the culture broth, the supernatant obtained by cell separation (sedimentation, centrifugation) has been used for the hydrolysis of cellulose (Wilke et al., 1976).

10.1.7 Formation of Ethanol

10.1.7.1 Classical Fermentation Process

The actual formation of ethanol takes place during alcoholic fermentation. Under practical conditions, 1 kg of sugar (sucrose) gives about 0.6 L of ethanol, and 1 kg of starch about 0.65 L (about 90% of theory).

In the classical process, the fermentation of worts (e.g., molasses) or mashes takes place in fermentation vessels suitable for the purpose (tanks, vats) as a **batch process**. The yeast necessary for fermentation is cultivated in a separate process step. In the fermentation of molasses, the continuous multiplication of the working yeast takes place in a prefermentation tank in sterilized molasses and it is distributed in the necessary amount over the main fermentation tanks. After distillation, the yeast that was present in the fermented wort remains in the slop (stillage) (see Fig. 10-1 and Fig. 10-4). In the case of clear fermentation media such as molasses, the yeast can be separated off before distillation and be used to inoculate (pitch) the substrate arising for fermentation (Fig. 10-6). In this way a high concentration of cells and their rapid fermentation (24 to 36 h) can be achieved. However, this mode of operation opens up the possibility of infection.

The sugar content of the molasses is adjusted to 14 to 16% which permits an alcohol

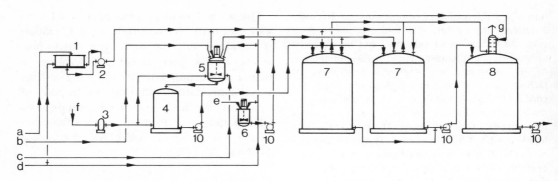

Fig. 10-4. Scheme of a unit for fermenting molasses by the classical process (Misselhorn, K. and Starcosa GmbH, 1980).

1 = molasses mixing station	a = molasses
2 = mixing pump	b = sulfuric acid
3 = blower	c = steam
4 = prefermentation tank	d = process water
5 = molasses boiler and pure culture container	e = nutrient salts
6 = preparation of nutrient salts	f = air
7 = main fermentation tank	g = carbon dioxide
8 = intermediate container	h = fermented molasses to distillation
9 = carbon dioxide washer	
10 = pump	

content of 8 to 10 vol% in the fermented wort (Kretzschmar, 1955).

In the case of mashes from starch-containing raw materials, because of its solid-matter content the recovery of the yeast from the fermented mash is impossible. A separate yeast mash ("artificial yeast") must be processed. The amount of amylolytic enzymes used for the saccharification of the starch affects not only the concentration of yeast cells but also the time of fermentation (36 to 72 h). Depending on the initial raw material, the extract content of the mashes ranges between 16% and 19%. Of the total extract about 80 to 90% is fermentable.

The **course of fermentation** is essentially characterized by three part-sections which pass into one another. During the first 12 to 24 hours, a pronounced multiplication of the yeast takes place with the consumption of the oxygen present. By the introduction of additional oxygen, the multiplication of the yeast and, therefore, fermentation can be forced, with a simultaneous protection against infection. In the middle phase (12 to 48 h), there is a predominant formation of alcohol with the postsaccharification of oligosaccharides, and the multiplication of the yeast falls off. The following stage (48 to 72 h) is characterized by an asymptotically decreasing formation of alcohol and insignificant multiplication of the yeast. The fermentation activity of the yeast liberates heat, particularly during the phase of alcohol formation so that the temperature of the fermentation substrate rises to 40 °C (removal of heat by cooling). Typical curves for alcohol, extract, pH and temperature, are shown in Fig. 10-5. Ethanol entrained by the carbon dioxide arising in fermentation is recovered by a special washing process ("car-

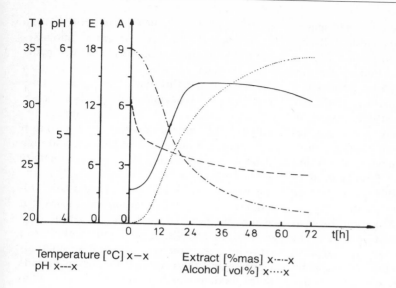

Temperature [°C] x—x
pH x---x

Extract [%mas] x----x
Alcohol [vol%] x····x

Fig. 10-5. Typical curves of various parameters in classical fermentation.

bon dioxide wash", see Fig. 10-1 and 10-4). A shortening of the time of fermentation to 36 to 48 h can be achieved in the case of mashes by means of a higher pitching temperature and a larger amount of yeast mash (Kreipe, 1972, 1981).

Propagation of Yeast

Normally, in potato and cereal distilleries the mash is inoculated with compressed yeast (about 0.3 kg YDM/m³ of mash; YDM = yeast dry matter) or with pure-culture yeast only at the beginning of the working period. Subsequently, pitching is carried out with **"artificial yeast,"** a part-mash which is cultivated as yeast mash. From the main mash pitched first, about 5 to 10% is taken as yeast mash and after the simplified sulfuric acid process at pH 2.5 to 3.5 it is treated first under quasi-pure-culture conditions. After an incubation time of about 24 h, it is used again to inoculate a new main mash from which, again the yeast mash is diverted off. The "artificial yeast propagation" ensures that on each working day a well matured powerfully fermenting, and infection-poor yeast is available (Kreipe, 1972, 1981; Goslich, 1981). The process originally developed by Delbrück using cultures of lactic acid bacteria is of no importance today.

10.1.7.2 Semi-Continuous Fermentation Processes

A continuous stream of mash (wort) can be fermented and fermented mash (or wort) can be distilled continuously by means of the **cyclic filling and emptying** of a battery of fermentation vessels. In this case, the pitching of fresh fermentation substrate is carried out with material from the main fermentation stage. Such a procedure harbors the risk of the introduction of infection.

10.1.7.3 Continuous Fermentation Processes

Fermentation processes in which a suitable system is supplied continuously with fermentation substrate and fermented substrate is run off in equal amount (and which permit the expectation of an improvement in the space-time yield) have not yet been successfully introduced because of infections and degeneration of the yeast. Their use is limited to a few cases e.g., sulfite waste liquors, wood-sugar worts (Reiff et al., 1961, 1962) (Fig. 10-6), and whey. However, very recently efforts have been made to ferment molasses and mashes continuously, as well. In addition to multistage processes such as are envisaged in wood sugar fermentation and the fermentation of brewers worts (Bishop, 1970), single-stage processes stand out as the most suitable.

The principle of the fermentation tower as it has come into use to a small extent in the brewery industry, has also been investigated, in modified form, and so have other systems, e.g., stirred tanks, loop reactors, etc., (Rehm, 1980; Mössner et al., 1979). Basic criteria for a continuous process of fermenting molasses and mashes from starch-containing raw materials have been given by Goslich (1972) and by Dellweg et al. (Engelbart, 1978). If the requirement for **economic efficiency** is to be satisfied, simple and robust systems (fermenters) with suitable microorganisms must ensure a high output, a high yield of alcohol, and high alcohol concentration. The total productivity of a plant is decisively affected not only by the specific rates of fermentation (and alcohol tolerance) of the fermentation organisms but also by the local concentration situation (concentrations of cells, sugars, and alcohol) as a consequence of the sedimentation of microorganisms and the evolution of carbon dioxide (back-mixing) which makes definite flow con-

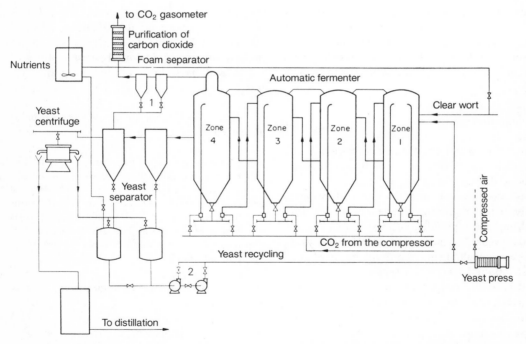

Fig. 10-6. Flow sheet for the continuous manufacture of ethanol from wood sugar solution (after Reiff et al., 1961, 1962).
1 = Foam separator; 2 = centrifugal separators

ditions necessary. Other prerequisites are optimum relationships between nutrient, temperature, pH, and oxygen concentration (0.2 to 5 mg O_2/g YDM), and limited concentrations of sugar (0.5 to 1 g/L) in the fermentation substrate. The achievement of the necessary cell concentration (g YDM/L), to which the rate of fermentation is directly related, can be realized in clear fermentation substrates with the preferential use of flocculating yeasts and suitable retention or recycling systems (sedimentation, centrifugation).

The **principle of yeast recycling** can be realized only if mashes obtained from cereals, potatoes, or fruits which contain solid matter (up to 10%) are liquefied totally or crude fibers, etc., are separated by decantation or filtration. In contrast to classical ideas, in aerobiosis with the strict limitation of glucose high yields of alcohol can be obtained. The rapidly growing populations arising under these conditions are, moreover, less susceptible to infection (Fiechter, 1979; Engelbart, 1979a, 1979b). In the case of typical distillers' yeasts, a maximum specific rate of fermentation of about 1 mL A/g YDM·h can be observed. It falls off when the concentration of alcohol in the fermentation substrate is about 6%. The **maximum rate of fermentation** corresponds to the differential at the point of inflection of the alcohol curve of a batch fermentation. The productivity of a plant is defined as the amount of alcohol formed referred to a definite time and amount of fermentation substrate (L A/m³·d) for a desired concentration of alcohol. In addition to the throughput of substrate (of the input of sugars) and the required productivity, the specific rate of fermentation and the concentration of cells (which determine the rate of fermentation) form essential characteristics in the dimensioning of fermenter systems.

Misselhorn (1979) has described a two-stage unit consisting of two prefermenters and one tower for the fermentation of molasses. The yeast from the tower can be returned to the fermenter. It has been operated with an ordinary distillers' yeast and a flocculating yeast. A suitable concentration of yeast in the prefermenter proved to be 30 to 40 g YDM/L of fermentation substrate. A mean residence time of the yeast in the system (avoidance of overageing of the population), of 7 to 8 cycles (= 50 to 100 h) was found, 15 to 30% of the effluent yeast having to be removed. At 30 g YDM/L in the system and 9 g YDM/L (about 30%) in the effluent, this gives for 9 vol% A a yield of only 80% of theory (Fig. 10-7). The flow sheet of a single-stage process with yeast recycling for the fermentation of sugar-containing raw materials has been given by Faust, Präve, and Sukatsch (1979). A flocculating strain of yeasts with a high cell density (about 50 to 60 g YDM/L) is present in an airlift loop reactor. Because of the spontaneous fermentation of the sugar added (sugar content of the fermentation substrate 14 to 16%, pH = 5), the concentration of free sugar remains below 0.1% (about 0.2 g/L). The process is carried out under aerobic conditions, and the yeast entrained in the effluent from the reactor is substantially retained in a special separating vessel (sedimenter) so that it can be returned to the fermenter. The bulk of the yeast-free fermented wort (ethanol content up to 8.5 vol%, pH = 4) then flows to the distillation section (Fig. 10-8). The use of a Waagner-Biró submerged reactor for the fermentation of molasses and cereal worts has been reported by Meyrath (1979). The system works with flocculating yeast. The yeast entrained from the fermenter is retained in a sedimentation vessel and is returned to the reactor via a homogenizing device. The gassing system, which is connected with the yeast recycling device permits a high utilization of the atmospheric oxygen. Alcohol concentrations of up to 10 vol% can be achieved in one step. Advantages of the system that have been mentioned are small reactor volumes, no tendency to con-

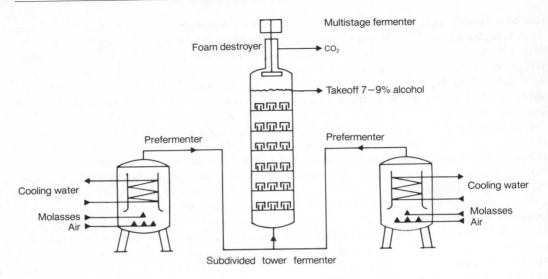

Fig. 10-7. Plant for the continuous fermentation of molasses (after Misselhorn, 1979).

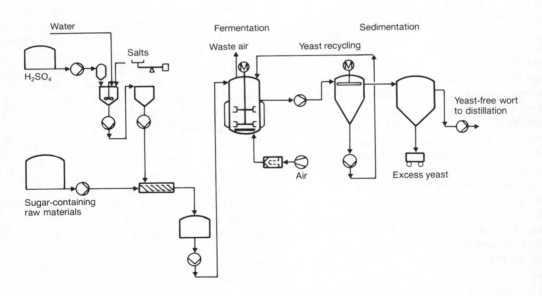

Fig. 10-8. Flow sheet of a one-stage process with yeast recycling for the continuous fermentation of clear fermentation substrates (Faust et al., 1979).

tamination, and a higher quality of the crude alcohol.

10.1.7.4 By-products of Fermentation

In alcoholic fermentation, in addition to the main products ethanol and carbon dioxide, a number of other metabolic products are produced which are combined under the term by-products of fermentation. The most important of them include methanol, higher alcohols such as propyl, butyl and amyl alcohols (so-called fusel oils), glycerol, acetaldehyde, esters (mainly of acetic acid), and various acids, of which succinic acid, in particular, contributes to the fall in the pH during fermentation. Fusel oil alcohols arise mainly in the metabolism of the yeast from amino acids which, after decarboxylation and deamination are hydrogenated to the alcohols having one C atom less. Crude spirits may contain up to 0.5% of fusel oil.

10.1.8 Recovery of Ethanol (Distillation)

The separation of the ethanol from the fermented substrate is currently performed exclusively by distillation (Kirschbaum, 1960; Klisch, 1981). Distillation and rectification are **thermal processes for separating** mixtures of liquids that are based on the fundamental operations of evaporation and condensation. Separation takes place here as the result of **different boiling behaviors** (boiling points and vapor pressures) of the individual components (e.g.; ethanol = readily boiling; water = difficultly boiling). On evaporation, the vapor contains more of the readily boiling components than the liquid mixture. A measure of the enrichment of the low-boiling component in the vapor of a liquid mixture is the relative volatility, which is expressed as the ratio of the saturated vapor pressures (or boiling points) of the **pure** components at a given temperature of the mixture. The greater the relative volatility is, the more readily can the mixture be separated

by distillation. In a boiling liquid mixture, at constant pressure an equilibrium between liquid and vapor exists, since the same number of liquid molecules passes into the vapor phase (evaporates) in unit time as vapor molecules return to the liquid phase (condense). Such a boiling equilibrium also exists when only **one** component (e.g., ethanol) is considered. Figures 10-9a and b show graphically the boiling and condensation curves and the liquid-vapor equilibrium curve for the ethanol-water binary mixture at 1013.25 hPa (760 torr). The **boiling and condensation curves** show the relationship between boiling point (or condensation point) and vapor or liquid concentration. The boiling point of the mixture (= mash) falls with increasing concentration of alcohol X. When the liquid and vapor phases are in equilibrium, the **equilibrium curve** gives the alcohol content in the vapor Y and therefore the theoretically possible increase in concentration $s_{theor} = Y/X$ as a function of the alcohol content of the mixture X. On the 45° line (X = Y), the molar concentrations in the vapor and liquid are equal and no enrichment of the alcohol in the vapor takes place. For ethanol-water this is the case at 97.2 vol% (= 89.5 mol%). The point of intersection between the equilibrium curve and the 45° line is known as the **azeotropic point**, and here the boiling temperature reaches its lowest value of 78.15°C (boiling point of pure ethanol = 78.4°C). Only one of the components of a binary mixture that forms an azeotrope can be separated in the pure state on distillation (bottom product: water).

In the case of **simple distillation**, the mixed vapor is condensed without reflux, giving a distillate. No further enrichment of alcohol in the vapor takes place in the connecting conduit between the evaporator (stillpot, boiler) and the condenser (liquefier). If, in distillation, in addition to the distillate condenser a reflux condenser (dephlegmator) is used, the vapor of the high-boiling component con-

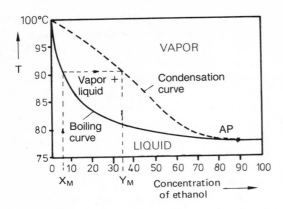

Fig. 10-9 a. Boiling and condensation curves for a liquid mixture of ethanol and water (Klisch, 1981).
X   = ethanol in the liquid
Y   = concentration of ethanol in the vapor
AP = azeotropic point
X and Y in mol/100 mol

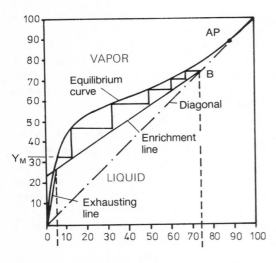

Fig. 10-9 b. Liquid-vapor equilibrium curve for ethanol-water at atmospheric pressure (Klisch, 1981).

denses in the latter and flows back as a condensate so that the low-boiling components are further enriched in the vapor. If the low-boiling components are to be obtained at higher concentration, the distillate must be subjected to a further distillation (**rectification**). The enrichment of the low-boiling components in the mixed vapor and of the high-boiling components in the liquid is achieved by a continuous countercurrent of vapor and condensate in a vertical exchange column (rectifying column) with appropriate separating stages (plates). By the continuous supply of heat to the evaporator (boiler) and continuous cooling in the dephlegmator, a circulation of material through rising vapor and the reflux of the condensate is achieved throughout the column. At each separating step (e.g., bubble tray) an exchange of mass and heat takes place. High-boiling material condenses from the vapor and is enriched in the liquid, the temperature of which increases continuously in the direction of flow. Low-boiling material evaporates because of the heat of condensation being liberated from the liquid and becomes enriched in the vapor, the temperature of which decreases continuously in the direction of flow. Rectification can be performed only when part of the vapor (overhead product) is liquefied in the dephlegmator (mainly the high-boiling components) and the condensate (reflux) is fed back to the head of the column. In the dephlegmator, the reflux heat to be removed is used for preheating the mash (heat exchange).

The **reflux number** (reflux ratio) gives the ratio of the amount of reflux to the amount of distillate produced. With an infinitely large number of theoretical **separating steps** (theoretical limiting case), a minimum reflux ratio v_{min} is obtained which depends on the concentration of the distillate X_{dist} and the concentration of the mixture (alcohol content of the mash) X_M.

$$v_{min} = \frac{X_{dist} - Y_M}{Y_M - X_M}$$

Y_M is taken from the equilibrium curve (Fig. 10-9).

So that a finite number of theoretical separating steps can be realized in practice, the minimum reflux ratio must be increased by a finite amount (v = practical reflux ratio).

To prepare a distillate of the desired strength (X_{dist}) from a mixture of given concentration (X_M), a definite number of separating steps (or concentrating plates) is necessary. By a **theoretical separating step or plate** is understood the height of a unit of the separating column within which the vapor and the liquid reach boiling equilibrium by mass exchange. With the aid of the equilibrium curve and the enrichment line [it is derived from v and X_{dist} and lies between the points A ($Y_{oi} Y_o = X_{dist}/(v+1)$) and B], the number of theoretical **concentrating plates** can be determined graphically from the representation of the lines of the individual slopes. Each corner point from the equilibrium curve corresponds to a theoretical plate n_{theor} (see Fig. 10-9b). The enrichment curves give the theoretically possible enrichment in each case. In practice, the various factors, such as the reflux ratio, the constructional arrangement of the plates (depth of penetration of the vapor, exchange processes), and the velocity of the vapor (loading of the vapor with liquid), cause a decrease of the theoretically possible enrichment ratio. The actual enrichment ratio s is therefore below s_{theor} for which ideal mass and heating exchange behavior is presupposed.

The number of rectifying plates necessary in practice, n_{pract}, is determined on the basis of the mean enrichment ratio $s_m = s/s_{theor}$ (≈ 0.6 to 0.8); $n_{pract} = n_{theor}/s_m$. The mean enrichment ratio is called the efficiency $\eta = s_m \cdot 100 [\%]$ of a plate. The number of plates (**boiling plates** $n_{pract} \approx 15$) of the beer still (mash or exhausting column) and the rectifying column is determined by the exhausting line (see Fig. 9b).

An important relationship exists between the reflux ratio and the number of separating steps. The smaller the reflux ratio, the larger is the number of plates necessary and the smaller is the demand for heat energy of the distillation-rectification plant.

Crude spirits usually have an ethanol content of more than 85% and include a (certain) amount of fermentation by-products. This is the form in which they arise in grain and potato distilleries with 20-tray beer stills. An energy of 5 to 6.5 M J/L A must be used for this distillation and concentration in 1- or 2-step distillation units.

The **purification of crude spirits** (separation of fermentation by-products by a process for high quality alcohol) in a distillation-rectification unit (50- to 55-tray rectifying column [B, D], 45-tray aldehyde column [C]) according to Fig. 10-10, requires an energy consumption of about 9 MJ/L A. The alcohol content of the main fraction **(Primasprit)** is close to that of the azeotrope. With an improved interconnection of the individual columns, the consumption of energy can be lowered to about 6 MJ/L A (Misselhorn, 1979).

Absolute alcohol (more than 99% A) is obtained by the addition of a so-called entraining agent, e.g., cylohexane, to the azeotrope, whereupon the minimum boiling point disappears (Fig. 10-11). The entraining agent can be recovered in a special recovery column. The dehydration is carried out in a 50 tray dewatering column. Dehydration consumes about 4 MJ/L A.

A reduction in the consumption of energy in the manufacture of absolute alcohol can be achieved only by multistage distillation in columns with different pressures or by using the heat pump principle.

A two-pressure distillation and dehydration unit with a total consumption of energy of about 5.5 MJ/L A has been described by Misselhorn (1981).

10.1.9 Utilization of Slop (Stillage)

By slop (stillage) is understood essentially the by-products from which the alcohol has been

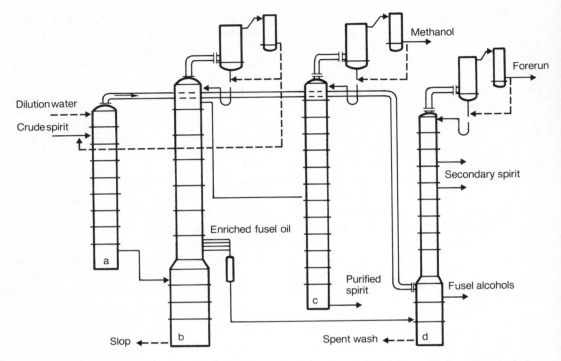

Fig. 10-10. Scheme of a rectification plant for the purification of crude spirit to a high-quality alcohol (Acker et al., 1970).

removed by distillation (beer still bottoms product) arising in the manufacture of alcohol. Slop separated from its solid matter can be reused in the process as dilution water for cerals or cassava. With the direct heating of a distillation unit (column), i.e., the feed of steam into the mash, 1 m³ of mash gives about 1,1 m³ of slop while with indirect heating the figure is about 0,9 m³. The slop contains all the unfermented constituents of the mash, particularly the nutrient materials protein, fat, crude fiber, and minerals. It forms a valuable **cattle feed.** Slops from clear solutions (sugar cane, molasses), as also the slops from cereals or potatoes, contain the whole of the amount of yeast used, provided that it has not been separated off. The last-mentioned slop in particular, can be used, with the appropriate ad-

ditives, for the production of **biomass.** To solve the problem of effluents, the yeast fermentation of the slop alone, for instance, is inadequate, for only part of the BOD (biological oxygen demand) load is decomposed in the yeast fermentation. Slop and also pomace can be digested: the anaerobic degradation of the organic matter gives rise to about 0.5 to 0.6 m³ of **biogas** per kg of BOD_5. The biogas so obtained has a net calorific value of 20 to 25 MJ/m^3.

10.1.10 Potable Alcohol

Spirituous beverages include two main categories, the spirits and the liqueurs (Wüstenfeld, 1964). **Spirits** are always direct products

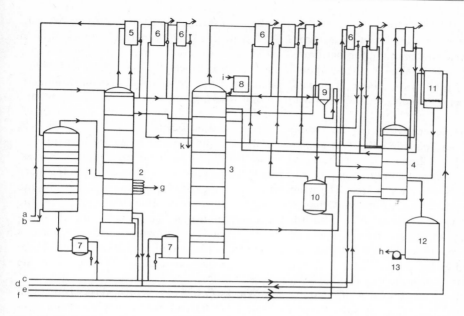

Fig. 10-11. Scheme of plant for the production of absolute alcohol (after Misselhorn, K. and Starcosa GmbH, 1980).

1 = mash column (beer still)
2 = rectification column
3 = dewatering column (azeotropic distillation)
4 = recovery column
5 = preheating condenser
6 = condenser
7 = forced circulation evaporator
8 = entraining agent reservoir
9 = decanter
10 = alcohol cooler
11 = washer
12 = storage tank
13 = pump

a = mash (beer feed)
b = slop (stillage)
c = steam
d = slop (stillage)
e = process water
f = cooling water
g = fusel oil
h = absolute alcohol (pure ethanol)
i = entraining agent
k = aldehydes

of the distillery which, after rectification, are simply diluted with water to drinking strength if necessary. They are sometimes stored for a certain time and occasionally contain aroma-imparting or improving additives. Also to be included here are those products which consist of highly concentrated industrial spirit, water, and aromatic substances determining their particular nature, together with small amounts of sugars or extracts.

In contrast to this, **liqueurs** are products with a comparatively high sugar content of at least 22 g/100 mL and with minimum alcohol contents which are laid down for the individual varieties.

Spirits are extract-free or extract-poor spirituous beverages with or without taste ingredients. The alcohol content must be at least 32%. Spirits are classified as: wine brandy, schnapps, rum, arrack, grain brandy, whisk(e)y, fruit brandy (from stone fruits, berries, and variety-pure apples and pears, fruit spirits, and pomaceous brandy), juniper brandies (Steinhäger, gin, wacholder, Geneva) and special spirits (spirits from roots, fruit and wine residues, yeast brandies, Enzian, aquavit, vodka, bitters).

Cognac is a wine brandy which, according to French law, can be made only from grapes of an accurately delimited area (Charente, Dordogne, Deux Sèvres) and only by the producers themselves in the given area. The wine must not be sugared and no material change after its import is impossible. Today, the still yeast-containing wines are mainly distilled from simple direct-fired copper pot-stills using only a head giving a weak reflux. All the alcohol is driven over in the first firing, giving a brouillis with 25 to 35 vol% of alcohol. About three brouillis are then subjected to fine distillation together in the same or, better, a special but similarly constructed still.

Armagnac enjoys the same legal protection in relation to the name of its origin as Cognac and comes from the south of France, Gascony and its departments. Since not as much yeast is left in the wine for distilling, Armagnac is usually not so "soapy" as Cognac but it has a full ester and aromatic, and sometimes tart, flavor.

German brandy is made mainly from foreign wines, the importation of which is favored by the Customs regulations. The imported wines for distillation, usually turbid with yeast, are tested for their suitability for importation. Both the wine proper and also the wine distillate used for strengthening must correspond to the regulations of the wine law. In contrast to the manufacture of Cognac and Armagnac, German brandy is manufactured overwhelmingly by column distillation in order to obtain a comparatively mild final distillate.

Every brandy is stored in oak barrels (Limousin oak), in Germany for at least six months. During this time the distillate "ages",

taking up extractives from the wood. After dilution to drinking strength (38 to 44%), as a rule, certain aroma-imparting ingredients are added for characterization e.g., wine-distillate extracts from chips of Limousin wood, almond shells, green walnuts, and dried plums, and also caramel, dessert wine, and sugar syrup or caramel syrup.

Rum is spirits obtained by the fermentation and distillation of sugar cane juice, molasses, or syrup or other materials arising in the manufacture of crude sugar and obtained by the manufacturing processes customary in the country of origin. Rum distilleries are operated in countries growing sugar cane, such as Jamaica, Cuba, Haiti, and Puerto Rico. There are extraordinary quality differences in the case of rum.

Whisky (whiskey): **Scotch whisky** is distilled from a mash that must be obtained from cereals saccharified with malt diastase. It must mature in the barrels for at least three years. A distinction is made between malt whisky and grain whisky. The former is produced exclusively from barley malt in pot stills, while the latter has as the starting material various species of cereals, primarily rye, but also unmalted barley, corn, and oats and is almost always distilled in column apparatuses (patent stills). The barley is malted in the usual way and the malt grains are exposed directly to the smoke of burning peat or even of coal. Storage is carried out in wooden barrels, mainly of American oak, or in sherry barrels that have previously been used for the export of sherries; occasionally, internally charred barrels are also used. Scotch whisky is marketed almost exclusively as a mixture of malt and grain whiskies (blended).

Irish whiskey is a pure pot-still whisky from 30 to 50% of barley malt together with unmalted barley, rye, oats, and wheat.

American whiskey (whisky) consists essentially of two types, rye whiskey and Bourbon whiskey. The starting material for rye whiskey must consist of at least 51% of rye. The starting material for Bourbon whiskey contains at least 51% of corn (maize), with some rye, and barley malt is used for saccharification.

Canadian whisky is comparable in its types with US whiskey; it is stored in charred oak barrels for 2 to 8 years.

Kirsch is the first among the **fruit brandies.** The cherries are harvested without stalks and are usually mashed without grinding. As a rule, the breaking of the pits leads to a pungent bitter almond taste. After fermentation, taking place spontaneously or brought about by the addition of pure-culture yeast, the mashes are distilled in fruit stills (Pieper, 1977).

Plum brandy, mirabelle brandy, and apricot and peach brandies are obtained similarly. The production of "fruit spirits" by steeping fruit in brandy is permitted only in the case of peaches and apricots.

In addition to these brandies from stone fruits, **pomaceous brandies** produced from variety-pure pears and apples enjoy great popularity. In contrast to stone fruit, the pomaceous fruit must be macerated well before fermentation. The process is otherwise the same.

Berry brandies are produced from rowanberries, currants, gooseberries, elderberries, bilberries, and rose hips. Here, in otherwise similar processes, the so-called berry spirits play a large part. The ripe, fresh, and, so far as possible, unfermented fruit is treated in the still or in other containers with undiluted alcohol (40 to 100 L per 100 kg of fruit). The charges are allowed to stand for about a day and are then distilled. Raspberry spirit, blackberry spirit, blackcurrant spirit, and bilberry spirit are known.

Among **juniper brandies** are included Steinhäger, gin, wacholder, and geneva. Wacholder is a brandy manufactured from spirits and/or grain distillate with the addition of juniper distillate and/or juniper low wine. Steinhäger is a brandy which is produced exclusively by distillation using juniper singles from fermented juniper mash. Gin is a spirit produced with the use of distillates from juniper berries and herbs.

Under **grain brandy** and other cereal brandies (apart from whisky) are included products from barley, wheat, rye, oats, and buckwheat. Here, in the preparation of the mash, the starch must be broken down by mechanical destruction of the cell walls (bruising), gelatinization at 70 to 80°C, and saccharification with the aid of technical enzymes or through the addition of granulated barley malt. After mashing, fermentation is carried out with the addition of yeast, and distillation as already described.

Vodka (Russian: little water) is a spirit produced from the middle run after two rectifications of potato spirit or from spirit and/or grain distillate according to a special process, possibly with small amounts of additives. The processes and the additives must, in particular, emphasize the characteristic feature of vodka, the mildness of the taste. The extract content must not exceed 0.3 g in 100 mL. Coumarin-containing grasses, such as buffalo grass and holy grass, are used for imparting aroma. The alcohol content must be at least 40 vol%.

10.1.11   Literature

Acker, L., Bergner, K.-G., Diemair, W., Heinemann, W., Kiermeier, F., Schormüller, J. and Souci, S. W.: *Handbuch der Lebensmittelchemie.* Vol. VII. Springer-Verlag, Berlin, Heidelberg, New York 1965/70, p. 530.

Anderle, G., "Die Herstellung von 1,2 Mio. Liter Alkohol/Tag. Beispiel des Brasilianischen Alkoholplanes". 5. *Symp. Techn. Mikrobiol.* Verlag Versuchs- und Lehranstalt f. Spiritusfabrikation, Berlin 1982, p. 435.

Aunstrup, K., "Enzymes of industrial interest; traditional products", *Annu. Rep. Ferment. Processes* **2,** 125 (1978).

Bellamy, W. D., Schenectady, N. Y. (USA): Herstellung von Ethanol aus Cellulose. D.O.S. 2,808,932 (1978).

Bernhardt, W., Menrad, H. and König, A., "Ethanol aus Biomasse als zukünftiger Kraftstoff für Automobile", *Starch/Stärke* **8,** 254 (1979).

Bernhardt, W. and Menrad, H., "Äthanol aus Biomasse als Kraftstoff für Automobile", *4. Symp. Techn. Mikrobiol.* Verlag Versuchs- und Lehranstalt f. Spiritusfabrikation, Berlin 1979, p. 18.

Bishop, L. R., "A system of continuous fermentation", *J. Inst. Brew.* **76,** 172 (1970).

Borud, O. J., "Verwertung von Abfällen der kartoffelverarbeitenden Industrie", *Starch/Stärke* **23,** 172 (1971).

Bruchmann, E.-E., Betsch, E., Ghafuri, M., Knupfer, H., Lauster, M., Layer, P. and Schmid, S., "Beitrag zur Kenntnis des Einflusses funktioneller Gruppen in Cellulose auf ihre Spaltbarkeit durch ein mikrobielles Cellulase-System", *3. Symp. Techn. Mikrobiol.* Verlag Versuchs- und Lehranstalt f. Spiritusfabrikation, Berlin 1973, p. 533.

Bruchmann, E.-E., "Verfahrensoptimierung auf biochemischer Grundlage – erläutert an der enzymatischen Celluloseverzuckerung", *Z. Lebensmitteltechnol. Verfahrenstech.* **30,** 240 (1979).

Cysewski, G. R. and Wilke, C. R., "Rapid ethanol fermentation using vacuum and cell recycle", *Biotechnol. Bioeng.* **19,** 1125 (1977).

Dellweg, H., "Verwendung cellulosehaltiger Rohstoffe in der Fermentationsindustrie", *Branntweinwirtschaft* **118,** 101 (1978).

Drawert, F., In: "Biokonversion", *2. BMFT-Statusseminar „Bioverfahrenstechnik"*, Berlin 1979.

Engelbart, W., Offer, G. and Dellweg, H., "Beitrag zur Entwicklung kontinuierlicher Verfahren für die Erzeugung von Alkohol aus stärkehaltigen Rohstoffen", *3. Symp. Techn. Mikrobiol.* Verlag Versuchs- und Lehranstalt f. Spiritusfabrikation, Berlin 1973, p. 157.

Engelbart, W., "Kontinuierliche Vergärung von Maischen aus stärkehaltigen Rohstoffen", *Branntweinwirtschaft* **118,** 17, 57 (1978).

Engelbart, W., "Vergärung von Zuckersäften", *4. Symp. Techn. Mikrobiol.* Verlag Versuchs- und

Lehranstalt f. Spiritusfabrikation, Berlin 1979 a, p. 57.

Engelbart, W., "Hefevermehrung bei mikroaerober alkoholischer Gärung", *4. Symp. Techn. Mikrobiol.* Verlag Versuchs- und Lehranstalt f. Spiritusfabrikation, Berlin 1979 b, p. 85.

Faust, U., Präve, P. and Sukatsch, D. A., "Kontinuierliche Äthanolherstellung durch ein Gärverfahren der Hoechst/Uhde-Biotechnologie", *4. Symp. Techn. Mikrobiol.* Verlag Versuchs- und Lehranstalt f. Spiritusfabrikation, Berlin 1979, p. 37.

Fiechter, A., "Zur Regulation der Aethanolbildung in Hefe", *4. Symp. Techn. Mikrobiol.* Verlag Versuchs- und Lehranstalt f. Spiritusfabrikation, Berlin 1979, p. 75.

Gauss, W. F., Suzuki, Sh., Takagi, M. and Toda, S.: Herstellung von Alkohol aus Cellulose. D.O.S. 2,541,960 (1979).

Ghose, T. K. and Kostick, M., "Enzymatic saccharification of cellulose in semi- and continously agitated systems", *Biotechnol. Bioeng.* **12,** 921 (1970).

Goslich, V., "Versuche zur Entwicklung eines Verfahrens zur kontinuierlichen Vergärung von Melasse", *Branntweinwirtschaft* **112,** 285 (1972).

Goslich, V., "Kontrolle der Hefesatzführung". *Brennerei-Kalender* 1981, p. 307.

Gutcho, S. J., "Microbial enzyme production", *Chem. Technol. Rev.* **28,** Noyes Data Corporation, London 1974.

Karlson, P.: *Lehrbuch der Biochemie.* Thieme-Verlag, Stuttgart 1977.

Kirschbaum, E.: *Destillier- und Rektifiziertechnik.* Springer-Verlag, Berlin, Göttingen, Heidelberg 1960.

Klisch, W., "Betrachtungen über den Destillationsprozeß". *Brennerei-Kalender* 1981, p. 285.

Klisch, W. and Drawert, F., *Branntweinwirtschaft* **122,** 102–105 (1982).

Kreipe, H., *Technologie der Getreide- und Kartoffelbrennerei.* Verlag Hans Carl, Nürnberg 1972.

Kreipe, H.: "Getreide- und Kartoffelbrennerei". In.: *Handbuch der Getränketechnologie.* Ulmer Verlag, Stuttgart 1981.

Kreipe, H., "Wird das „Kaltmaischverfahren" wieder interessant?", *Branntweinwirtschaft* **120,** 354 (1980).

Kretzschmar, H.: *Hefe und Alkohol.* Springer-Verlag, Berlin, Göttingen, Heidelberg 1955.

Linko, P., "Über die Herstellung von Cellulasen und die enzymatische Spaltung von Cellulose", *Chem. Ing. Tech.* **9**, 655 (1978).

Meyrath, J., "Das ALCO-FLOC-System, eine kontinuierliche und zuverlässige Methode zur Äthanolproduktion mit extrem hoher Produktivität", *4. Symp. Techn. Mikrobiol.* Verlag Versuchs- und Lehranstalt f. Spiritusfabrikation, Berlin 1979, p. 107.

Misselhorn, K., "Äthanolherstellung unter energiewirtschaftlichem Aspekt – Stand der Technik", *4. Symp. Techn. Mikrobiol.* Verlag Versuchs- und Lehranstalt f. Spiritusfabrikation, Berlin 1979, p. 47.

Misselhorn, K. and Brückner, H., "Flüchtige Maillardprodukte und ihre Wirkung auf die Atmung der Hefe", *4. Symp. Techn. Mikrobiol.* Verlag Versuchs- und Lehranstalt f. Spiritusfabrikation, Berlin 1979, p. 95.

Misselhorn, K. and Starcosa GmbH, Braunschweig, "Äthanol als Energiequelle und chemischer Rohstoff", *Branntweinwirtschaft* **120**, 2 (1980).

Misselhorn, K., "Ethanol als biotechnologische Energiequelle", *Chem. Ing. Tech.* **53**, 47–50 (1981).

Mössner, G., Ramspeck, W. and Sittig, W., "Bioreaktoren im Vergleich mit chemischen Reaktoren", *Chem. Tech. Heidelberg* **8**, 329 (1980).

Nagai, S., Onodera, M. and Aiba, S., "Kinetics of extracellular cellulase and amylase production from Trichoderma sp.", *Eur. J. Appl. Microbiol.* **3**, 9 (1976).

Pathak, A. and Ghose, T. K., *Process Biochem.* **4**, 35 (1973).

Pieper, H. J., "Aktuelle Forschungsergebnisse der Alkoholtechnologie", *Z. Lebensmitteltechnol. Verfahrenstech.* **5**, 200 (1980).

Pieper, H. J., "Aspekte zum gegenwärtigen Stand brennereitechnologischer Entwicklung". *Brennerei-Kalender* 1981, p. 257.

Pieper, H. J., Bruchmann, E.-E. and Kolb, E.: *Technologie der Obstbrennerei.* Ulmer-Verlag, Stuttgart 1977.

Pieper, H. J.: "Betrachtungen zur Produktion von Gärungsalkohol als Energieträger". *Die Kleinbrennerei,* **33**, 1, 14 (1981).

Prescott, S. C. and Dunn, C. G.: *Industrial Microbiology.* McGraw-Hill Book Company, Inc. New York, Toronto, London 1949.

Projektierung Chemische Verfahrenstechnik GmbH, Düsseldorf, D.O.S. 2,732,327 (1978).

Rehm, H. J.: *Industrielle Mikrobiologie.* Springer-Verlag, Berlin, Heidelberg, New York 1980.

Reiff, F., Kautzmann, R., Lüers, H. and Lindemann, M.: *Die Hefen,* Vol. I, II. Verlag Hans Carl, Nürnberg 1961, 1962.

Scheller, W. A., "The production of ethanol by the fermentation of grain", *Intern. Symp. on Alcohol Fuel Techn.,* Vol. III. Volkswagenwerk AG, Wolfsburg, 1977.

Schmid, S.: *Beitrag zur Cellulosefermentation durch aerobe, mesophile Bakterien, insbesondere Wirkung von Spurenelementen auf Celluloseabbau und Biomasseproduktion.* Dissertation, Universität Hohenheim, 1977.

Schreiber, W., "Enzymtechnologie – ein Zweig der technischen Biochemie", *Z. Lebensmitteltechnol. Verfahrenstech.* **6**, 252 (1980).

Schreier, K., "Praktische Erfahrungen beim Bau und Betrieb großer Äthanolanlagen in Brasilien", *Branntweinwirtschaft* **120**, 82 (1980).

Stegemann, J., "SUPRAMYL – ein Verfahrensschritt für die Herstellung von Energiealkohol", *Alkohol-Industrie* **11**, 272 (1980).

Wilke, C. R., Stockar, U. V. and Yang, R. D., "Process design basis for enzymatic hydrolysis of newsprint", *AIChE Symp. Ser.,* No. 158, Vol. **72**, 104 (1976).

Wüstenfeld, H. and Haeseler, G.: *Trinkbranntwein und Liköre.* Paul Parey-Verlag, Berlin, Hamburg 1964.

Yamane, K., Suzuki, H., Hirotani, M., Ozawa, H. and Nishizawa, K., "Effect of nature and supply of carbon sources in cellulase formation in Pseudomonas fluorescens var. cellulosa", *J. Biochem. Tokyo* **67**, 9 (1970).

10.2   *Wine*

Friedrich Drawert and Werner Klisch

10.2.1   *General Observation*

The technology of wine preparation is characterized world-wide both by the production of high-quality wines (e.g., France, Germany) and also ordinary wines (France, Italy, Spain, etc.).

In EG-VO (EC marketing order) No. 3282/73, Art. 3, the preparation of wine is described generally as the processing of fresh wine grapes or mashes, grape must, concentrated grape must, grape juice, concentrated grape juice, or young wine to form wine by complete or partial alcoholic fermentation. The possibilities mentioned already indicate a pronounced technical intervention in wine preparation, the critical question to be posed being whether sufficient facts are known about essential constituents, e.g., the fermentation substrate, resulting from individual technological measures. Since in the preparation of wine, continuous processes are known only in experimental setups but hardly in practice, it is very much a question of optimizing the current techniques or technologies with the aim of improving quality.

The composition and therefore the quality of the wine can best be represented and understood if wine is regarded as the end product of a **biotechnological sequence** (Drawert and Rapp, 1969) (Fig. 10-12).

The biological stages of this series contribute in a definite way and manner to the linkage of biochemical and chemical reactions through specific metabolic processes to bring about a modification of the constituents in which the particular importance is attached to the **biogenesis** of certain substances or groups of substances. The influence of variety, climate, and soil on the constituents of the grapes expressed in the first member of the series sketched, which leads to a definite **variation in the constituents of the grapes,** is important. The second member of the sequence, particularly in relation to the ripeness and the state of the grapes (sound, or infected by rot or noble rot) is also of great influence on the composition of the aroma substances. Little attention has so far been devoted to variations in the constituents due to **technological** factors involved in the crushing, mashing and pressing of the grapes. At the moment of destruction of the cell structure – and this applies quite generally to fruit –, depending on the ripeness, temperature, pH, and atmospheric oxygen, enzymatic processes are initiated to a greater or smaller degree that lead, for example, to a hydrolytic cleavage of esters under the action of enzymes and, which is still more serious, to the very rapid formation of hexanal and hexenals from C-18 unsaturated fatty acids as the result of enzymatic oxidative processes, particularly in the case of unripe

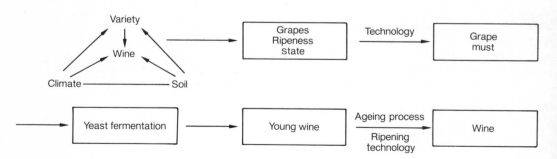

Fig. 10-12. Biotechnological series of wines.

grapes, these aldehydes being responsible for the grassy smell or taste of musts from unripe grapes that sometimes unpleasantly appear (Drawert et al., 1965, 1966, 1969, 1973, 1974, 1978). The formation of such unpleasant nuances of odor and taste can largely be avoided by rapidly raising the temperature up to the inhibition point of the enzymes concerned and rapid cooling (Drawert et al., 1976), as shown in Fig. 10-13. Factors such as the time for which the mashes stand as a function of the temperature, the treatment of the mash such as, for example, the use of sulfur dioxide or the introduction of pectolytic enzymes in order to improve the yield of juice, the nature of the pressing of the mashes and

the treatment of the press must, such as desliming filtration or desliming precipitation, have a great influence on the final quality.

What must be particularly emphasized here is that valuable aroma substances have a tendency to bind more or less firmly to fragments of the cells or to particles of turbidity so that, for example, when the turbidity is sufficiently removed 40 to 70% of the aroma material, estimated on parallel examples, can be lost together with the solid matter of the mash (pomace). Finally, the yeast fermentation leads to a far-reaching change in the pattern of constituents of the fermentation substrate. Thus, for example, amino acids enter the metabolism of the yeast with quasi-biochemical value in relation to the formation of fermentation by-products (Drawert and Rapp, 1964).

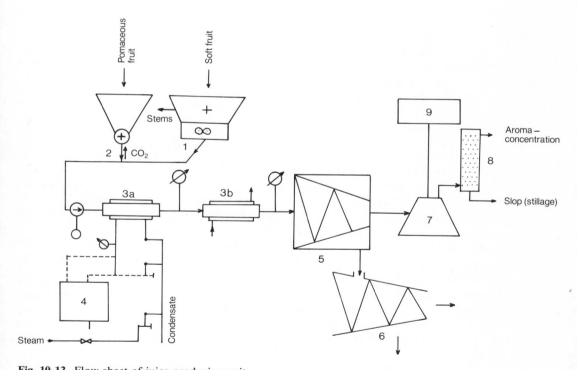

Fig. 10-13. Flow sheet of juice-producing unit.
1 = squeezing-roll mill; 2 = fruit cutter; 3 a = Thermalizer TH 10; 3 b = Thermalizer TH 35; 4 = steam pressure regulator; 5 = decanter; 6 = worm press; 7 = evaporator; 8 = packed column; 9 = concentrate reservoir (Drawert et al., 1976).

Of particular importance for quality of the wine is the **variety of grapes.** In practical wine growing, about 46 varieties for white wine and about 23 varieties for red wine are being cultivated. Among these, as hitherto, the "old" white wine varieties such as Riesling, Müller-Thurgau, Silvaner, Ruländer, white Burgundy, red Traminer and, among the red wine varieties, blue late Burgundy, blue Portugese, Limberger, and blue Trollinger play a large part. In addition to these, new varieties are under cultivation in Germany, such as Scheurebe, Siegerrebe, Huxel-Rebe, Faber, Morio-Muscat, Bacchus, Optima, Kerner, Ehrenfelser, Rieslaner, Perle, and Ortega, among which it is particularly the aroma-rich white-wine varieties that are playing an increasing role. In terms of areas of cultivation, only three varieties stand out: Müller-Thurgau (27% of the total planted grape area), Riesling (21%), and Silvaner (17%). Among the countries of the European Community, Germany is the classical country of white wines with numerous quality gradations. The production of red wine is low and is limited to a few particularly suitable places (Hillebrand, 1978).

For the purposes of the production of high-quality wines, wine grapes should be harvested in the state of full ripeness, which, unfortunately, is frequently not the case because of weather influences or misjudgement. As with any other types of fruit, the ripening of wine grapes is characterised by a lively **acid-sugar metabolism.** During the growth of the grapes, the acid content rises, but it falls again during the ripening period. The maximum on the acid curve is generally designated the beginning of ripening; it can frequently be recognized from the change in the color of the berries, which is accompanied by a simultaneous rise in the concentration of sugars.

The beginning of the ripening phase coinciding with the turning down of the acid curve also appears otherwise to be a very decisive phase in the growth of the berries. After this moment, the increase in the number of cells ceases and further growth must be explained solely by the enlargement of the cells (Drawert, 1967). The temporal position and quantitative level of the acid maximum depend on the variety of grape and, to a large extent, on environmental influences. If the course of the ripening of the berries is shown graphically on the basis of the sugar and acid levels, so-called ripening curves with a point of intersection are obtained. As Husfeld (1962) has described in detail, the ripening curves and their points of intersection express certain output properties of the varieties of grape. For example, early-ripening varieties have an early point of intersection; if the position of the point of intersection is still high, this means that sugars (mainly glucose and fructose) are being intensively decomposed. A close relationship exists between the metabolism of the acids and sugars taking place in the grapes and the metabolism of the constituents such as amino acids.

The (German) **wine law** of 1971 distinguishes the following quality classes: 1) Deutscher Tafelwein (German table wine); 2) Qualitätswein bestimmter Anbaugebiete, Q. b. A (high-quality wine from definite growing areas); and 3) Qualitätswein mit Prädikat, Prädikatswein (high-quality wine with grade, graded wine) with the grades Kabinett (cabinet), Spätlese (late vintage), Auslese (selected-bunch), Beerenauslese (selected-grape), and Trockenbeerenauslese (selected-partially-dried-grape), and the speciality Eiswein (ice wine) from grapes affected by frost. The second and third quality classes are also given a control number on the label and in the tender. The official test number guarantees the high quality. Testing is carried out basically on the bottled wine. In contrast to the high-quality wines, table wine [Landwein (local wine), Tischwein (dinner wine) or Konsumwein (ordinary wine)], as Deutscher Tafelwein, need have no place names and no official testing numbers. On the other hand, – like the high-quality wines –, it is produced from permitted varieties of grape and definite weights of must (minimum requirement).

If the berries in the unripe state are damaged, e.g., by **fungal attack** (Peronospora, Oidium) or by hail, rot may arise, which often makes premature picking necessary. From about 70° Oechsle*, depending on the state of the skins of the berries and weathering, the so-called **noble rot** arises, which is the result of attack by the noble rot fungus *Botrytis cinerea*. This attack is characterized by a shrinkage of the berries in which the loss in weight may amount to about 40%. Simultaneously, however, the amounts of sugars and also that of glycerol and also the concentration of so-called extractive substances as a whole, rise more or less intensively. This means that must densities of 100 to 200° Oechsle and more are reached, which are the bases for the production of, in particular, Auslese, Beerenauslese, and Trockenbeerenauslese wines. The production of such wines sets high demands on the vintner, since here a special preparation technique of the berries subjected to noble rot and a particularly careful performance of the fermentation is necessary. In the case of varieties with a bouquet, such as, for example, Gewürztraminer, Muskat, or Scheurebe, the bouquet typical of the variety may be very greatly masked by the so-called Botrytis note.

10.2.2 Harvesting of the Grapes and Pressing

The **grape harvest** must be preceded by a thorough overhaul and cleaning of all the necessary instruments and containers. The grape harvest is still carried out overwhelmingly by hand and includes a number of individual operations

- The cutting off of the bunches with grape scissors and collection in small back-baskets or tubs; the cutting out of bunches or berries attacked by noble rot and their separate collection can be carried out simultaneously (Auslese).

- Emptying into carrying containers (baskets, boxes).

---

* 1° Oechsle = 1° Oe ≈ 1000 · (specific gravity [20°C] − 1)

- Carrying or sending the receiving containers to the vehicles with the transport containers; here the crushing of the bunches can already take place through their weight.

- Transport of the gathered material to the press-house.

In the German wine growing regions, completely mechanized harvesting is still under trial. (On the various systems, see Troost, 1980). Troost has characterized the individual steps in the technology of the preparation of white wine in a flow sheet. (Fig. 10-14).

The **presshouse** has to deal with pronounced peaks of activity, and because of the sensitivity of the mashes to change, the following basic law must be followed: everything gathered on one day should be pressed on the same day. The rational way of working in the presshouse is responsible for technical requirements such as the ready transport of grapes, mashes, must, and pomace, and efficient pressing. For this purpose, the grapes are tipped into a sunken grape crusher and the mash is pumped into stock or juice-extraction containers.

In the case of white wine grapes, a distinction must frequently be made about whether they are or are not **stripped** or **destalked.** By this is understood the separation of the berries from the stalks or stems before they are crushed. In fact, particularly in the unripe state under relatively high pressures or in fermenting mashes, stalks introduce undesired substances such as phenolic or tannin-like compounds or even pesticides into the press must. The previous removal of the stalks undoubtedly leads to cleaner and purer musts and therefore to wines with corresponding properties. The question of whether white wine grapes should be picked separately or not depends on the variety of grape, its state of ripeness, and the proposed subsequent processing of the mash. The principles of the various grape-picking machines (Troost, 1980) are based on the beating off of the bunches from the stems and partially also from the stalks by a beater, a toothed shaft with wooden or plastic teeth, and the forcing of the strip-

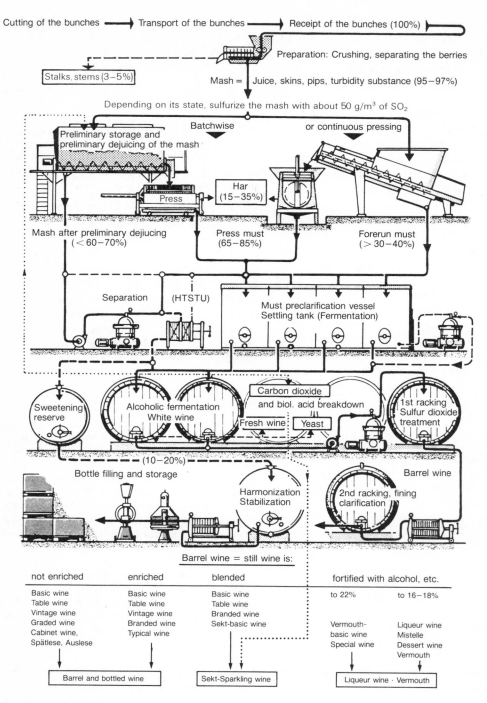

Cutting of the bunches ⟶ Transport of the bunches ⟶ Receipt of the bunches (100%)

Preparation: Crushing, separating the berries

Stalks, stems (3–5%)

Mash = Juice, skins, pips, turbidity substance (95–97%)

Depending on its state, sulfurize the mash with about 50 g/m³ of SO₂

Batchwise   or continuous pressing

Preliminary storage and preliminary dejuicing of the mash

Press

Har (15–35%)

Mash after preliminary dejuicing (< 60–70%)   Press must (65–85%)   Forerun must (> 30–40%)

Separation   (HTSTU)   Must preclarification vessel Settling tank (Fermentation)

Sweetening reserve   Alcoholic fermentation White wine   Carbon dioxide and biol. acid breakdown   Fresh wine   Yeast   1st racking Sulfur dioxide treatment

(10–20%)

Bottle filling and storage   Harmonization Stabilization   Barrel wine   2nd racking, fining clarification

Barrel wine = still wine is:

not enriched	enriched	blended		fortified with alcohol, etc.
			to 22%	to 16–18%
Basic wine	Basic wine	Basic wine		
Table wine	Table wine	Table wine		
Vintage wine	Vintage wine	Branded wine		
Graded wine	Branded wine	Sekt-basic wine	Vermouth-basic wine	Liqueur wine
Cabinet wine,	Typical wine		Special wine	Mistelle
Spätlese, Auslese				Dessert wine
				Vermouth

Barrel and bottled wine   Sekt-Sparkling wine   Liqueur wine · Vermouth

Fig. 10-14. Flow sheet for the preparation of white wine (after Troost, 1980).

ped bunches through a sieve-drum or a perforated cylinder; the stalks from which the grapes have been removed are discharged. The grapes may subsequently be fed directly into a mill or a mill of suitable design can be placed before the destalking step.

The **mills** consist as a rule of squeezing rolls of various profiles in which the surfaces that come into contact with the grapes either have a protective coating of lacquer or are provided with rubber or plastic profiles. Hard wood rollers are also used.

After greatly differing mash standing times, with or without preliminary removal of juice and possibly after treatment with sulfur dioxide, the material is fed to **presses.** The pressing process and the outflow of juice can be substantially facilitated by the addition of pectinolytic enzymes particularly if, depending on variety and ripeness, the grapes contain increased amounts of mucilaginous components. It is true that the addition of **pectinolytic enzymes** prolongs the standing time of the mash (Maurer, 1973), but it gives the advantages of a higher yield of juice, a faster settling and clarification of the must, a modification of the fermentation process, and, probably, also an increase in the degree of oxidation of the must. On the addition of pectinolytic enzymes, however, it must be borne in mind that these enzymes, particularly in the applied form of technical enzymes, include many side activities which, for example, lead to the cleavage of depsides (Burkhardt, 1977) or of bouquet materials such as esters (esterases), depending on the prevailing conditions such as pH, temperature, etc. With this may be associated a loss of the variety bouquet, freshness, and the characteristic properties (Urlaub, 1979). Combination with the **warm fermentation of the mash** at temperatures up to about 45°C is also used, but here it must be observed that, as a rule, the so-called tannin content of the musts rises, which may lead to

adverse qualitative effects, particularly with inexpert handling.

Figure 10-15 gives a review of the various **press systems.**

According to Troost (1980), the rate of outflow of the juice and the yield of juice are the better the larger the number of disintegrated cells in the fruit tissue. In the pressing process it is more a matter of the turning over of the mash or of the press cake by relatively frequent collisions than of high pressures. The pressing process is affected by the thickness of the layer of the press cake at any given moment. Of less importance is the time for which the pressure is maintained and the level of pressure. Also of importance for the **pressing time** and the **pressing yield** is the direction in which the pressure is applied in relation to the direction of outflow of juice. For example, in the case of the bladder press 16 in Fig. 10-15, the direction of pressing of the bladder, which can be blown up internally, is approximately parallel to the direction of outflow of the juice, while, on the other hand, with other pressing systems there is a deviation by 90°. Horizontal presses are frequently used. Because of the perforated cylinder arranged horizontally, their rotary motion causes a more copious outflow of juice; furthermore the mash within the press basket can be loosened (turned over) by a chain-ring system when the press plates move away from one another. In the various designs, the press baskets consist either of wooden rods or of slit sieve-like stainless steel plates. The highly turbid must is stated to be a certain disadvantage of modern horizontal presses. Comparatively large amounts of turbidity lead to a faster or even violent fermentation; they may also introduce undesirable constituents into the wine through the fermentation process. On the other hand, it must be borne in mind that, as stated at the beginning of this section, with the aroma-rich varieties a considerable proportion of the aroma typical of the variety is associated with the turbidity which, in combination with the alcoholic fermentation, is dissolved to a greater or smaller extent and then contributes to the variety bouquet of the wine. The correct treatment of highly turbid musts requires much experience and knowledge and can be carried out with complete success only in small to medium-sized wineries. So-called **pressing aids** such as, for example, sil-

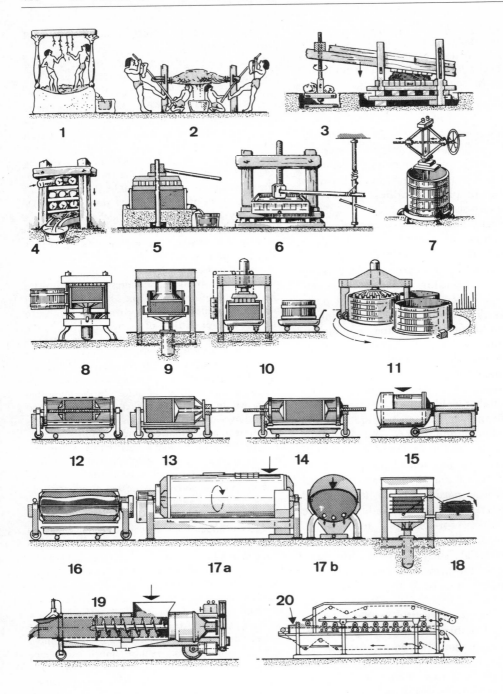

1

2

3

4

5

6

7

8

9

10

11

12

13

14

15

16

17a

17b

18

19

20

ica gel, perlite, and cellulose fibers (Solcaflox, Trubex, etc.) have been used for some time. On continuous pressing systems (worm presses, centrifugal separators, belt presses, eccentric presses), see Troost, pp. 111-127 (1980).

10.2.3 Fermentation

After the appropriate pretreatment or clarification, the pressing musts pass into the fermentation vats. Table 10-1 gives a review of

Fig. 10-15. Review of the development and design of old and current presses (after Troost, 1980).

1–7 = historic presses (preindustrial epoch):

 1 = Egyptian treading vat with grape treaders and brickwork trough with wooden frame and supporting ropes, run-off pipe, and juice basins

 2 = Egyptian torsion press. The trodden-out grapes are pressed in woven sacks (wringing press). The sacks are either pulled out or rung out as at 2. Still used today in Amazonas as the "Tipiti" manioc press

 3 = beam press (lever press, "Torkel", from Roman times up to today)

 4 = Roman wedge press, less suitable apparatus.

 5 = "low-pressure" press in section with stone base and wooden spindle, which was later made of iron

 6 = yoke press ("high-pressure press") with rectangular (wooden) and later round basket and base (Middle Ages until today)

 7 = toggle-lever press (mainly Austrian) up to the end of the 19th century

8–11 = hydraulic vertical basket presses, since 1835, disappeared about 1955. First tippable, then moving on rails, and later freely removable base and baskets:

 8 = bottom-pressure press with one or two swivelling baskets

 9 = bottom-pressure press with top-pressure nature, i.e., in pressing the mash remains in contact with the base (short pathway for the juice)

10 = top-pressure press, freely removable

11 = top-pressure press, three-basket carousel, common in France.

12–15 = present-day horizontal presses, moving freely or stationary:

12 = Inner spindle rotating in the opposite direction with two press plates, spindle present in the mash, basket rotating

13 = spindle extending upwards with one press plate and juice cloth

14 = spindle extending outwards with two press plates (stationary)

15 = oil-hydraulic piston press with juice bowl. Pressures 8 to 15 bar

16–20 = pneumatic presses, since 1951:

16 = horizontal compressed-air press (bladder press, pressure up to 6 bar) with axially-arranged extensible rubber bladder, pressing the mash outwards radially and expanding

17a = tank press, large press for compressed air (operating pressure 2 bar) with closed press jacket, juice-discharging perforated areas, and nonextensible press membrane

17b = cross-section through the pressing chamber

18 = packed press with two or three cages, swivellable, works fast with pressures of up to 30 bar, very labor-intensive

19 = horizontal worm screw press, dia. 600 to 800 mm with outputs of up to 14 tons/h. Works together with berry-picking machine and juice preextractor in large wineries

20 = double-belt press for fruit difficult to press

Table 10-1 Review of the Wine Containers Customary in Germany, their Nature and Application (according to Troost, 1980).

Material	Designation	Capacity, liters	Shape	Surface, m²/hl	Internal protection Cladding	Preservation	External protection Coating	Purpose
1	2	3	4	5	6	7	8	9
Wood (Oak)	Hektofass	100	round	1.1–1.6	usually none	periodically by sulfur dioxide, On long standing empty, filling with 25 g/hl of SO_2 (wet preservation)	impregnating oil, possibly a priming coat of impregnating salt solutions, no paint or varnish and even linseed oil only to a limited extent	vessels for transport and for the settling of turbidity and residues
	Ohm (Rheingau)	150	round					
	Ohm (Mosel)	160	round					
	Doppelhekto	200	round	0.8–1.3	impregnation with Mammut-Ventur DO, Steramit vino, Durolit or Defalit spez., polyamide, epoxide resin, etc.			as above; also fermentation vessels
	Viertelstück	300	round, oval	0.7–0.85				transport
	Zulast (Mosel)	480	round	0.6–0.7				fermentation, and storage
	Halbfuder (Saar)	500	round	0.6–0.7				
	Halbstück (Rheingau)	600	round, oval	0.5–0.6				
	Fuder (Mosel, Saar)	960 (1000)	round	0.6–0.66				vessels
	Stückfass (Rhein)	1200	round, oval	0.4–0.6				
	Doppelstück	2400–2600	round, oval	0.4				fermentation and storage vessels
	2–10 fudr. Fässer	2000–10000	round, oval	0.3–0.2				
	3-n Stück Fässer	3600–9600	round, oval	0.22				fermentation, storage and blending vessels
Metal a) Open-hearth steel (composite material)	Tank, storage tank, pressure tank pressureless up to 0.5 bar pressure tank up to operating pressure of 8 bar	optimum capacity 6000–20000 and more, 1000000	cylinder or cone, horizontal or vertical, tower type D:h = 1:2 to 1:6		a) **vitreous enamel** hard, brittle **plastics** cold-hardening epoxide resin	not needed	in damp rooms special tank or boat varnish reaction-varnish	fermentation and storage vessels
b) Stainless steel (chromium-nickel steel, chromiummolybdenum nickel steel)	tanks, mostly pressure-less	as in a)	horizontal and vertical tanks, round or dished, also with flanged walls or shells		b) none	not needed, ventilation	usually hot needed	juice-extracting, fermentation, and storage vessels for dry rooms; fermentation and storage tanks, filling reservoirs, nozzle containers, etc.

GRP plastic Polyester resin with glass fiber	Erka, Juno, Rexoplast, Staffelstein, Speidel, etc. pressureless	300–100000	cylindrical, stock tanks, oval, box shape, horizontal and vertical tanks	polyester, epoxide resin steamable up to 115°C	not needed, ventilation	not needed, but possible	fermentation, storage, and transport containers, also blending and filling tanks
Reinforced concrete	concrete and cement vessels cisterns	5000–20000 upwards to 300000, etc.	depending on space utilization, prismatic, rectangular, polygonal, also vertical cylindrical vessels	a) glass plates with luting or cement joints b) epoxide coating, joint-free	not needed ventilation	cement plaster; better, clinker	blending and storage vessels; also fermentation vessels; more rarely juice-extracting vessels, preclarification containers, fermentation vessels for red wine mash
Glass Bottles	Korbflasche (basket bottle) Literflasche (liter bottle) Ganze Flasche (whole bottle) Tokajer-Flasche (Tokay bottle) Halbe Flasche (half bottle) Viertelflasche (quarter bottle) 0.2-Literflasche (0.2-liter bottle) Achtelflasche (eighth bottle) Probenflasche (sample bottle)	5–50 1 and 2 0.7 and 0.75 0.5 0.35 and 0.375 0.25 0.2 0.1 0.08	carboys and cylindrical bottles distinctions are made between: Schlegel, Bocksbeutel-, Burgunder-, Bordeaux- and Likörflasche, etc.; and light- and medium-weight glass, etc., of various colors	colors of the glass: greenish, colorless, brown (blue)	cleaning and sterilisation, otherwise furnace-sterile, cooling-oven packed one-trip bottles	basket, laths, sugar reserve, residues and turbidity containers, Styropor beds, folded cardboard, framework cardboard, trays, corrugated board, etc.	draft wine, bottled wine, white and red wines, liqueur wine, and the like

Red wine grapes ➝ Receipt of bunches = 100% mass

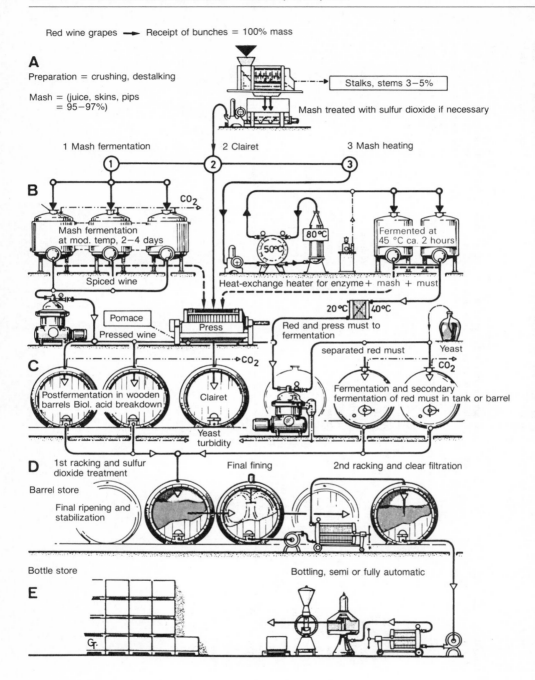

A

Preparation = crushing, destalking

Mash = (juice, skins, pips
    = 95–97%)

Stalks, stems 3–5%

Mash treated with sulfur dioxide if necessary

1 Mash fermentation   2 Clairet   3 Mash heating

B CO_2

Mash fermentation
at mod. temp, 2–4 days

80 °C   50 °C

Fermented at
45 °C ca. 2 hours

Spiced wine

Heat-exchange heater for enzyme + mash + must

20 °C ⊠ 40 °C

Pomace

Pressed wine   Press

Red and press must to
fermentation

separated red must   Yeast

CO_2

C CO_2

Postfermentation in wooden
barrels Biol. acid breakdown

Clairet

Fermentation and secondary
fermentation of red must in tank or barrel

Yeast
turbidity

D   1st racking and sulfur
     dioxide treatment

Final fining   2nd racking and clear filtration

Barrel store

Final ripening and
stabilization

Bottle store   Bottling, semi or fully automatic

E

GT.

Fig. 10-16. Flowsheet for red wine preparation technology (after: Troost, 1980).

the most common wine vats and their properties and applications. **The wooden vat** is sensitive and requires much maintenance. Its interaction with the contents is considerable. The wooden vat is unsuitable for the amounts which it is desired to treat in the larger wineries. For large containers when the storage area is limited, metal tanks with capacities of up to about 250 000 L are preferred. These may be arranged vertically (tower tanks) or horizontally. If they are not made of stainless steel, the most diverse internal coatings may be used (see Table 10-1). Apart from their possible size and the saving of storage space, steel tanks have advantages such as simple cleaning, capability of being used for the storage of white and red wines successively, low amount of leakage and loss of gas, and also the possibility of applying pressure. **Glass-reinforced polyester** (GFP) tanks also exhibit the advantages mentioned. They are being used to an increasing degree in small and medium-sized wineries. The various staple forms, in particular, are very advantageous.

The **technique of fermentation** in the preparation of white wine (see Fig. 10-14) is simple in comparison with that for red wine. Apart from the preparation of the so-called clairet, the **preparation of red wine** has the special feature that the pigment localized in the cells in the grape skins must be released in order to impart the characteristic color to the wine. The pigments (anthocyanins) cannot be brought into solution mechanically, but they can be by heating the mash, or by enzymatic digestion, or, more simply and more certainly, by means of the alcohol that forms on fermentation. Figure 10-16 shows the flow sheet giving the technique of the preparation of red wine. The red mashes can now be allowed to ferment in open vats whereupon the so-called **pomace cap** or "**hat**" collects on the surface which, without further precautions extends out of the fermenting liquid and is highly susceptible to infection or oxidation. For this rea-

son, here perforated bottoms are used which force the pomace cap down or move to leach it better. The closed fermentation of the mash with the mechanical treatment of the pomace cap with or without pressuring with carbon dioxide or with tempered fermentation with the release of pressure according to Klenk et al. (1954) is more satisfactory. At an optimum fermentation temperature of 20 to 26°C, here the treatment of the mash cake is carried out by **pressure variation.** On rapid release of the pressure, the compressed carbon dioxide is suddenly liberated, rises, and mixes the mash. In **Defranceschi's process** (1955), the cap of the mash is removed mechanically from the top and is recirculated from the bottom. The **Padovan system** (Gervasi 1965) works similarly.

For large vessels, the **Ducellier-Isman fermentation process** has proved satisfactory in a number of countries (Fig. 10-17).

As in other processes, here fermentation can be kept in check by cooling. The fermentation carbon dioxide that is evolved automatically forces part of the liquids through the cooling channel E. This cooled part collects in section G of the vat about 30 cm deep and flows back into the mash at predetermined time intervals.

Overflows brought about by the buildup of carbon dioxide pressure are also used in the **Vinomat principle** of Waagner-Biró with an airtightly sealed overflow chamber and in the MWB (Metallwerk Buchs) fermentation tank (Haushofer and Bayer, 1967; Lemperle and Kerner, 1968; Schobinger and Schneider, 1975).

Among the continuous large-scale fermentation processes for the manufacture of red wine, those of **Cremaschi** and **Ladousse** (1963) must be singled out. The Ladousse process (Foulonneau, 1968; Nègres, 1967) corresponds in principle to that of **Cremaschi.** No recirculation of the mash during fermentation takes place in a single-tower continuous vessel. The mash rises in an annular external vessel with a predetermined velocity so that the fermentation is complete at the top, and the pomace is removed by a rotating worm and pressed out. In the inner part, the fermenting young wine moves downwards and

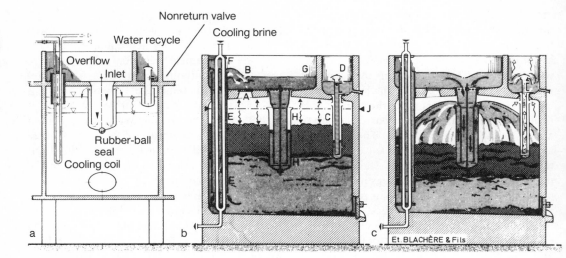

Fig. 10-17. Automatic turning over of the red-wine mash and periodic coverage of the mash with the aid of carbon dioxide formed, with simultaneous temperature control (cooling) (L'autovinificateur, BSGDG "Ducellier-Isman" system) (after: Troost, 1980).

a = new form of a fermentation block for 15 to 30 000 L of mash with the fermentation elements

b = stage of rising pressure: the mash is forced down from filling level J by the carbon dioxide forming; the arrows show the pressure expansion. The fermenting wine rises through the bundle of cooling tubes E at F into the vat G

c = stage of pressure equilization and overflowing of the mash with the aid of the pressure valves C and D operating automatically and inevitably.

A = Filling aperture; B = cover; C = pressure valve with D = sealing water; E = tube cooler; F = conduit for cooling brine; G = receiver for the rising red must; H = return pipe (syphon) with distributor.

is taken off at the bottom. The daily throughput is given as 150 to 180 tons of mash.

There are now numerous processes for **heating the mash** or its **warm fermentation** in which temperatures between about 45 °C and 80 °C are used with fermentation times between 2 and 12 hours with or without the addition of enzymes. At higher temperatures, it is true, the color yield is better, but the danger exists of a more or less pronounced change in the color and the taste sensation. Since the yield of color is comparatively greater above 60 °C, for large wineries the short-time heating process has been developed for red wine mash.

In Bucher's **Roto process** (Haushofer et al., 1971; Lemperle et al., 1973), the fermentation of the mash is carried out in a rotating tank (periodic immersion of the pomace cap), the mash being heated to 45 to 50 °C in a countercurrent process.

In the plant technique of W. Schmidt KG, the high-temperature short-time heating of red wine mashes takes place in stages, beginning with the heating of the destalked mash to 45 to 50 °C as it passes through a spiral heat exchanger, then its heating to 80 to 85 °C in a double-tube heater with residence times in the heater of 1.5 to 2 min followed by the recooling of the heated mash to 45 °C during its return passage through the heat exchanger (Maurer, 1976; Maurer et al., 1974; Steinhilper, 1976; Meidinger, 1975; Schobinger, 1976) (Fig. 10-18).

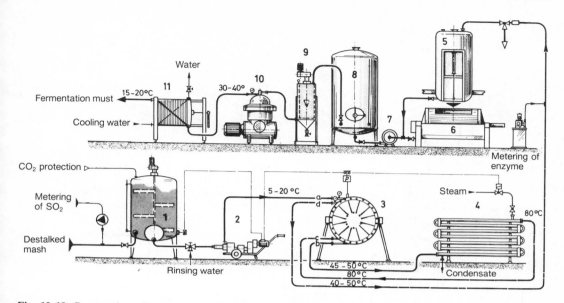

Fig. 10-18. Preparation of red wine by the short-time high-temperature process. Scheme of plant according to Maurer, Steinhilper, and Knoll (1974).
1 = Mash buffer tank with incorporated stirrer for destalked mash; 2 = Mohno pump for the transport of the mash; a–b = forerun; c–d = return flow; 3 = Schmidt/Bretten spiral heat exchanger; 4 = double-tube heater; 5 = residence tank for warm fermentation of the mash; 6 = horizontal press; 7 = juice pump; 8 = intermediate tank for evening out a nonuniform flow of red must; 9 = rotating-brush sieve; 10 = self-discharging separator; 11 = plate apparatus used as cooler for the fermentation of the must at about 20 °C.
Example for an economic use of energy by the recovery of 50% of the heat without cooling water in the back-cooling of the mash.

In the continuous **Imeca-Sick** mash heating process (Lemperle et al., 1973), the stripped red wine mash passes into a worm-type preliminary dejuicer, and the partially dejuiced mash passes into the mash heater where the desired temperature is adjusted by means of a double-tube heater in the liquid circuit and the spraying of the mash (Fig. 10-19).

10.2.4 Wine Finishing

Towards the end of fermentation or after fermentation, the yeast and particles of turbidity settle on the bottom of the fermentation vessel. The yeast sediment undergoes an autolysis, which can lead to its rising from the bottom and to turbidity phenomena difficult to eliminate. In addition, through decomposition processes in the autolyzing yeast, hydrogen sulfide and mercaptans are given off, causing the so-called yeast taint, which disappears again only slowly in the young wine or on storage.

For this reason, the young wines must be drawn off or racked. Racking is also carried out for the purpose of eliminating crusts of tartar and yeasts in the cask or to suppress postfermentation in order to keep a certain residual sweetness. A yeast accumulation of 3 to

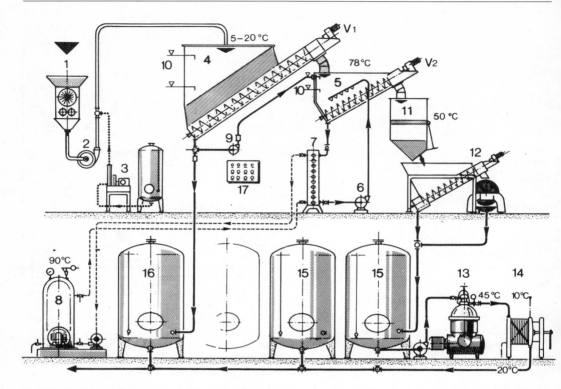

Fig. 10-19. Scheme of the Imeca-Sick red-wine mash heating unit with partial juice extraction and heating to 72°C with a high-temperature residence time of 35 min. Output 10–30 tons/h, according to Lemperle, Trogus, and Frank, 1973.

1 = mill with destalking machine; 2 = mash pump; 3 = sulfur dioxide metering apparatus for the continuous treatment of the mash; 4 = draining tank (clairet) with worm discharge; 5 = mash tank, double-walled, for heating the mash, with must spraying device; 6 = must pump; 7 = tube heater; 8 = hot-water producer; 9 = level pump for tank (5) with level control switch = 10; 11 = receiver, self-discharging (high-temperature residence time); 12 = draining tank with discharge worm and press; 13 = separator; 14 = cooling device; 15 = fermentation tanks; 16 = fermentation for clairet; 17 = electrical control unit; V_1 and V_2 adjustable drives for the worms.

5 L of a viscous fluid yeast sediment per hL of wine must be reckoned with or, in the case of wines the musts of which were preclarified, about 1.5 to 2 L/hL. The wine still adhering to the yeast can be recovered in part by separate storage (settling), but this is associated with the danger of further autolysis and a deterioration of the taste. The yeast may also be carefully pressed out in so-called yeast bags or be subjected to intensive filtration. The centrifugal separation of the yeast is less successful. It is true that yeast-pressing wine is wine, but it cannot be sold as such. It may be used as make-up wine in the same winery if it contains not more than 10 L of pure alcohol per 100 kg and at least 25 wt% of dry matter. The yeast can also be processed to give yeast brandy, which is highly prized by connoisseurs.

The **biochemical oxygen demand** (BOD$_5$) of the **effluents** from wineries may assume considerable values. While in the case of domestic sewage a BOD$_5$ of about 350 mg/L is to be reckoned with, that of the must pre-clarification turbidity (desliming turbidity) and the separator discharge in the clarification of must fluctuates around 54 000 mg/L; old, decomposed yeast sediment around 500 000 mg/L; and the turbidity from the first racking about 82 000 mg/L. In view of the considerable taxes to be expected after the Effluent Discharge Tax Laws, it is recommended that all separable components should be composted or returned to the vineyards.

As a rule, wines are treated with **sulfur dioxide** itself, or with preparations which yield sulfur dioxide, in order to achieve a reductive medium. The consumption of sulfur must be monitored continuously. From 25 to 75 mg/L of free sulfur dioxide is permitted in all wines, while the total amount of sulfurous acid for normal wines up to and including cabinet wine may be 175 to 275 mg/L, for Spätlese 300 mg/L, for Auslese and Eiswein 350 mg/L, and for Beerenauslese and Trockenbeerenauslese 400 mg/L. However, W. Walter of the Walthari-Hof at Edenkoben (Federal Republic of Germany), has shown that attractive and wholesome wines can be finished without the addition of sulfur dioxide by a special process. It is also possible to add ascorbic acid (vitamin C) in order to keep a wine reductive.

A fundamental role, particularly in the case of red wines, is played by the **biological breakdown of acids,** during which malic acid is decomposed and the actual acid content of a wine therefore falls. In climatically unfavorable years in which the full ripening of the berries is not achieved, on an average white wine musts introduce more than 10 ‰ of total acid, and red wine musts up to 8 to 10 ‰ of acid, into the fermentation process. Particularly in the case of red wine, however, an acid content of 4.5 to 6 ‰ is desired in order to obtain mild wines. Bacteria such as Leuconostoc or Pediococcus develop, particularly in the postfermentation phase, if the cell density of the yeast is diminished by sedimentation, in a kind of symbiosis with the yeasts or their secretion products, and they then break down malic acid more or less completely to lactic acid (Mayer, 1979; Mayer and Vetch, 1973; Meyer et al., 1971; Radler, 1969).

Musts or wines may also be **deacidified** by the addition of calcium carbonate, when calcium tartrate or the calcium double salt of malic and tartaric acids is said to be formed. The so-called calcium double salt deacidification process has found rapid introduction into practice.

Since, as a rule, wines separate out organic and inorganic turbidities (salts of fruit acids, protein-tannin compounds, polyphenols, pectins) and biological turbidities, **filtration** with filter aids (Kieselguhr) is necessary in order that the wines may be bottled in the clear bright state. In order to avoid renewed turbidity after bottling, wines are "fined" with the agents summarized in Table 10-2. The fining turbidity must also be removed by racking and filtration.

10.2.5 *Improvement Processes*

Processes exist for improving a poor quality and low sales value of a wine that are due essentially to the inadequate ripening of the berries and consequent low concentration of sugar and high concentration of acids. According to, e.g., the new German wine law the wet addition of sugars (sucrose, dextrose, glucose) will be permitted only up to 1984 (10-15%). The improvement may be carried out as early as the must stage, or during or after fermentation (refermentation). In addition to the wet addition of sugars, dry addition is also known. For both types of addition of sugars, so-called sugaring tables are used. The wine law of 1971 and the EC marketing order of 1970 also envisage the use of grape

Table 10-2. Review of the Permitted Fining and Treating Agents (after Troost, 1980).

No.	Fining agent (Trade Mark)	El. ch. in the wine	State in the wine	Is the wine affected?	Application
1.	**Isinglass** (sturgeon, sheatfish) in leaves or strips	+	colloidally dissolved	no	*clarification* of sensitive tannin-poor white wines with sufficient acid, preclarification
2.	**Protein**	+			
	a) egg protein (white of egg)	+	colloidally dissolved	no	*clarification* of red wine, Auslesen, when they are
	b) ovalbumin, dried (perishable)	+	colloidally dissolved	scarcely	rough. With stalky white wines, taste-improving through elimination of tannins
3.	**Gelatin** (edible gelatin), acid-digested, low Bloom No. (about 60–100)				*clarification* of red and white wines, color-lightening and taste-improving in tannin-rich wines
	a) dry	+	colloidally dissolved	scarcely	
	b) liquid	+	colloidally dissolved	scarcely	
4.	**Casein,** dry **potassium caseinate**	+	colloidally dissolved	yes yes	treatment of highly colored beet wines. *Elimination of tannins* and pigments
5.	**Tannin** various types acid. Tanic. DAB 6	–	dissolved	no	*addition* to gelatin fining in tannin-poor white wines
6.	**Silica sol** 15–30% silicic acid silica (gel)	–	colloidally dissolved	no	*additive* in gelatin fining, preclarification, errors of taste
7.	**Spanish earth kaolin**	–	solid, slurry	somewhat somewhat	*protein stabilization,* fining of heavy sweet wines or slimy viscous wines
8.	**Bentonite**		powder or		*protein stabilization.*
	a) Na bentonite highly swellable	–	granulate to be preswollen	yes	adsorption of protein after heat or
	b) Ca bentonite weakly swellable	–	in water or wine and	yes	bentonite test
	c) mixed bentonite	–	stirred in	yes	

Amount per hectoliter	Possible combination	Moment of application	Contact time	Moment of racking early	late
0.5–2 g	alone or after blue fining	young and finished wine	15–30 min	4 days	3–6 weeks
a) 2–3 b) 8–16 g	alone	young and finished wines	15–30 min	4 days	3–6 weeks
a) 5–30 g b) 20–150 mL	alone or after tannin or silica sol and possibly bentonite, blue fining	must, young wine before 2nd racking	4–6 h	4 days any excess of gelatin removed by bentonite	3–6 weeks
6–50 g	alone or before gelatin	as required young wine	2–3 h stirring	about 1 week, depending on rate of settling	
2–10 g limit 10 g/hL	to be added before gelatin in a ratio of 1:1	as required	as for gelatin	as for gelatin	
10–15 times the amount of gelatin	to be added before the gelatin in a ratio of 1:1.5 to 1:10	as required	as for gelatin	as for gelatin	
100–400 g 200–600 g	postfining with isinglass or gelatin	as required	20–30 min with thorough mixing	after settling, as desired	
a) 50–250 g b) 80–400 g as required	following blue fining or gelatin or isinglass	as required, must and young wine	20–30 min with thorough mixing	after 1 week, depending on settling	

Table 10-2. Review of the Permitted Fining and Treating Agents (after Troost, 1980).

No.	Fining agent (Trade Mark)	El. ch. in the wine	State in the wine	Is the wine affected?	Application
9.	**Yeast,** wine yeast thick fluid from preclarified must (young wine)	–	slurry "liquid"	no, if yeast sound	*refreshing* tired wines, elimination of small errors. Not in wines with residual sugars or acid-poor wines
10.	**Carbon,** permitted only in the form of activated carbon up to 1 g/L and only in white wine		solid, finely ground or granulate	yes	elimination or modification of *errors of taste, smell, and color* in must and wine, clarification of spirits
11.	**Blue fining** Potassium hexacyanoferrate(III) Möslinger fining		dissolved	scarcely, has ripening effect	*removal of heavy metals* in wine, *clarifying agent,* ripeness-promoting together with gelatin allowed only in wine
12.	**Calcium phytate** (formerly aferrin) permitted from Sept. 1, 78 for red wine		colloidally dissolved	no	elimination of *iron(III) compounds* without preliminary trial, instead of blue fining
13.	**Gum arabic** permitted by EG-VO 337/79 of Feb. 5, 79		colloidally dissolved	no	acts as protective colloid, short-term prevention of precipitation of tartar and copper turbidity (masking) and the precipitation of red wine pigment
14.	**Polyclar AT** (PVPP) permitted up to 1978		powder, solid	scarcely	adsorbs interfering *tannins* or polyphenols; lightens the color
15.	**Silver chloride** Sulfidex, Ercofid still permitted for domestic wine up to 1979		insoluble powder, slurry	no	*eliminates rank tastes* (due to sulfur and mercaptans)
16.	**Copper sulfate** Preliminary trial		dissolved	somewhat (bouquet)	*eliminates rank sulfur tastes* and related taste faults

Amount per hectoliter	Possible combination	Moment of application	Contact time	Moment of racking early	late
up to 5 liters, limit = 5%	if required with carbon, then yeast as postfining	about January after 1st racking	1–2 days stir several times	soon after settling, filtration, or centrifugation	
must: 50–200 g wine: 2–10 g limit 100 g/hL	postfining with yeast or gelatin. Clear filtration	must, young wine, wine	15 min with thorough mixing	soon after settling or centrifugation	
must be determined accurately by preliminary trial	under certain circs. Carbon or bentonite beforehand, gelatin afterwards	at the 2nd racking and also with older wines. Not with unfermented grape must	immediately, sometimes subsequent flocculation after another 2–3 days	1 weeks over K5, in the case of must, kieselguhr after 1 day	3
8 g (limiting value)	none, gelatine postfining after 3 days	red wine before bottling	3 days	1–3 weeks traces of iron must be detectable	
10–20 g	none (stabilize with SO_2)	before bottling	–	–	
30–70–100 g limiting amount 250 g/hL	none	must, wine	stir for 1–2 h	after settling, filtration, posttreatment with sulfur dioxide	
50–200 g	postfining by blue fining, permitted residual silver 0.1 mg/L	young wine	stir well for 3 h or more	postfining by blue fining or with bentonite	
up to 2 g (limiting amount)	postfining by blue fining, limiting amount of Cu 1 mg/L	young wine	3 h	after action fine out residual Cu, blue fining	

must concentrates, which can be obtained by various evaporating apparatuses, by freeze-concentration, or by reverse osmosis.

Today, the filling of wines is carried out preferentially into bottles through various filter systems, very diverse filling systems and filling techniques being used (Troost, 1980).

10.2.6　Literature

Burkhardt, R., *Dtsch. Lebensm. Rundsch.* **72,** 417 (1976); **73,** 189 (1977).

Defranceschi, F., *Mitt. Klosterneuburg, Rebe u. Wein* **1955,** 340.

Drawert, F.: "Wein". In: *Ullmanns Encyklopädie der technischen Chemie,* Vol. 18, 3rd Ed. Verlag Urban u. Schwarzenberg, München, Berlin, Wien 1967.

Drawert, F., "Chemistry of Winemaking", *Adv. Chem. Ser.* **137,** 1 (1974).

Drawert, F.: *Symp. Aromastoffe in Früchten u. Fruchtsäften.* Int. Fruchtsaft-Union, Juris-Verlag, Bern 1978.

Drawert, F., Heimann, W., Emberger, R. and Tressl, R., *Liebigs Ann. Chem.* **694,** 200 (1966).

Drawert, F., Kuchenbauer, F., Brückner, H. and Schreier, P., *Chem. Mikrobiol. Technol. Lebensm.* **5,** 27 (1976).

Drawert, F. and Rapp, A., *Vitis* **4,** 262 (1964).

Drawert, F. and Rapp, A., *Vitis* **5,** 351 (1966); *Brauwissenschaft* **22,** 169 (1969).

Drawert, F., Rapp, A. and Ulrich, W., *Vitis* **5,** 195 (1965).

Drawert, F., Tressl, R., Heimann, W., Emberger, R. and Speck, M., *Chem. Mikrobiol. Technol. Lebensm.* **2,** 10 (1973).

Foulonneau, C., *Vignes et Vins* **1968,** 12.

Gervasi, E., *Vini Ital.* **1965,** 93.

Haushofer, H. and Bayer, E., *Mitt. Klosterneuburg, Rebe u. Wein* **1967,** 344.

Haushofer, H., Meier, W. and Bayer, E., *Mitt. Klosterneuburg, Rebe u. Wein* **1971,** 389.

Hillebrand, W.: *Taschenbuch der Rebsorten,* 5th Ed. Zeitschriftenverlag Dr. Bilz u. Dr. Fraund K.G., Wiesbaden 1978.

Husfeld, B., *Dtsch. Weinbau* **7,** 539 (1952); „Reben", In: *Handbuch der Pflanzenzüchtung,* Vol. VI, 2nd Ed. Verlag Paul Parey, Berlin-Hamburg, 1962, pp. 723–773.

Klenk, K., Villforth, E. and Fuhrmann, R., *Mitt. Klosterneuburg, Rebe u. Wein* **1954,** 1.

Ladousse, G., *Vignes et Vins* **1962,** 11; abstract in: *Weinberg Keller* **10,** 180 (1963).

Lemperle, E. and Kerner, E., *Wein Wiss.* **23,** 281, 408 (1968).

Lemperle, E., Trogus, H. and Frank, J., *Wein Wiss.* **28,** 181 (1973).

Maurer, R., *Mitt. Klosterneuburg, Rebe u. Wein* **1973,** 290.

Maurer, R., *Allg. Dtsch. Weinfachztg.* **109,** 579 (1973); *Dtsch. Weinbau* **31,** 663 (1976).

Maurer, R., Steinhilper, W. and Knoll, P., *Dtsch. Weinbau* **29,** 1040 (1974).

Mayer, K., *Schweiz. Z. Obst- Weinbau* **110,** 291 (1974); **112,** 372 (1976).

Mayer, K., *Weinwirtschaft* **115,** 223 (1979).

Mayer, K., Pause, G. and Vetsch, U., *Mitt. Geb. Lebensmittelunters. Hyg.* **62,** 397 (1971).

Mayer, K. and Vetsch, U., *Schweiz. Z. Obst-, Weinbau* **109,** 635 (1973).

Meidinger, F.: *Weinbaujahrbuch 1975,* p. 209.

Nègre, L., *Prog. Agric. Vitic.* **1967,** 503.

Radler, F., *Vitis* **3,** 136, 144 (1962); *Wein Wiss.* **24,** 418 (1969).

Schobinger, U. and Schneider, R., *Schweiz. Z. Obst-Weinbau* **111,** 503 (1975).

Schobinger, U., *Schweiz. Z. Obst-, Weinbau* **112,** 498 (1976).

Steinhilper, W., *Dtsch. Weinbau* **31,** 661 (1976).

Troost, G., *Technologie des Weines,* 5th Ed. Verlag E. Ulmer, Stuttgart 1980.

Urlaub, R., *Weinwirtschaft* **115,** 839 (1979).

10.3 Beer

Gert Sommer

10.3.1 Definition of the Term

Beer is a beverage containing alcohol and carbon dioxide that is prepared by the fermentation of an aqueous extract from malt or malt substitutes that has been treated with hops. In the Federal Republic of Germany, its manufacture is subject to strict legal requirements (§ 9 of the Beer Control Law of 1971). According to this, bottom-fermented beer is manufactured only from **barley malt, hops,** and **water** with the use of **yeast.** Any addition of foreign matter that could remain in the beer is forbidden. Regulations permitting exceptions exist for top-fermented beers, for which wheat malt and, with the exception of Bavaria and Baden-Württemberg, technically pure cane, beet, or invert sugar and starch sugar, as well as caramel prepared from them, may be used. As an exception to this, for the manufacture of export beers other brewing and auxiliary materials may also be used.

The manufacture of beer is composed of the areas of the **malting** of the barley, **brewing, fermentation,** and **storage,** together with **filtration** and **filling.**

10.3.2 Raw Materials

10.3.2.1 Brewing Barley

Barley has always been the main raw material for beer. The seedling is protected by the husks, and at the same time the husks act as a natural filtering layer in the purification of the worts. In continental Europe, **two-rowed spring barley** is used almost exclusively. In the USA and Canada, six-rowed barleys are used on the large scale for malting, and in England both spring and winter barleys are used.

The varieties and their origins play an overwhelming role for the malting process and the quality of the beer.

To judge brewing barley, both external characteristics such as color, smell, fineness of the husks, formation of the grain, contamination, and attack by pests, and also objective methods of investigations are used.

Variety: The batches of brewing barley should, above all, be pure varieties. Recently, it has become possible to determine the varieties by gel electrophoresis.

Water content: When its water content is above 16%, the barley can be stored for only a short time and must be dried before storage.

Germination capacity and germination power: Germination capacity is defined as the percentage of all grains with intact blastoderm, and germinating power as the percentage of the grains germinating under natural conditions in three and five days. The germinating capacity should be at least 96%.

Grading: The barley is graded through a standardized set of sieves with slit widths of 2.8, 2.5, and 2.2 mm. Brewing barley should contain the highest possible proportion with a size greater than 2.5 mm (bold barley).

Protein content: For technological reasons, the lowest possible protein content is desirable.

When the protein content rises by 1%, under otherwise identical conditions the extract yield of the malt falls by 0.8%, the extract difference rises by 0.5, and the Kolbach index[*] falls by 2.5. Corresponding changes arise with an alteration in the amount of bold barley (Table 10-3).

In addition to this, attempts are made by determining the structure of the grain such as, for example, the β-glucan content and the hardness of the grain or by determining the husks, to characterize the malting quality of the barley more thoroughly. Because of analytical difficulties, these methods have

---

[*] Kolbach index: soluble protein as a percentage of the wort protein.

Table 10-3. Barley Properties – Malt Quality.

Barley	Yield of extract	Extract difference (cell wall dissolution)	Kolbach index (protein dissolution)
+ 1% of protein	− 0.8%	+ 0.5	− 2.5
+ 10% of whole barley	+ 0.4%	− 0.1	+ 0.7

not yet been generally adopted. Table 10-4 lists the composition of brewing barley.

Table 10-4. Chemical Composition of Barley (Water-free).

Component	%
Starch	63
Sugars	2
Pentosans	9
Cellulose	5
Protein	11
Fats	2.5
Mineral matter	2.6
Other substances	4.9

10.3.2.2 Hops

The hop flowers or inflorescences contain the **bitter substances** and **essential oils** that are of interest for the preparation of beer. The chemistry of the bitter substances is an extraordinarily extensive and complex field; thus, so far more than 900 compounds have been isolated from the hop.

The bitter substances of the hop are classified as follows:

α-acids (humulones)   β-acids (lupolones)
                    + O₂
             soft resins
             hard resins

The **β-acids** are not soluble in either wort or beer, so that they possess no brewing value. The **α-acids** are slightly soluble in wort but not at the pH of beer. In the boiling of the wort they are converted

into so-called iso-α-acids. These **iso-α-acids** form the really valuable bitter substances of the beer. The oxidation products of the bitter acids – the soft resins and hard resins – are, on the other hand, readily soluble but they possess only a considerably smaller intensity of bitterness.

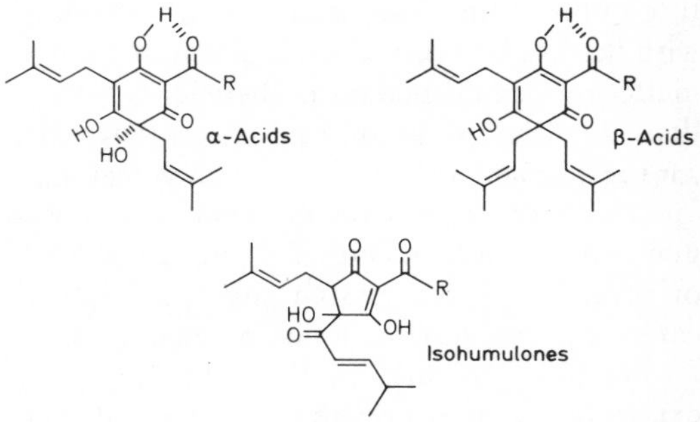

Fig. 10-20. Bitter acids of the hop.

The most important bitter acids are shown by the formulas in Fig. 10-20.

The hop inflorescences exhibit a characteristic and intensive aroma. The **aroma materials** include many chemical compounds such as aliphatic terpene and sesquiterpene hydrocarbons, aliphatic and terpene esters, aldehydes, ketones, alcohols, epoxides, lactones, ethers, and sulfur-containing compounds. The brewing value of the whole oils is, however, disputed, particularly since at the present time it has not yet been unambiguously determined which of this group of substances brings about a hop aroma in the beer and how this can be affected by technological measures.

Because of their sensitivity to oxidation, hops can be stored for only a limited time. In order to decrease the loss in value during storage and to increase the yield of bitter substances in brewing, to-day hops are frequently processed into **extract** or **powder pellets.** In the manufacture of the extract, the bitter principles are extracted with methylene chloride or, more recently, with carbon dioxide and, after the solvent has been evaporated off, the concentrate is packed into airtight cans. For the preparation of hop pellets, the hops are first dried more intensively than usual and are then ground and the powder is molded into pellets either immediately or after the removal of part of the leaves. Packaging is again carried out with the substantial exclusion of atmospheric oxygen.

10.3.2.3   Water for Brewing

The composition of the water used in brewing has a substantial influence on the quality or on the type of beer. In fact, the types of beer that are renowned through the world, such as Pilsner, Münchner, Dortmunder, and Wiener beers, originally owed their nature primarily to the water used for their brewing. Today, however, we are in a position to prepare any water in such a way that it can be used to manufacture the desired type of beer. In Germany, the Drinking Water Decree applies to the composition and preparation of water for brewing. The main point of interest for the brewer is the concentration of bicarbonate. The reaction during mashing of the bicarbonates with the H^+ arising from the malt displaces the pH of the mash into an unfavorable region. The consequences are poorer yield of extract, darker color, and a tart, rough, taste of the beer.

On the other hand, by reaction with phosphates or proteins in accordance with the equation

$$3\,Ca^{++} + 2\,HPO_4^{--} \rightarrow Ca_3(PO_4)_2 + 2\,H^+$$

calcium and magnesium ions have an acidity-promoting action in the mash. For this reason, calcium chloride or calcium sulfate is often added to the water for brewing in an amount corresponding to up to 350 mg of CaO/L.

Magnesium salts are less desirable in water for brewing, since, on the one hand, the preparation of water containing magnesium bicarbonate is more difficult and, on the other hand, an excessive magnesium content may lead to a deterioration of the taste.

In the last few years, it has often been shown that the nitrate content of water is rising. Nitrate contents exceeding 25 to 50 mg/L may, by reduction to nitrite, cause damage to the yeast and disturbances of the fermentation process.

The preparation of the water for brewing has fundamentally the task of removing the bicarbonates that are harmful for the brewing process. This is mainly carried out by precipitation processes with milk of lime or ion exchange. An acid treatment is also occasionally used.

10.3.3   Preparation of the Malt

The task of the malting process is, by germination, to form the enzymes necessary for the mashing process and to achieve a certain loosening of the structure of the grain.

10.3.3.1   Steeping of the Barley

In order to activate the vital processes, the grain must take up water. At a water content as low as about 25%, an irregular **germination** sets in. The optimum water content for germination is about 36%, while the optimum water content for the **formation of enzymes** and the modification of the grain is about 45 to 48%. In the newer **steeping processes** steeping is first carried out to a water content of 34 to 36% in order to achieve a rapid uniform germination. After this, the water content is raised in steps to the necessary level. During the whole steeping period, care must be taken that the material undergoing steeping has an adequate supply of oxygen.

In this process, the rate of uptake of water depends on the time, the temperature, and the state of the grain (size of the grain, variety, year). In the steeping process, in general, temperatures of between 12 and 18°C are preferred. Below 12°C, the uptake of water and germination take place too slowly and at excessive temperatures in the case of large units there are often difficulties in supplying an adequate and uniform amount of oxygen. In addition, the losses of extract rise because of increased respiration. In practice, the operation is carried out mainly with large **conical steeping vessels,** equipped with a ring nozzle system for aeration and also with a suction device for the removal of the carbon dioxide that arises through respiration in the so-called air rests during the steeping process. Most steeping processes are arranged in accordance with the basic scheme of Table 10-5.

Table 10-5. Steeping Processes.

Type of steeping	Time	Temperature	Water content
	h	°C	%
Immersion steeping	6– 8	12–14	35
Air rest	16–20	14–16	36
Immersion steeping	4– 6	14–16	42
Air rest	15–20	16–18	42
Immersion steeping	1– 2	16	45

The minimum consumption of water in such a steeping process is 2.5 to 3.4 m^3/ton of barley, while the actual uptake of water is only about 0.7 m^3/ton. In order to save water, in some cases steeping is carried out for a shorter time and the remainder of the water is sprayed on during germination.

10.3.3.2 Germination of the Barley

The process of germination and the modification of the malt can be controlled by the degree of steeping, of the water content of the green malt, the germination temperature, and the germination time. Since, in general, the steeping times are fixed by the malthouse equipment, in practice the modification process can be changed by means of the time parameter to only a limited extent.

An increasing water content in germination has a favorable effect on the yield of extract, on the modification of the cell wall, and on proteolysis, and also on the formation of enzymes. With rising germination temperature, it is true, the modification of the cell wall can be improved but the malting loss rises greatly, while the yield of extract, the solubility of the proteins, and the formation of enzymes diminish. It follows from this that the germination should be carried out at a temperature as low as possible and the modification process should be governed exclusively through the water content.

In practice, water contents of 44 to 50% and germination temperatures of 12 to 17°C have proved to be the optima. Today, germination is carried out almost exclusively in **pneumatic units.** The rectangular or circular vessels are provided with a perforated bottom under which there is an air channel. The material for germination forms a layer about 1 to 2 m high in these vessels and must be loosened at regular intervals (12 to 24 hours) in order to avoid felting. This is done by special helical turners or by transport from germination unit to germination unit. In order to remove the heat and carbon dioxide arising during its respiration, the germination material must be continuously aerated. The amount of air required is about 500 m^3/ton of barley. In the warmer seasons of the year, the germination air must be cooled. In order to save energy, part of the waste air, depending on the external air conditions, is reused. However, when this is done the carbon dioxide content of the germination air should not rise above 1 to 3%. In order to prevent excessive drying out of the green malt by the continuous aeration (about 0.5 to 1% per day), the germination air is partly humidified, or, when it is turned, the green malt is sprayed with water.

Today the average steeping and germination time amounts to 7 to 8 days. It can be shortened to 1 or 2 days by the addition of gibberellic acid (0.1 g/ton) with simultaneously better dissolution, but this is not permitted in Germany.

10.3.3.3 Kilning

The aim of kilning can be summarized as follows: **Drying of the green malt** from a moisture content of about 45% to 4% in order to stop the enzymatic and chemical reactions and, in the final kilning phase, to form the taste and aroma materials. In order to retain the enzymes and to avoid the formation of color in the case of a light-colored malt, the predrying process must be carried out gently at low temperatures (50 to 60°C). Only in the final phase is the temperature raised in order to bring the residual water content down from 10 to 15% to 4%. The curing temperature has a large influence on the color and aroma of the malt. For light malt, a curing of 4 to 5 hours at 80 to 85°C is regarded as the optimum for the taste and foaming properties of the beer.

In the preparation of dark "Munich malts", on the other hand, one must attempt to achieve a substantial formation of sugars and amino acids in the malt. This is done by heating the green malt, when it still has a high moisture content, to 40 to 45°C in the kiln and keeping it this temperature for several hours. After this, the malt is first dried and is subjected to curing at 100 to 110°C.

Drying is carried out on so-called kilning floors made from perforated sheets in a layer height of 60 to 120 cm. At the present time, the heating of the drying air is carried out predominantly by the direct mixing of flue gases with the drying air. Recently, however, it has been established that, particularly in gas burners with a high flame temperature, excessive amounts of NO_x are formed which, with the amines of the malt, produce dimethylnitrosamine. The NO_x content of the drying air can be controlled by lowering the flame temperature and, within certain limits, by sulfurizing (combustion of sulfur). The safest – but also most expensive – method is probably indirect heating. A level of 0.15 ppm is regarded as the limiting value for the NO_x content of the drying air.

10.3.3.4 The Evaluation of the Brewing Malt

In order to characterize the material changes caused by malting, the malt is milled and investigated in the laboratory by means of a standardized mashing process (Congress mashing process). The most important analyses are the water content (4.0 to 4.5%), the extract yield of the Congress mash (80.5%), and the soluble protein in the wort (4.4 g/100 g of malt), the Kolbach index or degree of solubility of the protein (soluble protein in the Congress wort as a percentage of the wort protein, 40%), color of the boiled Congress wort [5.0 EBC (European Brewery Convention) units], viscosity of the Congress wort (1.60 mPa s), pH of the Congress wort (5.8), and the extract difference (difference of yields between the Congress process with malt flour and a coarse meal, 2.3%) as a measure of the modification of the cell wall. In addition to this, there is a number of determinations such as the determination of enzymes, the β-glucan content and friability, and mashing at various temperatures which, however, have not come into general use for normal commercial analysis.

10.3.4   Preparation of the Beer

10.3.4.1 Technology of the Brewery (Fig. 10-21)

Malt contains only about 19% of water-soluble substances, and by far the greater part of it is, therefore, insoluble. The task of brewery operations is to obtain the malt extract as completely as possible in a short time and at

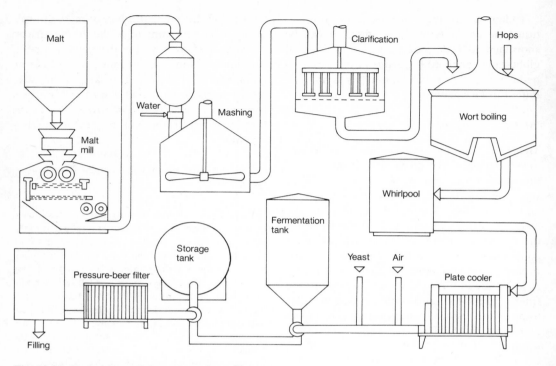

Fig. 10-21. Technology of the preparation of beer.

low cost. The brewery operations can be divided into the following areas:

Milling

The formation of the extract in mashing takes place fastest when flour is used. In practice, the processing of flour has not come into general use up to the present time because of the difficult problems of separation. The grists must therefore not be too fine and form a compromise between extract formation and extract recovery in mashing. In no case should the husks be disintegrated too greatly in the milling process, since otherwise on extraction the filter bed packs too tightly and retards the lautering process. In practice, there are two systems today, **dry milling** with conditioning

of the husks and **wet milling.** In dry milling with conditioning, the malt is slightly moistened with steam or water immediately before milling, and in wet milling the malt is steeped more or less intensively before milling. This leads to a substantial retention of the husks. Both systems have advantages and disadvantages, so that in the choice of the method of milling the characteristics of the particular brewery are decisive.

Mashing

The aim of mashing is to convert the constituents of the malt substantially into a soluble form and, in addition to this, to achieve a definite composition of the wort. The mashing operation is determined essentially by the three parameters time, temperature, and concentration. If one bears in mind the four most important enzymatic reactions in mashing, – namely, degradation of β-glucan, degradation of the protein, formation of maltose, and degradation of starch to products reacting negatively with iodine (Table 10-6) –, the mashing process is practically preprogrammed.

The optimum temperatures for α- and β-amylases are about 10 to 15°C below those given here. Since the gelatinization temperature of malt starch is 60 to 70°C, however, higher temperatures must be used in mashing.

The individual temperature ranges in mashing are observed in accordance with the malt solution and the type of beer desired. With a barely modified malt, in general, mashing will be carried out at a temperature at 40 to 50 °C, but with a very substantially modified malt this will be done at a temperature of 55 to 60°C. However, a malting procedure that is faulty in relation to the degradation of β-glucan and of protein can only be partially corrected on mashing in the brewery. In Germany, it is permitted to correct the pH of the mash only by an appropriate preparation of the water, by the addition of sour malt, or by using a wort soured with the aid of lactic acid bacteria.

The simplest, shortest, and most rational mashing process is an infusion process with rising temperature.

Such a process is characterized by its simplicity and lower consumption of energy and gives beers with a somewhat lighter color and also a better head retention. Disadvantageous features are that higher demands must be placed on the malt solution for this purpose, the extract yields are somewhat lowered, and there is a higher loss of bitter substances, and a lower colloidal stability of the beer must be taken into account. Today, decoction mashing processes in which one or more parts of the mash are boiled and the increase in temperature is achieved by recycling the hot mash are still used overwhelmingly. Mashing is carried out in circular or angular copper or stainless steel vessels with heating surfaces and stirrers.

Lautering

After mashing, the extract-containing wort must be separated from the undissolved constituents, the draff. In this process, the draff forms a natural filtering layer, so that a relatively clear wort can be obtained, which is advantageous for technological reasons. In practice, hitherto only two extraction systems have succeeded in gaining wide acceptance, the **lauter tun** and the **mash filter.**

The lauter tun is a cylindrical vessel with a flat or slightly conical bottom. Above this there is a perforated bottom upon which the draff is retained. The issuing wort runs into a

Table 10-6. Enzymatic Reactions in Mashing.

pH	Temperature °C	Action	Enzyme
4.8–5.0	40–50	degradation of gums	glucanases
4.5–4.7	50–60	formation of protein degradation products	proteolytic enzymes
5.3	60–64	formation of maltose	β-amylase
5.8	70–74	degradation of starch	α-amylase

collecting pipe and is dumped into the wort copper. In order to prevent a solidification of the filter bed, in the clarification process the draff is loosened at irregular intervals with a rake consisting essentially of vertical knives. After the first wort has run off, the filter bed is extracted by being sparged with hot water.

The **mash filter** is a frame filter in which the filtering layer is retained by polypropylene cloths. After mashing, the mash is pumped at a low pressure into the filter frames. When the pumping of the mash has finished, the first wort is also run off. For final extraction, hot water is run through each second outlet through the filter bed into the chambers in order to obtain the residual extract.

Wort Boiling

The aims of the boiling of the wort can be summarized as follows:

- Dissolution and isomerization of the bitter substances
  The optimum time of boiling of the hops for the utilization of the bitter substances is about 90 minutes. For this reason, it is also advantageous on economic grounds to add the bulk of the hops at the beginning of the boiling process. To the extent that a certain hop aroma is required in the beer, part of the hops is added during boiling or after completion of the process. The average amount of hops added for a Pilsner beer is about 9 to 10 g of α-acid per hL. The yield of bitter substances in the beer amounts to only about 30 to 35%.

- Coagulation of protein
  During the mashing and sparging, part of the protein (albumin and globulin) passes into solution. An excessive amount of coagulable nitrogen in the beer can interfere with the filtration of the beer and causes a lowering of its colloidal stability. In gener-

al, a level of 20 mg/L is sought, but this is often not achieved because of differences in the construction of the coppers.

- Elimination of undesirable aroma substances
  For reasons of taste, the bulk of the readily volatile hop oils must be driven off during the boiling of the wort. In addition, in the boiling process a multiplicity of carbonyl compounds with intensive flavors arise which would to some extent have an unfavorable influence on the aroma of the beer. For the reasons given, an evaporation level of 5 to 10% is to be aimed at.

- Concentration of the wort
  The sparging of the filter bed to obtain extract lowers the concentration of the wort. In earlier years, the highest possible rate of evaporation was aimed at in order to increase the brewhouse yield. Because of the drastic rise in the cost of energy in recent years, evaporation solely for the purpose of obtaining an extract would be uneconomic.

- Formation of reducing substances and aroma substances
  The reaction of reducing sugars and amino acids gives rise to numerous oxygen, nitrogen, and heterocyclic compounds which are known to be characteristic aroma constituents of foodstuffs.

- Inactivation of the enzymes
  A further degradation of the substrate by the malt enzymes after the brewery is undesirable for technological reasons. An exception is formed by diet beer to which a malt extract is added in the fermentation cellar.

- Sterilization of the wort
  Although, after boiling, the wort is not absolutely sterile, it contains no germs that are harmful for the preparation of beer.

10.3.4.2 Cooling of the Wort

The boiled wort must first be substantially separated from the spent hops and the turbidity formed on boiling (protein-tannin compounds). If natural hops are used, the **separation of the spent hops** takes place in a straining vessel, the hop back, which in some cases is also provided with a worm press. The other hop residues and the turbidity are generally removed today by means of **settling vats** (whirlpools) or **centrifuges.** The wort is then cooled. Cooling is carried out either in two stages with 1.2 times the amount of brewing water being heated to about 80°C in the first stage and the wort being cooled to the pitching temperature by means of a coolant in the second stage, or the brewing water is previously cooled to a temperature which is sufficient for the pitching temperature of the wort to be reached. In the cooling of the worts, substances causing turbidity, the so-called cold break, are again formed. The necessity for removing cold break is disputed in breweries. In some breweries, the cold break is completely or partly removed by settling, flotation, or filtration.

10.3.4.3 Fermentation

Yeast

Apart from certain exceptions, the fermentation of the wort is carried out with pure cultures of yeast. The brewers' yeasts belong to the genus Saccharomyces. The brewer distinguishes top and bottom yeasts. The obvious difference is that the **top yeasts** rise to the top at the end of fermentation, and the **bottom yeasts** sink to the bottom. This property of the yeast is not, however, absolutely fixed. Thus, it has been observed that when fermentation is carried out in closed tanks top yeasts often no longer rise but settle to the bottom, while bottom yeasts become top-fermenting under certain conditions. Analytically, the yeasts are distinguished by their **fermentation of raffinose.** Top yeasts contain no melibiase and can therefore ferment raffinose only to a degree of $\frac{1}{3}$.

In addition, another distinction is made between powdery and flocculating yeasts. The **flocculating yeasts** exhibit a pronounced flocculation behavior at the end of fermentation, while **powdery yeasts** settle only very slowly. In general, flocculating yeasts give a better quality of the beer but it is difficult in practical operation to achieve a uniform flocculation. A premature flocculation prevents adequate postfermentation, while flocculation that is to late means an excessive concentration of yeast on storage and can lead to difficulties in filtration and to an autolysis taste.

Fermentation and Storage

The fermentation and metabolism of the yeast is affected basically by the composition of the wort (α-amino nitrogen, oxygen content, mineral substances, fermentable sugars), the concentration of yeast, the temperature of fermentation, agitation, and pressure (carbon dioxide content).

Fermentation is initiated by the pitching of the wort with yeast. The average amount of yeast added is about 1 L of yeast in the form of a thick pulp per hL or, more accurately, 15 to 20 million yeast cells per mL. An **adequate supply of oxygen** to the yeast is important for its multiplication and rapid fermentation. Since, on the other hand, depending on the operating conditions, the oxygen has a considerable influence on the formation of metabolic products of the yeasts, no generally valid guideline can be given for the aeration of the wort. In the majority of cases, an oxygen concentration of 6 to 8 mg/L is aimed at. In the filling of large tanks over a long period the aeration is often decreased during the last few hours. In the conventional fermentation processes, pitching is carried out at at temperature of 6 to 8 °C, the fermentation temperature is allowed to rise to 8 to 10 °C, and towards the end the material is cooled again, to 4 to 6 °C. The fermentation time amounts to about seven days. During the main fermentation, about 90% of the fermentable extract is fermented, after which the young beer is transferred into the storage cellars where a slow secondary fermentation and maturation of the beer takes place in four to six weeks. Here the temperature is lowered to about − 1 °C in order to precipitate turbidity-forming materials.

Forced fermentation processes take place at higher temperatures (14 to 18 °C) in closed tanks under counterpressure. The counterpressure brings about an enrichment of the carbon dioxide in the beer and it again inhibits the multiplication of the yeast and the metabolism of the yeast which is intensified at higher temperatures. In warm pressure fermentation processes, fermentation is basically carried out to completion in the fermentation tank and the maturation of the beer is awaited at relatively high temperatures. Then the beer is cooled either in the fermentation tank or in the storage cellar. Since the maturation of the beer has already been concluded at this time, the cold storage phase now has only the aim of precipitating the turbidity materials and can therefore be shortened to 7 to 14 days.

Present knowledge concerning the **biochemical transformations** during the maturation phase still contains gaps. In the main, volatile sulfur compounds, such as hydrogen sulfide, dimethyl sulfide, diethyl sulfide, and ethyl mercaptan, lower fatty acids, aldehydes, and α-acetolactate or the biacetyl arising from it are made responsible for the young bouquet formed during the main fermentation. The formation and reduction of biacetyl and pentanedione has been investigated the most thoroughly. α-Acetolactate and α-acetohydroxybutyrate are intermediate products that arise during amino acid synthesis by yeast. By oxi-

dative decarboxylation they form biacetyl and pentanedione, respectively. The taste threshold level of biacetyl in beer is 0.2 to 0.15 mg/L. Biacetyl imparts to the beer an oppressive slightly sweetish smell and taste. During the maturation phase, the biacetyl formed is reduced by the yeast. In practice, the reduction of the biacetyl is often regarded as an indication of the maturation of the beer.

The same features apply to top fermentation, but here considerably higher fermentation temperatures (18 to 25 °C) are used. The fermentation time is now only one to three days and the time of storage 7 to 21 days. In general, top yeasts form more aroma substances, this being favored by the high fermentation temperature.

Filtration

After maturation and storage, the beer is filtered. Here, the **slurrying filters** with kieselguhr or mixtures of kieselguhr and perlite have come into general use. In addition, the beer may be filtered through **sterilizing layers.** A normally manufactured beer has a colloidal stability of about 6 to 8 weeks. If a longer keepability is to be guaranteed, the beer must be additionally stabilized. In Germany, only adsorption agents such as bentonites, silica gels, and xerogels (adsorption of proteins) and also PVPP (adsorption of polyphenols) are permitted for this purpose. In other countries, tannin and proteolytic enzymes are frequently added. The preparation of beers retaining their taste for a long period still presents difficulties. In any case, any uptake of oxygen during filtration and filling must be substantially avoided.

10.3.4.4   Chemical Composition of Beer

The beers in the Federal Republic of Germany are placed in classes according to their **original wort strength** (extract content of the

Table 10-7. Classification of German Beers.

Beer	Original wort %	Proportion of the (German) market in 1979 %
Einfachbiere (small or table beers)	2–5.5	0.1
Schankbiere (draft beers)	7–8	0.2
Vollbiere (full-strength beers)	11–14	98.9
Starkbiere (strong beers)	over 16	0.8

wort in g/100 g before fermentation) (Table 10-7.)

The analytical composition of beers depends more on the original wort strength than on the other production conditions. The analytical composition of an average Pilsner beer with an original wort strength of 11.9% can be found in Table 10-8.

Table 10-8. Composition of Beer.

Component	Content
Original wort	11.9 g/100 g
Extract	42.0 g/L
Alcohol	39.0 g/L
Carbohydrates	29.0 g/L
Protein	5.1 g/L
Mineral substances	1.5 g/L
Organic acids	591 mg/L
Glycerol	1617 mg/L
Higher aliphatic alcohols	88 mg/L
Bitter substances	34 mg/L
Polyphenols	185 mg/L
Vitamins	
Thiamine	33 μg/L
Riboflavin	410 μg/L
Pyridoxine	650 μg/L
Pantothenic acid	1632 μg/L
Niacin	7875 μg/L
Biotin	13 μg/L
Calorific value	1828 kJ/L

Particular special beers are **diet beer** and **alcohol-free beers.** Diet beers may contain only 7.5 g/L of metabolizable carbohydrates and must therefore be extremely highly fermented. This is achieved by the addition of an enzyme-rich malt extract in the fermentation cellar. Diet beers therefore necessarily contain about 25% more alcohol than the corresponding normally fermented beers.

Alcohol-poor or alcohol-free beers are generally manufactured by a retarded fermentation or by distilling off the alcohol.

10.3.5   Literature

Clerck, J. de: *Lehrbuch der Brauerei,* Vol. I, 2nd Ed. Versuchs- und Lehranstalt für Brauerei, Berlin 1964.

Hough, J. S., Briggs, D. E. and R. Stevens: *Malting and Brewing science.* Chapman and Hall, London 1971.

Narziss, L.: *Abriß der Bierbrauerei.* 4th Ed. Ferdinand Enke Verlag, Stuttgart 1980.

Piendl, A., "Deutsches Pilsener Lagerbier", *Brauwelt* **120** (15), 518–532 (1980).

Schuster, K., Weinfurter, F. und L. Narziss: *Die Bierbrauerei,* Vol. 1: Die Technologie der Malzbereitung. 6th Ed. Ferdinand Enke Verlag, Stuttgart 1976.

Rinke, W.: "Das Bier". In: *Grundlagen und Fortschritte der Lebensmitteluntersuchung,* Vol. 10. Paul Parey, Berlin, Hamburg 1967.

Chapter 11

Primary Metabolites

Karl Buchta

11.1   Introduction

The list of metabolic products that can be obtained by means of suitable microorganisms has grown to a considerable size, and future research will certainly extent it further. Of course in reviewing the situation one must be clear about the fact that although these products can indeed all be obtained, at the present time for a large number of them this cannot be done **economically**. There may be various reasons for this: thus, many fermentation products are in competition with cheaper natural or synthetic substances, or their use and, therefore, the demand for them is not yet large enough for them to be produced economically.

The summary in this chapter can, of course, not go into detail. Rather, a brief account and references to further literature will be given, with a somewhat more exhaustive account of the products that appear to be the most important at the present time.

The technical processes that can be used for recovery are the same for many products. In the following section, these will be briefly shown schematically (see also Chapters 6 and 12).

11.2   Technical Processes

11.2.1   Surface Processes on Solid Substrates

Today, on the industrial scale this mode of operation no longer plays more than a subordinate role. It had its origin in the history of the preparation of foodstuffs in East Asia, where, for example, in the koji process moistened rice grains in heaps were subjected to a microbial fermentation. This process, very similar in its industrial version to the surface processes on liquid substrates discussed below, is mentioned here only for the sake of completeness, since it is not used in the production of primary metabolic products.

11.2.2   Surface Processes on Liquid Substrates

These processes, which are still practised today on the industrial scale, are also very ancient. The prepared sterile nutrient solution is filled into open metal trays 2 to 20 cm high and inoculated on the surface by being sprayed with suspensions of spores.

The whole arrangement is placed in a room which can be kept aseptic. The supply of oxygen and the regulation of the temperature are carried out by aerating the room with sterile, conditioned air. Since in this process the organisms used take up the necessary oxygen via diffusion but this is affected in uncontrollable manner by the growth of the microorganisms on the surface of the nutrient solution, such fermentations are very difficult to control and their course remains obscure.

11.2.3   Submerged Processes, Anaerobic

From the point of view of apparatus, these are the least expensive processes, since no aeration devices and often no stirrer, either, are necessary. Furthermore, the geometric proportions of the fermenter space play only a small part, so that all shapes of vessel can be used. In the technical performance of these processes, depending on the size of the end stage it must be preceded by one or more **preliminary stages for the multiplication of the microorgan-**

isms. The duration and size of such a preliminary cultivation must be determined for each microorganism and varies between a few hours and several days, and the same applies to the size ratio of the successive steps, which may amount to from 1:100 to 1:10.

The dissolution or suspension of the nutrients and auxiliary materials in water and the sterilization of the nutrient solution are carried out either in the fermentation vessel itself or in a preparation vessel provided for this particular purpose from which the sterile medium is then transferred aseptically into the separately sterilized containers. While, in the apparatus described previously, after starting up it is hardly possible to intervene further in the fermentation once it has begun, here it is possible to carry out **control measures** and to make **additions** during the fermentation. The most important measure is, for example, the maintenance of the **optimum process temperature,** which can be done by passing heating or cooling media through outer jackets or built-in coils. The course of the fermentation in relation to these parameters can readily be followed by taking samples for analysis and by built-in measurement sensors and be corrected if necessary.

11.2.4 Submerged Processes, Aerobic

The development of the technical equipment necessary for these processes began with the start of the production of antibiotics on the large technical scale. They are the most common in the fermentation industry today.

For this type of fermentation, as already described for anaerobic processes, several vessels of different sizes are connected in series in order to make it possible to grow the bio-mass necessary for inoculating the production stage (Blakeborough, 1967). The **size** of these fermenters, which are usually made of stainless steel, ranges up to a capacity of 100 m^3, and even still larger capacities are possible. Because of the aeration with sterile compressed air or mixtures of gases that are always required here and the resulting formation of foam during fermentation, these fermenters cannot be completely filled. Chemical and/or mechanical **foam suppressing arrangements** must be provided. The nature of the **stirrers** used and also their geometry and that of the vessels are of great importance for the optimum course of these fermentations. The economy of the process is considerably affected both by the energy demand and by mass transport (Calderbank, 1967; Finn, 1967). (See also Chapters 6 and 18).

In these units, almost every parameter can be modified. Provided that the biochemical course of the process is known, it is possible today with the aid of the most modern developments in the field of electronics to intervene in the subsequent course of the process in the shortest possible time so that the fermentation can always be kept under the optimum conditions. These systems also permit an almost complete **automation** of the total process so that even for large plants only a minimum number of personnel is necessary for their operation.

All the methods described so far belong to the so-called **batch** or **individual processes.** In contrast to these are the **continuous processes** in which the microorganisms can be kept for a long time by various provisions in a physiological state which corresponds to the optimum production phase. Even though continuous processes are theoretically applicable for many products – and can be performed technically with both submerged processes – they are not, with a few exceptions, used in practice.

11.3   Products

11.3.1   Organic Acids

Acetic Acid

CH₃—CO₂H   **MW:[1]   60.05**
                      mp:[2]   16.6

[1] MW = molecular weight (= molecular mass)
[2] mp = melting point (in °C)

The manufacture and use of vinegar has come down to us from prehistoric times. Conner and Allgeier (1976) have given a very good review of the history of the preparation of vinegar. It is known by tradition today that the Babylonians had a commercial manufacture of vinegar as long as 5000 years ago. The starting materials were palm juice and date syrup, and later beer and wine from raisins were also used.

Nothing has changed in the method of production today: alcohol is obtained by fermentation from a cheap readily available source of sugar, and this is converted into acetic acid in a second step.

The fundamental advances have appeared in the technological field. But even here the decisive advance was achieved very early, since the manufacture of acetic acid by the **generator principle** which belongs to the surface processes, was described as early as 1670. Here, the stems of the bunches of grapes (the system of stalks, upon which the berries hang) were used for filling the fermentation vessels, while today birchwood shavings are used. The acetic acid bacteria colonize these and are then "immobilized" so that they are not appreciably washed off by the wine that is trickled over the packing. This trickling operation, moreover, fulfils two essential conditions: the temperature is kept in the optimum range and the **supply of oxygen** necessary for the oxidative stage is ensured. Today, additional aeration is used and the consequence is a series of designs of special fermenters (Vaughn, 1954).

Of course, the apparatuses developed for aerobic submerged fermentation can also be used for this purpose. They have the advantage that no filling with wood shavings is necessary, so that tank room is saved and shorter fermentation times are achieved. The yields of acetic acid are 85 to 94%, referred to the alcohol fed.

The **taxonomy** of the microorganisms involved in the formation of acetic acid presented difficulties for a long time, on the one hand, since mixed cultures were present and, on the other hand, since the Acetobacter species, which form the most important group, readily tend to undergo mutations (Greenshields, 1978).

Propionic Acid

HO₂C—CH₂—CH₃   **MW: 74.08**
                          mp: −22.0

Propionic acid can be obtained in a similar manner to the production of lactic acid by fermentation (p. 443). The microorganisms that may be used are various species of the genus Propionibacterium. Which of the species is taken depends on the type of carbon source to be fermented. Thus, *Propionibacterium freudenreichii* and *Propionibacterium jensenii* form propionic acid only from sugars, while *Propionibacterium technicum* can also ferment starch, dextrin and glycogen.

The temperature optimum of the fermentation is 30°C and the pH optimum is 6.8 to 7.2. These conditions and the fact that the fermentation lasts 7 to 12 days, are, according to Rehm (1967), the reasons why there is a great susceptibility to infections with other microorganisms, especially bacteria.

In addition to propionic acid, relatively large amounts of **acetic acid** are also formed; in the case of *Propionibacterium arabinosum,* the ratio is 2:1. The total yield is 75 to 85%, referred to the sugar used, 15 to 20% being converted into carbon dioxide by respiration.

The **amount** of propionic acid manufactured by biotechnological processes is only small since, on the one hand, the demand is not large and, on the other hand, there are also **chemical** processes of manufacture.

In addition to the propionic acid bacteria, *Clostridium propionicum* also forms propionic acid – by a different synthetic pathway according to Wilkinson and Rose (1963).

Butyric Acid

$$HO_2C—(CH_2)_2—CH_3$$
MW: **88.10**
mp: **−7.9**

Clostridium butyricum forms considerable amounts of butyric acid, together with acetic acid, from glucose. The gaseous end products consist of a mixture of carbon dioxide and hydrogen.

Oxalic Acid

$$HO_2C—CO_2H$$
MW: **90.04**
mp: **189.5**

No *ad hoc* fermentation for the production of oxalic acid is practised. Depending on the process used, this acid is formed **as a by-product** in larger or smaller amount in the fermentative manufacture of citric acid (Section 11.3). A high phosphate content and a pH in the weakly acid region, in particular, lead to an increased formation of oxalic acid.

Today, the careful choice of the strain and improved fermentation conditions keep the formation of oxalic acid as a by-product in citric acid fermentation so low that the recovery of the oxalic acid is not economically feasible.

However, its isolation is fairly simple since the solubilities of the calcium salts of oxalic and citric acids differ very widely. If, after the separation of the mycelium, sufficient calcium is added to the filtrate, insoluble calcium oxalate precipitates at low temperatures while calcium citrate precipitates only at temperatures around 100°C.

Fumaric Acid

(trans-Butenedioic acid)
$$HO_2C—CH＝CH—CO_2H$$
MW: **116.07**
mp: **286-7**

The biological production of fumaric acid was previously carried out on the industrial scale with the aid of *Rhizopus nigricans*. Today, fumaric acid is obtained by chemical synthesis, a method which at the present time is even cheaper than the biological process.

Sucrose, glucose, or starch is used as the raw material for the **submerged process**; a **neutralizing agent** must also be present in adequate amount. The yields in 4 to 7 days at 30°C and above amount to more than 65%, referred to the sugar consumed.

Normal paraffins can also be used as the raw material. In this case, Candida is used as the microorganism, giving an 84% yield in 7 days (Miall, 1978; Rehm, 1967).

Itaconic Acid

(Methylenesuccinic acid)
$$HO_2C—C(＝CH_2)—CH_2—CO_2H$$
MW: **130.10**
mp: **161-2**
D:[1] **1.6**

[1] D = density at 20°C (in g/L)

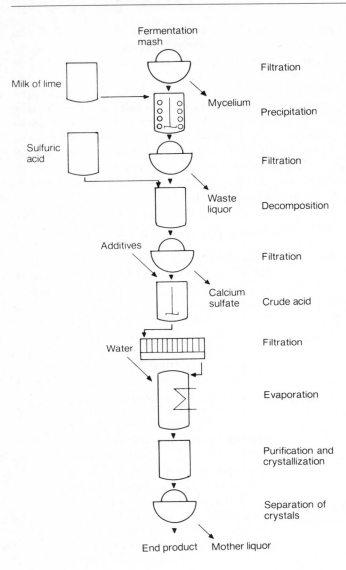

Fermentation
mash

Milk of lime

Sulfuric
acid

Additives

Water

Filtration

Mycelium

Precipitation

Filtration

Waste
liquor   Decomposition

Filtration

Calcium
sulfate   Crude acid

Filtration

Evaporation

Purification and
crystallization

Separation of
crystals

End product   Mother liquor

Fig. 11-1. Production of citric acid by the precipitation method.

Itaconic acid, which is used in the **paint** and **plastics industries,** can be obtained both by the surface process and by the submerged method with the aid of *Aspergillus terreus* or *Aspergillus itaconicus.*

In the **surface process,** a **sugar solution** is converted into itaconic acid in a thin layer in aluminium trays at 30 to 32 °C (Lockwood and Ward, 1945).

The submerged method works better, and in this, apart from **glucose, molasses** can be used. In 3 to 4 days at a cultivation temperature of 40 °C, 50 to 60 g of itaconic acid is formed per 100 g of sugar consumed (Pfeifer et al., 1952;

Kinoshita and Tanaka, 1960; Nubel and Ratajak, 1966). It has proved to be particularly advantageous partially to neutralize the acid formed. Its isolation is simple and is achieved by concentrating the filtrate and allowing the cooled concentrate to crystallize out.

Lactic Acid

(2-Hydroxypropanoic acid)
CH_3—$CH(OH)$—CO_2H

MW:	**90.08**
mp:	**25-6**
	(L(+)-acid)
	18
	(DL-acid)
$[\alpha]_D^{20}$ [1] =	**+3.3°**
	(c[2]=5; H_2O)
	(L(+)-acid)
D:	**1.294**

[1] $[\alpha]_D^{20}$ = specific rotation (α) at 20°C (20) of the D line of sodium (D) (in °)
[2] c = concentration (in g/100 mL solution)

The methods for the technical production of lactic acid by fermentation can be divided into two types: the **homofermentative,** in which only lactic acid is formed and the **heterofermentative,** in which, in addition to lactic acid, considerable amounts of **acetic acid** and **alcohol** are formed (Franke and Buchta, 1960). Since the latter is of no interest for the industrial process here we shall describe only the homofermentation.

The process is an **anaerobic submerged method** (see Section 11.2.3). Diluted molasses can be used as the starting material, but sugar solutions are better. Since lactic acid exists in a L(+) and a D(−) form and can therefore also appear as the **racemate,** the **choice of organism** and of **suitable fermentation conditions** is decisive for determining which of the forms

is produced. For use in the foodstuffs industry, the L(+) form must be preferred, since the human organism is adapted only to dissimilation of this form. But the optically pure forms are also necessary for certain technical applications [e.g., polylactide (Nielsen and Veibel, 1967)].

The lactic acid bacteria (Lactobacillus spp.) are oxygen-sensitive and exhibit full efficiency only in a weakly acid pH range. For the latter reason, calcium carbonate is added to neutralize the acid formed; the carbon dioxide produced also drives the residual oxygen out of the fermentation solution and maintains anaerobic conditions. An advantage for the aseptic performance of fermentation is that some lactic acid bacteria have their optimum temperature range at 45 to 50°C in which most microorganisms forming possible sources of infection are incapable of multiplication.

After the acid has been liberated from its salt, isolation is carried out either by solvent extraction or via alcohol esters. Where the fermentation solutions are pure, ion-exchangers and subsequent concentration can also be used (Buchta, 1974) (Fig. 11-2).

L(−)-Malic Acid

(Hydroxysuccinic acid)
HO_2C—CH_2—$CH(OH)$—CO_2H

MW:	**134.09**
mp:	**100**
$[\alpha]_D^{18}$ =	**−2.3°**
D:	**1.595**

This acid can easily be obtained chemically, but the fermentative possibilities could one day gain greater importance.

The raw material is fumarate, which is converted enzymatically into L(−)-malate. For this purpose it is possible to use the isolated

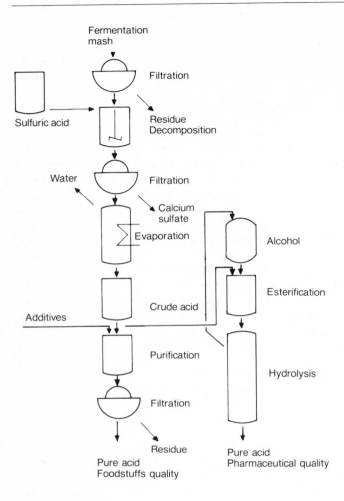

Fig. 11-2. Production of lactic acid.

Fermentation mash

Filtration

Sulfuric acid

Residue
Decomposition

Water

Filtration

Calcium sulfate

Evaporation

Alcohol

Crude acid

Esterification

Additives

Purification

Hydrolysis

Filtration

Residue

Pure acid
Foodstuffs quality

Pure acid
Pharmaceutical quality

enzyme fumarase or the complete cells of microorganisms that contain this enzyme. The reaction takes place almost quantitatively in 20 hours (Kitahara, 1969; Degen et al., 1974; Morisi et al., 1974; Chibata et al., 1975). The microorganisms that are cultivated aerobically in the presence of fumaric acid belong to the genera Brevibacterium, Corynebacterium, Escherichia, Microbacterium, Proteus, Pichia, Paracolobactrum, etc.

A fumarase of animal origin may also be used for this process.

D(+)-Tartaric Acid

$$HO_2C—CH(OH)—CH(OH)—CO_2H$$

MW: 150.09
mp: 170 (d.)[1]
$[\alpha]_D^{20} =$ $+14°$ (20%, H_2O)
D: 1.759

[1] d. = decomposition

This acid was originally obtained from **tartar**, but today it is also accessible by fermentation.

If, in fact, the 5-ketogluconic acid fermentation is carried on beyond the end point, this compound is transformed further into D(+)-tartaric acid (Minoda et al., 1972; Yamada et al., 1969; Kotera et al., 1972).

On the basis of new knowledge, the designation of natural tartaric acid hitherto customary as the L(+) form is no longer tenable (Buchta, 1974).

Another **starting material** that can be used for the microbial production of tartaric acid is cis-epoxysuccinic acid, which is manufactured chemically from **maleate** (Kamatani et al., 1976). The microorganisms that can bring about this transformation belong to the genera Acinetobacter, Agrobacterium, Rhizobium, and Pseudomonas. With aeration and stirring at 20°C, up to 40% of the starting material is 55 to 93% converted into tartaric acid in 2 to 4 days, particularly when small amounts of non-ionic surface-active agents are added to the reaction medium.

Citric Acid

(2-Hydroxy-1,2,3-propanetricarboxylic acid)
$$HO_2C—CH_2—C(OH)(CO_2H)—CH_2—CO_2H$$

MW:	**192.12**
mp:	**153**
D:	**1.542**

Both the surface process on liquid media (see Section 11.2.2) and the aerobic submerged method (see Section 11.2.4) are used for the manufacture of this acid. The microorganisms are usually selected strains of the fungus *Aspergillus niger* (Buchta, 1974; Miall, 1978).

The starting material used for the **surface process** is diluted **beet sugar** or **cane sugar molasses.** Because of the sensitivity of the fungus to heavy-metal ions, the nutrient solution must undergo suitable pretreatment, e.g., pre-cipitation with potassium ferrocyanide or ion exchange.

On the surface that is inoculated with spores, the fungus forms a closed mycelial mat, and in 8 to 10 days it converts the sugar supplied into citric acid in a yield of 60 to 80%. The formation of oxalic acid as a by-product can be prevented by the choise of suitable strains and appropriate pH conditions (Johnson, 1954; Rudy, 1967; Rehm, 1971; Rose, 1961).

In the **aerobic submerged process,** in which, besides molasses, **sugar solutions** may also be used, the maximum yield is reached after a fermentation time of only 6 to 8 days. Here, in addition to strains of *Aspergillus niger,* yeasts are also employed (Roberts, jun., 1974; Miall and Parker, 1977; Jungbunzlauer, 1978).

More recently, processes have also been described in which **hydrocarbons** are used as starting material. The microorganisms performing these fermentations are yeasts of the genera Hansenula and Candida. These fermentations, likewise performed by the aerobic submerged method, require considerable amounts of oxygen and reach their maximum after only four days (Hustede and Siebert, 1975; Hustede and Siebert, 1977a, b; Iizuka et al., 1978).

Likewise using C_{14}–C_{16} normal paraffins as raw material, a **continuous process** has been described (Miall and Parker, 1978) in which, after a discontinuous initial cultivation phase of, for example, 71 h, in the subsequent continuous process running for 233 h, 4.2 kg of citric acid monohydrate can be obtained from 3.3 kg of normal paraffins. A small amount of isocitric acid is also formed. *Candida lipolytica* ATCC 20 228 (ATCC=American Type Culture Collection) has been used as the microorganism in this process.

When hydrocarbons are used as substrate and yeasts as the organisms in citric acid fermentation, there appears to be an increased tendency to the formation of **isocitric acid as** by-product. Miall and Parker (1978) have described processes in which almost equal amounts of citric and isocitric acids are formed and in one case actually isocitric acid alone. However, by **selection from mutations,** strains can be obtained which form substantially less isocitric acid and therefore more citric acid. Additions of aconitate hydratase inhibitors, such as sodium fluoroacetate and methanol, can also help to overcome this trouble.

The recovery of the citric acid formed is generally carried out by a process in which it is precipitated as the calcium salt followed by purification (Fig. 11-1).

D-Gluconic Acid

$$HO_2C-\underset{\underset{H}{|}}{\overset{\overset{OH}{|}}{C}}-\underset{\underset{OH}{|}}{\overset{\overset{H}{|}}{C}}-\underset{\underset{H}{|}}{\overset{\overset{OH}{|}}{C}}-\underset{\underset{H}{|}}{\overset{\overset{OH}{|}}{C}}-CH_2OH$$

MW:	196.15
mp:	125-6
$[\alpha]_D^{10} =$	$-6.7°$

The production of gluconic acid by acid fermentation was one of the first fermentation processes used technically but is no longer of any importance, since gluconic acid is more readily available by the electrochemical or enzymatic transformation of glucose (Baker, 1953; Walon, 1970).

Both the surface process and also the submerged method can be used for this fermentation. While the **surface processes** are uneconomic because of the small layer height and the long fermentation times, in **stirred** and **aerated fermenters** glucose concentrations of up to 30% can be converted by *Aspergillus niger* at 30°C in a yield of 97% in about 40 h (Buchta, 1974; Miall, 1978).

A process that probably gives the highest conversion feeds only part of the glucose to be transformed at the start. Further amounts of glucose are added in the course of fermentation. The gluconic acid formed is partially neutralized. In this way, in a running time of about 60 hours the fungus *Aspergillus niger* can process so much glucose, with almost complete conversion, that a concentration of more than 600 g/L of sodium gluconate equivalents is present, about half as the free acid (Miall, 1978).

α-Ketoglutaric Acid

(2-Oxoglutaric acid)
$$HO_2C-CO-CH_2-CH_2-CO_2H$$

MW:	146.10
mp:	112-4

With **stirring** and **aeration** at 27°C, *Pseudomonas fluorescens*, in particular, but also other species of bacteria such as Serratia, Kluyvera, Bacillus, and Gluconobacter, form α-ketoglutaric acid from various carbohydrates in a yield of 16 to 17%, referred to glucose, in 3 to 5 days (Lockwood and Stodola, 1946; Lockwood and Stodola, 1948). With a new bacterium, strain No. 84C, it has been possible, with the addition of 10% of sugar, to obtain yields of up to 56% (Asai et al., 1955).

α-Ketoglutaric acid can also be obtained in a yield of 50% in 1 to 2 days from glutamic acid as the starting material (Borel, 1962).

Its **isolation** is carried out via the calcium salt at an elevated temperature, since the solubility becomes lower with rising temperature. The free acid can be obtained by decomposing the calcium salt and be further purified (Berger and Witt, 1958), and an extraction with solvents is also possible (Koepsell et al., 1955).

2-Oxo-D-gluconic Acid

(D-*arabino*-2-Hexulosonic acid)
HO₂C—CO—CH(OH)—CH(OH)—
—CH(OH)—CH₂OH

MW: 194.14

In aerobic submerged cultures, Pseudomonas species such as *Pseudomonas fluorescens* and *Pseudomonas fragi* form 2-oxogluconic acid from glucose in yields of up to 92% (Hall, 1963).

Misenheimer et al. (1965) have described a process in which by means of *Serratia marcescens* NRRL B-486 a 12% glucose nutrient solution is 95 to 100% converted into calcium 2-oxo-D-gluconate in 16 h. The process is performed in 20 liter-fermenters at 30°C with a rate of aeration of 0.75 v/v/min and a stirrer speed of 400 rpm. If further amounts of glucose are added during the fermentation, yields of 95-100% in 24 h can be obtained from 180 g/L of glucose, and yields of 85 to 90% in 32 to 40 h from 240 g/L of glucose.

5-Oxo-D-gluconic Acid

(D-*xylo*-5-Hexulosonic acid)
HO₂C—CH(OH)—CH(OH)—CH(OH)—
—CO—CH₂OH

MW: 194.14

The conversion of glucose into 5-oxogluconic acid is brought about by *Acetobacter suboxydans*. This process takes place in two phases: first the glucose is converted into gluconic acid, and the latter is then oxidized further. Here again, the acid formed must be neutralized, so that calcium carbonate is used as an ingredient of the medium (Hall, 1963). In aerobic submerged culture, up to 90% of theory of calcium 5-oxo-D-gluconate can be obtained in 5 to 6 days (Stubbs et al., 1940, 1943).

2,5-Dioxo-D-gluconic Acid

(D-*threo*-3,4,6-Trihydroxy-2,5-dioxohexanoic acid)
HO₂C—CO—CH(OH)—CH(OH)—
—CO—CH₂OH

This acid has been detected as a fermentation product in cultures of *Acetobacter melanogenum* and *Gluconobacter liquefaciens*. However, it is **not a stable end product,** since part is slowly oxidized further to 3,5-dihydroxy-4-oxopyran (rubiginol). Its decomposition products subsequently give the brown pigments that are typical for the microorganism. The bulk is reduced to gluconate and metabolites (Hall, 1963).

Kita and Hall (1979) have now found in *Acetobacter cerinus* a bacterium which does not have the above-mentioned disadvantage and gives 2,5-dioxo-D-gluconic acid in yields of more than 95%, referred to glucose. Cultivation is carried out in a medium containing 2.5% of glucose, 0.5% of corn steep liquor, 0.05% of primary potassium phosphate, 0.05% of secondary potassium phosphate, 0.02% of magnesium sulfate, and 0.63% of calcium carbonate at pH 6.2 and 28°C for 24 h on the shaking machine. After sterilization, the pH is 5.0, and inoculation is carried out with 0.5% (vol/vol) of a suspension from an agar culture. 5% of this **starter culture** is used for inoculating the **production medium.** This contains 11% of glucose, 0.05% of corn steep liquor, 0.058% of secondary ammonium phosphate, 0.015% of primary potassium phosphate, 0.05% of magnesium sulfate, 0.05% of urea, 1 mg/L of copper sulfate, and 300 μg/L of nicotinic acid. After a fermentation time of 20 h sterile glucose is added in an amount of 55 g/L. The pH is kept at 5.5 with sodium hydroxide solution and the fermentation is continued to completion. Stirring is carried out at the rate of 1700 rpm and aeration at 0.5 v/v/min. The maximum yield is reached after about 40 h.

2-Oxo-L-gulonic Acid

(D-*xylo*-2-Hexulosonic acid)
HO₂C—CO—CH(OH)—CH(OH)—
   —CH(OH)—CH₂OH

MW: 194.14
mp: 171(d.)

This acid is of interest to the extent that it forms an intermediate stage in the biological production of ascorbic acid.

Gray (1945a, b) obtained two US patents for the apparently complicated process. According to these, calcium 5-oxo-D-gluconate, after liberation of the acid and its chemical reduction, is fermented in admixture with glucose and nutrients by means of *Acetobacter suboxydans* with stirring and aeration. The calcium 5-oxogluconate re-formed here is returned to the process, and the calcium L-idonate present in the filtrate, after being supplemented by a sugar-containing nutrient solution, is inoculated with a culture of *Pseudomonas mildenbergii*. With stirring and aeration, calcium 2-oxo-L-gulonate arises in a yield of about 50% of the sugar originally used.

In an alkaline medium at room temperature, the methyl ester of 2-oxogulonate is rapidly converted into ascorbic acid, and by adding trypsin the yield can be raised from 50% to about 80% (Monzini, 1952).

Epoxysuccinic Acid

(L-trans-1,2-Oxiranedicarboxylic acid)

MW: 132.08
mp: 180-5(d.)

According to Miall (1978), Paecilomyces sp. and *Aspergillus fumigatus* form epoxysuccinic acid as a metabolic product. In submerged cultures, 39% yields can be obtained from sucrose.

This acid can serve as an intermediate in the production of tartaric acid; however, so far, biological conversions with various microorganisms have given only mesotartaric acid and not the natural form.

D-Erythorbic Acid

(Isoascorbic acid)

MW: 176.12
mp: 174

This acid, which is also called **isoascorbic acid** and **D-araboascorbic acid** does not have any biological vitamin C (ascorbic acid) action, but like vitamin C it acts as an **antioxidant** and **stabilizing agent** in foodstuffs.

Two methods are possible for obtaining erythorbic acid microbially. On the one hand, 2-oxogluconic acid can be converted chemically into its methyl ester which is then saponified. According to Miall (1978), however, there is a second pathway – a direct biological process: in a medium with 8% of glucose and nutrient salts, a mutant of *Penicillium notatum* gives a yield of 40% in 5 days, and when the medium contains 12% of glucose the same yield is obtained in 12 days.

Kojic Acid

(5-Hydroxy-2-(hydroxymethyl)-4-pyrone)

MW: 142.11
mp: 152-4

Aspergillus sp, mainly the *flavus oryzae* group, form kojic acid from glucose, arabinose, ethanol, or glycerol. According to Miall (1978) the yields in cultures by the surface method are better than those obtained in submerged cultures, but in more recent Japanese publication yields of more than 75% in this type of fermentation, as well, have been described.

Lockwood (1954) gives the following **medium** as suitable for the **surface fermentation:** 20% glucose, 0.0054% phosphoric acid, 0.01% potassium chloride, 0.05% magnesium sulfate, and 0.1125% ammonium nitrate. A significant increase in yield is said to be found if 0.01% of ethylene chlorohydrin is also added to the medium. In a fermentation lasting 12 days, 45 g of kojic acid was obtained from 100 g of initial glucose.

After the concentration of the culture filtrate, the kojic acid readily crystallizes out. In order to obtain a colorless product, however, **iron ions** must carefully be excluded, since the smallest traces of them give a deep red color with kojic acid.

Kojic acid, which is easily obtainable by fermentation, has so far found **no application.**

11.3.2 Amino Acids

In recent years, the production of amino acids by fermentation has made considerable advances. A series of microorganisms, often **special mutants,** has been found which are capable, by overproduction under certain conditions, of making amino acids technically accessible.

Table 11-1 lists the amino acids that can be obtained, at least on the laboratory scale, together with a selection of microorganisms that are capable of forming them. When information on the yield of end product was available, this is also given.

The processes by which the amino acids listed are manufactured are fermentations in aerated and stirred fermenters i.e., typical **aerobic submerged processes.**

However, the **methods of growing the culture** are very diverse. While with some amino acids only one medium is necessary for all stages of cultivation, with others the initial production of cell mass must be carried out on media the compositions of which differ greatly from those of the true production media. Some **typical production media** are listed in Table 11-2.

Another possibility for obtaining amino acids by fermentation consists, in the case of some microorganisms, of pretreating the cells that have been bred and bringing them, as a kind of **crude enzyme,** into contact with a reaction solution, in which the desired end product is then produced.

In many cases, however, not just **one** amino acid is formed but **several,** usually in different amounts which again can be controlled within limits by certain additives.

The diversity of the special fermentation conditions that are clearly shown by what has been said above does not permit us to give details here. Those interested must therefore be recommended to obtain these from the numerous monographs.

11.3.3 Polysaccharides

As **natural nutrient reserves** and **skeletal materials,** this group of substances is widespread in the plant kingdom. While polysaccharides from **higher plants** and **algae** have already been used intensively on the technical scale for a long time, it is only recently that more attention has been devoted to similar compounds formed by **microorganisms.** A prerequisite for economic production is, however, that the polysaccharide is formed extracellularly in relatively large amounts.

Lawson and Sutherland (1978) have given a good review of the technical application and economic importance of plant polysaccharides. According to Righelato (1976), fermentation has been developed both in **batch** and in **continuous processes** up to the 1000 liter-scale. The greatest difficulty consists in the transfer of oxygen in these highly viscous liquids. Because of their non-Newtonian flow behavior, no direct relationship exist between the stirring energy introduced and the transfer of oxygen, so that the optimization of stirring and aeration must be carried out from the aspect of cost.

Table 11-1. Amino Acids that can be Produced Biotechnologically with the Aid of Microorganisms.

Amino acid	Microorganisms	Sources of C	Yield	Concentration	Time	Literature source
L(−)-Alanine $CH_3{-}CH(NH_2){-}CO_2H$	Corynebact., Brevibact., Bacillus	carbohydrates	40%			Kinoshita et al. (1978)
L(+)-Arginine $H_2N{-}C(NH){-}NH{-}(CH_2)_3{-}CH(NH_2){-}CO_2H$	Brevibact. flavum, Bacillus subtilis	glucose		29 g/L	72 h	Kinoshita et al. (1978)
L(+)-Aspartic acid $HO_2C{-}CH_2{-}CH(NH_2){-}CO_2H$	Escherichia, Pseudomonas	fumaric acid				Kinoshita et al. (1978)
L(+)-Citrulline $H_2N{-}CO{-}NH{-}(CH_2)_3{-}CH(NH_2){-}CO_2H$	Bacillus subtilis, Corynebact. glutamicum	glucose n-paraffins		26 g/L		Kinoshita et al. (1978)
L(−)-DOPA (Dihydroxyphenylalanine) $OH{-}\text{[ring]}{-}CH_2{-}CH(NH_2){-}CO_2H$, HO	Pseudomonas maltophila, Erwinia herbicola	L-tyrosine glucose	68%	14-15 g/L 3.55 g/L		Kinoshita et al. (1978) Florent et al. (1974)
	Vibrio tyrosinaticus					Ogata et al. (1973)
L(+)-Glutamic acid $HO_2C{-}(CH_2)_2{-}CH(NH_2){-}CO_2H$	Corynebact. glutamicum group, Nocardia erythropolis group, Brevibact. flavum	carbohydrates n-paraffins acetic acid	65% 48%	84 g/L 98 g/L	48 h 48 h	Tanaka et al. (1969) Kinoshita et al. (1978)
L(−)-Histidine $\text{[imidazole ring, } N{=}\backslash NH]{-}CH_2{-}CH(NH_2){-}CO_2H$	Corynebact. glutamicum	glucose saccharose cane sugar molasses		15 g/L		Kinoshita et al. (1978) Kubota et al. (1971)
L-Homoserine $HO{-}(CH_2)_2{-}CH(NH_2){-}CO_2H$	Corynebact. glutamicum	glucose n-paraffins		13-15 g/L 6- 7 g/L 14-17 g/L		Kinoshita et al. (1978)
L(+)-Isoleucine $CH_3{-}CH_2{-}CH(CH_3){-}CH(NH_2){-}CO_2H$	Serratia marcesens, Brevibact. flavum	carbohydrates		14-17 g/L	44-72 h	Kinoshita et al. (1978) Zhdanova et al. (1979)

Amino acid	Microorganisms	Substrate	Yield (%)	Concentration	Time	Reference
L(−)-Leucine $(CH_3)_2CH-CH_2-CH(NH_2)-CO_2H$	*Serratia marcescens,* *Corynebact. glutamicum,* *Brevibact. flavum*	carbohydrates		19 g/L	48 h	Kinoshita et al. (1978)
L(+)-Lysine $H_2N-(CH_2)_4-CH(NH_2)-CO_2H$	*Corynebact. glycinophilum,* Nocardia	cane sugar molasses carbohydrates acetic acid	30–40% 29%	44 g/L 3.2 g/L 75 g/L	60 h 96 h 48 h	Kinoshita et al. (1978) Nakayama et al. (1972) Tanaka et al. (1969)
L(+)-Ornithine $H_2N-(CH_2)_3-CH(NH_2)-CO_2H$	*Corynebact., Brevibact.,* *Arthrobact., Bacillus,* *Escherich., Streptomyces*	carbohydrates	36%			Kinoshita et al. (1978)
L(−)-Phenylalanine $C_6H_5-CH_2-CH(NH_2)-CO_2H$	*Corynebact. glutamicum,* *Brevibact. flavum*	carbohydrates cane sugar molasses		9 g/L		Kinoshita et al. (1978)
L(−)-Proline (structure)	*Corynebact. glutamicum*	cane sugar molasses		31 g/L		Kinoshita et al. (1978)
L-Serine $HO-CH_2-CH(NH_2)-CO_2H$	*Corynebact. glycinophilum,* Nocardia	glycine glucose		10 g/L 0.5 g/L	72 h	Kinoshita et al. (1978) Nakayama et al. (1978)
L(−)-Threonine $CH_3-CH(OH)-CH(NH_2)-CO_2H$	*Escherichia coli*	fructose, molasses glycerol, acetic acid	14%	14 g/L 27 g/L	120 h 48 h	Kinoshita et al. (1978)
L-Tryptophan (structure)	*Hansenula anomala,* *Candida utilis,* *Bac. subtilis,* *Proteus rettgeri,* *Corynebact. glutamicum*	carbohydrates		12 g/L	48 h	Kinoshita et al. (1978)
L(−)-Tyrosine (structure)	*Corynebact. glutamicum*	carbohydrates		17 g/L		Kinoshita et al. (1978)
L(+)-Valine $(CH_3)_2CH-CH(NH_2)-CO_2H$	Aerobacter, Escherichia	carbohydrates		23 g/L		Kinoshita et al. (1978)

Table 11-2. Typical Production Media for Obtaining Amino Acids.

Constituent of the medium	DOPA	Glutamic acid	Histidine	Homo-serine	Iso-leucine	Leucine	Lysine	Phenyl-alanine	Threo-nine	Trypto-phan	Tyrosine	Valine
Glucose	1.1%	10%		10%	13%	8%	3%		10%			7.5%
Saccharose			9%									
Cane sugar molasses[a]			6%					10%		10%	10%	
Acetic acid							0.7%					
KH_2PO_4		0.1%	0.2%	0.1%	0.15%	0.1%	0.2%	0.05%	1.5%	0.05%	0.05%	0.05%
K_2HPO_4			0.1%					0.05%		0.05%	0.05%	
$MgSO_4 \cdot 7H_2O$	0.055%	0.025%	0.05%	0.03%	0.05%	0.04%	0.04%	0.025%	0.04%	0.025%	0.025%	
$CaCO_3$			3%	2%	4%	5%		2%	5%	2%	2%	1%
$(NH_4)_2SO_4$	0.22%		4%	2%	3%	4%		2%	3%	2%	2%	1.5%
$FeSO_4 \cdot 7H_2O$						2 mg/L	0.001%		2 mg/L			
$MnSO_4 \cdot 4H_2O$						2 mg/L	0.001%		2 mg/L			
Leucine				400 mg/L								40 µg/L
Threonine												
Methionine						40 mg/L						
Isoleucine						20 mg/L						
Tyrosine	0.4%											
Corn steep liquor	0.55%	0.25%								1%		
Meat extract			0.75%									
NZ amines		0.25%						0.25%				
Urea		0.5%	0.2%									
Soybean meal							3.5%		4 mL/L[b]			
Ascorbic acid	0.15%											
Biotin			80 µg/L	30 µg/L	200 µg/L	50 µg/L	50 µg/L		200 µg/L			1 µg/L
Thiamine-HCl			1 mg/L	300 µg/L	300 µg/L	300 µg/L	40 µg/L		300 µg/L			
Temperature	30°C	30–35°C	30°C		30°C		33°C		31°C			
pH	6.6/5.5	7–8						7.2	7.2	7.2	7.2	
pH-control with	NH_4OH/HCl	NH_4^+							KOH			

[a] Amount given as glucose
[b] Hydrolysate

Dextran

Of the exopolysaccharides formed by microorganisms, dextran is of great importance because of its use as a **blood plasma extender.** The discovery of this polysaccharide took place over 150 years ago, but more than 100 years had to pass before the chemical nature of this substance was accurately known and the taxonomic classification of the microorganisms responsible for its production was carried out, these microorganisms being pests of the sugar industry, as shown in detail by Behrens and Ringpfeil (1964) in the historical review of their monograph.

Since this macromolecule with its α-1,6-glucosidic bonds is not split by the β-amylase of the body, an English group considered its use as blood plasma extender possible as early as 1937, but the problem was not solved until 1943 by Ingelman and Grönwall by partial hydrolysis and fractionation (Behrens and Ringpfeil, 1964).

The industrial production by directed fermentation that is now coming into use was faced with a number of problems which also occur with other microbial polysaccharides. The formation of these substances greatly raises the **viscosity of the fermentation solutions.** Because of this, a powerful energy installation is required for the stirrers and, in spite of this, it is possible to work only with relatively low concentrations of product. This means again, that the process can be performed **economically** only by using very large fermenters (with capacities of up to 200 m^3) with high consumptions of water and solvents in the recovery stage.

The microorganism mainly used for the production of dextran is *Leuconostoc mesenteroides,* but *Betacoccus arabinosaceus, Betabacterium vermiformi, Streptobacterium dextranicum, Streptococcus viridans, Streptococcus viscosum,* and others, have also been mentioned (Behrens and Ringpfeil, 1964). The nutrient solution is very simple, containing 10% of sucrose, 0.1% of peptone, 0.1% of potassium chloride, and 0.2% of secondary sodium phosphate in mains water at pH 8.0. The sucrose is substantially broken down and the formation of dextran reaches a maximum within 24 h. After separation of the cell mass, which has its problems because of the increase in viscosity which has been mentioned, the extract can be recovered by solvent precipitation (alcohol, acetone). The molecular size appropriate to the particular proposed use is achieved by suitable methods such as mild acid hydrolysis or controlled partial enzymatic degradation.

Because of the technical problems that have been mentioned several times, an early search was made for **enzymatic processes of synthesis,** and these have actually been found (Behrens and Ringpfeil, 1964).

Xanthan

In the series of economically interesting biopolymers xanthan ranks directly after dextran. Because of its special physical properties, this polysaccharide is used mainly in the **technical sector** but is now beginning to make inroads into the **foodstuffs** and **fodder industry** (Lawson and Sutherland, 1978).

This polymer was first detected in 1961 in cultures of *Xanthomonas campestris* NRRL B-1459 (NRRL = Northern Regional Research Laboratories), a causative agent of plant diseases, and the same authors studied it in detail (Slodki and Cadmus, 1978). It is based on a β-1,4-linked D-glucosyl basic skeleton with side chains of three units of D-mannose and D-glucuronic acid in a ratio of 2:1.

The starting material used is glucose or hydrolyzed starch with the addition of sodium salts and organic nitrogen. 40 to 70% of the source of carbohydrate is converted into xanthan in 36 to 84 h, the best yields being obtained when the pH is kept constant. The fermentation conditions affect not only the amount but also the quality of the product.

Other Xanthomonas species form polysaccharides similar to xanthan but with different sugar compositions.

These fermentations must be performed with particular care, since Xanthomonas species are **plant pests.** All material must be treated in such a way that no viable microorganisms can pass into the environment.

Pullulan

The fungus *Aureobasidium pullulans* (syn.: *Pullularia pullulans, Dematium pullulans*) forms the polysaccharide pullulan in a yield of up to 22% from glucose, fructose, sucrose, or maltose. The addition of thiamine raises the yield to 32%, and more recent publications even speak of yields of up to 75% (Slodki and Cadmus, 1978). Chemically, pullulan is an α-D-glucan with 1,4- and 1,6-bound glucosyl residues in a ratio of 2:1. In their review, Slodki and Cadmus (1978) give a series of publications in which fermentation conditions to increase the yield and control the degree of polymerization are described. These show that the chemical composition of the product depends greatly on the manner of performing cultivation.

As in the case of dextran, here the **increase in viscosity** of the medium due to the formation of the product is the main problem in its isolation and purification. Kato and Nomura (1976) have proposed diluting the culture solution to such an extent that the cells of the microorganisms can easily be separated by **filtration** or **centrifugation.** Since it is likewise necessary to eliminate the **pigments** formed during fermentation, a treatment with activated carbon can be carried out at this stage. Finally, the solution is concentrated to a pullulan content of about 30 g/100 mL. In place of the otherwise used methanol as precipitant,

of which up to three times the volume of the filtrate must be added, Kato and Nomura add alcohols, ester, or ethers with three or more carbon atoms. Because of the lower water solubility, only 20 to 30% of these, referred to the aqueous concentrate, is necessary to achieve complete precipitation. The precipitated pullulan is separated off and dried in the usual way.

Glucans with β-1,3 Bonds

a) Scleroglucan

The fungus *Sclerotium glucanicum* forms a β-1,3-glucan which is on the market for technical applications under the trade name Polytran® (Lawson and Sutherland, 1978). In addition to 65 to 75% of 1,3-bonds, this scleroglutan also contains 1,6-bonds.

Its microbial production can start from numerous carbohydrates, and organic sources of nitrogen, such as yeast extract, appear to be necessary. According to Slodki and Cadmus (1978), about 1 g of polysaccharide can be obtained from 3 to 15 g of carbohydrate in aerobic submerged fermentation at 25 to 30°C in 2 to 5 days.

Plectania occidentalis, an ascomycete, also forms from glucose a glucan containing up to 60 to 70% of β-1,3 bonds in 10 days.

The glucan from cultures of a Helotium species has a somewhat more complex structure. Starting from 3 to 4% glucose, a yield of up to 65% is obtained in 64 h. In addition to organic sources of nitrogen, mineral salts, phosphate, and thiamin are necessary (Slodki and Cadmus, 1978).

b) Curdlan

The biopolymer curdlan is formed by a mutant of *Alcaligenes faecalis* var. *myxogenes.* It is an almost pure β-1,3 glucan. On being heated in aqueous solution, it irreversibly forms a gel the solidity of which is between those of agar and gelatin gels (Lawson and Sutherland, 1978).

According to Slodki and Cadmus (1978), the best yields – 4 g/100 mL – are obtained from glucose. The circumstance that curdlan is insoluble in water means that the fermentation solutions do not become more viscous through the formation of the product. It also makes the recovery procedure simpler. The suspended polymer is dissolved by the addition of caustic soda, the bacterial cells are filtered off, and after neutralization with hydrochloric acid the water-swollen polysaccharide reprecipitates. The end product is obtained by centrifugation and spray-drying.

c) Succinoglucan

The polysaccharide succinoglucan has likewise been isolated from cultures of *Alcaligenes faecalis* var. *myxogenes*. It consists of glucose, galactose, and succinic acid in a ratio of 7:1:1.5. It has been possible to obtain 1,9% of succinoglucan from a medium containing 4% of glucose. Manganese and iron ions appeared to be necessary for the formation of the polysaccharide. Calcium carbonate is the best buffering agent (Slodki and Cadmus, 1978). 28°C was the optimum temperature for the formation of the products, and the time of fermentation was about 5 days.

Microbial Alginate

Alginates, which are widely used in the **foodstuffs, pharmaceutical, textile,** and **paper industries** came originally from the marine algae Laminaria. Marked fluctuations in quality and an incipient shortage of the raw material led to the search for equivalent biopolymers of **microbial** origin with the aim of industrial manufacture.

Subsequently, exopolysaccharides very similar to the algal products were found in cultures of *Pseudomonas aeruginosa* and *Azotobacter vinelandii*. These also consist of esters of mannuronic and guluronic acids, but the ratio is shifted towards a higher proportion of mannuronic acid than is the case for alginate.

Lawson and Sutherland (1978) have given a summary of the most recent literature in this field. According to this, the type of **source of carbohydrate** for the bacteria, which may be mannitol, sucrose, or other sugars, has no influence on the composition of the biopolymer. Low nitrogen contents and a low temperature of 12°C appear to be decisive for a high yield. Since *Pseudomonas aeruginosa* is not complete unobjectionable for man, the development work has concentrated on *Azotobacter vinelandii*. Through various changes in the parameters it has been possible to increase the yield of polysaccharide from the original 5% to 25% of the sugar used (2%). Simultaneously, the viscosity behavior has been improved to such an extent that the bacterial product corresponds to the algal products of the lower and medium viscosity ranges.

Other Bacterial Polysaccharides

Erwinia tahitica forms a polymer consisting of glucose, galactose, uronic acid, and fucose residues in an approximate ratio of 3:2:1.5:1, with an acetyl content of 4.5% (Lawson and Sutherland, 1978). Its physical properties resemble those of xanthan.

In a medium consisting of 3% of partially hydrolyzed starch, 0.5% of enzymatically digested soybean meal, 0.09% of ammonium nitrate, 0.5% of primary potassium phosphate, and 0.01% of magnesium sulfate at pH 6.0 to 6.5, the formation of 1.6% of polysaccharide took place at 30°C in 64 to 72 h. The final viscosity of the fermentation solution was 4600 mPa·s (Slodki and Cadmus, 1978).

Another heteropolysaccharide has been isolated from cultures of *Azotobacter indicus* var. *myxogenes*. It consists of glucose, rhamnose, and galacturonic acid residues (6.6:1.5:1) with an acetyl content of 8 to 10%. A good production medium contains 2% of glucose, 0.05% of enzymatically digested soybean meal, 0.09% of ammonium nitrate, 0.5% of secondary potassium phosphate, and 0.01% of magnesium sulfate. At pH 6.5 to 7.5 and 30°C, with stirring and aeration, the fermentation lasts 37 to 48 h. The final viscosity is 5000 to 7000 mPa·s (Slodki and Cadmus, 1978).

Slodki and Cadmus (1978) have given a summary of investigations on the formation of a polymer in cultures of *Arthrobacter viscosus*. This water-soluble polysaccharide consists of glucose, galactose, and mannuronic acid residues in equimolecular ratio and is 25% acetylated. The biopolymer is readily precipitated from aqueous solutions by means of ethanol or methanol in the presence of an electrolyte. In the presence of salts, the viscosity rises, and at high temperatures it is stable over a pH range of 5 to 10.

Good yields are obtained on a medium containing 3% of glucose, 0.3% of enzymatically hydrolyzed casein, 0.4% of secondary potassium phosphate, 0.04% of magnesium sulfate (anhydrous), and 0.001% of manganese sulfate at pH 7. In a fermentation time of 4 days, 40 to 50% of the glucose was converted into polymer, and the viscosity of the culture solution was about 12000 mPa·s. The concentration of magnesium sulfate is very important in this fermentation. 0.04% was the optimum, at 0.01% the yield fell by 4%, and in the absence of this salt no polymer was formed although satisfactory growth took place.

11.3.4 *Vitamins and Provitamins*

Vitamin B₁₂

Although the therapeutic action of liver preparations in pernicious anemia had been known since 1926, the active principle (vitamin B₁₂) was discovered only in 1948. Since **liver** was economically of no interest as a raw material for its production, other sources were

sought. In this connection it was found that a series of microorganisms form this vitamin and contain it in relatively large amounts (Hester and Ward, 1954).

In sewage sludge, especially in activated sludge, and in antibiotic fermentations cyanocobalamin (vitamin B₁₂) arises as a by-product and can be obtained from the material concerned. However, it is more economic, particularly if pure products are to be obtained, to perform **directed fermentations.** Cultures of Propionibacterium and Pseudomonas species are most suitable for this purpose (Perlman, 1978).

19 to 23 mg/L of vitamin B₁₂ is obtained from glucose, corn steep liquor, and cobalt salts as medium. The fermentation by means of *Propionibacterium freudenreichii* or *Propionibacterium shermanii* is carried out anaerobically for three days and then aerobically for another three or four days.

The total amount of cobamids (including the coenzym form of vitamin B₁₂) formed remains in the cells of the microorganisms. The separation and drying of this cell mass yields a product which can find use directly as a **fodder additive.**

However, the vitamin B₁₂ activity can be liberated from the cells by various methods of treatment in which the coenzyme form is transformed into cyanocobalamin. This can be isolated from the solution by various methods.

Vitamin B₂ Group

Vitamin B₂ (riboflavin, lactoflavin) can also be obtained by fermentation with several microorganisms. According to the choice of microorganisms, anaerobic or aerobic submerged processes are involved.

Clostridium acetobutylicum represents the anaerobic type that was originally used for this process. It is still of some interest since riboflavin arises as a by-product during the acetone-butanol fermentation (Section 11.3.5). Hickey (1954) has described a process of this type in which the distillation residue contains 50 to 60 µg/g of riboflavin and can be used as a fodder additive. With this bacterium, the yield of riboflavin is very highly dependent on the iron content of the nutrient solution, the best yields being obtained with small amounts of iron.

The processes of the **aerobic type** that are customary today make use of the yeasts Debaryomyces and Candida or the fungi *Ashbya gossypii* and *Eromothecium ashbyii*. It is true that Candida yeasts exhibit a still greater sensitivity to iron ions than the Clostridium mentioned above, but their yields of riboflavin are good. Hickey (1954) gives 100 to 103 µg/mL for *Candida guilliermondii* and more than 500 µg/mL for *Candida flareri* in glucose solutions in 5 to 7 days. A typical medium has the following composition: 4% glucose, 0.184% urea, 0.02% magnesium sulfate, 0.05% secondary potassium phosphate, 1 µg/L biotin, 140 µg/L zinc, and 20 µg/L each boron, manganese, copper, and molybdenum. The prepared medium should not contain more than 40 to 50 µg/L of iron.

There are fewer difficulties with the iron content in the case of ascomycete cultures. For *Ashbya gossypii,* Perlman (1978) reported a concentration of more than 4000 mg/L if suitable organic nitrogen sources and selected mutants were used. Nitela et al. (1971) have described a process with *Eromothecium ashbyii* strains in which collagen of various grades of purity makes a substantial contribution to the riboflavin yield of 4500 to 5000 µg/mL. This process, which has been described for a production level of 25 to 30 m^3, involves a somewhat complicated cultivation of the material for inoculation and a production medium containing 0.5 to 5% of crude plant lecithin, 1 to 5% of crude collagen, 1 to 5% of corn (maize) extract, 5 to 10% of unrefined

plant oil or hydrogenated oil, 1.5% of glucose, 0.1 to 0.5% of primary potassium phosphate, and 1 to 10 mg% of trace elements (cobalt, manganese, magnesium, and zinc). At pH 7 to 8 and 32°C, the fermentation lasts 7 to 8 days with stirring and aeration at the rate of 1 to 3 v/v/min. During fermentation, ammonia is fed in from time to time.

According to Perlman (1978), the optimum conditions for fermentation with *Ashbya gossypii* are an aeration rate of 0.33 v/v/min, a cultivation temperature of 28°C, and an energy input for stirring of 0.74 kW for 1 m^3 of medium. Foaming is controlled at the beginning with a silicone antifoaming agent and later with soybean oil, which simultaneously acts as a nutrient.

If the riboflavin is not to be used directly as a crude product in the form of a fodder additive, according to Perlman (1978) it can also be obtained in crystalline form from this crude product.

Fukui (1971) has reported on developments in Japan on the recovery of flavin adenine ribonucleotide directly from fermentations with *Eromothecium ashbyii*. This product is still obtained on the industrial scale by chemical synthesis at the present time.

β-Carotenoids

β-Carotene is important as a **precursor of vitamin A** and can also be used as a **foodstuff pigment.**

Some microorganisms form this compound and similar substances in large amounts, so that production by fermentation is possible. According to Perlman (1978), however, this method is not being followed at the present time, since β-carotene manufactured synthetically is substantially cheaper.

In **biosynthesis, stimulators** play an important role for the yield. Such stimulators have been found in β-ionone, deodorized kerosine, and waste products from the refining of plant oils ("autoclave oil"). The choice of microorganisms also has a great influence, particularly the use of + and − strains in the case of *Blakeslea trispora*.

Pazola et al. (1971) inoculated a medium containing 3% of dry brewers' yeast, 2.5% of ground maize, 3% of soybean meal, 4% of kerosine, 0.2 mg% of thiamin hydrochloride, and 4.6% of "autoclave oil" with the + and − strains of *Blakeslea trispora* grown separately. After cultivation at 26 to 28°C for 4 to 6 days, 0.0935% of β- or α-ionone was added and cultivation was continued for another five days. The mycelium formed contained the carotene, which could be extracted from it. The yield of carotene was about 100 mg/100 mL of medium. Other constituents of the medium may be citrus molasses, cottonseed kernel meal, and combinations of them. According to Perlman (1978), a rise in the viscosity of the medium to about 600 mPa·s, which can be brought about by starch, carboxymethylcellulose, or plant mucilages exerts a substantial influence on the growth and the formation of the end product.

Becker et al. (1972) used *Rhodotorula gracilis* for their microbial process. This takes place in two stages: **the first** serves for the growth of the inoculation stage and the production of biomass, and in the **second stage** the biomass formed is enriched. The growth of the inoculation stage and the production of biomass take place in a simple medium containing 8% of sugar beet molasses and 0.2% of secondary ammonium phosphate at pH 5 and 30°C. The time of cultivation in the individual stages is given as 24 to 72 h, and the rate of aeration rises from 8 mg of oxygen/L/min to 100 mg of oxygen/L/min. The end stage in a volume of 2000 L is likewise carried on at 30°C and 120 mg of oxygen/L/min for 24 h. After this time, 20 g/L of yeast dry matter has formed. From this, in a centrifugal separator, 400 L of a yeast milk containing 100 g/L of

dry matter is obtained which, after being transferred to another fermenter, is post-treated at pH 5.5 and 30°C with aeration at the rate of 130 mg of oxygen/L/min for 48 h. In this second stage, additions of sucrose, common salt and trace elements (cobalt, copper, manganese, zinc, iron, iodine, and molybdenum), individually, or in combinations, give substantial improvements in the yield of end product. In this way, 35 to 40 kg of yeast dry matter containing 120 to 150 mg/g of carotenoids can be obtained by spray-drying.

Fukui (1971) found suitable fermentation conditions for the accumulation of carotenoids in media containing hydrocarbons and various bacteria, including *Mycobacterium smegmatis, Nocardia lutea,* and *Nocardia corallina*. In this case, the bulk of the carotenoids was found in the medium itself, the main products being 4-oxo-β-carotene and xanthophyll derivatives; it was possible to obtain 1.5 to 2.0 mg/L of the substance. It is true that the xanthophylls are not active as provitamins, but they can be used for coloring foodstuffs.

Ascorbic Acid

Ascorbic acid or vitamin C is not in fact directly a fermentation product, but **precursors** for its **chemical synthesis** can be obtained by biological methods.

Thus, a series of Acetobacter species is capable of converting sorbitol into L-sorbose, which is then converted chemically via 2-oxo-L-gulonic acid into ascorbic acid.

According to Lockwood (1954), **surface fermentations** of sorbitol solutions last seven days and give yields of 80 to 90%.

On the other hand, yields of 98% can be achieved in intensely aerated **submerged fermentations** (0.33 v/v/min, 2 bar gauge pressure), the fermentation times being 14 h with 10% sorbitol solutions, 24 h with 20% solutions, and 40 h with 29% solutions.

On the **technical scale,** it is advantageous to start with 10 to 15% of sorbitol solution to which 0.5% of corn steep liquor has been added and to feed in further sorbitol. Fermentation takes place in the optimum manner at 30 to 35°C, but considerable amounts of heat are liberated and an adequate possibility of cooling must be available.

Since the microorganism *Acetobacter suboxydans* is sensitive to nickel, corresponding care must be taken in the choice of the material of the fermenter.

Recovery is carried out by filtration, vacuum concentration, and crystallization in a similar manner to the sugar recovery processes. The yields in this stage amount to 80 to 90%.

Another method consists in obtaining 2-oxo-L-gulonic acid (Section 11.3.1) by fermentation from 5-oxo-D-gluconic acid (Section 11.3.1) and then converting it chemically into ascorbic acid.

Ergosterol

(5,7,22-Ergostatrien-3 β-ol)

MW: 396.63
mp: 168.0

Ergosterol, which must be included among the **provitamins** can be found fairly frequently in microorganisms. Van Lanen (1954) has given the following amounts:

Bacteria	0 to 0.49%
Yeasts	0.14 to 2.9%
Fungi	0.02 to 2.3%

Ergosterol can be recovered as a by-product from the cells of bakers' yeast or from the mycelia in the manufacture of citric acid or antibiotics. However, processes are also known which permit higher yields of ergosterol with specially bred yeasts. Ergosterol is converted into biologically active vitamin D_2 by UV irradiation in any of the recovery stages.

11.3.5 Alcohols and Solvents

Acetone–Butyl Alcohol–Isopropyl Alcohol

This **anaerobic form of fermentation** was discovered and utilized industrially very early on. McCutchan and Hickey (1954) have compiled a good historical review from which only a few points will be reproduced.

Pasteur was probably the first to recognize **butanol** as an end product of microbial metabolism, in 1861. **Acetone,** which is also formed in considerable amounts, was first discovered by Schardinger in 1905. While butanol, starting material for butadiene for **synthetic rubbers** first got the corresponding fermentation industry going, during the First World War interest turned to the by-product acetone as a raw material for the explosive **cordite.** When, later, butyl acetate was used in large amounts as a solvent for **nitrocellulose lacquers,** interest turned once more to butanol. Although, today, this alcohol is in vigorous competition with synthetic butanol, large fermentation plants are still in operation.

The question of what source of carbohydrate can be used depends, on the one hand, on the price and, on the other hand, very greatly on the choice of microorganism. Thus, there are species which can only utilize invert sugar and there are also those which assimilate sucrose and for which, therefore, molasses can be used without pretreatment. To an overwhelming extent, these are species of the genus Clostridium. Organic nitrogen is not necessary, but ammonium salts and phosphate must be present in small amounts. A little calcium carbonate as buffer is also important. Molasses from sugar manufacture or cereal mashes can be used as the sources of carbohydrate. The optimum temperature is between 30 and 37°C.

While the risk of infection with bacteria hardly raises any problems, **bacteriophages** can cause such difficulties that manufacturing plants are forced to shut down.

With an initial feed of 5 to 7% of sugar, 29 to 33% of alcohol is formed in 48 to 56 h. The classical ratio of butanol to acetone to alcohol is 6:3:1. This ratio can be displaced to 74:24:2 by the use of new strains and changes in the propagation of the culture.

It must also be mentioned that part of the converted raw material escapes in the form of a **gas** containing 60% of **carbon dioxide** and 40% of **hydrogen** which is explosive with air. Since for this reason it must be trapped, it can also be separated and the products be marketed as other by-products, particularly since these gases are at high purity (Hastings, 1978). It should also be observed that the distillation residues form a good source for riboflavin (Section 11.3.4).

The influence that the **choice of strain** has on the composition of the end product has been shown by Wilkinson and Rose (1963) in a table. Thus, the fermentation mentioned above must be ascribed to strains of the species *Clostridium acetobutylicum,* while *Clostridium butylicum* forms butanol as the main product, together with butyric and acetic acids, and, although it forms no acetone or ethanol, it does, in return, produce isopropyl alcohol.

Butane-2,3-diol

CH$_3$	CH$_3$	CH$_3$
HCOH	HOCH	HCOH
HCOH	HCOH	HOCH
CH$_3$	CH$_3$	CH$_3$
meso-form	**D(−)-form**	**L(+)-form**
mp: 34.4	mp: 19.0	
$[\alpha]_D^{20} = 0.0°$	$[\alpha]_D^{20} = -13.34°$	

Butane-2,3-diol was discovered as a fermentation product as early as the end of the last century, but only during the 40's did intensive research and development work in this field begin. As Ledingham and Neish (1954) have observed in their exhaustive review on these investigations, in spite of everything this fermentation has never progressed beyond the semitechnical scale to a process used industrially.

The bulk of the development work was carried out with *Aerobacter aerogenes, Serratia marcescens, Bacillus polymyxa,* and *Bacillus subtilis.* The fermentation may always, depending on the strain, be carried out aerobically or anaerobically. The raw materials used are sugars, starch, molasses, and other carbohydrate-containing waste products, to which nitrogen-containing materials are added. A typical medium for the **anaerobic process** contains 7.5% of maize starch, 0.5% of maize gluten, 0.006% of potassium permanganate, and 0.5% of calcium carbonate. In 48 h at 30°C, *Bacillus polymyxa* forms 26.8% of the diol and 14.8% of ethanol from the starch present. Whether the starch-containing raw materials should be pretreated and what other additives must be introduced depends substantially on the strain used.

In the **aerobic process,** in which sugars or molasses are usually used as the raw materials, the yields are considerably higher. With 5 to 20% of initial sugar, 85% of theory, corresponding to about 40% of the sugar used, of butane-2,3-diol, with only small amounts of ethanol as by-product, can be obtained in 24 h.

For **isolation,** the filtrate is acidified and treated with formaldehyde and is then distilled. The oily phase contains 98 to 100% of the butanediol in the form of the formal, from which the free diol can be obtained in 95% yield with acidified methanol. Extraction of the diol from the filtrate with diethyl ether or n-butanol is also possible.

Which of the three stereoisomers is formed preferentially depends primarily on the choice of strain, as well as the nature and amount of by-products worth mentioning, which may be ethanol, formic acid, acetic acid, lactic acid, and hydrogen.

Polyhydric Alcohols

Polyhydric alcohols are formed in amounts worthy of mention by some microorganisms, particularly those that tolerate high concentrations of sugars and salt. These are mainly yeasts and yeast-like microorganisms which are associated in nature with flowers, fruits, and honey-collecting insects. They are also known as **sources of infection** in jams, honey, and pickling liquors.

The microbially formed polyhydric alcohols are glycerol, mannitol, arabitol, erythritol, and xylitol.

Glycerol, which was formerly obtained on the large scale by fermentation, is mainly obtained today from petrochemistry. While mannitol can be obtained more easily from other sources – it occurs in a number of plants –, access to erythritol, xylitol, and arabitol in an economically manner is possible only by microbial processes.

Glycerol

$$HO—CH_2—CH(OH)—CH_2—OH$$

MW: 92.09
mp: 18.18

A very good historical summary of glycerol as a metabolic product has been given by Underkofler (1954). Pasteur found long ago that in the preparation of wine and beer the yeast forms 2.5 to 2.6 g of glycerol for each 100 g of sugars fermented. After further elucidation of the mechanism of alcoholic fermentation, Neuburg at the beginning of this century succeeded in substantially increasing the accumulation of glycerol by fixing the acetaldehyde in the course of fermentation by means of sulfite. Subsequently a multiplicity of publications appeared on this subject and a series of production processes were developed and put into practice.

The so-called **"German process"** used 4% of sodium sulfite in a fermentation solution with 10% of sucrose, 0.5% of ammonium nitrate, and 0.075% of secondary potassium phosphate, inoculated with 1% of yeast. The end product after 48 to 60 h at 30°C consisted of 20 to 25% of glycerol, 30% of ethanol, and 5% of acetaldehyde, referred to the sugars fermented. Because of the nonsugar solids, especially when molasses were used as the raw material, only poor yields, seldom exceeding 50%, were obtained in the recovery procedure. According to Spencer and Spencer (1978), this problem has still not been solved today.

In addition to yeasts, certain strains of *Bacillus subtilis* have been found that form considerable amounts of glycerol, usually together with other products such as butane-2,3-diol, acetoin, ethanol, and lactic acid. From a mash containing 3% of glucose, 1% of yeast extract, and 1% of calcium carbonate with pH 6.2 to 6.8 at 30°C, under anaerobic conditions, the yields of the main end products were

28.2% of butane-2,3-diol and 20.4% of glycerol. If highly productive strains are bred, this process may have a good chance of success.

Until now, the production of glycerol by fermentation had little prospect in comparison with the chemical method, but the shortage of crude oil and its increasing cost could give another impulse to this direction of fermentation.

D-Mannitol

$$HO-CH_2-\overset{\overset{\displaystyle H}{|}}{C}-\overset{\overset{\displaystyle H}{|}}{C}-\overset{\overset{\displaystyle OH}{|}}{C}-\overset{\overset{\displaystyle OH}{|}}{C}-CH_2-OH$$
$$\underset{OH\;OH\;H\;\;\;H}{}$$

MW: 182.17
mp: 166

The microbial production of D-mannitol by means of *Candida lipolytica* from paraffins with 12 to 18-carbon atoms has been described by DeZeeuw and Tynan (1972). The inoculum, in an amount of up to 5% of the production medium, is added in two stages in a **submerged aeration process.** The production medium contains 0.2% of urea, 0.1% of ammonium sulfate, 0.1% of calcium sulfate, 0.05% of potassium sulfate, 0.025% of magnesium sulfate, 0.25 mg-% of iron sulfate, and 1.0 mg-% of manganese sulfate, and also 500 μg/L of thiamine hydrochloride and 1 mL/L of a solution of trace elements (100 μg each of copper, cobalt, zinc, molybdenum, and boron, and 1 mg of calcium chloride). After adjustment of the pH to 3.5 and sterilization, 20% of a mixture of paraffins is added and, after inoculation, fermentation is carried out at 24 to 25 °C with stirring (1750 rpm) and aeration at 1.0 v/v/min for 8 to 9 days. After this time, 12 g/L of D-mannitol is present, and this can be crystallized from the filtered and concentrated fermentation broth.

D-Arabitol

$$HO-CH_2-\overset{\overset{\displaystyle H}{|}}{C}-\overset{\overset{\displaystyle OH}{|}}{C}-\overset{\overset{\displaystyle OH}{|}}{C}-CH_2-OH$$
$$\underset{OH\;H\;\;\;H}{}$$

MW: 152.14
mp: 103

Ueda (1970) used *Pichia ohmeri* in order to obtain D-arabitol from glucose solutions.

The nutrient medium contained 2% of glucose, 0.1% of yeast extract, 0.2% of urea, 0.1% of primary potassium phosphate, 0.1% of magnesium sulfate, and 0.5% of calcium carbonate. After sterilization, inoculation was carried out with 5% of preculture, and the whole was fermented at 30 °C with aeration at the rate of 1.0 v/v/min and stirring at the rate of 200 rpm for 120 h. During the first 95 h, a sufficient amount of 70% glucose solution was added continuously to maintain the concentration at 4 to 5%. The consumption of glucose was 15 g/100 mL. The yield amounted to 8.6 g of D-arabitol/100 mL, corresponding to 50%.

After filtration, treatment of the filtrate with calcium hydroxide in the hot, treatment with carbon, separation of the solids, and concentration it was possible to obtain the end product as a crystalline mass which was recrystallized from ethanol for further purification.

Xylitol

$$HO-CH_2-\overset{\overset{\displaystyle OH}{|}}{C}-\overset{\overset{\displaystyle H}{|}}{C}-\overset{\overset{\displaystyle OH}{|}}{C}-CH_2-OH$$
$$\underset{H\;\;\;OH\;H}{}$$

MW: 152.14
mp: 61–61.5 (metastable)
         93–94.5 (stable)

Using xylulose as substrate and yeast strains of the genera Candida, Monilia, Pichia, Hansenula, Saccharomyces, Zygosaccharomyces, and Debaryomyces, which can assimilate xylulose, Onishi and Suzuki (1969, 1970) succeeded in obtaining yields of xylitol of up to 48%, referred to xylulose.

Since, however, xylulose is not a generally available source of carbon, it must first be obtained from glucose, which is possible by a microbial method. The whole process is therefore a **multistage** one.

In the **first stage,** arabitol is obtained by fermentation from glucose (see above and Onishi and Suzuki, 1970).

The unfiltered arabitol-containing nutrient solution is sterilized for the **second stage,** inoculated with *Acetobacter suboxydans,* and kept at 30°C under aerobic conditions. Xylulose is formed in high yield from the arabitol present and can be recovered by extraction of the dry residue with hot ethanol.

The production of xylitol takes place in the **third stage.** For this purpose, either the isolated xylulose can be used as a source of sugar in a nutrient medium or the fermentation solution from the production of xylose is taken, sterilized, and used further for the xylitol fermentation.

Summarizing, the process runs as follows:

Debaryomyces sake ATCC 20 212 is inoculated into a nutrient medium containing 15% of glucose, 4% of corn steep liquor, 0.1% of primary potassium phosphate, 0.05% of magnesium sulfate, 0.01% of calcium chloride, and 0.01% of sodium chloride with a pH of 6.0, and is cultivated with shaking at 30°C for 4 days. During this period, 5.34 g/100 mL of D-arabitol is formed.

The nutrient medium is then adjusted to pH 6 with sodium hydroxide and is sterilized at 120°C for 15 min. *Acetobacter suboxydans* ATCC 621 is inoculated into it and cultivation is carried out with aeration for 2 days. 5.0 g of D-xylulose/100 mL accumulates.

Without the isolation of the D-xylulose from the fermentation mash, 4% of corn steep liquor are added. After adjustment of the pH to 6.0 and sterilization at 110°C for 5 min., *Candida guilliermondii* var. *soya* ATCC 20 216 is inoculated into it and cultivation is carried out with shaking at 30°C for 3 days. With complete consumption of the sugar, 2.0 g of xylitol/100 mL is formed. The yield of xylitol referred to the amount of glucose originally used is 13.3%.

Erythritol

$$HO-CH_2-\overset{\overset{\displaystyle OH}{|}}{\underset{\underset{\displaystyle H}{|}}{C}}-\overset{\overset{\displaystyle OH}{|}}{\underset{\underset{\displaystyle H}{|}}{C}}-CH_2-OH$$

MW: 122.12
mp: 119.5; 126

According to Spencer and Spencer (1978), erythritol can be obtained by means of *Candida zeylanoides* from normal alkanes and with the aid of *Trigonopsis variabilis* from glucose or glycerol as substrate.

In the case of normal alkanes as substrate and *Candida zeylanoides,* citric acid is normally formed. If, however, the pH is brought down to 3.0 and below, the formation of acid is suppressed and the production of erythritol begins. The phosphate content is also critical: at amounts of 0.1 to 0.2% of primary potassium phosphate, mannitol formed instead of erythritol. The formation of the polyol starts at the end of the growth phase, about 20 h after inoculation. Only inorganic compounds should be used as sources of nitrogen. Under optimum conditions, yields of 180 g/L of erythritol can be obtained after cultivation for 160 h.

Dihydroxyacetone

HO—CH$_2$—CO—CH$_2$—OH

MW: 90.08
mp: 65–71 (monomer)
          117 (dimer)
          ~ 80 (equilibrium mixture)

Dihydroxyacetone can be obtained from glycerol with strains of *Acetobacter xylinum, Acetobacter suboxydans, Acetobacter aceti, Bacterium orleanse,* and other species that have previously been adapted to glycerol as substrate. According to Rehm (1967), the greatest problem in this fermentation consists in the shortening of the normally very long time of fermentation. Additions of yeast extract or corn steep liquor appear to effect this. Octadecanol and other antifoaming agents which, because of the intense aeration necessary, must be added in any case, also shorten the fermentation time. Thus, at pH 5.2 and 28 °C, 95 to 96 % of the glycerol added is oxidized in 96 h. In another case, *Acetobacter suboxidans* formed 90 g/L of dihydroxyacetone from 110 g/L of glycerol in only 72 h.

The initial concentration of glycerol appears to have an essential influence on the yield. Hall (1963) mentions a process in which 10 % glycerol is used initially and further glycerol is added during the fermentation. In this way, yields of 175 g/L of dihydroxyacetone could be obtained.

According to a Japanese patent, a mutant of *Brevibacterium fuscum* is capable of forming dihydroxyacetone directly from glucose.

11.3.6   Miscellaneous Products

Fats and Fatty Acids

A detailed account of the world situation for the supply of fats and oils of plant and animal origin has been given by Ratledge (1978). The good supply position and the legal limitations on the use of substitutes have not exactly promoted the developments directed to opening up microbial sources in this field. In times of shortage, however, such as during the two World Wars, endeavors of this type were made which had some success but were never transformed into practice. From a present-day point of view, a development in this field is only desirable if it is carried out with quite definite aims. It should either allow expensive products to be produced microbially at lower cost or substances should be found in this group of products which open up special possibilities of application.

Since for the sake of economy in the case of products already obtainable from other sources the necessary criteria are the highest quality in the largest possible yield in the shortest possible time, bacteria and algae are excluded right away, and therefore only the **yeasts** and **fungi** remain. The microorganisms that, on suitable cultivation, give more than 30 % of fat in the dry matter may be given in tabular form from the above-mentioned literature source (Table 11-3).

The composition of the microbially produced fat also, of course, plays a deciding role. Ratledge (1978) also gives a tabular summary for this aspect (Table 11-4).

The processes described in the literature include **static surface processes** as well as **aerated submerged processes.** Since the formation of fat is an optimum only in nitrogen-poor media in which, however, growth hardly takes place, the microorganisms must be bred with sufficient nitrogen in a **precultivation stage.** In the case of *Rhodotorula gracilis* this lasts 12 to 14 h according to Rehm (1978). In the following production stage, which requires about 50 h, 14 g of fat can be obtained from 100 g of glucose. The yeast mass contains about 42 % of fat and 23 % of protein. It is rarely possible to use the whole cells but the fat must be sep-

Table 11-3. Yeasts and Mold Fungi that have been Investigated since 1959 as Potential Fat Producers. It has been Reported that they Possess a Minimum Fat Content of about 30%. After Ratledge (1978).

Organisms	Substrate	Fat content (% dry weight)	Fat coefficient (g fat prod./100 g substrate)	Lipid/ fatty acid analysis given
Yeasts				
Candida guilliermondii	n-alkanes	30	–	no
Candida intermedia	n-alkanes	20	–	no
Candida tropicalis	n-alkanes	32	–	no
Candida sp. no. 107	glucose	42	22.5	yes
Candida sp. no. 107	n-alkanes	15–37	25	yes
Cryptococcus terricolus	glucose	55–65	21	no
Hansenula anomala	glucose	17	–	no
Hansenula ciferrii	molasses	22	–	no
Hansenula saturnus	molasses	20	–	no
Hansenula saturnus	glucose	28	8	no
Lipomyces lipofer	glucose	38	–	yes
Lipomyces lipofer	peat hydrolysate	48	–	yes
Lipomyces sp.	glucose	67	20	no
	xylose	48	17	no
	various wastes and molasses	66	up to 24	no
Lipomyces starkeyi	lactose	31	10	no
Lipomyces starkeyi	glucose	31–38	9–15	yes
Rhodotorula gracilis	molasses	40	44 (only briefly)	yes
Rhodotorula gracilis	glucose	64	–	no
Rhodotorula gracilis	cane sugar syrup	67	21	no
Rhodotorula gracilis	glucose	64	15 (transiently) 44 (only briefly)	yes
Rhodotorula gracilis	ethanol	62	15	yes
	synthetic ethanol	60	14	yes
	glucose	66	17	yes
	alkanes	32	–	yes
Mold fungi				
Aspergillus fischeri	saccharose	32–53	12–20	no
Aspergillus fumigatus	maltose and other sources	20	–	no
Aspergillus nidulans	glucose	27	9	no
Aspergillus nidulans	glucose	15	7	no
Aspergillus ochraceus	saccharose	48	13	yes
Aspergillus terreus	saccharose	51–57	10–13	yes

Table 11-3. (continued)

Organisms	Substrate	Fat content (% dry weight)	Fat coefficient (g fat prod./100 g substrate)	Lipid/ fatty acid analysis given
Aspergillus terreus	starch	18–24	6	no
Aspergillus ustus	lactose	36	12.7	no
Chaetomium globosum	glucose	54	–	yes
Cladosporium fulvum	saccharose	22–14	7	no
Cladosporium herbarum	saccharose	20–29	7–11	no
Gibberella fujikuroi (*Fusarium moniliforme*)	glucose	45	7.8	no
Malbranchea pulchella	glucose	27	–	yes
Mortierella vinacea	acetat	28	–	no
	glucose	66	18	no
	maltose	34	–	no
Mucor miehei	glucose	24	–	yes
Mucor pusillus	glucose	26	–	yes
Myrothecium sp.	not given	30	–	yes
Penicillium funiculosum	n-alkanes	22	–	yes
Penicillium gladioli	saccharose	32	5.7	no
Penicillium javanicum	glucose	39	9	no
Penicillium lilacinum	date extract	23	–	no
Penicillium lilacinum	saccharose	35	25	no
Penicillium soppi	n-alkanes saccharose	11–25	–	yes
Penicillium soppi	molasses	19	–	no
Penicillium spinulosum	molasses and saccharose	25–64	6–16	no
Pythium irregulare	glucose	30–42	–	yes
Pythium ultimum	glucose	48	–	yes
Rhizopus arrhizus	glucose + maltose	20	–	yes
Rhizopus sp.	glucose	27	–	yes
Stilbella thermophila	glucose	38	–	yes

Table 11-4. Fatty Acid Compositions of the Lipids of Fat-Producing Microorganisms that can be Cultivated on Carbohydrates. After Ratledge (1978).

Organisms	Substrate	Relative fatty acid content (%, w/w)											
		12:0	14:0	14:1	16:0	16:1	17:0 and 17:1	18:0	18:1	18:2	18:3	20:0 and 22:0	20 and un-saturated
Yeasts													
Candida sp. no. 107 (batch culture)	glucose	–	1	–	22	2	–	8	31	26	–	3	7
Candida sp. no. 107 (continuous culture)	glucose	–	1	–	37	1	–	14	36	8	–	–	4
Hansenula anomola (triglycerides)	glucose	–	tr.	–	20	2	1	2	49	26	–	–	–
Hansenula anomala	glucose	–	–	–	12	10	–	–	28	24	19	–	–
Hansenula anomala	glucose	tr.	3	tr.	35	2	2	36	3	–	3	–	–
Lipomyces lipofer	glucose	–	tr.	–	17	4	–	10	48	16	3	–	–
Lipomyces lipofer (triglycerides)	glucose	–	tr.	–	12	3	–	6	77	3	tr.	tr.	–
Lipomyces lipofer (triglycerides)	glucose	–	2	–	16	7	–	3	62	9	1	tr.	–
Lipomyces starkeyi (triglycerides)	glucose	–	–	–	40	6	–	5	44	4	–	–	–
Rhodotorula gracilis	glucose	tr.	1	–	24	2	1	11	45	12	3	2	–
Rhodotorula gracilis	glucose	–	1	–	20	2	4	1	42	21	8	–	–
Rhodotorula gracilis	glucose	–	1	–	31	–	–	9	53	1	5	–	–
Rhodotorula gracilis	ethanol	–	1	–	35	–	–	11	46	1	6	–	–
Rhodotorula graminis	starch and glucose	1	4	1	32	tr.	–	3	37	10	5	–	3
Rhodotorula glutinis	glucose	–	1	–	12	2	1	7	50	21	6	–	–
Mold fungi													
Aspergillus nidulans	glucose	–	1	–	21	1	–	16	40	17	tr.	1	2
Aspergillus niger	glucose	1	2	–	22	3	–	5	7	46	11	1	1
Aspergillus niger	lactose	3	5	–	50	2	2	10	11	14	2	–	–
Aspergillus ochraceus	saccharose	–	tr.	–	38	–	–	tr.	15	45	2	–	–
Aspergillus terreus	saccharose	tr.	2	–	23	tr.	–	tr.	14	40	21	–	–
Chaetomium globosum	glucose	–	–	–	58	3	4	8	27	–	–	–	–
Fusarium moniliforme	glucose	–	1	1	14	–	–	11	30	42	1	–	–
Malbranchea pulchella	glucose	–	–	–	11	–	11	27	51	–	–	–	–
Mucor globosus	glucose	2	8	–	26	8	7	26	8	16	–	–	–
Mucor ramannianus	glucose	–	2	–	19	3	–	4	28	14	31[a]	–	–
Penicillium chrysogenum	sucrose	tr.	tr.	–	18	1	tr.	9	11	53	–	6	tr.
Penicillium chrysogenum	glucose	–	–	–	13	1	–	5	14	61	7	–	–
Penicillium chrysogenum	glucose	tr.	tr.	–	24	3	tr.	9	5	48	–	5	4
Penicillium lilacinum	glucose	–	tr.	–	16	3	–	2	40	13	–	–	1
Penicillium soppi	glucose	–	1	–	20	2	1	5	9	50	13	tr.	–
Penicillium soppi	lactose	2	2	–	41	1	tr.	8	12	32	3	tr.	–
Penicillium spinulosum	glucose	–	tr.	–	18	4	–	12	43	21	tr.	1	tr.
Pythium irregulare	glucose	3	7	2	15	13	–	3	30	4	2[a]	13	8
Pythium ultimum	glucose	–	8	–	23	9	–	7	22	15	2[a]	5	11
Rhizopus arrhizus	glucose	–	–	–	21	4	–	9	42	17	8[a]	–	–
Rhizopus sp.	glucose	–	1	–	21	2	–	5	30	29	12[a]	–	–
Stilbella thermophila	glucose	–	2	–	43	2	14	25	14	–	–	–	–

[a] γ-Linolenic acid

arated by extraction and, if necessary, be purified further. The protein-rich residue can be used as cattle fodder.

5'-Nucleotides

Inosine 5'-Monophosphate:	**R = H**
Guanosine 5'-Monophosphate:	**R = NH₂**
Xanthosine 5'-Monophosphate:	**R = OH**

In addition to the **pharmacological** action of nucleotides, the **taste-enhancing** action of the 5'-nucleotides is a particularly interesting phenomenon. The compounds themselves are tasteless, but in combination with glutamic acid they give a taste-enhancing effect by synergism (Demain, 1978; Fritsche, 1978).

Of the four 5'-nucleotides, guanosine 5'-monophosphate had a taste-enhancing action three times greater than that of inosine 5'-monophosphate, while adenosine 5'-monophosphate and xanthosine 5'-monophosphate had hardly any action in this direction (Ogata, 1975, 1971).

In addition to a series of **enzymatic production processes,** there are also **fermentation methods** for the production of guanosine 5'-MP (MP = monophosphate) or inosine 5'-MP. Abe et al. (1966) have shown that a series of

bacteria (Micrococcus, Brevibacterium, Bacillus) exhibit an overproduction of purine ribonucleosides. In glucose nutrient solutions, to which small amounts of guanine and biotin must be added, 5 to 7 g/L of xanthosine 5'-MP can be obtained in aerobic submerged fermentations in about 3 days. Since, as already mentioned, this compound does not exhibit the desired action or scarcely does so, it must be converted into guanosine 5'-MP. This can be brought about by a special mutant of *Bacillus ammoniagenes* (Ogata, 1975). By using a mixed culture of the microorganism accumulating xanthosine 5'-MP with that which converts this substance, the process can be reduced to a single stage. However, it goes without saying that such a mixed culture requires a very careful harmonization in the ratio of the inoculating material of the two strains and in the supply of glucose and urea. The maximum concentration of guanosine 5'-nucleotide amounts to more than 9 g/L.

11.4   Literature

Abe, S., Udagawa, K., Nara, T. and Misawa, M.: Verfahren zur Herstellung von 5'-Xanthylsäure. D.A.S. 1,215,638 (1966).

Asai, T., Aida, K., Sugisaki, Z. and Yakeishi, N., "On α-ketoglutaric acid fermentation", *J. Gen. Appl. Microbiol.* **1**, 308–346 (1955).

Baker, D. L.: Enzymatic process for producing gluconic acid. US-Pat. 2,651,592 (1953).

Becker, M. J., Krause, L. J., Seile, M. K., Wiestur, U. E., Tschazkij, P. A. and Kluna, G. W.: Mikrobiologisches Verfahren zur Herstellung von Konzentraten, die Karotinoide enthalten. D.O.S. 2,059,387 (1972).

Behrens, U. and Ringpfeil, M.: *Mikrobielle Polysaccharide.* Wissenschaftl. Taschenbücher, Vol. 19. Akademie-Verlag, Berlin 1964.

Berger, C. and Witt, E. E.: Process for the recovery of α-ketoglutaric acid. US-Pat. 2,841,616 (1958).

Blakeborough, N.: "Industrial Fermentation". In: Blakeborough, N. (ed.): *Biochemical and Biological Engineering Science*, Vol. 1. Academic Press, London 1967, pp. 25–48.

Borel, E. A.: Biosynthesis of α-ketoglutaric acid. US-Pat. 3, 022, 233 (1962).

Buchta, K., "Die biotechnologische Gewinnung von organischen Säuren", *Chem. Ztg.* **98**, 532–538 (1974).

Calderbank, P. H.: "Mass Transfer in Fermentation Equipment". In: Blakeborough, N. (ed.): *Biochemical and Biological Engineering Science*, Vol. 1. Academic Press, London 1967, pp. 102–180.

Chibata, J. S., Tosa, T., Sato, T. and Yamamoto, K.: Verfahren zur Herstellung von L-Äpfelsäure und immobilisierter Fumarase-produzierender Mikroorganismen zur Durchführung des Verfahrens. D.O.S. 2,450,137 (1975).

Conner, H. A. and Allgeier, R. J.: "Vinegar: its History and Development". In: Perlman, D. (ed.): *Advances in Microbiology*, Vol. 20. Academic Press, New York 1976, pp. 81–133.

Degen, L., Odo, N. and Olivieri, R.: Verfahren zur Herstellung von L-Äpfelsäure durch mikrobiologische Fermentation und Mittel zur Durchführung des Verfahrens. D.O.S. 2,363,285 (1974).

Demain, A. L., "Production of nucleotides by microorganisms", *Econ. Microbiol.* **2**, 187–208 (1978).

DeZeeuw, J. R. and Tynan, III, E. J.: Fermentative Verfahren zur Herstellung von D-Mannit. D.O.S. 2,203,467 (1972).

Finn, R. K.: "Agitation and Aeration". In: Blakeborough, N. (ed.): *Biochemical and Biological Engineering Science*, Vol. 1. Academic Press, London 1967, pp. 69–99.

Florent, J., Lunel, J. and Renaut, J.: Verfahren zur Herstellung von L-β-3,4-Dihydroxyphenylalanin durch Fermentation. D.A.S. 2,102,793 (1974).

Franke, W. and Buchta, K.: "Die Milchsäuregärung". In: *Handbuch der Pflanzenphysiologie* Vol. XII/1. Springer Verlag, Berlin 1960, pp. 844–1008.

Fritsche, W.: *Biochemische Grundlagen der industriellen Mikrobiologie.* VEB Gustav Fischer Verlag, Jena 1978, pp. 97–98.

Fukui, S., "Fermentative procedures for vitamin production", *Biochem. Ind. Aspects Ferment.* **1971**, 71–90.

Gray, B. E.: Preparation of 2-keto-gulonic acid and its salts. US-Pat. 2,421,611 (a), US-Pat. 2,421,612 (b) (1945).

Greenshields, R. N., "Acetic acid: vinegar", *Econ. Microbiol.* **2**, 121–186 (1978).

Hall, A. N., "Miscellaneous oxidative transformation", *Biochem. Ind. Microorg.* **1963**, 607–628.

Hastings, J. J. H., "Acetone-butyl alcohol fermentation", *Econ. Microbiol.* **2**, 31–45 (1978).

Hester, A. S. and Ward, G. E., "Vitamin B_{12} feed supplement", *Ind. Eng. Chem.* **46**, 238–243 (1954).

Hickey, R. J.: "Production of Riboflavine by Fermentation". In: Underkofler, L. A. and Hickey, R. J. (eds.): *Industrial Fermentations,* Vol. 2. Chemical Publishing Co., New York 1954, pp. 157–190.

Hustede, H. and Siebert, D.: Verfahren zur Herstellung von Citronensäure. D.A.S. 2,264,763 (1977 a).

Hustede, H. and Siebert, D.: Verfahren zur Herstellung von Citronensäure. D.A.S. 2,212,929 (1977 b).

Hustede, H. and Siebert, D.: Verfahren zur Herstellung von Hefemutanten mit hohem Citronensäurebildungsvermögen. D.O.S. 2,264,764 (1975).

Iizuka, H., Shimizu, J., Ishii, K. and Nakajima, Y.: Verfahren zur biotechnologischen Herstellung von Zitronensäure und ihren Salzen durch Mikroorganismen. D.A.S. 1,812,710 (1978).

Johnson, M. J.: In: Underkofler, L. A. and Hickey, R. J. (eds.): *Industrial Fermentation,* Vol. 1. Chemical Publishing Co., New York 1954, p. 420.

Jungbunzlauer Spiritus- und Chem. Fabrik AG: Verfahren zur Herstellung von Zitronensäure durch submerse Gärung. D.A.S. 2,118,361 (1978).

Kamatani, Y., Okazaki, H., Imai, K., Fujita, N., Yamazaki, Y. and Ogino, K.: Verfahren zur Herstellung von Weinsäure. D.O.S. 2,600,589 (1976).

Kato, K. and Nomura, T.: Verfahren zur Reinigung von Pullulan. D.O.S. 2,504,108 (1976).

Kinoshita, S. and Nakayama, K., "Amino acids", *Econ. Microbiol.* **2**, 210–261 (1978).

Kinoshita, S. and Tanaka, K.: Verfahren zur Erzeugung von Itakonsäure durch Gärung. D.A.S. 1,086,654 (1960).

Kita, D. A. and Hall, K. E.: Verfahren zur Herstellung von 2,5-Diketogluconsäure. D.O.S. 2,849,393 (1979).

Kitahara, K.: Verfahren zur Herstellung von L-Äpfelsäure. D.O.S. 1,417,033 (1969).

Koepsell, H. J., Stodola, F. H. and Sharpe, E. S.: Preparation and recovery of α-ketoglutaric acid. US-Pat. 2,724,680 (1955).

Kotera, U., Kodama, Y., Minoda, Y. and Yamada, K., "Microbial formation of tartaric acid from glucose V", *Agric. Biol. Chem.* **36**, 1315–1325 (1972).

Kubota, K., Shiro, T. and Okumura, S., "Fermentative production of L-histidine I", *J. Gen. Appl. Microbiol.* **17**, 1–12 (1971).

Lawson, C. J. and Sutherland, I. W., "Polysaccharides", *Econ. Microbiol.* **2**, 327–392 (1978).

Ledingham, G. A. and Neish, A. C.: "Fermentative Production of 2,3-butanediol". In: Underkofler, L. A. and Hickey, R. J. (eds.): *Industrial Fermentations*, Vol. 2. Chemical Publishing Co., New York 1954, pp. 27–93.

Lockwood, L. B.: "Ketogenic Fermentation Processes". In: Underkofler, L. A. and Hickey, R. J. (eds.): *Industrial Fermentations*, Vol. 2. Chemical Publishing Co., New York 1954, pp. 1–23.

Lockwood, L. B. and Stodola, F. H.: Fermentation process for production of α-ketoglutaric acid. US-Pat. 2,443,919 (1948).

Lockwood, L. B. and Stodola, F. H., "Preliminary studies on the production of α-ketoglutaric acid by Pseudomonas fluorescens", *J. Biol. Chem.* **164**, 81–83 (1946).

Lockwood, L. B. and Ward, G. E.: "Fermentation process for itaconic acid", *Ind. Eng. Chem.* **37**, 405 (1945).

McCutchan, W. N. and Hickey, R. J.: "The butanol-acetone fermentations". In: Underkofler, L. A. and Hickey, R. J. (eds.): *Industrial Fermentations*, Vol. 1. Chemical Publishing Co., New York 1954, pp. 347–388.

Miall, L. M., "Organic acids", *Econ. Microbiol.* **2**, 48–119 (1978).

Miall, L. M. and Parker, G. F.: Verfahren zur Herstellung von Zitronensäure aus Kohlenwasserstoffen. D.A.S. 2,323,106 (1978).

Miall, L. M. and Parker, G. F.: Kontinuierliches Verfahren zur fermentativen Herstellung von Zitronensäure. D.A.S. 2,429,224 (1977).

Minoda, Y., Kodama, T., Kotera, U. and Yamada, K.: Fermentative manufacture of L(+)-tartaric acid. Jap. Pat. 7,233,154, Ref. in: C.A. **77**, 138, 350 k (1972).

Misenheimer, T. J., Anderson, R. F., Lagoda, A. A. and Tyler, D. D., "Production of 2-ketogluconic acid by *Serratia marcescens*", *Appl. Microbiol.* **13**, 393–396 (1965).

Monzini, A., "Transformation of the methyl ester of 2-oxo-L-gulonic acid into vitamin C", *Ric. Sci.* **22**, 1601–1607 (1952).

Morisi, F., Mosti, R. and Bettonte, M.: Verfahren zur enzymatischen Herstellung von L-Äpfelsäure. D.O.S. 2,415,310 (1974).

Nakayama, K., Araki, T. and Tanaka, Y., "Fermentative production of L-serine", *Jpn. Kokai Tokkyo Koho* **78**, 118, 589 (1978).

Nakayama, K. and Araki, K.: Verfahren zur biochemischen Herstellung von L-Lysin. D.A.S. 2,034,406 (1972).

Nielsen, J. J. and Veibel, S., "The reactivity of lactic acid and some of its simple derivatives", *Acta Polytechnica Scandinavica* Serie No. Ch 63, Copenhagen (1967).

Nitela, J., Hurduc, M., Ardelean, V., Alupei, G., Bostan, R., Paffala, M., Ionescu, S., Lewin, R. and Buiuc, M.: Biosynthese von Riboflavin. D.O.S. 2,028,355 (1971).

Nubel, R. C. and Ratajak, E. J.: Verfahren zur biochemischen Herstellung von Itakonsäure. D.A.S. 1,225,585 (1966).

Ogata, K.: "Industrial production of nucleotides, nucleosides and related substances". In: Sagaguchi, K., Uemura, T. and Kinoshita, S. (eds.): *Biochemical and Industrial Aspects of Fermentation.* Kodanska Ltd., Tokyo 1971, pp. 37–59.

Ogata, K., "The microbial production of nucleic acid-related compounds", *Adv. Appl. Microbiol.* **19**, 209–247 (1975).

Ogata, K., Yamada, H., Enei, H. and Okumura, S.: Fermentatives Verfahren zur Herstellung von L-Dihydroxyphenylalanin. D.A.S. 1,960,524 (1973).

Onishi, H. and Suzuki, T., "Microbial production of xylitol from glucose", *Appl. Microbiol.* **18**, 1031–1035 (1969).

Onishi, H. and Suzuki, T.: Verfahren zur Herstellung von Xylit auf mikrobiologischem Wege. D.A.S. 1,939,035 (1973).

Pazola, Z., Switek, H., Janicki, J. and Michnikow-ska, W.: Verfahren zur mikrobiologischen Herstellung von Carotinen. D.O.S. 1,642,687 (1971).

Perlman, D., "Vitamins", *Econ. Microbiol.* **2**, 303–326 (1978).

Pfeifer, V. F., Vojnovich, Ch. and Neger, E. N., "Itaconic acid by fermentation with *Aspergillus terreus*", *Ind. Eng. Chem.* **44**, 2975–2980 (1952).

Ratledge, C., "Lipids and fatty acids", *Econ. Microbiol.* **2**, 263–302 (1978).

Rehm, H.-J.: *Industrielle Mikrobiologie.* Springer Verlag, Berlin 1967, pp. 375–377.

Rehm, H.-J.: *Einführung in die industrielle Mikrobiologie.* Heidelberger Taschenbücher No. 804, Springer Verlag, Heidelberg 1971, p. 51.

Righelato, R. C., "Fermentation", *Chem. Ind. London* **1976**, 261–262.

Roberts jun., F. F.: Biotechnisches Verfahren zur Herstellung von Zitronensäure. D.A.S. 1,808,615 (1974).

Rose, A. H.: *Industrial Microbiology.* Butterworth, London 1961, p. 181.

Rudy, H.: *Fruchtsäuren.* Dr. A. Hüthig Verlag, Heidelberg 1967, p. 67.

Slodki, M. E. and Cadmus, M. C., "Production of microbial polysaccharides", *Adv. Appl. Microbiol.* **23**, 19–54 (1978).

Spencer, J. F. T. and Spencer, D. M., "Production of polyhydroxyalcohols by osmotolerant yeasts", *Econ. Microbiol.* **2**, 393–425 (1978).

Stubbs, J. H., Lockwood, L. B., Roe, E. T. and Ward, G. E.: Ketogluconic acids from glucose. US-Pat. 2,318,641 (1943).

Stubbs, J. J., Lockwood, L. B., Roe, E. T. and Ward, G. E., "Ketogluconic acids from glucose. Bacte-rial production", *Ind. Eng. Chem.* **32**, 1626–1631 (1940).

Takenaka, Y., Yoshii, H. and Hirose, Y., "Fermentative production of L-glutamic acid", *Jpn. Kokai Tokkyo Koho* **78**, 121, 994 (1978).

Tanaka, K., Ohshima, K., Tokoro, Y. and Okii, M.: Verfahren zur Herstellung von L-Lysin durch Gärung. D.O.S. 1,807,621 (1969).

Ueda, K.: Mikrobiologisches Verfahren zur Herstellung von D-Arabit. D.A.S. 1,926,178 (1970).

Underkofler, L. A.: "Glycerol". In: Underkofler, L. A. and Hickey, R. J. (eds.): *Industrial Fermentations,* Vol. 1. Chemical Publishing Co., New York 1954, pp. 252–270.

Van Lanen, J. M.: "Production of vitamins other than riboflavin". In: Underkofler, L. A. and Hickey, R. J. (eds.): *Industrial Fermentations,* Vol. 2. Chemical Publishing Co., New York 1954, pp. 191–216.

Vaughn, R. H.: "Acetic acid – Vinegar". In: Underkofler, L. A. and Hickey, R. J. (eds.): *Industrial Fermentations,* Vol. 1. Chemical Publishing Co., New York 1954, pp. 498–535.

Walon, R. G. Ph.: Verfahren zur enzymatischen Herstellung von Gluconsäure. D.O.S. 2,003,732 (1970).

Wilkinson, J. F. and Rose, A. H., "Fermentation processes", *Biochem. Ind. Microorg.* **1963**, 379–414.

Yamada, K., Minoda, Y., Kodama, T. and Kotera, U.: "Microbial formation of tartaric acid from glucose", *Ferment. Adv. Pap. Int. Ferment. Symp. 3rd* **1968**, 541–560 (pub. 1969).

Zhdanova, N. I., Leonova, T. V. and Kozyreva, L. F.: L-Isoleucin. D.O.S. 2,828,387 (1979).

Chapter 12

Enzymes

Maria-Regina Kula

12.1   Basic Concepts

Enzymes are the **catalysts of biological systems.** They accelerate the course of chemical reactions by several orders through a substantial decrease in the activation energy. The catalytic activity of the enzyme secreted by the cells or isolated from them is maintained under suitable conditions and permits the use of these enzymes as catalysts outside the cells. All enzymes are proteins. As catalysts, they are characterized by high substrate and functional specificities. The **substrate specificity** means that the enzyme catalyzes the reaction of only one chemical compound or a group of chemically very similar compounds. The **functional specificity** is expressed by the fact that an enzyme catalyzes only one definite reaction and the substrate undergoes a definite conversion with high stereo- and regiospecificities. In accordance with the types of reactions which they catalyze, enzymes are classified in six main classes (Enzyme Nomenclature, 1979).

a) Oxidoreductases
   catalyze oxidation and reduction reactions by the transfer of hydrogen and/or electrons;

b) Transferases
   catalyze the transfer of certain groups from a donor molecule to a suitable acceptor molecule;

c) Hydrolases
   catalyze hydrolytic reactions;

d) Lyases
   catalyze cleavage reactions nonhydrolytically, leaving a double bond, or catalyze the addition of groups to double bonds;

e) Isomerases
   catalyze reversible transformations of isomeric compounds;

f) Ligases (synthetases)
   catalyze the covalent linkage of the molecules with the simultaneous cleavage of an energy-rich bond (e.g. in ATP).

The **systematic name** of an enzyme is formed of two parts. The first part is based on the equation of the chemical reaction and the second part, with the ending "-ase" shows the type of reaction. The number given to an enzyme in the EC (Enzyme Commission) system identifies the catalytic activity according to international agreement. This number is composed of four groups of figures. The first figure is the number of the main class, the second and third figures relate to further subdivisions within a main class, and the last figure is the current number of the enzyme in the group defined by the first three figures, for example:

main class 3 – hydrolases
subclass 3.2 – hydrolases acting on glycosyl compounds
subgroup 3.2.1 – hydrolases hydrolyzing O-glycosyl compounds
enzyme 3.2.1.1 – 1,4-α-D-glucan glucanohydrolase.

In addition to the systematic names, **trivial names** are still frequently used. The enzyme named in the above example is better known as α-amylase or, in the older literature, as diastase. In clinical chemistry, in particular, abbreviations for frequently studied enzymes in a two- or three-letter code are also used. These abbreviations have not yet been made official.
   The **mechanism** of an enzymatically catalyzed reaction can be represented by individual steps. The **first** step consists in the formation of an enzyme-substrate complex. This raises the reactivity of the substrate. In the **second** step, the enzyme-bound substrate is converted into the product. The **third** step consists in the dissociation of the resulting product-enzyme complex into enzyme and product. In this way, the enzyme is liberated and can react again with the next substrate molecule. This scheme can be extended if more than one substrate is in-

volved in the reaction. The rate of the reaction can be deduced from these relationships, and in the simplest case Michaelis and Menten (1913) obtained the following equation:

$$v = \frac{V[S]}{K_m + [S]}$$

v = rate of the reaction (in min^{-1})
V = maximum rate, at $[S] \to \infty$ (in min^{-1})
$[S]$ = concentration of the substrate (in mol/L)
K_m = Michaelis constant (in mol/L).

The **Michaelis constant** is equal to that substrate concentration for which

$$v = \frac{V}{2}$$

This constant characterizes the affinity between enzyme and substrate and is an important parameter in enzymology. A low K_m value corresponds to a high affinity. At substrate concentrations $< 0.01\ K_m$, the rate of the reaction is directly proportional to the concentration of the substrate, while for high concentrations ($[S] > 100\ K_m$), on the other hand, the rate of the reaction is of zero order and no longer depends on the concentration of the substrate. In the intermediate range of 0.01 to $100\ K_m$, mixed orders are observed. A compilation of kinetic and molecular parameters of enzymes has been published by Barman (1969).

The formation of the enzyme-substrate complex takes place stereospecifically. The binding ability depends on the structure of the protein and is lost on denaturation. Many enzymes have in their active centers so-called prosthetic groups or bind coenzymes reversibly. The **prosthetic groups** and **coenzymes** are low-molecular-weight compounds some of which are known as vitamins. Table 12-1 lists the most important coenzymes. An enzyme is best characterized by its **catalytic acivity**, which is usually given as a measure of the amount of enzyme. According to the recommendations of the IUB (International Union of Biochemistry), the unit of enzyme activity, the **katal** (kat), is defined as that amount of enzyme which, under the conditions laid down for the particular enzyme, at 30°C catalyzes the conversion of one mole of substrate/sec (Bergmeyer, 1977). In the biochemical literature, activities are also frequently given in units of μmol/min. In addition to the basic unit of catalytic activity, the following derived units are determined: the **volume activity** (kat/L), the **specific activity** (kat/kg), and the **molar**

Table 12-1. Prosthetic Groups and Coenzymes.

Compound	Function
NAD/NADH	redox reactions and hydrogen transfer
NADP/NADPH	redox reactions and hydrogen transfer
FAD	redox reactions and hydrogen transfer
FMN	redox reactions and hydrogen transfer
Heme	electron Transfer
Coenzyme A	acyl transfer
ADP	sugar transfer
UDP	sugar transfer
ATP	source of energy, phosphate-pyrophosphate transfer, adenylation
Pyridoxal phosphate	transamination, amino acid decarboxylation
Biotin	CO_2 group transfer
Tetrahydrofolic acid	C_1-group transfer
S-Adenosylmethionine	methyl group transfer
Vitamin B_{12}	isomerization

activity (kat/mol). For practical reasons, decimal multiples or fractions of these units are also frequently used. In the case of many enzymes employed industrially, however, the substrate is a polymer occurring in nature with variable and sometimes unknown structure. Here the definition of enzyme activity given above fails (Aunstrup, 1979). For characterization in such cases, reactions under standard conditions are taken which permit the most relevant possible statement with respect to the particular use, e.g., the milk clotting activity of acid proteases. As with all chemical reactions, the rate of the enzyme-catalyzed reactions rises with the temperature. However, this rise is not possible without limit, since at higher temperatures the enzymes are rapidly denatured. Every enzyme therefore has its **temperature optimum,** which, as a rule, is between 40 and 80°C. Values outside this range are known. The **pH** also affects enzyme activity, since the hydrogen ion concentration affects the charge and state of dissociation of the whole protein molecule. At certain pH values, the substrate is no longer bound, and at extreme pH values the enzyme is usually irreversibly denatured. The pH optimum depends on the composition of the medium, the temperature, and the pH stability of the enzyme. The latter need not necessarily coincide with the pH optimum of the rate of the reaction. Many enzymes are activated by certain **inorganic ions** such as, for example, calcium ions (Ca^{2+}), magnesium ions (Mg^{2+}), or chloride ions (Cl^-). Substances that lower enzymatic activity are known as inhibitors. Irreversible inhibitors react with the enzyme in a way that destroys the active site. **Reversible inhibitors** react with the enzyme up to a characteristic equilibrium. This type of inhibition may be competitive, noncompetitive, or uncompetitive, and its effects on the K_m value and the maximum rate of the reaction are summarized in Table 12-2. In technical reactions, particular atten-

tion must be paid to a possible product inhibition of the enzyme used (Kula et al., 1980). **Allosteric enzymes** possess, in addition to the active center, an allosteric center. The latter binds reversibly, but with high affinity, certain ligands that affect the enzymatic activity. These ligands can act either as inhibitors or as activators. This possibility is frequently used in nature for regulating the metabolism (see Chapters 3 and 7).

12.2   Production of Enzymes

12.2.1   Sources of Enzymes

Enzymes are obtained from animal, plant, and microbial starting material. In the last 30 years, microorganisms have achieved a paramount importance, but enzymes from animal and plant material are nevertheless still important for special applications. As a rule, this relates to enzymes which have so far not been detected in microorganisms, especially those upon the specificity of which such high demands are placed that corresponding enzymes of microbial origin are not available as substitutes (e.g., papain) or in those cases where the activity of individual enzymes in the plant or animal tissue is so high that it appears more economic to extract the enzyme from this source than to carry out a fermentation. Here, suitable measures must be taken to ensure that the enzymatic activity is retained after harvesting or in the slaughterhouse. Of course, in extraction from plant tissues production is highly season-dependent.

12.2.2   Selection of Suitable Strains and Mutants of Microorganisms

The following aspects are decisive for the selection of a microorganism as the source of an

Table 12-2. Effect of Inhibitors on the Michaelis Parameters.

Type of inhibition	V_{max}	K_m
competitive	unchanged	increased
noncompetitive	lowered	unchanged
uncompetitive	lowered	lowered

enzyme: the organism must give high yields of enzyme in the shortest possible fermentation time. Extracellular enzymes are preferred, since their isolation is relatively simple and expensive processes for disintegrating the cells can be avoided. However, as a rule, only enzymes of class 3 occur extracellularly, especially those that can hydrolyze polymers occurring in nature to smaller fragments. A production strain must not produce toxic substances and antibiotics and should grow on cheap nutrients; in addition, the smallest possible amount of interfering by-products (such as pigments, slime, and possibly proteases) should arise. At the present time, most of the technical enzymes are obtained from two genera, namely Bacillus and Aspergillus.

In the case of strains of Bacillus, mutants are selected that can no longer form spores. Since Aspergillus cultures are frequently inoculated with conidia, in these processes great value is placed on good spore formation. The improvement of strains is a permanent task of industrial microbiology. Since most of these organisms have not been very well investigated genetically, empirical methods still have to be relied on to a substantial extent. However, genetic engineering is expected to play a major role in the future. A process of strain improvement with respect to the production of enzymes will seek, especially, the following properties:

a) mutants that produce the enzyme constitutively, i.e., without an inductor;

b) the production of the desired enzyme in the mutants is not inhibited by repressors; and

c) the yield of enzyme is considerably increased by multiplication of the gene copies, and/or changes in the signal sequences preceding the structural gene to bring about high expression.

12.2.3   Nutrient Media

Production media can be composed of synthetic or natural raw materials. As a rule, the latter are cheaper and frequently also more effective if the demands for trace substances are not adequately known. The media must contain sources of carbon and energy, and also of nitrogen, together with the necessary mineral substances and growth factors when auxotrophic microorganisms are used. If inducible enzymes are to be produced, the **inductor** must be present in the medium. On the other hand, the medium should not contain substances that cause the repression of enzyme production. Constituents of the fermentation media themselves may cause a catabolic repression or an induction (Wang et al., 1979). Typical inductors are substrates such as, for example, starch for amylase, urea for urease, and xylose for xylose isomerase. Some substances act in small amounts as inductors but in higher concentrations as repressors; e.g., cellobiose for cellulases. A highly inductive effect is often shown by substrate analogs, such as isopropyl β-D-thiogalactoside for β-galactosidase, or by substrate derivatives that can be degraded only slowly, such as sucrose palmitate for invertase (Reese et al., 1969). **Coenzymes** may also have inductive effects. Thus, thiamine increases the production of pyruvate carboxylase (Witt and Neufang, 1970). Products of the enzyme-catalyzed reactions may also act as inductors; e.g., maltodextrins in the production of α-amylase, and maltose for pullulanase. On the other hand, the formation of some **catabolic enzymes** is inhibited by the direct or indirect products of their activity; e.g., the production of protease in Bacillus species by amino acids. In the production of **biosynthetic enzymes,** an end-product inhibition is frequently observed; e.g., glutamate dehydrogenase in *B.licheniformis* by glutamate and casein hydrolysate, and tryptophan synthase by tryptophan. In the case of the so-called catabolite repression, the choice of the source of carbon is very critical. If high concentrations of easily assimilable sugars, such as glucose, lead to repression of the formation of the enzyme, the actual concentration in the fermenter can be kept very low by slow feeding during growth. Also important for the **yield of enzyme** is a correct choice of the source of nitrogen (organically bound nitrogen, ammonium or nitrate ions), and a balanced ratio of mineral substances and trace elements. In the **optimization of the medium,** one must also take care that the subsequent purification of the enzyme is not affected and that at the end of the fermentation the medium has been substantially consumed. The **most important ingredients** of media used technically are summarized in Table 12-3. Usually the nutrient media used for maintaining the strain and for the production of spores are different from those for the cultivation of the inoculum and for produc-

tion. Like inoculum media, strain-maintaining media should, furthermore, exert a selection pressure on the population in order to suppress undesirable mutants. Because of the danger of infection, the number of necessary passages before the main fermentation should be kept to a minimum.

12.2.4 Fermentation

Two general procedures are used: surface cultures (= solid-substrate cultures) and submerged cultures (= liquid cultures) (see Chapters 6 and 11). Solid-substrate cultures are of minor importance today, although a number of enzymes are still produced in this way from Aspergillus, Mucor, or Rhizopus.

Surface Cultures

Table 12-3. Complex Constituents of Technical Media for the Production of Enzymes.

Carbohydrates as sources of carbon and energy	cereal meal soybean meal potato starch wheat and rice bran molasses
Organic nitrogen (amino acids)	fish meal gelatin casein soybean meal bran distillers' solubles peptones
Growth substances and trace elements	yeast extract corn steep liquor plant oil meal of oil-bearing seeds bran

The cultivation of microorganisms is carried out on a **basic substrate** with a high content of nutrients and a large surface such as, for example, wheat bran and/or rice bran and cereal meal, with the addition of mineral substances and salts (Vetter et al., 1975; Hesseltine, 1972; Ruttloff et al., 1979). The low water content of the medium suppresses bacterial infections. The growth of fungi and the production of enzyme on the technical scale is carried out either by the **tray process,** where the substrate is spread in a thin layer (1 to 10 cm) and is surface-aerated in climatized incubation rooms or cabinets, or by the **drum process** in horizontally rotating drums. In the **high-heap process** (height 60 cm and more), a continuous stream of air is forced from below through the nutrient substrate. In this way a better removal of the heat of reaction (as compared with the above-mentioned processes) is achieved in fast-growing cultures, and also a better supply of oxygen which reaches the inner layers. Solid-substrate cultures are inoculated exclusively with **spores.** Depending on the production strains used, the growth phase lasts 1 to 7 days. Critical points in this type of fermentation are the control of the moisture content (Nishio et al., 1979) and of the temperature in the nutrient substrates and also the avoidance of foreign infections. After cultivation has been completed, the fungi are homogenized and dried to a moisture content of 10 to 12%. The powder obtained after milling can be used directly for many purposes, or the fungal mycelium is extracted with water or salt solution in countercurrent mode and worked up further as described in section 12.3. In this case, a substantially more concentrated enzyme solution is obtained than in the submerged process.

Submerged Cultures

In principle, the same fermenters and general methods are used for the production of enzymes by the submerged process as for the production of antibiotics or single-cell protein, but the nutrient media (compare Section 12.2.3) and sometimes the fermentation conditions are different (Lilly, 1979; Aunstrup, 1979; Aunstrup et al., 1979). Production usually takes place in mechanically stirred tanks with capacities of 10 000 to 100 000 liters in **batch operation.** Depending on the enzyme and the microorganisms used, the main fermentation lasts 50 to 150 h. **Continuous fermentations** on the industrial scale have been described for glucose isomerase (Diers, 1976). Due to the instability of highly mutated production strains and the difficult sterilization of technical media, continuous fermentations have so far found only limited use for the production of enyzmes. The rich media make an effective sterile control essential for success in

the production of enzymes. The rates of synthesis of an enzyme may differ in the individual phases of growth. If it is the highest in the exponential phase, the specific rate of synthesis of the enzyme corresponds to the rate of growth of the microorganism. However, in inducible systems with catabolic repression, a maximum enzyme synthesis is frequently observed in the stationary phase, when the growth of the microorganisms has fallen practically to zero. Operation in a **two-stage cascade,** in which a high concentration of cell mass is first produced and the production of the enzyme can be carried out in a second reactor under different conditions, is possible (Mitra and Wilke, 1975; Ryu et al., 1979). In addition to the influences of the **nutrient medium,** the amount of inoculum, and the physiological state of the cells in the inoculum, **operational parameters** such as the pH, the partial pressure of oxygen and, sometimes, of carbon dioxide in the liquid, and the influence of shearing forces that result from the type and intensity of **aeration** must be taken into account for optimizing the production of enzymes. Additions of surface-active agents can lead to increased excretion of extracellular enzymes and thereby to higher yields (Faith et al., 1971). Physical parameters can be used for monitoring the cultivation process and for determining the moment of harvesting. However, the automated determination of the enzyme content would be more important. This has previously been possible only off-line and with a relatively large time delay. Application of membrane techniques improves this situation (Kroner and Kula, 1984).

At the moment of harvesting, the fermenter is cooled and then the culture liquid is separated from the cell mass, and also, if necessary, from the remaining solid ingredients of the nutrient medium, by centrifugation and/ or filtration. In the case of **extracellular enzymes,** the major portion of the enzyme is found in the culture filtrate. In this case, the biomass is discarded. **Intracellular enzymes** are concentrated with the biomass. In these cases, the culture filtrate is discarded.

12.3   *Isolation of Enzymes*

12.3.1   *Disintegration of Biological Material*

Generally, for the recovery of enzymes from **animal tissue,** only certain organs – e.g., pancreases – are used. These organs, after the trimming of fat and connective tissue, are macerated in the fresh or deep-frozen state. Machines from meat technology such as cutting mills or frozen meat grinders are used for this purpose. A subsequent passage through a colloid mill leads to the extensive disintegration of the cell structure. The same purpose is achieved by treating the cell homogenate with acetone at subzero temperatures. The enzymes are extracted with buffers from the dry acetone powder or directly from the cell homogenate (see Chapter 8).

The disintegration of **plant material** for the production of enzymes follows the technology used in the manufacture of fruit and vegetable juices. The raw material is macerated with chopping or shredding machines, hammer mills, hackers, etc., treated with buffer if necessary, and pressed out hydraulically. A pretreatment with lytic enzymes to break down the cell walls is frequently indicated (see Chapters 5 and 8).

To obtain intracellular enzymes from **microorganisms,** the mechanically stable cell wall must be broken open or made permeable. The desired enzyme must not be denatured in the disintegration process. In this connection, particular attention must be devoted to thermal stress, to changes in the pH due to metabolic activities, and to the liberation of proteases (see Chapter 8). Mechanical processes of disintegration have proved particularly satisfactory for working on the large scale. High-pressure homogenizers and agitator bead mills are used for this purpose.

High-pressure Homogenizer

Detailed investigations on the disintegration of *Saccharomyces cervisiae* with the Manton-Gaulin **high-pressure homogenizer** have been published (Follows et al., 1971; Hetherington et al., 1971; Brookman, 1974) (see Chapter 8).

The disintegration of microorganisms – measured as the increase in the concentration of soluble protein in the supernatant solution – shows a significant dependence on the temperature and pressure. On the other hand, the disintegration is independent of the concentration of cells. The following equation describes the situation:

$$\log \frac{R_m}{R_m - R} = k \cdot N \cdot P^{2.9}$$

R_m = maximum amount of protein;
R = soluble protein;
N = number of passages through the homogenizer;
k = temperature-dependent rate constant;
P = working pressure.

The machine is operated at pressures of up to 560 kg/cm². Brookman (1974) has shown that the disintegration of the microorganisms depends on the absolute magnitude of the pressure drop and the speed with which this pressure drop can be realized in the machine. The steepness of pressure drop can be improved by a special valve seat (Hetherington et al., 1971). The efficacy of the disintegration of cells in the high-pressure homogenizer depends on the type of cell wall and, to some extent on the growth conditions of the organisms. The high-pressure homogenizer has been used for, among others, Saccharomyces, Candida, *E. coli, Pseudomonas aeruginosa, Bacillus megatherium,* and *Aspergillus niger.* In the disintegration of filamentous microorganisms, difficulties due to the blockage of the valve are observed, particularly at high cell concentrations.

Agitator Bead Mill

The **bead mills** used in the dyestuffs industry for grinding pigments can be adapted for the disintegration of microorganisms (Currie et al., 1972; Marffy and Kula, 1974; Limon-Lason et al., 1979; Rehacek and Schaefer, 1977; Schütte et al., 1983). Here, mills with horizontal shafts have advantages over mills with vertical shafts. The mill casing is filled with glass beads which are intensively agitated by rotating disks fixed to the shaft. The beads are retained in the casing of the mill by a sieve or friction gap, which permits a continuous performance of cell disintegration. The liberation of proteins and enzymes from the cells in this process follows first-order kinetics.

The development of heat in agitator mills is considerable. In the case of sensitive enzymes, the temperature of the suspension must be kept within limits by effective means of cooling. Mills with horizontal shafts have self-cleaning bead separators, so that these apparatuses do not tend to become blocked and are therefore also suitable for mycelia. A number of organisms that are difficult to break down by other methods, e.g., Streptococcus and Micrococcus species, algae, etc., have been successfully disintegrated in glass bead mills (Melling and Phillips, 1975a; Schütte et al., 1983).

Other Methods of Disintegration

On the laboratory scale, a number of other methods for the mechanical disintegration of cells are well established, such as **freeze-dispersion,** which was developed by Edebo (1969) and works in a particularly gentle and effective manner. **Ultrasonic treatment** is also used frequently on the laboratory scale for the disintegration of cells. However, its industrial application is opposed by difficulties in the transmission of power in large volumes, the development of heat, and the liberation of radicals which lead to the inactivation of enzymes (James et al., 1972).

Enzymatic methods of disintegration are generally burdened by the high costs of the process. In addition, the enzymes used for disintegration are mixed with the liberated protein and are lost in the process. **Immobilized enzymes** have not so far been used for disintegration, since the high molecular weight of the substrate lowers the effective action of the catalysts. Autolytic processes frequently lead to a liberation of proteases and to a decreased stability of the enzymes obtained. In individual cases, agents that affect the permeability of the cell membrane (e.g., organic solvents) or of the cell wall (e.g., penicillin in the case of Gram-negative bacteria) are also used for liberating enzymes.

12.3.2 Precipitation Processes

Precipitation of Proteins

The precipitation of a protein is frequently a rapid and efficient method for its concentration. Here, an increase in the specific activity is usually not aimed at. **Fractional precipitations** can be used for the separation of impurities and for raising the specific activity of a desired enzyme (Charm and Matteo, 1971). A special case is represented by **heat denaturation,** where in the case of heat-stable enzymes accompanying proteins are denatured at elevated temperatures and can be precipitated.

High **salt concentrations** remove the water of hydration from the protein molecule and thereby decrease its solubility. The precipitation process can be described by the equation

$$\log S = \beta - K \cdot \frac{\Gamma}{2},$$

where S is the protein solubility, $\frac{\Gamma}{2}$ is the ionic strength, and β and K are constants characteristic of the required protein. β depends both on the temperature and on the pH. A **precipitate** forms in a protein solution of known concentration when the ionic strength reaches the limiting value

$$\frac{\Gamma}{2} = \frac{\beta - \log S}{K}.$$

Foster et al. (1976) have shown, in addition, that the precipitation reaction depends critically on the performance of the process and different values are obtained when precipitation is brought about with saturated solutions or solid salts, or when investigations are made of batch-wise and continuous precipitations.

Sodium sulfate and **ammonium sulfate** are the main **precipitants** used. Precipitations with ammonium sulfate, on the technical scale cause problems because of the risk of corrosion, but they can be carried out at lower temperatures and even, because of the high solubility of this salt, around 0 °C. pH-Dependent precipitations at constant ionic strength are used more rarely, since the stability of enzymes is pH-dependent. Losses of activity must be reckoned with, particularly at acid pH values. At the isoelectric point, an enzyme reaches its lowest effective polarity and therefore shows its smallest solubility in a polar aqueous medium.

Organic solvents can also be used as precipitants. The solubility of proteins falls with the dielectric constant of the solvent. Because of the risk of **denaturing** proteins, the operations must be carried out at low temperatures, frequently below 0 °C. **Alcohols,** such as ethanol, methanol, and isopropanol, and occasionally also **acetone,** are the main precipitants used on the industrial scale. As a rule, **readily sedimenting flocs** are obtained by this method, which facilitates separation. Because of the high flammability of the solvents used and the danger of explosions, the operations must be performed with suitable safety measures. The ethanol fractionation of serum by Cohn et al. (1946) shows the potential of this method of precipitation. It also shows, simultaneously, how important and difficult is the control of the temperature in all stages of the process (Watt and Dickson, 1977).

A number of **polymers** have been tested as precipitants for proteins. **Polyethyleneglycol** and **polyethyleneimine** have found application in industrial processes. The solubility of proteins in the presence of polymers is affected by the temperature and the ionic strength, the pH, and the concentration of protein (Foster et al., 1973). In addition to this, both the molecular weight of the precipitant and the molecular weight of the desired protein are parameters of the precipitation process (Hönig and Kula, 1976; Kula et al., 1977). It is assumed that exclusion phenomena in polymer networks are responsible for the precipitation of protein. The precipitation is described by the equation

$$\log S = x - aC$$

where S represents the solubility of the protein and C the concentration of the polymer; while x and a are constants. x can be linked with the chemical potential of the protein by means of the following equation:

$$\frac{\mu - \mu^\circ}{RT} = \ln S + f S + a' C$$

In this equation,

μ = chemical potential of the protein,
μ° = standard chemical potential,
R = gas constant,
T = absolute temperature,
f = coefficient depending on the protein/protein interaction, and
a' = coefficient depending on polymer/protein interaction.

Fractional separations with polyethyleneglycol can be achieved only at low concentrations of protein (< 10 mg/mL), since otherwise interactions between proteins greatly affect the precipitation curves (Foster et al., 1973). In precipitations with polyethyleneimine, on the other hand, polymer/protein interactions have a greater effect because of ionic forces (Bergmeyer et al., 1970). Polyethyleneglycol, in particular, is arousing increasing interest as an alternative precipitant, since it is known that this hydrophilic polymer does not, as a rule, denature proteins and it is therefore possible to work at room temperature. Also advantageous is the fact that polyethyleneglycols are neither corrosive, nor poisonous, nor readily flammable.

Precipitation of Nucleic Acids

In the **purification** of intracellular enzymes, the removal of the soluble nucleic acids is desirable, since they impart a high viscosity to the solutions and interfere with the protein fractionations and chromatographic separations. Manganese(II) salts, streptomycin sulfate, protamine sulfate, cetyltriethylammonium bromide, and other salts are used as precipitants. Polyethyleneimine also leads to the precipitation of nucleic acids. It must be ascertained that the reagent used does not simultaneously precipitate the desired enzyme or lead to a decrease in its activity.

Coagulation and Flocculation

Coagulation is a process in which the surface charge of colloidal particles is neutralized by the addition of polyvalent ions with the opposite charge, which leads to coalescence. The formation of larger aggregates through a bridging process with a polyvalent polymer (see Chapter 8) is called flocculation.

In the production of extracellular enzymes, **carriers** such as starch, diatomaceous earth, etc., are added before the precipitant in order to give precipitates that are easier to handle. This procedure is particularly suitable for culture filtrates with relatively low concentrations of protein. When starch is employed as a carrier material for amylase and other starch-degrading enzymes, use is made simultaneously of its specific adsorption.

12.3.3 Separation of Solids

Solid-liquid separation (Table 12-4) is a central basic operation in the isolation of enzymes. This process step is necessary both in the separation of the cells from the culture broth and also in the clarification of the crude extract after the disintegration of the cells and the elimination of the cell fragments, in the separation of precipitates after precipitation operation, and, sometimes, in the separation of added adsorbents from protein-containing solutions. Two procedures are available for this task: **centrifugation** and **filtration** (Loncin, 1969) (see Chapter 8). The technical performance of solid-liquid separation in the production of intracellular enzymes is associated with more difficulties than in the separation of cells, since the particles are very small, the density difference and mechanical strength low, and the viscosity of the process solutions is usually relatively high. In many cases, therefore, a pretreatment is necessary.

Table 12-4. Summary of Methods and Equipment Used for Solid-Liquid Separation.

	Tubular bowl centrifuge	Chamber centrifuge	Disk separator	Nozzle separator	Self-cleaning separator	Filter press	Rotary vacuum filter	Decanter	Sieve centrifuge
Minimum difference in densities (%)	2	2	2	2	2	unimportant	unimportant	>2	unimportant
Solids concentration (%)	<2	<2	<1	<5	1–10	<10	>10	up to 40	>5
Separable particle size (μ)	0.5–500	1–500	0.5–500	0.5–500	0.5–500	1–100	0.5–100	2–$2\cdot10^4$	5–$1\cdot10^4$
Max. g-number (m/sec^2)	16000	7–11000	11000	6–9000	5–7500	–	–	2–5000	1500
Max. capacity (m^3/h)	3	10	200	200	60	4 m^3/h·m^2	5 t/h	5 t/h	up to 0.5 t
Volume in the system (L)	10	60	60	100	50	variable	up to 5 m^2	50–100	60–600
Installed energy (kW)	1.5	15	6	15	15	up to 10	12	15	25
Emptying	manual	manual	manual	automatic continuous	automatic at intervals	manual backflashing possible	automatic scraper system	automatic continuous	automatic manual
Cleaning interval	hours	hours	hours	weeks	weeks	weeks or less	weeks-months	500–700 h	hrs-weeks depending on operation
Time for cleaning	short	medium	medium	medium	medium	considerable	medium	medium	medium

The data have been compiled from the manufacturers' technical information

Centrifugation

The separation of solids by centrifugation is discussed in detail in Chapter 8, Section 8.2.3. The difficulties in the production of enzymes become clear on examination of the equations for throughput. Thus:

$$Q = \frac{d^2 \, \Delta\rho \, g}{18 \, \eta} \; \frac{r \, \omega^2}{g} \, F$$

where d is the diameter of the particles; $\Delta\rho$ is the difference in densities between the solid and the liquid; η is the kinematic viscosity, ω is the angular velocity, r is the radius; F is the effective clarification area; and g is the gravitational force (Hemfort, 1977).

The first part of the equation describes the influence of the properties of the suspension to be separated according to Stokes' law. The second part of the equation – the acceleration number and the effective clarification area F – show the dependence of the process on the parameters of the machine. The last two parts are combined under the term sigma factor.

For a given suspension, comparison of the sigma factors permits an estimate of the performance of different machines. Because of the uncertainties of many implied assumptions, however, preliminary trials are indispensible in practice. The capacity of industrial centrifuges is limited, since an increase in the radius is possible only within the limits of the mechanical strength of the materials available. The maximum permissible angular velocity falls with increasing volume of the rotor chamber and with continuous flow. It is therefore impossible on the industrial scale to achieve the separation efficiency of beaker centrifuges in the laboratory. As a consequence, in order to ensure acceptable yields in this step, a certain residual turbidity must be accepted (Naeher and Thum, 1974), which can lead to difficulties in the subsequent opera-

tions of enzyme purification. The following types of centrifuges have proved to be useful in working with biological material: tubular-bowl centrifuges, chamber centrifuges, and disk centrifuges. Sieve centrifuges are used particularly for the separation of adsorbents (hydroxylapatite, ion-exchange resins) in batch operation. A summary and comparison of the possible applications of various types of centrifuges and filters is given in Table 12-4.

The **tubular-bowl centrifuges** that are important for the separation of cell constituents possess clarification cylinders with relatively small diameters (5 to 15 cm), which permits high velocities in rotation. In this case, the acceleration number dominates the sigma factor. As a rule, the liquid is fed in at the bottom through a hollow shaft. The machine is driven from the top via belts (up to 20000 rpm) or, in a special form, by turbines (up to 55000 rpm). The sediment is thrown against the wall of the rotor, while the liquid rises to the top. In most of the tubular-bowl centrifuges used industrially, at the upper end of the rotor under the action of the centrifugal force the clarified liquid passes freely into a catcher, which can lead to pronounced foaming and the formation of aerosols and therefore to losses of enzyme activity. The clarified liquid is run off by gravity. Only a comparatively small space (0.2 to 8 L) is available for the separation of the sediment, so that the main disadvantage of these centrifuges is their low capacity. On the other hand, because of the low mass of the rotor fast brakings and accelerations are possible so that the down-time involved in changing the rotors can be reduced, with a consequent improvement in capacity.

The **tubular-bowl centrifuges** also include an air-driven **ultracentrifuge** which in continuous flow can give acceleration factors of up to 150000 g. This centrifuge is used mainly for zonal centrifugation in density gradients but it can also separate dissolved colloidal cell particles such as ribosomes, mitochondria, and microsomes, and also small amounts of fine precipitates from solutions of high density. Foam in the process solution is avoided by rotating seals and by the discharge of the clarified liquid under pressure.

The separation of cell debris and protein precipitates is difficult, and losses due to inadequate clarification or dewatering must be reckoned on even with considerably reduced throughputs (Wang et al., 1979). Thus, in the fractionation of plasma, throughputs of up to 1200 L/h are achieved in chamber centrifuges with a hydraulic capacity of 10 000 L/h (Hemfort, 1977).

Filtration

In the isolation of enzymes, **filtrations** can serve two purposes: either the recovery of the precipitate, or the separation of undissolved components from a process solution. Only in the latter case is the addition of filter aids relatively problem-free; otherwise the filter aid remains in the desired fraction and must later be removed separately. Filtrations with biological material are, as a rule, carried out at constant pressure. Therefore the time required for the filtration of a given volume after the accumulative filtration volume V has passed the filtering device is described by the following equation:

$$\frac{dt}{dV} = \frac{\eta\, r\, W}{A^2 p} V + \frac{R_m}{A_p}$$

η = viscosity of the liquid,
W = solids volume per unit volume of the feed solution,
r = cake-specific resistance constant per unit weight of cake,
R_m = resistance of the filtering layer,
A = the surface area of the filter,
p = applied (constant) pressure difference.

In the filter cake forming, the pressure drop is approximately proportional to $1/D^4$. The smaller the particles to be separated are, therefore, the more significant will be the effect of the cake resistance. In many cases, in fact, filtrations can be carried out only slowly, but more economically, when the stability of the enzyme permits longer process times. If the proportion of solids is small enough, **filter presses** are used. They are operated at positive pressure which is predetermined by the rated pressure of the pump used. Filter presses are also used, in particular, for sterile filtration in order to reduce the number of germs in the process solutions or liquid preparations. If the final volume of filtration is to be kept small, **vacuum drum filters** are used (see Chapter 8).

Extraction

The technological difficulties in solid-liquid separation which arise from the size of the particles can be overcome by **extraction processes** in which the diameter of the drops forms the deciding magnitude for the separation process. Here, multiphase aqueous systems are used (Albertsson, 1971), and by a suitable choice of the parameters it is ensured that cells or cell debris, on the one hand, and the desired enzyme, on the other hand, pass into different phases. The phases are separated in centrifugal separators (Kula, 1979). Multistage processes are also possible with the use of current technology. These processes are currently under trial on the pilot scale and are marked by high capacities and short residence times (Kroner et al., 1978; Hustedt et al., 1978; Kula et al., 1982; Kroner et al., 1984).

12.3.4 Purification

It is frequently impossible to **separate interfering activities** from enzyme preparations by single-stage processes such as precipitation. A series of **chromatographic processes** and **partition processes** are available for purification (Morris and Morris, 1976; Kula et al., 1982;

Janson and Hedman, 1982), some of which are also suitable for industrial processes (see Chapter 8, Section 8.5.2).

Adsorption and Ion-exchange Chromatography

The oldest chromatographic processes are based on **selective adsorptions** and desorptions of proteins on inorganic materials (see Chapter 8). Because of the high pressure drop and the low flow rates, these adsorbents are usually employed only in batch operation. **Ion-exchange chromatography** has gained greater importance for the separation of enzymes. The following requirements have to be met by the resins used: the matrix should be sufficiently hydrophilic to avoid the denaturation of the proteins and inert with respect to the eluents used, and it should, together with a rapid approach to equilibrium, have a high capacity for high-molecular-weight substances. From the technical point of view, a fast flow rate, a high separation power, a small change in volume on working with pH or salt gradients, and complete regenerability without loss or fall in quality are also required. Ion-exchange resins based on cellulose, dextran gels, agarose, or polyacrylamide gels have proved to be most suitable for the **chromatography of enzymes.** For anion-exchangers, the diethylaminoethyl group is introduced into the matrix, and carboxymethyl, phosphoryl, and sulfoethyl groups are common as cation-exchangers; a summary has been given by Melling and Phillips (1975b). Ion-exchangers are used for batchwise adsorption or, in multistage procedures, for increasing the sharpness of separation they are packed into columns as solid beds. Elution is carried out by stepwise increases in the ionic strength and/or changes in the pH or a gradual change of these parameters in a gradient. As a rule, gradient elution leads to purer products, but in return longer process times and greater dilution must be accepted.

Gel Filtration

In gel filtration, the **size and shape of the molecules** form the **criterion of separation.** Cross-linked polymers with definite pore diameters are used. Molecules that can penetrate through the pores into the interior of the gel are retained more strongly, since this increases the effective volume in a column. The exclusion limit and the range of fractionation can be selected in accordance with the pore diameter of the chromatographic material. Within the fractionation range, the elution volume is proportional to the logarithm of the molecular weight, on the assumption that globular proteins are involved (Andrews, 1970). Gel filtration is also frequently used on the industrial scale for the **desalting of protein solutions.** For this purpose, highly cross-linked materials with greater mechanical stability are preferred. Suitable chromatographic material can be manufactured on the basis of cross-linked dextrans, agarose, and polyacrylamide. A review of commercial products has been given by Melling and Phillips (1975b). For some time porous glass with definite pore diameters has also been available.

Affinity Chromatography

The name affinity chromatography covers processes which make use of a **biospecific binding** between enzymes and their ligands as the basis of separating processes (Jacoby and Wilchek, 1974). The specific ligands may be substrates or inhibitors. In addition to this, coenzymes can be used as group-specific ligands (Mosbach, 1978). The disadvantage of the affinity processes is that a specific resin must be developed separately for each enzyme. For this reason, **resins with group-specific reagents** such as NAD, AMP, lectins, heparins, etc., where a specific elution can be brought about by a suitable choice of eluent, are of interest (Graves and Wu, 1979). These methods have been well developed on the laboratory scale but hitherto have found industrial application only occasionally for analytical enzymes, particularly for the elimination of interfering activities.

Column Chromatography on the Technical Scale

Many of the commercial hydrophilic chromatographic materials that are used for the purification of enzymes are unsuitable for working on the large scale with columns having volumes of 10 to several hundreds of liters because of their physical properties and, in particular, their low mechanical strength. In the case of large columns, in addition, the problem of zone broadening arises so that the high resolution capacity of laboratory columns is not achieved (Janson, 1977). **Zone broadening** results from diffusion in the longitudinal direction, inadequate achievement of equilibrium, and imperfections in the packing of the columns. With increasing flow rate through the column, the influence of diffusion in the axial direction is decreased. On the other hand, the establishment of the equilibrium between the stationary and mobile phases is improved with decreasing flow rates. The optimum is achieved at very low flow rates. In an industrial process, the possible resolution must be renounced in favor of a reasonable throughput. Here the effect of the flow rate on the pressure drop in the column is frequently the dominating problem. A rise in the concentration of the protein solution is possible only within certain limits because it leads to a rise in the viscosity of the solution. As soon as the

zone boundary also represents a viscosity boundary the risk increases of a nonuniform flow profile at the zone front, where inhomogeneities of the packing will lead to the breakthrough of the front. **The size of the resin particles** is of interest in connection with the packing and resolution of columns. In theory, optimum resolution can be achieved with the smallest particle diameters. In industrial processes, the choice of particle size is dictated by the necessity for achieving reasonable flow rates and keeping the hydrodynamic pressure within limits. Because of the zone broadening, an improvement in the resolution of a column is proportional to the square root of the bed height. The height of the column cannot be increased at will, since the pressure drop rises greatly, mainly because of the increased flow resistance of the solid phase. An increase in pressure over a certain limiting value leads to a compression of the bed and to a drastic fall in the flow rates. These difficulties can be overcome to a certain extent by the use of **segmented columns.** Intensive work is being carried out on the improvement of the mechanical properties of enzyme-tolerating hydrophilic and porous matrices. Chromatographic separation processes may be very effective but they have the intrinsic disadvantage that they are batch processes. The procedure can be automated to a certain extent, and this is also being done on the industrial scale with success, particularly in the case of gel filtration (Duppel, 1977) and ion exchange (Janson and Hedman, 1982). Hitherto, however, no satisfactory continuous techniques for chromatography have been developed.

The **materials** used for the construction of chromatographic columns are, depending on the size and diameter, glass, plastics, and/or stainless steel. The construction of the endplates is of the greatest importance, as here the conversion of a flow of liquid from a relatively small tube into a uniform horizontal zone, or its collection from a large cross-section into a narrow tube, is of great importance for the resolution of the chromatographic column (Janson and Hedman, 1982). **Physical parameters,** such as the optical density at different wavelengths, conductivity, or volume flow can be monitored automatically and be utilized for the separate collection of the desired fractions (Jefferis and Kula, 1978). On the other hand, an on-line determination of the **enzymatic activity in the eluate** has not so far been possible. Suitable accessories such as fraction collectors, gradient formers, etc., for dealing with large volumes are becoming available commercially.

Electrophoretic Processes

The **differential rates of migration** of proteins in an electric field can be used for separation. Depending on the conditions, electrophoresis can be carried out as **zone electrophoresis** or **isotachophoresis,** or in **porosity gradients.** Here the removal of heat is of great importance. In order to suppress convection, viscous sugar solutions and polyacrylamide, agarose, or dextran gels are employed. Separations up to the gram scale are possible with enzymes but are used only in special cases (Radola and Graesslin, 1977).

12.3.5 Concentration

Extracellular enzymes occur in relatively dilute solutions and must be concentrated before their further use. In the isolation of **intracellular enzymes,** as well, concentration to reduce the volume of the process solution is frequently necessary. Both precipitation and absorption processes can be used for concentration purposes. On the industrial scale ultrafiltration has become the method of choice as a simple and efficient process step for concentration.

Ultrafiltration

Membranes with exclusion limits of 2000 to 300000 dalton are available for ultrafiltration (Strathmann, 1978; Staude, 1978). Here, as a rule, **anisotropic membranes** are used which consist of a very thin layer about 0.1 to 0.5 μ thick, which forms the filter proper, and which, by virtue of the manufacturing process, is supported on a relatively thick (20 μm to 1 mm) porous substructure that imparts mechanical strength to the filter. High rates of flow are achieved because of the extraordinarily thin filter layer. The blockage of the membrane can be virtually avoided. However, the formation of a secondary layer of retained molecules in front of the membrane can lead to considerable changes in the flow rates (concentration polarization). In ultrafiltration devices, attempts are made to keep the formation of a **polarization layer** to a minimum. For this purpose, the solution is pumped at high velocity in laminar or turbulent flow past the membrane so as to ensure the back-transport into the solution of the molecules collecting in front of the membrane. This gives rise to considerable shearing forces which, under certain circumstances, may lead to the inactivation of sensitive enzymes. In general, the losses of activity are relatively low. Concentration polarization also has a great influence on the retention characteristics of a membrane. The formation of a secondary layer and the different diffusion coefficients of molecules of different molecular weights have so far opposed the introduction of ultrafiltration as an effective separating technique, which would be theoretically conceivable. However, provided that the concentration of protein is not too high, in a concentration by ultrafiltration distinctly smaller molecules can be separated satisfactorily (Hatch and Price, 1978). The **stability** of a membrane is determined by its chemical structure. Useful service of up to 12 months can be achieved by regular cleaning. Membranes are used in the form of **flat membranes** in plate and cassette systems or as **hollow-fiber capillaries** and **tube membranes** in tube bundles. As a rule, flat membranes can be operated with a higher differential pressure and therefore permit the use of more viscous solutions and the achievement of a higher final concentration (Friedli and Kistler 1977; Guthöhrlein, 1977).

Engineering aspects and design of ultrafiltration processes are discussed in detail in a recent review, by Flaschel et al. (1983).

12.3.6 Desalting

Inorganic salts are frequently undesirable as materials accompanying enzymes for specific applications. Methods available for desalting or a definite exchange of salts are gel filtrations (compare Section 12.3.4), dialysis, and diafiltration.

Diafiltration

Diafiltration is the name given to an ultrafiltration process when the issuing permeate is continuously replaced by a supply of water or a buffer of known composition. The following equation describes the **decrease in the salt content** in the protein solution:

$$\ln \frac{C_o}{C_f} = \frac{V_f}{V_o}$$

C_o = salt concentration at the beginning,
C_f = salt concentration in the protein solution,
V_f = volume of the exchange liquid,
V_o = initial volume.

In the case of a salt exchange, the following equation is applicable:

$$\ln \frac{C_f}{C_f - C} = \frac{V_f}{V_o}$$

C_f = salt concentration in the feed solution,
C = actual salt concentration in the process solution.

It follows from these equations that, regardless of the initial concentration, 95% salt exchange is achieved when the permeate volume amounts to three times V_o. 99% exchange is reached after five residence times. A salt exchange can also be achieved in discrete steps of dilution and concentration. Then the following expression applies

$$C_e = \left(\frac{V_o}{V_d}\right)^n C_o$$

C_e = end concentration of the salt in the process solution,
C_o = initial concentration,
V_o = initial volume,
V_d = volume after dilution,
n = number of dilution steps performed.

In the case of low protein concentrations, the stepwise concentration and dilution of the solution is the fastest and most effective method.

Dialysis

The **elimination of impurities** with low molecular weights from a protein solution by dialysis is a long-known process. The **semipermeable membranes** used are generally cellulose acetate tubes. The transport of the molecules takes place here exclusively by diffusion, and therefore conventional dialysis is very time-consuming and, moreover, requires large amounts of water or buffer solution. Dialysis has the advantage of an uncomplicated mode of operation and very inexpensive apparatus. To accelerate the process more favorable ratios of surface to volume and adequate mixing of retentate and diffusate must be sought. This can be done, for example, by adapting the apparatus used for hemodialysis (Melling and Phillips, 1975b). However, the apparatus now becomes very much more expensive. The boundaries between dialysis and diafiltration are fluid.

12.3.7 Drying

The extracellular enzymes used in food technology are frequently added as **dry preparations**. The manufacture of dry free-flowing preparations can be carried out only with the aid of thermal processes. Here, the thermal stability of the enzyme must be carefully studied and, if necessary, be improved by the addition of stabilizers such as sugars, substrates of the enzymes, cofactors, reducing agents, or complex-forming agents (Schmid, 1979; Wiseman, 1978). The supply of heat must be controlled in such a way that a certain maximum temperature (frequently <40°C) is not exceeded in the material to be dried. Drying processes that may be considered are vacuum drying, freeze-drying, and spray-drying.

Vacuum Drying

In vacuum drying, pressures between 0.4 and 1.3 kPa must be used. The vacuum is produced and maintained with the aid of pumps of various designs. The vapors are condensed in a condenser that must be cooled in accordance with the desired vacuum. The heat exchange in vacuum dryers is usually carried out by direct contact on heated surfaces, e.g., the rollers of a vacuum roller dryer. During drying, an enrichment of dissolved substances in the liquid phase takes place, so that particular care must be taken to eliminate undesired salts before the vacuum drying process.

Freeze-drying

In freeze-drying, the liquid to be dried is frozen at temperatures below the eutectic point. Drying proper takes place by the sublimation of ice at pressures between 0.13 Pa and 13 Pa. The condenser must be cooled to temperatures below $-45°C$. Because of the necessary production of a high vacuum and of the cold for condensation, freeze-drying is an energy-intensive and expensive process step.

Spray-Drying

In spray-drying, the solution or suspension is sprayed into the drying chamber. Because of the highly increased surface obtained in this way, the water is evaporated in a very short time by the hot air blown in. The material for drying heats up only insignificantly during this process even with air inlet temperatures of 150 to 180°C. The air blown in is heated indirectly in a heat exchanger. The spraying device must be selected in such a way that a uniform atomization is achieved. Nozzle and rotating disk constructions are used for this purpose. Spray-drying units with evaporation capacities of more than 5000 kg of water/h are being constructed.

12.3.8 Storage and Transport

The possibilities for storing and transporting an enzyme preparation are of great importance for the use of enzymes as industrial catalysts, since the manufacturer is rarely the user. In order to save space and freight costs, dried powders or suspensions in ammonium sulfate, glycerol, or polyethyleneglycol solutions are preferred. The storage stability may depend on several process steps, but the last step is frequently of the greatest importance and must accordingly be carefully optimized. Depending on the intended use, care must also be taken here to reduce the germ number and, if necessary, to standardize the products.

12.4 Immobilization of Enzymes

The isolation of, in particular, intracellular enzymes is relatively expensive. Investigations were therefore carried out at an early period on the possibilities of **repeated use** of these catalysts and the possibilities of a **continuous reaction systems**. Both aims can be achieved with immobilized enzymes (Buchholz, 1979; Mosbach, 1976; Chibata, 1978b). As shown in Table 12-5, with immobilized enzymes a distinction is made between **entrapped** and **bound** enzymes. It must be borne in mind here that this classification does not take into account the fact that different processes may be used simultaneously or successively. In the individual preparations, however, either physical or chemical forces predominate. Both modes of operation have specific advantages and disadvantages. The most favorable form of immobilized enzyme in the individual case depends on the solubility and the molecular weight of the substrate, the stability of the enzyme, the necessity of cofactors for the desired reaction, and similar questions. A great multitude of natural and synthetic polymers has been used in the past for obtaining insoluble enzyme preparations, and Table 12-6 gives a selection of these. Only in the **membrane reactor** is the fixation of the enzyme basically renounced and the reaction space in the reactor sealed of

Table 12-5. Immobilization of Enzymes.

Entrapped enzymes	Support-bound enzymes
in polymeric networks	by adsorption
in semipermeable	by ionic binding
membranes (capsules	by covalent binding
or fibers)	
behind an ultrafiltra-	cross-linked with bi- or
tion membrane	multifunctional reagents

Table 12-6. Support Materials for the Immobilization of Enzymes.

Inorganic materials	Natural polymers	Synthetic polymers
Glass	cellulose	polyacrylamide
Silica gel	starch	nylon
Alumina	dextran	poly vinyl
Bentonite	agarose	alcohol
Hydroxylapatite	alginates	methacrylate
Nickel-nickel oxide	carragheenan	oxiranes
Titanium dioxide	collagen	
Zirconium dioxide		

by an ultrafiltration membrane (Wandrey and Flaschel, 1979). The possibilities of use are limited to products sufficiently small to pass through the membranes while the catalyst is retained. In the other forms of entrapped enzyme (polymeric network or microcapsules), both substrate and product must be able to pass through the pores of the network. Here increased resistances to mass transport must be expected. In the case of **bound enzymes,** macroporous carriers are preferred in order to create sufficiently large surface for adsorption or covalent binding. The covalent binding of enzymes to activated matrices is carried out essentially by methods in aqueous phase that are known in peptide or protein chemistry. The carrier must contain reactive groups that can enter into bonds with the side chains of the amino acids (Manecke et al., 1979; Schlünsen et al., 1979). It is particularly the ε-amino groups of lysine and the carboxy groups of the side chains of glutamic acid and aspartic acid that are used for this purpose. Linkages with aromatic amino acids are also possible via diazo couplings. The modification of the enzymes can change their activities and other properties. Attempts are frequently made to achieve a greater stability, solvent resistance, and pH tolerance in this way (Wiseman, 1978; Klibanov, 1979). In addition to losses of activity through denaturation during the immobilization of enzymes by covalent fixation, a decrease in the efficacy of the enzyme used must be taken into account, since film and pore diffusion limit mass transport. Corresponding investigations on reaction technique are necessary for designing a process (Wandrey and Flaschel, 1979a). For a continuous process, **column reactors,** and also **stirred tanks** and **cascades of stirred tanks** are used (Lilly, 1978). Here, product and/or substrate inhibition and the desired conversion play a decisive role in the selection (Carley-smith and Lilly, 1979). Depending on the value added and the operating costs of the process under consideration, the relative proportion of the costs of the catalysts may be between <1% and 50% of the total. It may therefore be important to take into consideration not only the reuse of the enzyme but also the **reuse of the support.** Inorganic supports can be subjected to rigorous purification steps. On the other hand, in the case of enzymes bound by ionic forces or by adsorption enzymes desorbed in the process can be replaced relatively easily. In evaluating the economic aspects of a process, information on the **efficiency** of a given catalyst and its **stability** under operating conditions are needed. Section 12.5 gives information on, and literature relating to, processes with immobilized enzymes that are performed commercially.

The isolation of the enzyme may also be avoided and the **microorganisms** used as catalysts **directly** for immobilization (Klein and Wagner, 1978). In these processes, care must be taken, in particular, that product and/or substrate are not further degraded or changed in an undesirable fashion.

12.5 Industrial Enzymes

Of the about 3000 enzymes known at the present time (Enzyme Nomenclature, 1978), only a comparatively few are produced on the large scale and used industrially. These are mainly extracellular hydrolytic enzymes which degrade naturally occurring polymers such as starch, proteins, pectins, and cellulose. A remarkable exception, however, is glucose isomerase. The most important enzymes produced industrially and their percentages in the total turnover are summarized in Table 12-7. General schemes for the production of intra- and extracellular enzymes are shown by Figs. 12-1 and 12-2. The industrial application of the enzymes is illustrated below. Further information is given by Reed (1975); Ruttloff et al., (1979); Vetter et al. (1975); Wiseman (1975); Godfrey and Reichelt (1983); and in the application reports issued by the enzyme manufacturers.

12.5.1 Proteases

Bacillus proteases

Measured by weight, **alkaline proteases** represent the greatest single item in enzyme production (see Table 12-7). The bulk of the alkaline proteases are used as **additives to detergents** in the form of granulates, prills, or Marumerizer pellets. Additions of enzymes lead to a distinctly better cleansing power of detergents, on the one hand through the hydrolytic degradation of difficult protein-containing soils such as blood, egg yolk, chocolate, etc., and, on the other hand, by increasing the detachment of the soil from the fibers, since the soil adheres more strongly in the presence of proteins.

In order to be active during the washing process, detergent proteases must satisfy the following prerequisites: they should exhibit a high activity but low specificity on the hydrolysis of peptide bonds and be capable of use at elevated temperatures. In addition, they must be stable in the presence of an alkaline

Table 12-7. Important Industrial Enzymes.

Enzyme	Most important micro-organisms	Reaction catalyzed	pH optimum	Temp. opt. °C up to	Annual prodn.* tons of enzyme prot.	Percentage of sales on the world scale
Bacillus protease	Bacillus sp.	Endohydrolysis of proteins	8–11	80	500	40
Fungal protease	Aspergillus sp. Mucor sp.	Endohydrolysis of proteins	4–6	60	20	8
Bacterial α-amylase	Bacillus sp.	Endohydrolysis of starch	5–7	110	300	12
Fungal α-amylase	Aspergillus sp.	Endohydrolysis of starch	4–5	60	10	3
Glucoamylase	Aspergillus sp.	Exohydrolysis of starch splitting off β-D-glucose	4–5	60	300	14
Pullulanase	Bacillus sp.	Hydrolysis of α-1,6 bonds	6–7	60	n.k.	<1
Glucose isomerase	Streptomyces sp. Actinoplanes sp. Bacillus sp.	Isomerisation of D-glucose to D-fructose	6.5–8.5	90	50	12
Pectinase (collective term)	Aspergillus sp	Hydrolysis of polygalacturonic acid and its methyl esters	4–5	50	10	10
Cellulase (collective term)	Trichoderma reesei	Hydrolysis of cellulose	4–5	50	n.k.	<1
Lactase	Aspergillus sp.	Hydrolysis of β-D-galactosides	3.5–6.6	55	n.k.	<1

Table 12-7. (continued)

Enzyme	Most important micro-organisms	Reaction catalyzed	pH optimum	Temp. opt. °C up to	Annual prodn.* tons of enzyme prot.	Percentage of sales on the world scale
Invertase	*Saccharomyces fragilis* Saccharomyces sp.	Splitting of sucrose into glucose and fructose	4.5	60	n.k.	
Glucose oxidase	Penicillium sp.	Oxidation of glucose to gluconic acid	5–7	40	n.k.	<1
Catalase	Aspergillus sp. *Micrococcus lysodeikticus*	Decomposition of H_2O_2	7	40	n.k.	<1
Lipase	Aspergillus sp. Rhizopus sp. Mucor sp.	Hydrolysis of fatty acid esters	5–7	40	n.k.	1

n.k. = not known, probably <10
* The values have been taken from Aunstrup (1979) and Aunstrup et al. (1979)

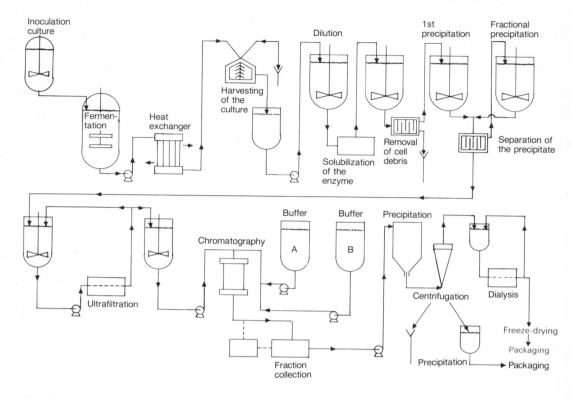

Fig. 12-1. Flowsheet for the manufacture of intracellular enzymes.

detergent liquor, complex-forming agents, bleaching agents, and surface-active agents. Of the various types of proteases, **microbial serine proteases** still satisfy these requirements best. **Subtilisins,** the serine proteases from *Bacillus licheniformis* and *Bacillus amyloliquefaciens,* show about 80% of their enzymatic activity in the pH range of 8 to 11, and can be used at temperatures up to 70°C. The stability of the subtilisins does not depend on metal ions, so that complexing additives in detergents, such as tripolyphosphates or EDTA do not greatly interfere. While the enzymatic activity decreases only slowly in the presence of perborate, H_2O_2 has a rapid deactivating effect. Consequently, proteolytic activity in en-

zyme-containing washing liquors can be expected only up to 55 to 60°C. Above this temperature the H_2O_2 liberated from perborates, together with the temperature itself, leads to a rapid loss of activity. The nature and blend of the surface-active agents used together with enzymes must be carefully optimized, since surfactants readily denature proteins. Nonionic surfactants have a denaturing effect only at higher concentrations than anionic surfactants.

Today, about 80% of the detergents offered on the market contain enzymes, the concentration of which, referred to active enzyme protein, is about 0.015 to 0.025%. The protease powder arising in production is not added to a

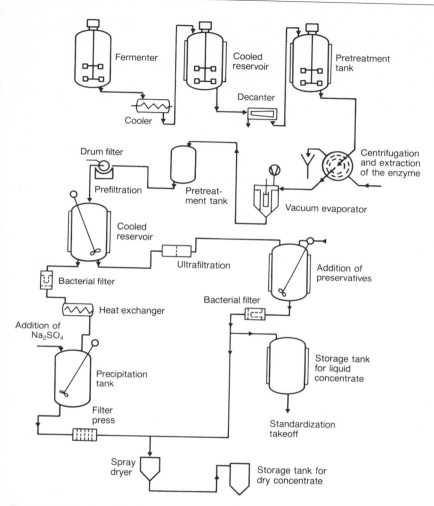

Fig. 12-2. Flowsheet for the manufacture of extracellular enzymes.

detergent directly, but is first brought into a substantially dust-free form. This is carried out by **embedding** (prill) the enzyme powder in or **coating** (Marumerizer) it with ethylene oxide adducts of fatty alcohols or with polyethyleneglycols melting at 50 to 70°C, etc., followed by shaping. In this way it has been possible substantially to eliminate the problem of dust, which, because of the risk of allergy associated with it caused public criticism of the

use of proteases in the 1970s and for a time led to a pronounced fall in production. The new form of manufacture also simultaneously improves the storage stability of the proteases.

The bulk of the proteases used in detergents is produced with *B. licheniformis*. The microorganism is cultivated in a medium rich in protein and protein hydrolysates at a neutral pH between 30 and 40°C.

It has proved to be advantageous to feed in carbohydrates in portions during the course of fermentation. The production of enzymes begins when the culture passes into the stationary phase (after 10 to 20 hours) and takes place an approximately constant rate for many hours so long as protein is still present in the medium.

Starch hydrolysates are degraded and assimilated by *B. licheniformis,* but at the end of the fermentation the serine protease is practically the only protein in the culture supernatant. The yields of commercial processes are, as a rule, high and can amount to more than 10% of the protein added to the medium.

The yields of proteases in the cultivation of *B. amyloliquefaciens* are not quite so high, and, in contrast to *B. licheniformis,* the culture supernatant contains other enzymes and, in particular, relatively large amounts of α-amylase. The serine protease from *B. amyloliquefaciens* is used for special washing and cleaning agents when the removal of carbohydrate-containing soil is important. Furthermore, in the last few years a serine protease has been obtained from culture supernatants from alkalophilic species of Bacillus. As compared with subtilisins, these proteases have a better stability at high pH values (up to pH 12). The proteases from alkalophilic strains exhibit better stability in detergents when the traditional complexing agent tripolyphosphate is replaced by citrate or gluconate. Their high alkali resistance also makes these proteases particularly suitable for the leather industry for the dehairing of skins and to reduce softening times.

Fungal Proteases

In general, fungal proteases are active in the acid pH range and are therefore also called **acid proteases.** The enzymes are produced mainly from the genera Mucor and Aspergillus. **Mucor proteases** from the thermophilic strains *M. pusillus* and *M. miehei* are used in the manufacture of cheese (see Chapter 9) and at the present time are displacing to an increasing extent the "calves' rennet" used for this purpose since ancient times. The microbial enzymes used for this purpose must exhibit a specificity similar to that of rennet since a limited hydrolysis of casein is of decisive importance for the production of cheese. In the fermentation of Mucor strains, lipases and esterases formed simultaneously, and also any nonspecific proteases present, must be eliminated from the enzyme solution, since they lead to undesirable by-products.

Acid proteases are also obtained from the Aspergillus strains *A. oryzae* and *A. niger.* Relatively large amounts of proteases are formed by Aspergillus species only when they are cultivated on solid substrates (wheat or rice bran). Additions of inorganic nitrogen improve the yield. In addition to proteases, relatively large amounts of α-amylase, glucoamylase, cellulases, and pectinases are formed. However, these side activities do not usually interfere with the application of the product.

Aspergillus proteases are used for the hydrolysis of soybean proteins in the production of soy sauce (see Chapter 9), as a constituent of enzyme preparations for the treatment of digestive disturbances, and in the baking industry. While soybean protein is degraded substantially to the amino acids, the addition of proteases to flour should bring about only a partial hydrolysis of the gluten present in the flour. This lowers the viscosity of the dough and shortens the kneading time. Additions of proteases to the flour also improves the quality of baked goods in storage. Since fungal proteases are deactivated at temperatures as low as 50°C, a rapid denaturation sets in at the beginning of the baking process and prevents a more complete hydrolysis of the proteins.

Aspergillus proteases find limited applications also in the manufacture of protein hydrolysates from slaughterhouse wastes and fish proteins.

12.5.2   α-Amylases

Bacterial α-amylase is an **endoenzyme** that cleaves α-1,4 bonds in amylose and amylopectin statistically, which leads to a rapid fall in the viscosity of gelatinized starch solutions. The process is therefore also known as the **liquefaction of starch.** The end products of the action of α-amylase are limit dextrins together with smaller amounts of glucose and maltose. Native starch is attacked by amylase only slowly or not at all, and an efficient use of this enzyme requires a previous **hydration** of the starch, which is carried out by heating in aqueous suspension. This process is called **gelatinization.** Depending on the origin of the starch, different temperatures are necessary for complete gelatinization. This has led to the demand for a high temperature stability of α-amylases.

The α-amylase from *Bacillus amyloliquefaciens* satisfies this requirement (active up to 90 °C) and has long been produced on the industrial scale. A further improvement was introduced by the α-amylase from *Bacillus licheniformis* developed by NOVO, which is deactivated only at 105-110 °C. α-Amylases are **metalloproteins** and are stabilized by calcium ions, while chelate-forming agents act as inhibitors. However, the activity and stability of the α-amylase from *B. licheniformis* is less dependent on the calcium content of the solution than the α-amylase from *B. amyloliquefaciens*. Both enzymes show their highest activities in the pH range of 6.5 to 7, i.e., in many applications the pH of the starch solution must be adjusted by the addition of alkali, for which purpose if desired, lime can be used. Bacillus amylases are rapidly deactivated below pH 6.

The liquefaction of starch with α-amylase can be carried out in **continuous** or **batch operations.** The extent of the desired hydrolysis of the starch is determined by the intended later use. If a colloidal starch solution with a given final viscosity is required, as, for example, for the surface sizing of paper or in the manufacture of coating compounds and paints, a limited, but reproducible, degradation of the starch is required. In the desizing of textiles or in the preparation of nutrient solutions based on starch in the fermentation industry, a more complete degradation of the starch is aimed at. If α-amylase is used as the first step of a combined enzymatic process for the production of glucose syrup, glucose-fructose mixtures with a high fructose content, or for the production of dextrose, degradation of the starch as far as 10 dextrose equivalents[1] is regarded as the optimum. In the distilling industry bacterial α-amylases have substantially replaced plant enzymes obtained from germinating cereals (malt). The increasing production of alcohol as a fuel from starch-containing raw materials is opening up greater possibilities of use for α-amylases and glucoamylases.

The production of the Bacillus amylases is carried out in **submerged culture** at temperatures between 30 and 40 °C at about neutral pH values. A rich medium of cereal meal and starch is used, together with an organic source of nitrogen. The formation of α-amylase starts when the culture passes into the stationary phase after 10 to 20 hours and continues for another 100 hours, until the source of carbon is exhausted. During the fermentation, the pH must be above 6, since otherwise amylase activity is lost through denaturation. The α-amylase is accompanied by other extracellular enzymes. *Bacillus licheniformis* produces a serine protease, while *B. amyloliquefaciens* produces,

---

[1] dextrose equivalents (DE) give the reducing power as a percentage of that of dextrose.

in addition, a neutral protease, and also β-glucanase and hemicellulase. Proteases interfere with the use of the amylases, since they contribute to the formation of colored by-products (melanin). Proteases are eliminated by adsorption on clay minerals or by a heat treatment of the extract making use of the extraordinary heat stability of the amylases. As a rule, commercial preparations no longer contain proteases.

Fungal α-amylases are obtained mainly from Aspergillus species *(A. niger, A. oryzae)*. They differ greatly from the bacterial α-amylases by their lower deactivation temperature, high saccharifying action, and low optimum pH value (pH 4 to 5). They are less suitable for the liquefaction of starch than bacterial α-amylases. They are used in the manufacture of baked products where this enzyme is added to amylase-poor flours in order to shorten and standardize the proof time of the dough. Fungal amylase is also used for the manufacture of maltose-rich syrups and in various areas of the foodstuffs industry where its activity in the degradation of starch at low pH values is utilized. The production of α-amylase can be carried out as a **solid-substrate culture** and also in **submerged processes** with selected strains of Aspergillus. Glucose acts as a repressor of the formation of amylase, and therefore the concentration of glucose in the fermentation broth must be controlled and kept low. In cultivation on solid substrates, more accompanying enzymes are formed. In particular, the protease content is higher than in α-amylases produced by the submerged process. In either case, the amount of glucoamylase is comparatively low.

12.5.3   Glucoamylase

Glucoamylase is the trivial name given to an **exoenzyme** which splits off glucose from starch and dextrins stepwise from the nonreducing end of the chain. The enzyme is formed extracellularly by some lower fungi and is obtained commercially from Aspergillus, Rhizopus, and Endomyces species. Because of its higher temperature stability (up to 60 °C), it is now preferred to use the enzyme from Aspergillus. Starting from maltose, the rate of the glucoamylase reaction rises with increasing chain length of the oligosaccharides and dextrins. α-1,4-Glucosidic bonds are rapidly cleaved by glucoamylase and α-1,6- and α-1,3-bonds considerably slower; nevertheless, under suitable conditions, an almost complete hydrolysis of starch to glucose is possible. If high concentrations of dextrin are used for saccharification with glucoamylase, the concentration of glucose passes through a maximum and then decreases again. This is caused (if transglucosidase activity can be excluded), by the reverse reaction of the enzyme, which leads to the accumulation of isomaltose, nigerose, panose, isomaltotriose, and other oligosaccharides in the sugar solution. For the technical saccharification process, depending on the starting material 27 to 40% starch suspensions are first liquefied with α-amylase (see 12.5.2), and after cooling to 60 °C and lowering the pH to 4 to 4.5 the product is hydrolyzed with glucoamylase at 60 °C for 48 to 96 hours. For further processing to fructose-rich syrups, the highest possible yield of glucose must be obtained in saccharification, since the di- and oligosaccharides affect the taste and are not degraded further in the subsequent isomerization process (see 12.5.5). An amount of 95 to 96% of glucose in the product solution must be achieved. Crystalline dextrose is also obtained from such starch hydrolysates. For the production of syrups with a dextrose equivalent of 60 to 70, glucoamylase is used at pH 5 and 55 °C together with fungal amylase. In distilleries and for the production of industrial alcohol, moreover, large amounts of glucoamylase are used for the saccharification of starch and the resulting mixture, with no isolation of the product, is fed to the fermenting yeast.

Immobilized glucoamylase has been studied intensively in the past but has not yet been successfully introduced into practice. The lowering of the operating temperature that becomes necessary and the lower glucose yield of the immobilized enzyme are the main obstacles to industrial use. Diffusional limitation contributes essentially to lowering the effective activity in the catalyst and to increasing the back-reaction. At the present time, the increase in productivity that can be achieved is insufficient to cover the cost for the support and immobilization. Since glucoamylase is a relatively cheap enzyme and the one-way process in solution has been well developed, increases in productivity are difficult to achieve.

For the **production** of glucoamylase, the Aspergillus species *A. niger, A. awamori, A. phoenices,* or *A. usamii* are cultivated under submerged conditions. Cultivation is carried out at 30 to 35 °C and lasts 4 to 5 days. A rich medium with a high starch content (up to 20%) is used for this purpose, the starch being liquefied with bacterial α-amylase before sterilization. In contrast to the α-amylase, the formation of glucoamylase is not repressed by glucose. During the fermentation, the pH drops to 3 to 4. The culture supernatant contains, in addition to glucoamylase, small amounts of other enzymes (protease, cellulase, lactase, α-amylase, and transglucosidase) together with considerable amounts of sugar alcohols and organic acids. Of the accompanying materials, transglucosidase, in particular, must be separated from the glucoamylase.

12.5.4 Pullulanase

Pullulanase is obtained from cultures of *Bacillus amylopullulyticus* or *Klebsiella pneumoniae*. The enzyme may occur in **cell-bound or extra-cellular form.** Pullulanase specifically hydrolyzes α-1,6-branches in amylopectins. Additions of pullulanase can shorten the saccharification times with glucoamylase and decrease the accumulation of isomaltose and panose. A maltose-rich syrup can be produced by the simultaneous action of pullulanase and β-amylase on the starch. A corresponding process is under industrial development in Japan (Maeda and Tsao, 1979). On the whole, at the present time, the use of pullulanase is still very limited.

12.5.5 Glucose Isomerase

The isomerization of glucose to fructose is the largest-scale technical process that is currently being performed with the aid of an immobilized enzyme. The process is based on the possibility of obtaining glucose-rich syrup by the **hydrolysis of starch** with α-amylase and glucoamylase (see Sections 12.5.2, 12.5.3), this being isomerized in a subsequent step to a mixture of glucose and fructose. This mixture, with a typical composition of 42% of fructose, 50% of glucose, and 8% of other mono- and disaccharides, is used as liquid sugar in food technology. In contrast to glucose, fructose has a greater sweetening power than the crystalline cane or beet sugar, sucrose, traditionally used for sweetening. Glucose isomerization has therefore made a full-value "sugar" available from starch. The production of fructose syrup on this basis has developed very rapidly, since 1967, particularly in the USA, where cheap corn starch is available. In 1978, $1.36 \cdot 10^6$ tons (dry weight) of high fructose syrup was produced there. The world production in 1980 was estimated at about $3.7 \cdot 10^6$ tons (Antrim et al., 1979). The amounts of enzyme given in Table 12-7 (p. 494) have now been far exceeded. The enzyme called glucose isomerase is, properly speaking, a **D-xylose**

Table 12-8. Glucose Isomerase Catalysts.

Source of enzyme	Immobilization technique and realization	Manufacturing firm
Streptomyces olivaceus	whole cells; cross-linked with glutaraldehyde in granulated particles	CAR-MI
Streptomyces wedmorensis	enzyme immobilized on DEAE-cellulose by ionic bonds, in fiber or granulate form	CLINTON
Streptomyces olivochromogenes	enzyme immobilized in aluminum oxide supports with standardized pore diameter	CORNING
Actinoplanes missouriensis	mycelium, enclosed in gelatin, cross-linked with glutaraldehyde	GIST BROCADES
Arthrobacter	enzyme immobilized in the cells with a flocculating agent; dried in the form of cylindrical particles	ICI
Streptomyces albus	fixed cells, amorphous	MILES KALI CHEMIE
Streptomyces phaeochromogenes	granulate	NAGASE
Bacillus coagulans	cross-linked enzyme mixed with inorganic diluent and extruded in solid form (cylinders)	NOVO
Streptomyces sp.	adsorption on ion-exchangers, granulate	SANMATSU

isomerase and occurs in a large number of microorganisms that can grow on xylose (Table 12-8). The enzyme requires bivalent cations, such as Co^{2+}, Mg^{2+}, and Mn^{2+}, but no other cofactors. Glucose isomerase is the first intracellular enzyme that has been used on the large scale. Technical processes run exclusively with **immobilized enzymes,** since the use of glucose isomerase in soluble form would be too expensive. Table 12-8 summarizes the preparations offered and the microorganisms used

to produce the catalysts. As a rule, glucose isomerase is produced by **submerged cultivation** in the pH range of 6.5 to 8.5 at 30°C, and the strains used are constitutive mutants and no longer require D-xylose or xylan as inductor. Nutrient media and fermentation conditions have been substantially optimized. As Table 12-8 shows, the isolation of the enzyme is generally omitted and whole or disintegrated cells are used. A large number of immobilized preparations of glucose isomerase have been investigated and described. For **technical application** a simple and cheap physical process such as adsorption or heat-treatment together with cross-linkage has been generally adopted. The catalyst is offered in amorphous or granulated form with different volume activities. Various types of reactor have been tested, and it has been found that a continuous mode of operation in **fixed-bed reactors** ist the best. The consumption of the enzyme in the fixed-bed reactor is smaller than in batch operation, and the substantially shorter residence times diminish the formation of by-products and permit, if desirable, higher operating temperatures, higher pH values, and allows to omit the addition of cobalt ions. Although the glucose isomerase catalysts used have been obtained from various microorganisms and have been produced by different processes, their operating parameters differ little. As a rule, isomerization is carried out in the pH range of 7.0 to 8.5 at 60 to 65 °C. The substrate solution used contains 40 to 50 % of glucose plus oligosaccharides (referred to dry matter) and exhibits a viscosity of 0.8 to 3 mPa · s. To **stabilize** and **activate** the enzyme, magnesium salts to a concentration of 0.5 to 5 mmol/L are added to the substrate solution. Since calcium acts as competitive inhibitor, the calcium content of the substrate solution must be monitored and, if necessary, be lowered with an ion-exchanger. Attempts are also made to keep the partial pressure of oxygen in the substrate solution low in order to avoid a deactivation of the glucose isomerase. Half-lives of 600 to 1500 hours have been found for individual catalysts with crystalline glucose as substrate. With the technical substrate, the half-lives are probably somewhat shorter. The **productivity** has been given as 1000 to 9000 kg (referred to dry matter) of 42 % fructose syrup per kg of catalyst. In order to avoid an alkali-catalyzed conversion of fructose into mannose and psicose, the pH of the the product solution is lowered and subse-

quently a purification is carried out by treatment with activated carbon and ion-exchangers. The fructose syrup obtained is concentrated to 71 % dry matter and is supplied to the consumer in this form (Fig. 12-3).

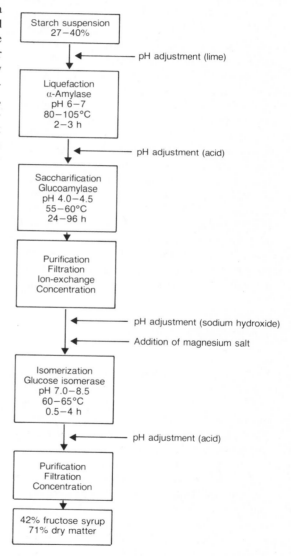

Fig. 12-3. Flowsheet for the hydrolysis of starch.

12.5.6 Pectinases

By the term pectinases is understood a mixture of endo- and exoenzymes, and also esterases, which take part in the **hydrolysis of pectin**. Pectinases are obtained, particularly, from Aspergillus species *(A. niger, A. wentii)*. The **type of cultivation** (submerged or on a solid substrate) affects the relative composition of the mixture of enzymes. Pectinases are used particularly in the technology of fruit and vegetable juices for depectinizing. The pectins contained in the pressed juices of fruit and vegetables lead to difficulties in filtration, to late turbidities, and to gelling. The pectin content varies according to the plant material, the degree of ripeness, the season, and the site, which makes it necessary to adapt the fermentation to the particular use. The pectins may also be hydrolyzed even before the juice is pressed out. The combined enzymatic treatment of the raw materials with pectinases and other enzymes, especially cellulases and hemicellulases, leads to an improvement in the yield and facilitates the processing of fruit and vegetables (Reed, 1975; Rombouts and Pilnik, 1978).

12.5.7 Cellulases

Cellulose is a polysaccharide composed of β-1,4-linked glucose units with a very pronounced secondary structure. Cellulose usually occurs in nature in the presence of lignin and other polysaccharides (hemicelluloses). Under the comprehensive term cellulases is understood a mixture of various endo- and exoenzymes. Aspergillus cellulases can be used for the **hydrolysis of cellulose derivatives** but exhibit no appreciable activity in relation to native cellulose. Today, *Trichoderma reesei* is largely used for the production of cellulase. The production of glucose from cellulose-containing wastes is not yet profitable but is being

intensively studied world-wide (Ghose and Ghosh, 1979). The **use** of cellulase preparations is therefore still limited today and extends to food technologies: improvement of the yield in juices, special nutrients (baby foods, instant products), the facilitated drying of plant products, etc.

12.5.8 β-Galactosidase

β-Galactosidase is formed intracellularly in yeasts and bacteria, but extracellularly in many fungi. The most important sources are the Aspergillus species *A. niger* and *A. oryzae*. The natural substrate of β-galactosidase is the milk sugar (lactose) that leads to pollution of the environment in the effluents of cheese factories and dairies. Since lactose is a sparingly soluble sugar, it crystallizes out in dairy products stored under cool conditions and in ice cream. Enzymatic hydrolysis leads to readily soluble sugars with improved sweetening power, and the further development of this process is investigated intensively in order to bring the **enzymatic degradation of lactose** to an economic cost structure. In Italy, a **cleavage of lactose in milk for drinking** is being carried out commercially with β-galactosidase from *Saccharomyces fragilis* because of the genetically determined lactose intolerance of certain sections of the population. Acid-stable β-galactosidases from Aspergillus are produced in relatively pure form as additives to digestive enzymes.

12.5.9 Other Enzymes

The use of other enzymes in industry is still limited. The reasons for this are either that the required enzymes are not available, or the technology for the performance of the enzyme-catalyzed process has not yet been satisfactorily developed, or the processes do not work profitably. There are enzymes which could be manufactured in large amounts fairly easily but nevertheless find little application, e.g., lipases. The hydrolysis of fats that they catalyze is used to a limited extent for accelerating the ripening of cheese and of milk chocolate. The addition of lipases to detergents has not so far been taken up, since surface-active agents also produce the desired effect. The **glucose oxidase/catalase system** has found some application in fruit and vegetable preserves. Glucose oxidase oxidises glucose to gluconic acid with the formation of hydrogen peroxide. The latter is split by catalase into water and oxygen. These reactions result in the binding of all the included oxygen, which leads to a stabilization of vitamin C in the preserves and to less corrosion in metal cans. In the absence of oxygen, for example, the shelf live of beer is also improved. In the manufacture of dried egg products, the elimination of glucose is sought in order to prevent the Maillard reaction. Glucose oxidase is also used for this purpose (Reed, 1975).

The steps catalyzed by immobilized enzymes in **organic synthesis** are acquiring ever greater importance. The manufacture of 6-aminopenicillanic acid from benzylpenicillin is very difficult to carry out chemically, since during acid hydrolysis the β-lactam ring will be cleaved to some extent. By enzymatic hydrolysis, 6-aminopenicillanic acid can be obtained almost without losses (Carleysmith and Lilly, 1979). From 6-aminopenicillanic acid semisynthetic penicillins are produced which differ in their respective activities and in their acid tolerance spectra. The stereospecific addition of water to fumaric acid is catalyzed by **fumarase** and leads to L-malic acid. A process for the manufacture of L-malic acid with immobilized microorganisms containing fumarase has been developed and brought into industrial practice in Japan (Takata et al., 1979). The possibilities to use enzymes for the **manufacture of amino acids** are also interest-

ing. The amino acids obtained by chemical synthesis are in the form of racemic mixtures. The separation of the D and L forms by chemical methods is frequently very difficult. A process developed by Chibata is based on the treatment of the N-acylated amino acids with the enzyme L-amino acid acylase from *Aspergillus oryzae* or hog kidneys. This deacylates the L-amino acid, which can readily be separated from the N-acyl-D-amino acid remaining in solution. The N-acyl-D-aminoacid is then chemically reracemized and returned to the process. By means of this process, using **immobilized acylase**, L-methionine, L-valine, L-alanine, and L-phenylalanine are manufactured industrially in a continuous process (Chibata, 1978a). Recently the enzyme membrane reactor has been successfully introduced for the same process (Wandrey et al., 1984). The production of L-aspartic acid is performed by the stereospecific addition of ammonia to fumaric acid catalyzed by the enzyme **aspartase** (Sato et al., 1975). There are proposals using specific enzymes as catalysts for a number of other amino acids. D-p-hydroxyphenylglycine, a building block of the semisynthetic penicillin amoxicillin is produced by a combined chemical and enzymatic process employing a D-hydantionase for the stereoselective cleavage of an intermediate (Yamada, 1982).

Enzymatic reactions also form the basis of transformation reactions used technically, e.g., in the **manufacture of L-sorbose** from D-sorbitol, a step in the synthesis of L-ascorbic acid, or the stereospecific **transformations of steroids** (see Chapter 14).

Enzyme-catalyzed processes with simple hydrolysis or isomerization steps have come into use in many areas, particularly when the cost of the enzyme, possibly in immobilized form, makes up a relatively small proportion of the manufacturing costs. Table 12-9 gives the proportional cost for the catalyst for different groups of products.

Table 12-9. Direct Enzyme Costs in Enzyme Processes (USA, 1977)*.

Product	Enzyme	Costs (US cents)
Additive to detergents	**protease**	2–4/kg of detergent
Liquefaction of starch	**amylase**	0.2–0.5/kg of starch
Saccharification of starch	**glucoamylase**	0.4–0.8/kg of starch
Glucose isomerization	**glucose isomerase**	1–1.5/kg of starch
Cheese manufacture	**microbial rennet**	0.1/L of milk
Alcohol by fermentation	**amylase**	0.2–0.5/L of alcohol
	glucoamylase	0.7–1.4/L of alcohol
Brewing	**amylase**	0.1/L of beer
	protease	
Baking	**amylase**	0.01/kg of flour
	protease	
Juice production	**pectinase**	0.01–0.2/L of juice
Winemaking	**pectinase**	0.1–0.2/L of wine
Dehairing of hides	**protease**	1–5/m² of hides

* The data have been taken over from Aunstrup (1979)

Many enzymes, however, need **coenzymes,** e.g., synthetases need ATP, and oxidoreductases need NAD/NADP. These coenzymes are converted in stoichiometric amounts and are very expensive. Consequently, possibilities of using coenzyme-dependent enzymes in future appear only when the coenzymes are either regenerated in the process, like, for example, pyridoxal phosphate, or they can easily be separated from the product and be regenerated. At the present time, such processes are still undergoing development on the laboratory and pilot scale (Wandrey et al., 1984).

Although the most important industrial enzymes today are of microbial origin, and microbial enzymes are currently becoming still more important, it should be realized that **enzymes from plant and animal sources** continue to be used in industry. The most important examples are **amylases** from germinated cereals (malt) in the brewing industry, **rennet** from calves' stomachs in the cheese industry, and **plant proteases** such as papain for tenderizing meat. So far, no microbial protease has been found the mode of action of which corresponds to that of papain in relation to the quality of meat.

12.6 Therapeutic Use of Enzymes

In the **medical field,** enzymes are playing an increasing role in the therapy, as well, although their use, particularly in the case of parenteral application, is associated with difficulties (Cooney and Rosenbluth, 1974). The **local application** of **proteinases, ribonucleases,** and **deoxyribonucleases** accelerates the degradation of necrotic tissue, masses of pus, secretions, or hematomas. **Hyaluronidase** brings about a hydrolysis of mucopolysaccharides. On external application, therefore, the deeper layers of the skin are loosened and the penetration of locally administered drugs into the tissues is improved. Oral administration permits the effects of enzymes to be exerted predominantly in the gastrointestinal tract. As a rule, the enzymes are not resorbed but undergo a rapid proteolytic degradation. The oral route is used preferentially for the treatment of digestive disturbances. To supplement the secretion of gastric juice, **pepsin** is given, and in pancreatic insufficiency enzyme preparations are used that contain **lipases, amylases,** and **proteases** of animal, plant, or microbial origin. A mixture of mammalian pancreas enzymes (pancreatin) is most frequently used for this purpose.

Enzymes for **parenteral injection** must meet high quality demands. They must be available in the highest purity, be free from endotoxins, and should not be immunogenic. The appearance and dissolution of blood clots, for example, are enzymatic processes. Here, an enzymatic treatment for thrombolysis has proved effective; the enzyme necessary for this purpose, **urokinase,** can be isolated from human urine or kidney cell cultures. Since the process of preparation makes this enzyme fairly expensive, a bacterial enzyme with a similar mode of action, **streptokinase** is also used for this indication. Specific proteases also play a role as activators of the system for the production of kinins – biologically active polypeptides – from their precursors, the α_2 serum globulins. The liberation of the kinins is catalyzed by **callicreins** and also by **trypsin.** Disturbances in the production of kinins are treated by injections of callicreins, mainly of animal origin. Particularly interesting are the possibilities of using enzymes in **tumor therapy.** Typical for some types of tumors is a metabolic defect which consists in the fact that the growth of the tumor cells is dependent on the supply of certain nonessential amino acids. Particularly good results are obtained in the treatment of some leukemias with **asparaginase.** This enzyme catalyzes the hydrolysis of L-asparagine to L-aspartic acid and ammonia.

The intravenous administration of asparaginase leads to a marked decrease in the asparagine level in the blood and to a cessation of the growth of asparagine-dependent tumors (Holcenberg and Roberts, 1977). Similar strategies are followed with **glutaminase** and **arginase** in tumor therapy. The enzymes used in these cases are mostly of microbial origin and can evoke immune reactions. Attempts are being made to suppress, or at least greatly to delay, the immune reaction by including foreign enzymes in liposomes (Gregoriadis, 1978) or by modifying the proteins with polysaccharides or polyethyleneglycols (Davis et al., 1978). The final success of these attempts cannot yet be evaluated. The results will also be of great importance for a possible enzymatic therapy in metabolic disturbances of genetic origin. In addition, the rapid progress in genetic engineering has changed the prospects of making human enzymes available for therapeutic purposes in future.

12.7 Enzymatic Analysis

By the term "enzymatic analysis" is understood the **determination of the concentration** of substrates, inhibitors, or activators which directly affect the rate of an enzyme reaction, the determination of **enzyme activities,** and the determination of **substances** with the aid of enzyme-labeled reagents (Bergmeyer, 1977). Use is made of the high substrate specificity of the enzymes, which permits the quantification of single substances in complex mixtures that could be determined chemically only with difficulty or would require a complicated process of separation. The determination of **metabolites** (glucose, triglycerides, cholesterol, urea, etc.) by enzyme-catalyzed reactions plays an important role in clinical chemistry and the foodstuffs industry (mono- and disaccharides, organic acids, alcohols, pyrophosphate, creatine, etc.). Where enzyme catalysts are used in industrial processes, the continuous **monitoring of catalytic activity** is a necessity. Here a suitable signal can be used to control the process. Further, in clinical chemistry the activities of certain enzymes in the serum and in the urine are measured. Diseased organs often release characteristic intracellular enzymes into the blood and the level of the enzymes in the serum can therefore be used for differential diagnosis and for monitoring treatments. **Enzyme immunoassays** that use enzymes as markers for immunological reaction partners are also of great importance for clinical chemistry. For example, the concentrations of hormones, immunoglobulins, pathogens and drugs can be determined comparatively rapidly and simply in this way.

Enzymes for analytical purposes must often be highly purified, since the solutions to be analyzed are usually mixtures of unknown composition, and undesired side-reactions may otherwise falsify the results (Naeher and Thum, 1974). Because of the high purity demands, analytical enzymes are frequently still fairly expensive but this is compensated by the simpler procedure and reduction in labor involved in enzymatic analysis, as compared with chemical methods. In addition, the relatively simple measuring technique permits a high degree of automation. In order to obtain a conveniently measurable signal, several successive enzyme-catalyzed reactions are frequently coupled with one another. In these methods, the **change in absorption** in NAD(P)-dependent reactions at 340 nm forms a very good and widely used signal for measurement. To determine ethanol, for example, the following reaction is employed:

$$\text{Ethanol} + \text{NAD}^+ \xrightleftharpoons{\text{ADH}} \text{Acetaldehyde}$$
$$+ \text{NADH} + \text{H}^+$$

ADH = alcohol dehydrogenase.

The increase in absorption measured at 340 nm is directly proportional to the ethanol content. The conversion and the rate of the reaction can be calculated directly from the known molar extinction coefficient of NADH. The determination of fructose may be given as an example of a **coupled assay**:

$$\text{Fructose} + \text{ATP} \xrightleftharpoons{\text{HK}} \text{Fructose 6-phosphate} + \text{ADP}$$
$$\updownarrow \text{PGI}$$
$$\text{Fructose 6-phosphate} \rightleftharpoons \text{Glucose 6-phosphate}$$
$$\updownarrow \text{G6P-DH}$$
$$\text{Glucose 6-phosphate} + \text{NADP} \rightleftharpoons$$
$$\text{Gluconate 6-phosphate} + \text{NADPH} + \text{H}^+$$

HK   = hexokinase
PGI   = phosphoglucose isomerase
G6P-DH = glucose 6-phosphate dehydrogenase

In this case, the measured signal is the absorption of the NADPH arising in the third reaction.

The hydrogen peroxide formed as a second product in the reactions of many oxidases can, under the action of the enzyme **peroxidase,** oxidize leucodyes to colored products. Glucose, for example, can be determined by this principle. The leucodyes used is usually o-dianisidine. The measured extinction is proportional to the concentration of glucose, which can be determined by comparison with a calibration curve. This reaction may also take place on strips of paper upon which the reagents are immobilized. After such a strip has been dipped into a glucose-containing solution, a color develops the intensity of which is compared with a reference. In this way it is possible to monitor process solutions in a simple manner and also, for example, to carry out precautionary investigations on diabetes in the public health service on a very large number of persons in a short time.

In addition to photometric methods, other properties, particularly **electrochemical** ones, are used for performing measurements. Here moreover, immobilized enzymes are frequently used (Bowers and Carr, 1980). **Conductometry, polarometry, potentiometry,** and **microcalorimetry** can be used to follow reactions in progress. Sensors, so-called **enzyme electrodes** and **thermistors,** have been developed as measuring devices. The most highly developed are glucose-sensitive electrodes using immobilized glucose oxidase. Here, either the decrease in the concentration of oxygen or the increase in the concentration of hydrogen peroxide in the reaction volume can be measured.

Other oxidases can be incorporated into enzyme electrodes on the same principle. Oligosaccharides that contain glucose residues can also be determined with glucose electrodes if, together with the glucose oxidase, suitable hydrolases are used that catalyze a specific hydrolysis of the oligosaccharide to glucose. Thus, for example, electrodes have been developed for the determination of lactose, sucrose, and maltose. The specific determination of ammonia by ammonia electrodes can be applied to the determination of amino acids with immobilized amino acid oxidase and to the determination of urea with urease. Electrodes that measure the partial pressure of carbon dioxide are employed for analytical determinations by means of decarboxylases. In the so-called **enzyme thermistors,** the **heat of the reaction** is used as the measurement signal. The solution to be analyzed is pumped through a column filled with immobilized enzyme and the rise in temperature is measured by means of thermistors. The heat of a reaction represents a universal measuring signal. If the absolute value of a reaction is too small, it can be amplified by subsequent reactions of the products formed with other immobilized enzymes (Mattiasson et al., 1978).

Development in the field of enzymatic analysis is in a state of rapid progress. With improved sensors and the use of microprocessors, numerous measuring and monitoring processes can be simplified and automated.

12.8   Literature

Albertsson, P. A.: *Partition of Cell Particles and Macromolecules,* 2nd Ed. Wiley-Interscience, New York (1971).

Antrim, R. L., Colilla, W. and Schnyder, B. J., "Glucose isomerase production of high-fructose syrups", *Appl. Biochem. Bioeng.* **2,** 98–155 (1979).

Andrews, P., "Estimation of molecular size and molecular weights of biological compounds by gel filtration", *Methods Biochem. Anal.* **18,** 1–53 (1970).

Atkinson, B. and Daoud, I. S., "Microbia flocs and flocculation in fermentation process engineering", *Adv. Biochem. Eng.* **4,** 42–124 (1976).

Aunstrup, K., "Production, isolation and economics of extracellular enzymes", *Appl. Biochem. Bioeng.* **2,** 27–69 (1979).

Aunstrup, K., Andresen, O., Falch, E. A. and Nielsen, T. K.: "Production of microbial enzymes". In: Peppler and Perlman (eds.): *Microbial Technology,* Vol. 1, 2nd Ed. Academic Press, New York 1979, pp. 281–309.

Barman, T. E.: *Enzyme Handbook.* Springer-Verlag, Berlin, Heidelberg, New York 1969.

Bergmeyer, H. U., Naeher, G., Thum, W. and Weimann, G.: D.B.P. 2,001,902,7 (1970).

Bergmeyer, H. U.: *Grundlagen der Enzymatischen Analyse.* Verlag Chemie, Weinheim, New York 1977.

Bowers, L. D. and Carr, P. W., "Immobilized enzymes in analytical chemistry", *Adv. Biochem. Eng.* **15,** 89–129 (1980).

Brookman, J. G., "Mechanism of cell disintegration in a high pressure homogenizer", *Biotechnol. Bioeng.* **16,** 371–383 (1974).

Buchholz, K. (ed.), "Characterization of immobilized biocatalysts", *DECHEMA Monogr.* **84** (1979).

Bucke, C., "Industrial Glucose Isomerase", *Top. Enzyme Ferment. Biotechnol.* **1,** 147–171 (1977).

Carleysmith, S. W. and Lilly, M. D., "Deacylation of benzylpenicillin by immobilized penicillin acylase in a continuous four-stage stirred-tank reactor", *Biotechnol. Bioeng.* **21,** 1057–1073 (1979).

Charm, S. E. and Matteo, C. C., "Scale-up of protein isolation", *Methods Enzymol.* **22,** 476–556 (1971).

Chibata, I., "Industrial application of immobilized enzyme systems", *Pure Appl. Chem.* **50**, 667–675 (1978 a).

Chibata, I. (ed.): *Immobilized Enzymes – Research and Developments*. Kodansha Ltd., Japan and John Wiley & Sons, New York (1978 b).

Cohn, E. J., Strong, L. E., Hughes, W. L., Mulford, D. J., Ashworth, J. N., Melin, M. and Taylor, H. C., "Preparation and properties of serum and proteins. A system for separation into fractions of the protein and lipoprotein components of biological tissues and fluids", *J. Am. Chem. Soc.* **68**, 459–475 (1946).

Cooney, D. A. and Rosenbluth, R. J., "Enzymes as therapeutic agents", *Adv. Pharmacol. Chemother.* **12**, 185–289 (1974).

Curie, J. A., Dunnill, P. and Lilly, M. D., "Release of protein from baker's yeast by disruption in an industrial agitator mill", *Biotechnol. Bioeng.* **14**, 725–736 (1972).

Davis, F. F., Abuchowski, A., van Es, T., Palcuk, N. C., Chen, R., Savoca, K. and Wieder, K., "Enzyme-polyethyleneglycol adducts:modified enzymes with unique properties". *Enzyme Eng.* **4**, 169–174 (1978).

Diers, I., *Contin. Cult. Appl. New Fields, Plenary Lect. Int. Symp. Contin. Cult. Microorg. 6th* **1975**, 208–225 (publ. 1976).

Duppel, W., "Gelfiltration im industriellen Maßstab", *GIT Fachz. Lab.* **8**, 689–692 (1977).

Edebo, L., "Disintegration of cells", *Ferment. Adv. Pap., Int. Ferment. Symp. 3rd* **1968**, 225–247 (publ. 1969).

Enzyme Nomenclature: *Recommendations (1978) of the Nomenclature Committee of the International Union of Biochemistry on the Nomenclature and Classification of Enzymes*. Academic Press, New York, San Francisco, London 1979.

Faith, W. T., Neubeck, C. E. and Reese, E. T., "Production and Applications of Enzymes", *Adv. Biochem. Eng.* **1**, 77–111 (1971).

Flaschel, E., Wandrey, Ch. and Kula, M.-R., "Ultrafiltration for the Separation of Biocatalysts", *Adv. Biochem. Eng.* **26**, 73–142 (1983).

Follows, M., Hetherington, P. J., Dunnill, P. and Lilly, M. D., "Release of enzymes from baker's yeast by disruption in an industrial homogenizer", *Biotechnol. Bioeng.* **13**, 549–560 (1971).

Foster, P. R., Dunnill, P. and Lilly, M. D., "The ki-netics of protein salting-out: precipitation of yeast enzymes by ammonium sulphate", *Biotechnol. Bioeng.* **18**, 545–580 (1976).

Foster, P. R., Dunnill, P. and Lilly, M. D., "The precipitation of enzymes from cell extracts of *Saccharomyces cerevisiae* by polyethyleneglycol", *Biochem. Biophys. Acta* **371**, 505–516 (1973).

Friedli, H. and Kistler, P.: "Concentration of human albumin solution by ultrafiltration". In: Sandberg, H. E. (ed.): *Proceedings of the International Workshop on Technology for Protein Separation and Improvement of Blood Plasma Fractionation*, Reston, VA, Sept. 7-9, 1977. DHEW Publication No. (NIH) 78-1422. U.S. Govt. Printing Office, Washington D.C. 1977, pp. 151–153.

Gasner, L. L. and Wang, D. J. C., "Microbial cell recovery enhancement through flocculation", *Biotechnol. Bioeng.* **12**, 873–887 (1970).

Ghose, T. K. and Ghosh, P., "Cellulase production and cellulose hydrolysis", *Proc. Biochem.* **14**, 20–24 (1979).

Godfrey, T. and Reichelt, J. (eds.): *Industrial Enzymology*. Macmillan Publishers, 1983.

Graves, D. J. and Wu, Y.-T., "The rational design of affinity chromatography separation processes", *Adv. Biochem. Eng.* **12**, 219–253 (1979).

Gregoriadis, G., "Liposomes as carriers of proteins: possible medical applications", *Enzyme Eng.* **4**, 187–192 (1978).

Guthöhrlein, G.: "Ultrafiltration methods used in blood plasma fractionation". In: Sandberg, H. E. (ed.): *Proceedings of the International Workshop on Technology for Protein Separation and Improvement of Blood Plasma Fractionation*, Reston, VA, Sept. 7-9, 1977. DHEW Publication No. (NIH) 78-1422. U.S. Govt. Printing Office, Washington D.C. 1977, pp. 146–150.

Hatch, R. T. and Price, J. D., "Staged ultrafiltration purification of enzymes", *AIChE. Symp. Series* **74** (172), 226–232 (1978).

Hemfort, H.: "Solid-liquid separation. The use of centrifuges in large-scale human blood fractionation processes". In: Sandberg, H. E. (ed.): *Proceedings of the International Workshop on Technology for Protein Separation and Improvement of Blood Plasma Fractionation*, Reston, VA, Sept. 7-9, 1977. DHEW Publication No. (NIH) 78-1422. U.S. Govt. Printing Office, Washington D.C. 1977, pp. 81–96.

Hemmingsen, S. H., "Development of an immobilized glucose isomerase for industrial application", *Appl. Biochem. Bioeng.* **2**, 157–183 (1979).

Hesseltine, C. W., "Solid state fermentation", *Biotechnol. Bioeng.* **14**, 517–532 (1972).

Hetherington, P. J., Follows, M., Dunnill, P. and Lilly, M. D., "Release of protein from baker's yeast in an industrial homogenizer", *Trans. Inst. Chem. Eng.* **49**, 142–148 (1971).

Hönig, W. and Kula, M.-R., "Selectivity of protein precipitation with polyethyleneglycol fractions of various molecular weights", *Anal. Biochem.* **72**, 502–512 (1976).

Holcenberg, J. S. and Roberts, J., "Enzymes as drugs", *Rev. Pharmacol. Toxicol.* **17**, 97–116 (1977).

Hustedt, H., Kroner, K.-H., Stach, W. and Kula, M.-R., "Procedure for the simultaneous large-scale isolation of pullulanase and 1,4-α-glucan phosphorylase from *Klebsiella pneumoniae* involving liquid-liquid separations", *Biotechnol. Bioeng.* **20**, 1989–2005 (1978).

Jacoby, W. B. and Wilchek, M. (eds.): *Methods in Enzymology,* Vol. 34. Academic Press, New York (1974).

James, C. J., Coakley, W. T., and Hughes, D. E., "Kinetics of protein release from yeast sonicated in batch and flow systems at 20 kHz", *Biotechnol. Bioeng.* **14**, 33–42 (1972).

Janson, J. C.: "Large Scale Chromatography of Proteins". In: Sandberg, H. E. (ed.): *Proceedings of the International Workshop on Technology for Protein Separation and Improvement of Blood Plasma Fractionation,* Reston, VA, Sept. 7–9, 1977. DHEW Publication No. (NIH) 78–1422. U.S. Govt. Printing Office, Washington D.C. 1977, pp. 205–220.

Janson, J. C. and Hedman, P., "Large scale chromatography of proteins", *Adv. Biochem. Eng.* **25**, 43–99 (1982).

Jefferis, III, R. P. and Kula, M.-R., "Application of computers to enzyme recovery", *Enzyme Eng.* **3**, 241–248 (1978).

Klein, J. and Wagner, F., "Immobilized whole cells", *DECHEMA Monogr.* **82**, 142–164 (1978).

Klibanov, A. M., "Enzyme stabilization by immobilization", *Anal. Biochem.* **93**, 1–25 (1979).

Kroner, K.-H., Hustedt, H., Granda, S. and Kula, M.-R., "Technical aspects of separation using aqueous two-phase systems in enzyme isolation processes", *Biotechnol. Bioeng.* **20**, 1967–1988 (1978).

Kroner, K. H., Hustedt, H. and Kula, M.-R., "Extractive enzyme recovery:economic considerations", *Proc. Biochem.* **19**, 170–179 (1984).

Kroner, K. H. and Kula, M.-R., "On-line measurement of extracellular enzymes during fermentation using membrane techniques", *Anal. Chim. Acta* **163**, 3–15 (1984).

Kula, M.-R., "Extraction and purification of enzymes using aqueous two-phase systems", *Appl. Biochem. Bioeng.* **2**, 71–95 (1979).

Kula, M.-R., Hönig, W. and Foellmer, H.: "Polyethylene glycol precipitation". In: Sandberg, H. E. (ed.): *Proceedings of the International Workshop on Technology for Protein Separation and Improvement of Blood Plasma Fractionation,* Reston, VA, Sept. 7–9, 1977. DHEW Publication No. (NIH) 78–1422. U.S. Govt. Printing Office, Washington D.C. 1977, pp. 361–371.

Kula, M.-R., Kroner, K. H. and Hustedt, H., "Purification of enzymes by liquid-liquid extraction", *Adv. Biochem. Eng.* **24**, 73–118 (1982).

Kula, M.-R., Wichmann, R., Oden, U. and Wandrey, C., "Influence of substrate or product inhibition on the performance of enzyme reactors", *Biochemie* **62**, 523–536 (1980).

Lilly, M. D., "Production of intracellular microbial enzymes", *Appl. Biochem. Bioeng.* **2**, 1–26 (1979).

Lilly, M. D., "Immobilized enzyme reactors", *DECHEMA Monogr.* **82**, 165–180 (1978).

Limon-Lason, J., Hoare, M., Orsborn, C. B., Doyle, D. J. and Dunnill, P., "Reactor properties of a high speed bead mill for microbial cell rupture", *Biotechnol. Bioeng.* **21**, 745–774 (1979).

Loncin, M.: *Die Grundlagen der Verfahrenstechnik in der Lebensmittelindustrie.* Verlag Sauerländer, Aarau, Frankfurt/M. 1969.

Maeda, H. and Tsao, G., "Maltose production", *Proc. Biochem.* **14**, 2–5, 27 (1979).

Manecke, G., Ehrenthal, E. and Schlünsen, J., "Chemical characteristics and properties of carriers", *DECHEMA Monogr.* **84**, 49–72 (1979).

Marffy, F. and Kula, M.-R., "Enzyme yields from cells of brewer's yeast by treatment in a horizontal disintegrator", *Biotechnol. Bioeng.* **16**, 623–634 (1974).

Mattiasson, B., Danielsson, B. and Mosbach, K., "Enzyme thermistor assays of cholesterol, oxalic acid, glucose and lactose in standard solutions and biological samples", *Enzyme Eng.* **3**, 453–460 (1978).

Melling, J. and Phillips, B. W.: "Large-scale extraction and purification of enzymes". In: Wiseman, A. (ed.): *Handbook of Enzyme Biotechnology.* Ellis Horwood Ltd., Chichester 1975 a, pp. 58–88.

Melling, J. and Phillips, B. W.: "Practical aspects of large-scale enzyme purification". In: Wiseman, A. (ed.): *Handbook of Enzyme Biotechnology.* Ellis Horwood Ltd., Chichester 1975 b, pp. 181–202.

Michaelis, L. and Menten, M. L., "Die Kinetik der Invertinwirkung", *Biochem. Z.* **49**, 333–369 (1913).

Mitra, G. and Wilke, C. R., "Continuous cellulase production", *Biotechnol. Bioeng.* **17**, 1–13 (1975).

Morris, C. J. O. R. and Morris, P.: *Separation Methods in Biochemistry,* 2nd Ed. Pitman Publishing, London 1976.

Mosbach, K., "Immobilized coenzymes in general ligand affinity chromatography and their use as active coenzymes", *Adv. Enzymol. Relat. Areas Mol. Biol.* **46**, 205–278 (1978).

Mosbach, K. (ed.), "Immobilized Enzymes", *Methods Enzymol.* **44** (1976).

Naeher, G. and Thum, W.: "Production of enzymes for research and clinical use". In: Spencer, B. (ed.): *Industrial Aspects of Biochemistry,* Vol. 1, Elsevier, New York 1974, pp, 47–64.

Nishio, N., Tai, K. and Nagai, S., "Hydrolase production by *Aspergillus niger* in solid-state cultivation", *Eur. J. Appl. Microbiol. Biotechnol.* **8**, 263–270 (1979).

Radola, B. J. and Graesslin, D. (eds.): *Electrofocussing and Isotachophoresis.* de Gruyter, Berlin, New York 1977.

Reed, G. (ed.): *Enzymes in food processing,* 2nd Ed. Academic Press, New York 1975.

Reese, E. T., Lola, J. E. and Parrish, F. W., "Modified substrates and modified products as inducers of carbohydrases", *J. Bacteriol.* **100**, 1151–1154 (1969).

Rehacek, J. and Schaefer, J., "Disintegration of microorganisms in industrial horizontal mill of novel design", *Biotechnol. Bioeng.* **19**, 1523–1534 (1977).

Reilly, P. J., "Starch hydrolysis with soluble and immobilized glucoamylase", *Appl. Biochem. Bioeng.* **2**, 185–207 (1979).

Rombouts, F. M. and Pilnik, W., "Enzymes in fruit and vegetable juice technology", *Proc. Biochem.* **13**, 9–13 (1978).

Ruttloff, H., Huber, J., Zickler, F. and Mangold, K.-H.: *Industrielle Enzyme.* Steinkopff-Verlag, Darmstadt 1979.

Ryu, D., Andreotti, R., Mandels, M., Gallo, B. and Reese, E. T., "Studies on quantitative physiology of *Trichoderma reesei* with two-stage continuous culture for cellulase production", *Biotechnol. Bioeng.* **21**, 1887–1903 (1979).

Sato, T., Mori, T., Tosa, T., Chibata, J., Furui, M., Yamashita, K. and Sumi, A., "Engineering analysis of continuous production of L-aspartic acid by immobilized *E.coli* cells in fixed beds". *Biotechnol. Bioeng.* **17**, 1797–1804 (1975).

Schlünsen, J., Ehrenthal, E. and Manecke, G., "Immobilization and efficiency of enzymes", *DECHEMA Monogr.* **84**, 145–168 (1979).

Schmid, R. D., "Stabilized soluble enzymes", *Adv. Biochem. Eng.* **12**, 41–118 (1979).

Schmidt-Kastner, G., "Methods of isolation and purification of enzymes", *DECHEMA Monogr.* **82**, 181–198 (1978).

Schütte, H., Kroner, K. H., Hustedt, H. and Kula, M.-R., "Experiences with a 20 litre industrial bead mill for the disruption of micro-organisms", *Enzyme Microb. Technol.* **5**, 143–148 (1983).

Staude, E.: "Membranen". In: *Ullmanns Enzyklopädie der technischen Chemie,* Vol. 16, 4th Ed. Verlag Chemie, Weinheim, New York 1978, pp. 515–535.

Strathmann, H., "Anwendung von Membranprozessen zur Trennung molekularer Gemische", *Chem. Tech. (Heidelberg)* **7**, 333–346 (1978).

Takata, J., Yamamoto, K., Tosa, T. and Chibata, J., "Screening of microorganisms having high fumarase activity and their immobilization with carrageenan", *Eur. J. Appl. Microbiol. Biotechnol.* **7**, 161–172 (1979).

Underkofler, L. A.: "Microbial Enzymes". In: Miller, B. M. and Litsky, W. (eds.): *Industrial Microbiology.* McGraw-Hill Inc., New York 1976, pp. 128–164.

Vetter, H., Grassl, M., Naeher, G., Böing, J., Uhlig, H., Thum, W., Jaworek, D., Michal, G., Wiesner K. and Pütter, J.: "Enzyme". In: *Ulmanns Enzyklopädie der technischen Chemie,* Vol. 10, 4th Ed. Verlag Chemie, Weinheim, New York 1975, pp. 475–561.

Wandrey, C. and Flaschel, E., "Process development and economic aspects in enzyme engineering. Acylase L-methionine system", *Adv. Biochem. Eng.* **12,** 147–218 (1979).

Wandrey, C., Wichmann, R., Kula, M.-R. and Bückmann, A. F., "Enzym – Membran – Reaktor", *Umschau* **84** (3), 88–91 (1984).

Wang, D. I. C., Cooney, C. L., Demain, A. L., Dunnill, P., Humphrey, A. E. and Lilly, M. D.: *Fermentation and Enzyme Technology.* John Wiley & Sons, New York, Chichester, Brisbane, Toronto 1979.

Watt, J. G. and Dickson, A. J.: "An interim report on the CSVM-fractionation process". In: Sandberg, H. E. (ed.): Proceedings of the International Workshop for Protein Separation and Improvement of Blood Plasma Fractionation, Reston, VA, Sept. 7–9, 1977. DHEW Publication No. (NIH) 78-1422. U.S. Govt. Printing Office, Washington D.C. 1977, pp. 245–258.

Wiseman, A. (ed.): *Handbook of Enzyme Biotechnology.* Ellis Horwood Ltd., Chichester 1975.

Wiseman, A., "Stabilization of enzymes", *Top. Enzyme Ferment. Biotechnol.* **2,** 280–303 (1978).

Witt, I. and Neufang, B., "Studies on the influence of thiamine on the synthesis of thiamine pyrophosphate–dependent enzymes in *Saccharomyces cerevisiae*", *Biochim. Biophys. Acta* **215,** 323–332 (1970).

Yamada, H., "Enzymatic processes for the synthesis of optically active amino acids". In: Chibata, J., Fukni, S. and Wingard jr., L. D. (eds.): *Enzyme Engineering,* Vol. 6. Plenum Press, New York 1982, pp. 97–106.

Chapter 13

Antibiotics and Other Secondary Metabolites

Hans Zähner

13.1   Introduction

Of the roughly 8000 microbial metabolites already described, only a few have come into comparatively wide use. The largest amounts of secondary microbial metabolites are used today in **plant protection** and **animal nutrition** while the market for antibiotics in **human medicine** is financially by far the most important.

The amounts of secondary metabolites that are formed per liter of culture by the **wild strains** fluctuate very widely but are generally less than 10 mg/L. However, yields of 5 g/L and more were necessary for an economically profitable fermentation. Without a substantial **rise in yield,** in many cases not even the amount necessary for evaluation can be prepared. Raising the yield and the processing of the metabolite to make it suitable for use must take place in parallel if one is not to be delayed by the other. Often the researcher faces difficulties in explaining to the production manager that enormous effort must be put into increasing yield and concentration for a given product (at the moment when no decision on its market introduction has yet been made).

Of the many investigations in quite different fields that must be carried out before a product can be introduced, only those of **biotechnological relevance,** i.e., those mainly serving to increase yields, will be mentioned here. They can be classified in three groups:

a) Optimization of the fermentation process through the composition of the nutrient solution, the temperature, the pH, pO_2, density of inoculation, preparation of the inoculum, speed of stirring, feeding system, etc.

b) Study of the biogenesis and biosynthesis of the metabolite in order to achieve appropriate improvements of the nutrient solu-

tion or feeding and in order to have a basis for a program of mutation at the same time.

c) Modification of the strain by
   – random search for mutants with higher yields;

   – search for mutants in the intermediate metabolism in those areas that are related to the biogenesis of the metabolite with the aim of increasing the availability of constructional units;

   – search for mutants that are resistant to high concentrations of their own metabolite;

   – search for permeation-damaged mutants;

   – search for mutants with other properties favorable for the fermentation process, e.g., the absence of undesired components, with higher osmotolerance, etc.;

   – construction of strains by crossing according to classical methods or by the fusion of protoplasts.

The methods of "genetic engineering" have so far found no application in raising the yield of secondary metabolites of microorganisms. On the one hand, the gap between what can be done today in the case of *Escherichia coli* and that which can be realized with these methods in the case of Penicillium or Cephalosporium, for example is still very large. On the other hand, the successes achieved by the classical methods are so significant that in the industry there have so far been relatively few research workers dealing with the genetics of microorganisms. However, a rapid change is taking place here. The "International Symposium on the Genetics of Industrial Microorganisms" that are held regularly have created the necessary contacts between scientists, and the recent investigations of Hopwood (1979) have made important advantage in the genetics of the streptomycetes available to a large circle.

Table 13-1 lists those secondary microbial metabolites that can (or could once) be obtained as **commercial products** and that have an importance beyond pure laboratory use. In the next few years the list will change greatly; in particular, other substances with uses other than human chemotherapy will be included in it. Some of the most important groups of antibiotics are discussed in more detail in the following sections. Unfortunately, for reasons of space, it has been possible to treat only some of the important antibiotics in more detail. In the case of others, reference must be made to the voluminous special literature (e.g., Korzybski et al., 1978; Bérdy et al., 1980 and 1982). This relates particularly to some antibiotics which have already been on the market for some time, such as chloramphenicol, griseofulvin, lincomycin, bacitracin, the nucleoside antibiotics (polyoxins, blasticidin S) and the polyene macrolides (nystatin, amphotericin), but also to some interesting new developments such as the bleomycins.

With the introduction of a product, however, its microbiological, biochemical and biotechnological treatment should not be broken off. On the one hand, biotechnological processes can always be improved further, even above yields of 30 g/L, and, on the other hand, the evaluation of practical experience may lead to modified products. In addition to the purely chemical **modification** that is first considered, there is a whole series of biochemical-microbiological methods which are still not generally known. Here is a brief list of them (after Whitefield, 1974, modified).

a) A substance is transformed **enzymatically,** for which purpose living cells, fixed cells, isolated free enzymes, or carrier-bound enzymes can be used. This field is known today as **biotransformation** (e.g., Kieslich, 1976) (see Chapter 14).

b) A producing strain is induced by the **addition of inhibitors** to form a **different spectrum of substances.**

c) A producing strain is supplied with **modified precursors** (e.g., in the production of penicillin V).

d) A strain is subjected to a **program of mutation,** and mutants are **selected** which form a different spectrum of secondary metabolites.

e) A strain is mutated in such a way that it can no longer synthesize certain precursors itself, and then modified precursors are supplied so that a modified end product is formed. This method, which is known as **mutasynthesis,** is being applied intensively to the aminoglycosides, among others (Daum and Lemke, 1979; Rinehart, 1979).

All antibiotics prepared technically today are obtained in **batch processes,** although there has been no lack of attempts to introduce continuous fermentation for the production of antibiotics, as well. The reasons are, on the one hand, the greatly increased cost of a multistage continuous fermentation in comparison with the batch process, while, on the other hand, the highly productive strains used today frequently represent reduced forms in relation to growth, and the probability that a spontaneously occurring **antibiotic-minus mutant** would multiply faster is very high. In continuous fermentation, the minus mutant would rapidly outgrow the reproductive strain, while this can be substantially avoided in the batch process by the use of special propagation media and production media differing from them.

Table 13-1. The Secondary Microbial Metabolites Manufactured for the Market (where derivatives are marketed, only the natural substance is given).

Name	Synonyms	Year of first description	Group	Producing agent	Application	Literature
Actinomycins		1940	chromopeptides	Streptomyces species	tumor therapy (limited)	Waksman, 1968; Kersten and Kersten, 1974; Meienhofer and Atherton, 1973; Mauger and Katz, 1978; Korzybski et al., 1978
Actinospectacin	spectino-mycin trobicin	1961	amino-glycoside	Streptomyces species	human and veterinary medicine, bacteria	see Aminoglycosides section
Adriamycin		1969	anthra-cyclines	Streptomyces species	tumor therapy	see Anthracyclines section
Amphomycin	glumamycin	1953	acylpoly-peptide	Streptomyces species	local, human medicine	Bodansky et al., 1973
Amphotericin B		1956	polyene heptaene	Streptomyces species	human medicine, fungi	Holz, 1974, 1979; Andreoli, 1974; Korzybski et al., 1978
Antimycin A-complex	A_3 = blast-mycin antipiriculin phyllomycin	1947		many streptomycetes	plant protection insects, fisheries	Leben and Keitt, 1947; Vezina et al., 1976; Sehgal et al., 1976; Lennon and Vezina, 1973
Bacitracins	ayfivin	1945	polypeptides	*Bacillus subtilis* *B. licheniformis*	human medicine, animal nutrition	Hickey, 1964; Katz and Demain, 1977; Storm and Toscano, 1979; Korzybski et al., 1978
Bicyclomycin	A 5879	1972		Streptomyces species	local, human medicine	Tanaka, 1979
Blasticidin S		1958	nucleosides	Streptomyces species	plant protection, fungi	Suhadolnik, 1979 a, b

Table 13-1. (continued).

Name	Synonyms	Year of first description	Group	Producing agent	Application	Literature
Bleomycins		1966	polypeptides	Streptomyces species	tumor therapy	Umezawa, 1973; Tanaka, 1977; Hecht, 1979; Haidle and Lloyd, 1979; Umezawa and Takita, 1980
Candicidins	trichomycin hamycin levorin	1953	polyenes heptaene	Streptomyces species	human medicine, fungi	Korzybski et al., 1978
Capreomycin	capromycin	1961	polypeptides	*Streptomyces capreolus*	human medicine, TB	Nomoto et al., 1977; Shiba et al., 1976, 1977
Carbomycins	magnamycins B = nidda-mycin	1952	macrolides	Streptomyces species	human medicine, Gram-pos. bacteria	see Macrolides section
Cellocidin	lenamycin aquamycin	1958		Streptomyces species	plant protection, fungi (limited)	Suzuki and Okuma, 1958; Suzuki et al., 1958
Carcinophylin		1954		*Streptomyces sahachiroi*	tumor therapy (limited)	Hata et al., 1954; Kamata et al., 1958 a, b; Onda et al., 1969, 1971
Cephalosporin C		1956	β-lactams	Cephalo-sporium strains, Streptomyces species	derivatives, human medicine, bacteria	see β-lactams section
Cephamycins	7-methoxy-cephalo-sporins	1971	β-lactams	Streptomyces species	derivatives, human medicine, bacteria	Albers-Schönberg et al., 1972; Miller et al., 1972 a, b, 1974; Onishi et al., 1974; Stapley et al., 1972
Chloramphenicol		1947		Streptomyces species	human medicine, bact. esp. typhus	Smith and Hinman, 1963; Malik, 1972; Vazquez, 1979

Table 13-1. (continued).

Name	Synonyms	Year of first description	Group	Producing agent	Application	Literature
Chlortetracycline	aureomycin	1948	tetracyclines	Streptomyces species	human medicine, Gram-pos. and -neg. bacteria	see Tetracyclines section
Chromo-mycin A_3	aburamycin	1955		Streptomyces species	tumor therapy	Gause, 1975; Kersten and Kersten, 1974; Korzybski et al., 1978
Clavulanic acid	MM-14151	1976	β-lactams	Streptomyces species	in combination with other β-lactams, human medicine	Brown et al., 1976 a, b; Bentley et al., 1977; Howarth et al., 1976
Cycloheximide	actidione naramycin A	1946	glutarimides	Streptomyces species	plant protection, fungi (limited)	Whiffen et al., 1946; Sisler and Siegel, 1967
Cycloserine	oxamycin P.A. 94 orientmycin	1952		Streptomyces species	human medicine, TB (limited)	Korzybski et al., 1978
Cyclosporins		1976	polypeptides	*Trichoderma polysporum, Cylindrocar-pum lucidum*	human medicine, immuno-suppression	Dreyfuss et al., 1976; Borel et al., 1976; Traber et al., 1977 a, b
Daunorubicin	daunomycin rubidomycin rubromycin C	1963	anthracyclines	Streptomyces species	tumor therapy	see Anthracyclines section
Destomycin		1965	aminoglycosides	*Streptoverti-cillium eurocidus*	veterinary medicine, anthelmintic	Kondo et al., 1965 a, b, 1975; see Aminoglycoside section
Enduracidins	enramycin	1968	acylpoly-peptides	*Streptomyces fungicidicus*	animal nutrition	Higashide et al., 1968; Asai et al., 1968; Mizuno et al., 1970; Matsuhashi et al., 1969

Table 13-1. (continued).

Name	Synonyms	Year of first description	Group	Producing agent	Application	Literature
Ergot alkaloids			alkaloids	*Claviceps paspali*	human medicine, various derivatives	Stadtler and Stütz, 1975; Gröger, 1978; Spalla and Marnati, 1978; Kobel and Sanglier, 1978; Berde and Schild, 1978
Ezomycins		1973		*Streptomyces kitizawaensis*	plant protection, fungi	Suhadolnik, 1979a, b
Erythromycin	ilotycin	1952	macrolides	Streptomyces species	human medicine, Gram-pos. bacteria	see Macrolides section
Ferrioxamine B		1960	sideramines	Streptomyces species	human medicine, iron storage diseases	Keller-Schierlein et al., 1964
Fumagillin	amebacilin fumidil fugillin	1951		*Aspergillus fumigatus*	human medicine, protozoa (limited)	Eble and Hanson, 1951; Tarbell et al., 1960, 1961; Corey and Snider, 1972
Fusidic acid	fucidin ramycin	1962	steroid	*Fusidium coccineum* other fungi	human medicine, Gram-pos. bacteria	v. Daehne et al., 1979; Haller and Löffler, 1969; Tanaka, 1975
Gentamicins		1963	amino-glycosides	Micromono-spora species	human medicine, Gram-pos. and -neg. bacteria	see Aminoglycosides section
Gibberellins		1934	plant growth factors	*Gibberella fujikuroi*	promotion of germination, malt, horticulture	Jefferys, 1970

Table 13-1. (continued).

Name	Synonyms	Year of first description	Group	Producing agent	Application	Literature
α-Glucosidase inhibitors		1970	oligosaccha-rides	Streptomyces and Actino-planes species	diabetes (not yet introduced)	Frommer et al., 1972, 1979; Puls et al., 1977; Schmidt et al., 1977
Griseofulvin	curling factor	1939	grisan	Penicillium species	human medicine, dermatophytes	Huber, 1967; Rhodes, 1963; Harris et al., 1976; Wagman and Weinstein, 1978
Hygromycin B		1958	amino-glycosides	*Streptomyces hygroscopicus*	veterinary medicine, anthelminthic	Mann and Bromer, 1958; Neuss et al., 1970 see Aminoglycosides section
Kanamycins		1957	amino-glycosides	Streptomyces species	human medicine, Gram-pos. and -neg. bacteria	see Aminoglycosides section
Kasugamycin		1965	amino-glycosides	*Streptomyces kasugaensis*	plant protection, fungi	Umezawa et al., 1965 a, b; Suhara et al., 1966, 1972
Lasalocide		1970	polyether	*Streptomyces lasaliensis*	veterinary medicine, animal nutrition	Westley, 1977; Hamill and Crandall, 1978
Leucomycins	kitasamycins josamycin = A₃	1953	macrolides	Streptomyces species	human medicine, Gram-pos. bacteria	see Macrolides section
Lincomycin		1962		*Streptomyces lincolnensis*	human medicine, Gram-pos. bacteria	Herrell, 1969; Chang, 1979; Eble, 1978
Lividomycins	quintomycin	1970	amino-glycosides	*Streptomyces lividus*	human medicine, Gram-pos. and -neg. bacteria	see Aminoglycosides section

Table 13-1. (continued).

Name	Synonyms	Year of first description	Group	Producing agent	Application	Literature
Macarbamycin	diumycin A	1970		*Streptomyces phaeo-chromogenes*	animal nutrition	Huber, 1979
Mithramycin	aureolic acid LA 7017	1953	chromomycins	Streptomyces species	tumor therapy	Gause, 1975; Kersten and Kersten, 1974; Korzybski et al., 1978
Mitomycins		1956		Streptomyces and Strepto-verticillium species	tumor therapy	Franck, 1979
Mocimycin	kirromycin, delvomycin	1972	kirromycin-efrotomycin group	Streptomyces species	animal nutrition	Vazquez, 1979
Moenomycin	flavomycin	1965		Streptomyces species	animal nutrition	Huber, 1979; Witteler et al., 1979
Monensin	monensic acid	1967	polyether	*Streptomyces cinnamonensis*	animal nutrition, veterinary medicine	Westley, 1977; Hamill and Crandall, 1978
Nanaomycin		1974	isochromane-quinone	*Streptomyces rosa var. notoensis*	veterinary medicine, fungi	Omura et al., 1974; Tanaka et al., 1975a, b, c
Neomycin	framycetin soframycin	1949	amino-glycosides	Streptomyces species	human medicine, bacteria local	see Aminoglycosides section
Nisins		1944	polypeptides	*Streptomyces lactis*	foodstuffs preservation	Lipinska, 1977; Mattick and Hirsch, 1944
Novobiocin	cathomycin PA 93 streptonivicin albamycin cardelmycin	1955	coumarin antibiotics	Streptomyces species	human medicine, Gram-pos. bacteria	Kominek and Sebek, 1974; Berger and Batcho, 1978; Ryan, 1979
Nystatin	fungicidin mycostatin	1950	polyenes tetraene	Streptomyces species	human medicine, fungi	Holz, 1974; Korzybski et al., 1978

Table 13-1. (continued).

Name	Synonyms	Year of first description	Group	Producing agent	Application	Literature
Oleandomycin	matromycin amimycin PA 105 Ro2-7638	1955	macrolides	Streptomyces species	human medicine, Gram-pos. bacteria	see Macrolides section
Oxytetracycline	terramycin	1950	tetracyclines	Streptomyces species	human medicine, Gram-pos. and -neg. bacteria	see Tetracyclines section
Paramomycin	aminosidin catenulin hydroxymycin gabbromycin humatin estomycin	1959 (1952)	amino-glycosides	Streptomyces species	human medicine, bacteria, amoebae (limited)	see Aminoglycosides section
Penicillins		1929/ 1941	β-lactams	various fungi	human medicine, bacteria	see β-Lactams section
Pentamycin		1958	polyenes pentaene	*Streptomyces penticus*	human medicine, fungi, trichomonads	Umezawa et al., 1958 a, b
Phosphono-mycin	fosfomycin	1969	phosphonic acid	Streptomyces species	human medicine, Gram-pos. and -neg. bacteria	Hendlin et al., 1969; Stapley et al., 1969; Christensen et al., 1969 Chaiet et al., 1970; Kahan et al., 1974
Pimaricin	natamycin	1958	polyenes tetraene	*Streptomyces natalensis*	human medicine, fungi, foodstuffs preservation	Raab, 1972
Pleuromutilin		1951		Pleurotus species	veterinary medicine, mycoplasmae	Högenauer, 1979
Polymyxins		1947	polypeptides	*Bacillus polymyxa*	human medicine, Gram-neg. bacteria	Benedict and Langlykke, 1947; Vogler and Studer, 1966; Paulus, 1967

Table 13-1. (continued).

Name	Synonyms	Year of first description	Group	Producing agent	Application	Literature
Polyoxins		1965	nucleosides	Streptomyces species	plant protection, fungi	Suhadolnik, 1979 a, b; Isono and Suzuki, 1979
Pyrrolnitrin		1964		*Pseudomonas pyrrocina*	human medicine, fungi	Arima et al., 1964, 1965; Nakano et al., 1966; Tripathi and Gottlieb, 1969; Gosteli, 1972; Floss et al., 1971
Resistomycin	heliomycin croceomycin	1951	quinones	Streptomyces species	human medicine, bacteria, local	Brockmann and Schmidt-Kastner, 1951; Brockmann and Reschke, 1968; Blinov et al., 1962
Ribostamycins	vistamycin SF-733 BU-1703-DA$_2$	1970	amino-glycosides	*Streptomyces ribosidificus*	human medicine, Gram-pos. and -neg. bacteria	see Aminoglycosides section
Rifamycins		1959	ansamycins	*Nocardia mediterranei*	human medicine, TB, bacteria	see Ansamycins section
Ristocetin	spontin	1956	glycoproteids	*Nocardia lurida*	human medicine, Gram-pos. bacteria	Grundy et al., 1956/57; Philip et al., 1956/57; Harris et al., 1975, 1978
Sagamycin	gentamicin C/2B XK-62-2	1975	amino-glycosides	Micromono-spora species	human medicine, Gram-pos. and -neg. bacteria	see Aminoglycosides section
Salinomycin		1973	polyethers	*Streptomyces albus*	veterinary medicine, animal nutrition	Westley, 1977; Hamill and Crandall, 1978
Sarkomycin		1953		*Streptomyces erythrochro-mogenes*	tumor therapy	Korzybski et al., 1978

Table 13-1. (continued).

Name	Synonyms	Year of first description	Group	Producing agent	Application	Literature
Siccanin		1962		*Helminthosporium siccans*	human medicine, fungi, local	Ishibashi, 1962; Hirai et al., 1967; 1971; Nose and Ende, 1971; Arai et al., 1969
Sisomycin	rickamicin dehydrogen tamicin	1970	amino-glycosides	Micromono-spora species	human medicine, Gram-pos. and -neg. bacteria	see Aminoglycosides section
Spiramycins	foromacidins	1954	macrolides	Streptomyces species	human medicine, Gram-pos. bacteria	see Macrolides section
Staphylomycins	virginiamy-cins, streptogram-ins, mikamycins, pristinamy-cins, etc. – each one part of the components	1955	A lactone B depsipep-tides	Streptomyces species	animal nutrition, human medicine (limited)	Crooy and DeNeys, 1972; Korzybski et al., 1978; Tanaka, 1975
Streptomycins		1944	amino-glycosides	Streptomyces species	human medicine, bacteria, TB	see Aminoglycosides section
Streptonigrin	bruneomycin	1960		Streptomyces species	tumor therapy	Mizuno, 1979
Streptovaricins		1957	ansamycins	*Streptomyces spectabilis*	human medicine, bacteria, TB	see Ansamycins section
Stendomycin		1963	polypeptides	Streptomyces species	plant protection, fungi	Thompson and Hughes, 1963; Bodansky et al., 1967, 1968, 1969
Tetranactan		1971	macrotetro-lides	*Streptomyces aureus*	plant protection, insects, mites	Ando et al., 1971a, b; Suzuki et al., 1971

Table 13-1. (continued).

Name	Synonyms	Year of first description	Group	Producing agent	Application	Literature
Thienamycin		1976	β-lactams	*Streptomyces cattleya*	human medicine, Gram-pos. and -neg. bacteria (not yet introduced)	Kahan et al., 1976; Albers-Schönberg et al., 1978
Thiopeptin		1970	polypeptides	*Streptomyces tateyamensis*	animal nutrition	Miyairi et al., 1970 Muramatsu et al., 1972, 1977
Thiostrepton	bryamycin	1955	polypeptides	Streptomyces species	veterinary medicine	Cundliffe, 1979
Tobramycin	nebramycin 6	1967 (1971)	amino-glycosides	*Streptomyces tenebrarius*	human medicine, Gram.-pos. and -neg. bacteria	see Aminoglycosides section
Tylosin		1960	macrolides	Streptomyces species	veterinary medicine, Gram-pos. bacteria	see Macrolides section
Tyrothricins		1939	polypeptides	*Bacillus brevis*	human medicine, local, bacteria	Katz and Demain, 1977; Hunter and Schwartz, 1967; Izumiya et al., 1979
Validamycin		1970	amino-glycosides	Streptomyces species	plant protection, fungi	Iwasa et al., 1970, 1971a, b; Horii et al., 1971a, b; Horii and Kameda, 1972
Valinomycin		1955	depsipeptides	Streptomyces species	constrn. of K-selective electrodes	Brockmann and Schmidt-Kastner, 1955; Shemyakin et al., 1963; Pinkerton et al., 1969; Wipf and Simon, 1970; Wipf et al., 1970

Table 13-1. (continued).

Name	Synonyms	Year of first description	Group	Producing agent	Application	Literature
Vancomycin		1956	glycoproteids	Streptomyces species	human medicine, Gram-pos. bacteria	Jordan and Reynolds, 1975; Smith et al., 1975; Williams and Kalman, 1977
Variotin		1959		*Paecilomyces varioti*	human medicine, fungi	Yonehara et al., 1959; Takeuchi and Yonehara, 1969; Tanabe and Seto, 1970
Viomycin	tuberactino-mycin vionactan celiomycin florimycin	1951	polypeptide	Streptomyces species	human medicine, TB	Korzybski et al., 1978
Zearalenone Zearalanol	ralon ralgro	1962	lactones	*Gibberella zeae*	animal nutrition (anabolics)	Hidy et al., 1977

13.2   β-Lactams

Even 50 years after the discovery of penicillin, the β-lactams form the **medically most important group** of antibiotics. The β-lactams discussed here – penicillins, cephalosporins, 7-methoxycephalosporins, thienamycins, and nocardicins – are characterized as a group not only by the fact that they all contain a β-lactam ring but also by their **common action mechanism,** the attack on the last stage of the synthesis of the bacterial cell wall (Hakenbeck et al., 1983; Morin and Gorman, 1982). However, other β-lactams with a different mode of action are known, e.g., clavulanic acid as an inhibitor of β-lactamases, the clavams with an activity against fungi, and wildfire toxin as a plant-harming agent.

13.2.1   Penicillins

The first publication (more about the biological effect than the substance) was made in 1929 by Fleming, the first description of the substance came 13 years later (Abraham et al., 1942), and today, 50 years later, the flood of publications is now impossible to overview (for review abstracts, see Abraham 1975, 1977, 1978; Flynn, 1972; Jung et al., 1980).

Penicillins have been detected in various fungi of the genera Penicillium, Aspergillus, Cephalosporium, Paecilomyces, Trichophyton, Epidermophyton, Gymnoascus, Thermoascus, Polypaecilum, and Malbranchea (Kitano et al., 1977; Mukherjee and Lee, 1978), and penicillin N also in a number of streptomycetes.

For the **technical manufacture** of the penicillins, highly specialized strains of *Penicillium chrysogenum* (auxiliary fruit form of *Talaromyces avellaneus*) are used exclusively. As a rule, wild strains form a mixture of various penicillins (see Table 13-2) in amounts of less than 1 mg/L, with the desired penicillin G making up only a small proportion. By adding phenylacetic acid it is possible to make **penicillin G** the main component and substantially to suppress the formation of other components. In a study lasting more than 30 years, it was possible to breed strains forming not 1 mg/L but more than 50 g/L of penicillin G. Even today development is not concluded, and advances in the genetics of Penicillium permit the expectation of further improvements (Ball, 1978). The economic aspects of the penicillin process have been discussed by Swartz (1979), and he also shows ways to possible further advances in which parameters other than the yield (time of fermentation, product recovery, ratio of antibiotics to other substances, etc.) are decisive today. The penicillin G manufactured in the batch process is either used in medicine directly as penicillin G salt or is cleaved to 6-aminopenicillanic acid (see Table 13-2) which, for its part, then serves as the starting material for the manufacture of **semisynthetic penicillins.** The modern penicillins – one speaks of the 3rd generation – are all **derivatives of 6-aminopenicillanic acid.** The splitting off of the side chain can be done chemically, which, however, is associated with great losses, or enzymatically. Initially, resting cells of *Escherichia coli* were used for this purpose, and then isolated enzymes were introduced and today carrier-bound penicillin acylases of various origins are offered. The advantage lies, on the one hand, in the fact that the purified penicillin is not recontaminated with bacterial cultures, and, on the other hand, in the shortening of the process, which reduces losses.

Penicillin V represents a biotechnological

Table 13-2. Natural Penicillins formed by *Penicillium chrysogenum.*

Name	Structure (R)
Penicillin G	$\bigcirc\!-CH_2-$
Penicillin F	$CH_3CH{=}CHCH_2CH_2-$
Dihydropenicillin F	$CH_3(CH_2)_4-$
Penicillin K	$CH_3(CH_2)_6-$
Penicillin X	$OH-\bigcirc\!-CH_2-$
Penicillin N	$HOOC-CH\ (CH_2)_3-$ $\quad\ \ NH_2$
Isopenicillin N	$H_2N-CH-(CH_2)_3-$ $\qquad\ \ COOH$

special case. If, instead of phenylacetic acid, phenoxyacetic acid is offered as the side chain to a normal penicillin producer, it incorporates the phenoxyacetic acid and forms penicillin V.

The **isolation** of the penicillin from the culture broth is carried out by extraction of the filtered broth with organic solvents at low pH values, and strict care must be taken that the aqueous penicillin solutions are kept at pH 2 to 4 for only seconds. After the extraction, the penicillin is returned to buffer and is again acidified and is reextracted with a smaller volume. The already highly concentrated penicillin is again brought into aqueous solution and is crystallized from this solution. The sensitivity of penicillin to heat, acids, and penicillinases makes it necessary to work rapidly with the avoidance of subsequent infections and at the lowest possible temperatures.

The **biogenesis** of penicillin is discussed exhaustively in Chapter 4, section 4.6. The synthesis of the L-α-aminoadipic acid, L-cysteine and L-valine takes place by the normal pathways of the intermediate metabolism, and a modification of these metabolic pathways by mutations also leads to a modification of the formation of penicillin. The three L-amino acids form a LLD-tripeptide from which isopenicillin N arises by a ring-forming process that has not yet been elucidated in detail. This stage is then followed by an exchange of side chains: aminoadipic acid is replaced by phenylacetic acid (O'Sullivan et al., 1979a, b; Demain et al., 1982).

A **total chemical synthesis** of the penicillin skeleton is possible (Sheehan and Henry-Logan, 1962; Baldwin et al., 1976; Nakatsuka et al., 1975a, b), but chemical synthesis is not economically competitive with the biotechnological process. The importance of chemical synthesis lies in the fact that today almost any conceivable modifications of the penicillin skeleton are accessible by this route (Jung et al., 1980). The possibility of carrying out many modifications in the penicillin skeleton has made it possible to draw up numerous structure-effect relationships (Pierce, 1977).

A gap still exists between the generally accepted observation that penicillin G and related β-lactams inhibit the last step or steps of the synthesis of the bacterial cell wall and a complete explanation of the mechanism of their action upon bacteria, in spite of a large amount of research (Spratt, 1978; Tomasz 1979; Moore et al., 1979; Boyd, 1979).

The **action** of penicillin (and to some extent also its relatives) is endangered by the appearance of the β-lactamases – penicillinases. For numerous strains, the genetic information for the β-lactamases is coded in the plasmid. The number of **penicillin-resistant bacteria** varies very widely, but can reach as much as 80% in the case of the Gram-negative bacteria. This resistance can be broken through by modifying the side chain or switching to other β-lactams (semisynthetic cephalosporins, 7-methoxycephalosporins), or by a combination of β-lactamase inhibitors such as clavulanic acid – until new β-lactamases appear (for a review, see Hamilton-Miller and Smith, 1979).

13.2.2 Cephalosporins and 7-Methoxycephalosporins

In 1956, Abraham and Newton reported on a new β-lactam with – as compared with the penicillins – a modified ring skeleton, **cephalosporin C,** which is formed together with cephalosporin N (penicillin N) and a steroid antibiotic (cephalosporin P) by *Cephalosporium acremonium.* They recognized that this gave a starting point for **overcoming penicillin resistance,** but their cephalosporin possessed an unfavorable side chain not leading to high efficacy. In cephalosporin C the sulfur-containing 5-ring of the penicillin is expanded to a 6-ring. The first publication on cephalosporin C raised a flood of further investigations, and today the cephalosporin derivatives are among the most used antibiotics, after the penicillins.

In the meantime, a fairly large number of fungi have been found which also form the basic skeleton of cephalosporin C (Kitano et al., 1977) (Table 13-3). Surprisingly, a number of Streptomyces strains of the most diverse types that synthesize the cephalosporin skeleton have also been found (see p. 18, Section 2.2). Some of them produced a derivative methoxylated in position 7.

The introduction of a methoxy group in position 7 leads to an increased stability against most β-lactamases and therefore to an even further improved (as compared with cephalosporin derivatives) action against penicillin-resistant bacteria.

None of the natural cephalosporins or 7-methoxycephalosporins (see Table 13-3) can be used medically in the **native form,** and therefore the **use of derivatives** is all the more widespread (for reviews, see Kanzaki and Fujisawa, 1976; Abraham, 1978; Jung et al., 1980).

Today two biotechnological pathways for obtaining the basic skeleton are open:

Table 13-3. Naturally Occurring Cephalosporins (after Hamill and Crandall, 1978 and Kitano et al., 1977).

Name	Producing agent	Structure		
		R	R'	R''
Cephalosporin C	*Cephalosporium acremonium*	—H	—H	—OCOCH₃
Deacetoxycephalosporin C	*Arachnomyces minimus Anixiopsis peruviana Spiroidium fuscum* many streptomycetes	—H	—H	—H
Deacetylcephalosporin C	*Cephalosporium sp.*	—H	—H	—OH
7-Methoxycephalosporin C	*Streptomyces lipmanii*	—H	—OCH₃	—OCOCH₃
Carbamoyl-7-methoxy-3-deacetylcephalosporin C (Cephamycin C)	*Streptomyces clavuligerus lactamdurans*	—H	—OCH₃	OCONH₂
Cephamycin A	*Streptomyces griseus*	—H	—OCH₃	—OCOC=CH—◯—OSO₂OH (OCH₃)
Cephamycin B	*Streptomyces griseus*	—H	—OCH₃	—OCOC=CH—◯—OH (OCH₃)
C 2081 X	*Streptomyces heteromorphus panayensis*	—H	—OCH₃	—OCOC=CH—◯—OH,OH (OCH₃)
N-Acetyldeacetoxy-cephalosporin C	*Cephalosporium acremonium*	—COCH₃	—H	—H

Table 13-3. (continued).

Name	Producing agent	Structure		
3-Methylthio-3-deacetoxycephalosporin C	*Cephalosporium acremonium*	—H	—H	—S—CH$_3$
3-O-Carbamoyl-3-deacetylcephalosporin C	*Streptomyces clavuligerus*	—H	—H	—OCONH$_2$
7-Methoxydeacetyl-cephalosporin C	*Streptomyces chartreusis*	—H	—OCH$_3$	—OH
7-Methoxydeacetoxy-cephalosporin C	*Streptomyces wadayamensis* 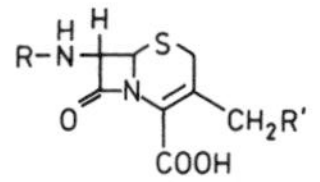	—H	—OCH$_3$	—H

Name	Producing agent	R	R'
7β-(4-Carboxybutanamido)-3-methyl-3-cephem-4-carboxylic acid	*Cephalosporium chrysogenum, C. acremonium, C. polyaleurum*	—CO(CH$_2$)$_3$COOH	—H
7β-(4-Carboxybutanamido)-3-hydroxymethyl-3-cephem-4-carboxylic acid	*C. chrysogenum, C. acremonium, C. polyaleurum*	—CO(CH$_2$)$_3$COOH	—OH
7β-(4-Carboxybutanamido)-3-acetoxymethyl-3-cephem-4-carboxylic acid	*C. chrysogenum, C.acremonium, C. polyaureum*	—CO(CH$_2$)$_3$COOH	—OCOCH$_3$
3-[(2-amino-2-carboxy-1,1-dimethylethylthio)-methyl]-7β-(D-5-amino-5-carboxyvaleramido)-3-cephem-4-carboxylic acid	Mutants of *Cephalosporium acremonium*	—CO(CH$_2$)$_3$CHCOOH, NH$_2$	—S—C(CH$_3$)$_2$—CH(COOH)(NH$_2$)

a) .**Fermentation of cephalosporin C,** in which a strain of *Cephalosporium acremonium* is usually used, or of 7-methoxycephalosporin with a streptomycete. The yields of cephalosporin C do not yet reach the level of the yields of penicillin, but great advances have been achieved here since *Cephalosporium acremonium* is accessible to a genetic treatment (Treichler et al., 1978; Nüesch et al., 1976, 1978). Before derivatives can be made, both in cephalosporin C and also in the 7-methoxycephalosporins, the side chains must be split off. In contrast to the investigations in the penicillin field, the enzymatic splitting off of these side chains has not yet been achieved. The transformation of isopenicillin N into penicillin N taking place in the course of biogenesis inhibits enzymatic cleavage. It is therefore necessary to split off the side chain by chemical methods, which, in spite of all efforts, still always causes considerable losses. Further derivatives can then be obtained at the 7-cephalosporanic acid stage.

b) Starting from a **microbiologically prepared basic skeleton** of penicillin, the ring can be expanded by **chemical methods.** The higher yields in the penicillin fermentation and the lower expense in the splitting off of the side chain partially compensate the expense on chemical ring expansion. Since their biogenesis leads to cephalosporins through an expansion of the penicillin skeleton, as well, this chemical method corresponds to the pathway to cephalosporin in the producing organism.

A **total chemical synthesis** of the cephalosporin skeleton is possible (Woodward et al., 1966; Nakatsuka et al., 1975a, b), but it is not competitive in spite of the great expense of the combined biotechnological-chemical process.

The **biogenesis** of the cephalosporins and 7-methoxycephalosporins is presented exhaustively in the section on secondary metabolism (see Chapter 4).

At the present time, the objects of intensive studies are both the formation of the LLD-tripeptide and also ring closure and ring expansion (Sawada et al., 1979; O'Sullivan et al., 1979c; Demain et al., 1982). The whole field of the **production of derivatives** of cephalosporanic acid and of 7-methoxycephalosporanic acid is in vigorous development. If the structure-activity relationships recognizable today in the penicillin series and in the cephalosporin series (Sassiver and Lewis, 1977; Weber and Ott, 1977) are compared, it may be assumed that it is easier to combine high resistance against β-lactamases with a broad spectrum, even including Gram-negative organisms, in the cephalosporin series than in the penicillin series.

13.2.3 New Basic β-Lactam Skeletons

After the discovery of the penicillins and the cephalosporin C related to them, it was for a long time (1956-1972) thought that all the basic β-lactam skeletons occurring in nature were known. The discovery of β-lactams in streptomycetes that was possible by the use of new test systems, however, showed a very much greater variation in β-lactams than was expected. Table 13-4 lists the new β-lactams. In spite of the length of this list, it may be assumed with certainty that we know only a proportion – possibly a small proportion – of the β-lactams occurring in nature. The introduction of new test methods for detecting β-lactams (e.g., β-lactam-supersensitive mutants, cell-free systems for cell wall synthesis, inhibition of β-lactamases) had introduced the new development, and an extension of the search to other producing agents – especially unusual actinomycetes – will reveal still other β-lactams.

Table 13-4. New Basic β-Lactam Skeletons.

Name	Formula	Producing agent	Activity	Literature
Clavulanic acid	(structure: OH, COOH)	*Streptomyces clavuligerus*	β-lactamase inhibitor weakly antibact.	Reading and Cole, 1977
β-Hydroxypropyl-clavulanic acid	(structure: OCO, OH, COOH)	*Streptomyces clavuligerus*	β-Lactamase inhibitor weakly antibact.	Beecham Ltd., 1977
Hydroxymethyl-clavam	(structure: CH_2OH)	*Streptomyces clavuligerus*	weak β-lactamase antifungal	Glaxo Ltd., 1977
Formyloxy-methylclavam	(structure: CH_2OCHO)	*Streptomyces clavuligerus*	weak β-lactamase antifungal	Glaxo Ltd., 1977
Carboxyclavam	(structure: COOH)	*Streptomyces clavuligerus*	weak β-lactamase antifungal	Glaxo Ltd., 1977
Thienamycin	(structure: $^+NH_3$, S, COO^-, OH)	*Streptomyces cattleya*	broad antibact.	Albers-Schönberg et al., 1978; Kahan et al., 1979
N-Acetyl-thienamycin	(structure: NH-Ac, S, COOH, HO)	*Streptomyces cattleya*	broad antibact.	Kahan et al., 1979; Albers-Schönberg et al., 1978
N-Acetyldehydro-thienamycin	(structure: NH-Ac, S, COOH, HO)	*Streptomyces cattleya*	broad antibact.	Kahan et al., 1979; Albers-Schönberg et al., 1978

Table 13-4. (continued).

Name	Structure	Organism	Activity	Reference
Epithienamycin A		*Streptomyces flavogrisiens*	broad antibact.	Merck Ltd., 1977
Epithienamycin B		*Streptomyces flavogrisiens*	broad antibact.	Merck Ltd., 1977
Epithienamycin C		*Streptomyces flavogrisiens fulvoviridis*	broad antibact. inhibitor	Pan Labs/Sanraku, 1978; Merck Ltd., 1977
Epithienamycin D		*Streptomyces flavogrisiens fulvoviridis*	broad antibact. inhibitor	Merck Ltd., 1977; Pan Labs/Sanraku, 1978
Olivanic acids: MM 4550 = MC 696-SY-A		*Streptomyces fulvoviridis olivaceus*	antibact. weak lactamase inhibitor	Maeda et al., 1977; Brown et al., 1977; Corbett et al., 1977
MM 13902 = 890 A_9		*Streptomyces fulvoviridis olivaceus*	broad antibact. lactamase inhibitor	Maeda et al., 1977; Brown et al., 1977; Corbett et al., 1977
MM 17880 = 890 A_{10}		*Streptomyces fulvoviridis olivaceus*	broad antibact. lactamase inhibitor	Maeda et al., 1977; Brown et al., 1977; Corbett et al., 1977
PS-5		Streptomyces sp.	broad antibact. lactamase inhibitor	Okamura et al., 1978

Table 13-4. (continued).

Name	Formula	Producing agent	Activity	Literature
Nocardicin A	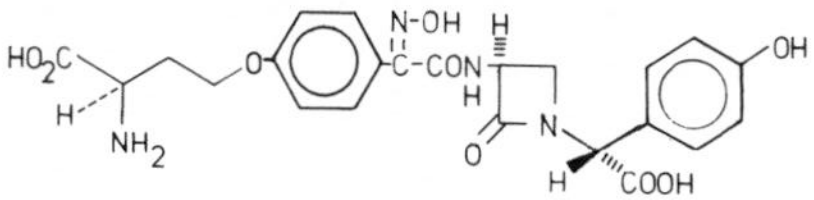	Nocardia uniformis var. tsuyamensis	weakly antibact.	Aoki et al., 1976, 1977
Nocardicin B (isomer of A)		Nocardia uniformis var. tsuyamensis	very weakly antibact.	Kurita et al., 1976; Aoki et al., 1977
Nocardicin C	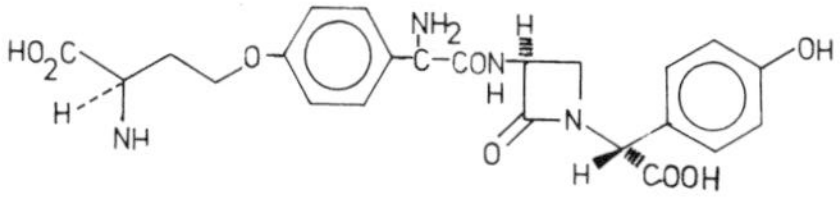	Nocardia uniformis var. tsuyamensis	only against β-lactam-supersensitive bacteria	Aoki et al., 1977
Nocardicin D	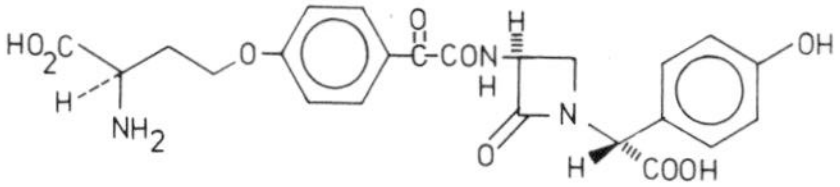	Nocardia uniformis var. tsuyamensis	weakly antibact.	Aoki et al., 1977
Nocardicin E	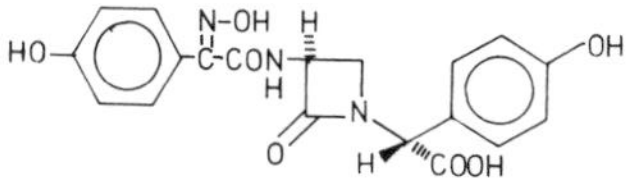	Nocardia uniformis var. tsuyamensis	not active	Aoki et al., 1977
Nocardicin F	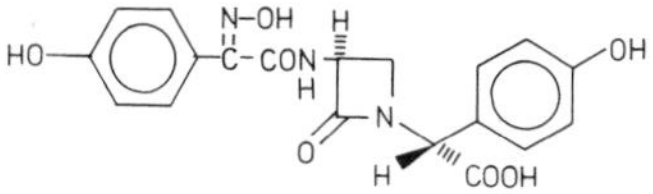	Nocardia uniformis var. tsuyamensis	none	Aoki et al., 1977
Nocardicin G	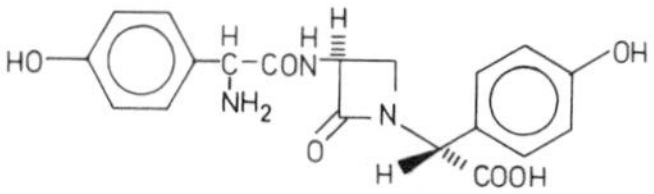	Nocardia uniformis var. tsuyamensis	active only against β-lactam-supersensitive bacteria	Aoki et al., 1977

Of the basic skeletons shown in Table 13-4, **thienamycin** and **clavulanic acid** appear suitable for rapid introduction. In favor of thienamycin is its high activity against Gram-negative and penicillin-resistant bacteria, provided that it is possible to improve its low stability, while in the case of clavulanic acid a combination with a semisynthetic penicillin appears interesting. A comprehensive account of the new β-lactams is given by Cooper (1979).

13.3   Aminoglycosides

Today, after the β-lactams, the aminoglycosides form the most important group of antibiotics. Since the discovery of the first representative of this group, **streptomycin,** by Waksman and his colleagues in 1944 (Schatz et al., 1944), this group of antibiotics has continuously expanded, first slowly – in 1949 came **neomycin** (Waksman and Lechevalier, 1949), and the **kanamycins** followed in 1957 (Umezawa et al., 1957) – and then at an increasing rate. The discovery of the **gentamicins** (Weinstein et al., 1963) led not only to a great advance in therapy but also to the knowledge that aminoglycosides occur outside the genus Streptomyces. Since then, development has taken place explosively. The number of naturally occurring aminoglycosides has exceeded 100. Table 13-5 shows a selection, and in addition there are the numerous derivatives and, recently, the **new aminoglycosides** obtained by **mutasynthesis** (Cox et al., 1977; Rinehart, 1979; Daum and Lemke, 1979). In addition to the unmodified aminoglycosides (streptomycin, neomycin, kanamycins A and B, gentamycin, tobramycin, and sisomycin), the first derivatives have been introduced into therapy – **amikacin** and **dibekacin,** two kanamycin derivatives, and **netilmicin,** a sisomycin derivative. **Kasugamycin** and the **validamycins** have been

introduced into plant protection. Comprehensive accounts of the aminoglycosides are given by Umezawa (1975). Nara (1977, 1978), and Reden and Dürckheimer (1979).

Aminoglycosides can be found in various Actinomycetes genera (Streptomyces, Nocardia, Micromonospora, Saccharopolyspora), and also various species of Bacillus and Pseudomonas.

There are many individual investigations on the **biogenesis** of the aminoglycosides, but only a few reviews (Rinehart and Stroshane, 1976; Rinehart 1979; Testa and Tilley, 1979). A short account of the regulation of the biogenesis of the aminoglycosides has been given by Demain (1979). The synthesis of individual constructional units – more or less directly from glucose – has been substantially elucidated, but the sequence of their assembly is not clear. Of special importance is the fact that mutants can be found of many aminoglycoside-producing agents that no longer synthesize individual constructional units but which when they are fed with the constructional units form aminoglycosides again. Such mutants are suitable for mutasynthesis since they also bring about the incorporation of modified constructional units. This takes place both with deoxystreptamine-minus and also with streptidine-minus mutants (Daum and Lemke, 1979; Rinehart, 1979). In connection with the biosynthesis of streptomycin, reference must also be made to factor A, which is not itself a precursor but appears to be necessary for the synthesis of the intact streptomycin (Kleiner et al., 1976; Khokhlov and Tovarova, 1979).

Factor A
Formula I

Table 13-5. Structures of the Most Important Aminoglycoside Antibiotics.

1. Streptomycin group

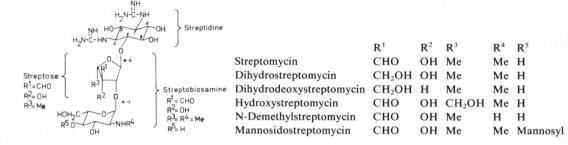

	R^1	R^2	R^3	R^4	R^5
Streptomycin	CHO	OH	Me	Me	H
Dihydrostreptomycin	CH$_2$OH	OH	Me	Me	H
Dihydrodeoxystreptomycin	CH$_2$OH	H	Me	Me	H
Hydroxystreptomycin	CHO	OH	CH$_2$OH	Me	H
N-Demethylstreptomycin	CHO	OH	Me	H	H
Mannosidostreptomycin	CHO	OH	Me	Me	Mannosyl

2. Neomycin group

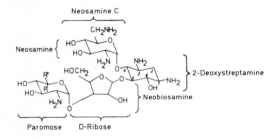

Neomycin B: R=CH$_2$NH$_2$, R′=H
Neomycin C: R=H, R′=CH$_2$NH$_2$

3. Paromomycins

Paromomycin I: R=CH$_2$NH$_2$, R′=H
Paromomycin II: R=H, R′=CH$_2$NH$_2$

4. Gentamicins and sisomycin

Gentamicin A

Table 13-5. (continued).

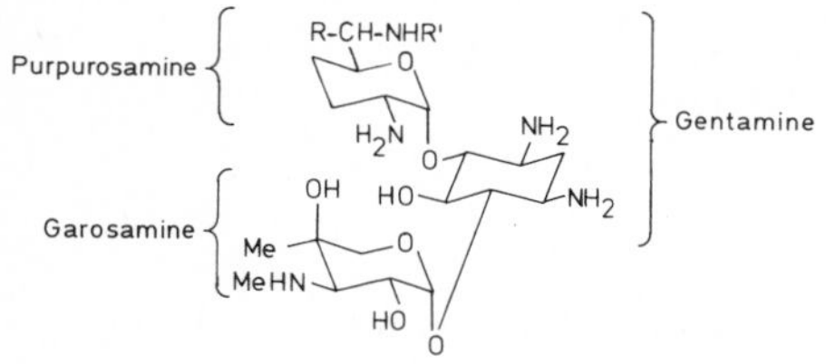

Purpurosamine / Garosamine — Gentamine

Gentamicin C_1: R = R' = Me
Gentamicin C_2: R = Me, R' = H
Gentamicin C_{1a}: R = R' = H

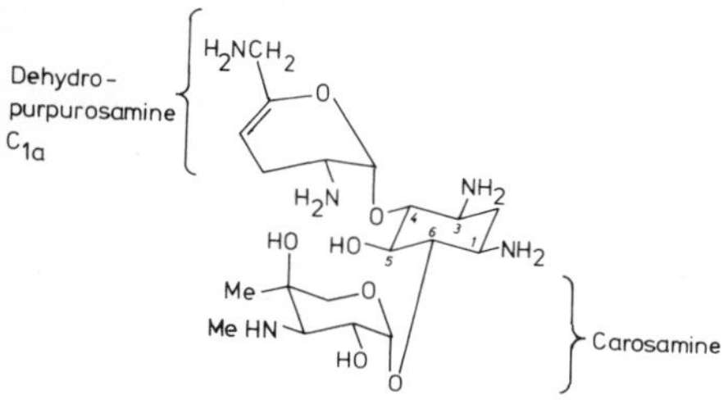

Dehydro-purpurosamine C_{1a} / Carosamine

Sisomicin

5. Kanamycin group

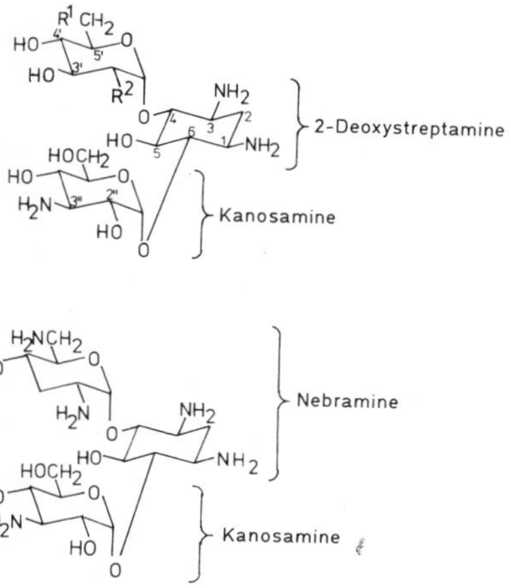

2-Deoxystreptamine / Kanosamine

Kanamycin A: $R^1 = NH_2$, $R^2 = OH$
Kanamycin B: $R^1 = NH_2$, $R^2 = NH_2$
Kanamycin C: $R^1 = OH$, $R^2 = NH_2$

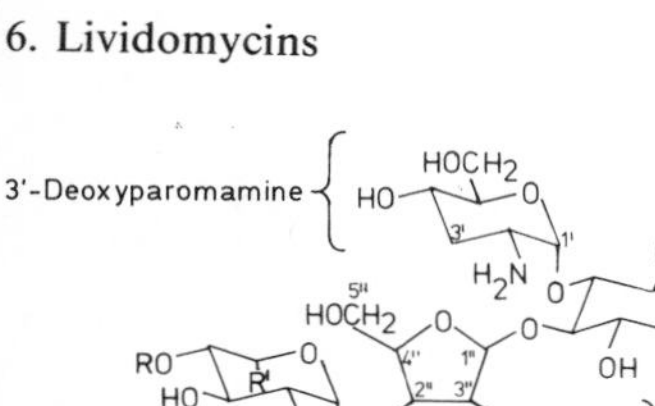

Nebramine / Kanosamine

Tobramycin (nebramycin factor 6) = 3'-deoxykanamycin B

6. Lividomycins

3'-Deoxyparomamine

Lividotriosamine:
R = mannosyl
$R' = CH_2NH_2$

Lividomycin A: R =

Lividomycin B: R = H

Table 13-5. (continued).

7. Ribostamycins

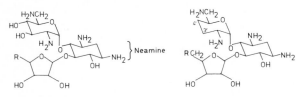

3',4'-Dideoxyribostamycin: R=OH
3',4',5''-Trideoxyribostamycin: R=H

Ribostamycin: R=CH$_2$OH

8. Hygromycin B and destomycin

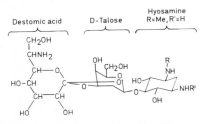

Hygromycin B: R=Me   R'=H
Destomycin A: R=H   R'=Me

9. Actinospectacin

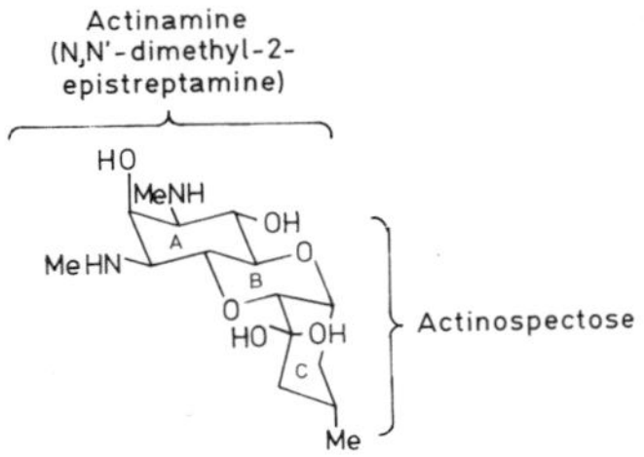

Actinamine
(N,N'-dimethyl-2-
epistreptamine)

Actinospectose

10. Kasugamycin

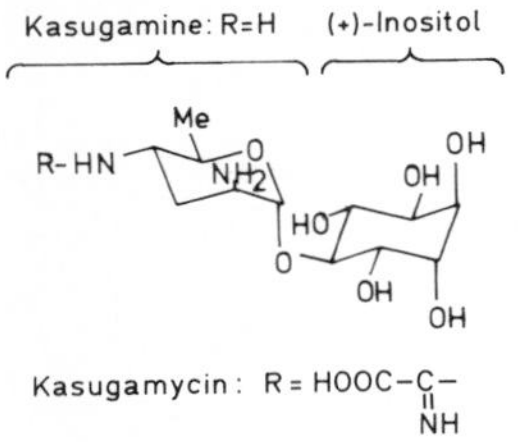

Kasugamine: R=H   (+)-Inositol

Me

R-HN

Kasugamycin: R = HOOC—C—
                         ‖
                         NH

Kasugamycin: R=HOOC—C—
                            ‖
                            NH

11. Validamycin

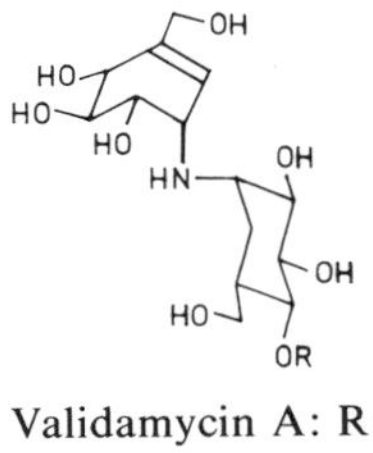

Validamycin A: R=β-D-Glucopyranosyl

The **fermentation yields** so far achieved with the aminoglycosides are distinctly below those for the penicillins and tetracyclines. Increasing the yields by mutation has proved to be very difficult. Since sugars, i.e., parts of the nutrient substrate, are converted into constructional units without first having to pass through large parts of the intermediate metabolism, there is no possibility of deliberately switching off regulation in the synthesis of the precursors, as is possible with the β-lactams, for example.

A special problem is presented by the **isolation of the individual components** since most strains form complex mixtures of aminoglycosides. Usually sufficient for isolating the main components is an absorption on cation-exchangers, elution with mineral acid, neutralization, and subsequent precipitation as a salt of an organic acid. Then the acid is removed by means of an anion-exchanger and the free base is recovered. Chromatographic methods must be used for the isolation of the auxiliary components. And in parallel to this, attempts are being made by the choice of suitable mutants to guide the fermentation in the direction of the desired components (Marquez and Kershner, 1978).

The **practical utilization** of the aminoglycosides is limited, on the one hand, by their neuro- and ototoxicities, even though this has been substantially lowered in the newer preparations, and, on the other hand, by the relatively rapid appearance of resistant strains. The clinically important glycoside resistance is based on a plasmid-coded inactivation (phosphorylation, adenylation, and acetylation, depending on the type of resistance and on the particular aminoglycoside). For a summary, see Umezawa (1979). Attempts are being made to overcome the resistance by modifying the aminoglycosides at the positions important for inactivation or by choosing aminoglycosides not containing the corresponding groups.

The aminoglycosides **inhibit the biosynthesis of protein** by procaryotes at the ribosomal level. In the case of streptomycin, action-site-resistant mutants can easily be selected. They have played an important role in connection with the elucidation of the biosynthesis of protein and the structure of the ribosome, but they play no part in the clinically important aminoglycoside resistance.

A polyamine transport system appears to be involved in the uptake of the aminoglycosides by the bacterial cell (Höltje, 1978, 1979a,b).

13.4 Tetracyclines

The tetracyclines belong to the antibiotics that were discovered at an early period and were rapidly commercialized. Table 13-6 shows the tetracyclines manufactured by fermentation, the first two being formed by wild strains and another two by mutants. Hitherto, tetracyclines have been found only in streptomycetes but appear to be widespread in this group. In the course of **biogenetic studies** (McCormick, 1967), numerous mutants were isolated which form the precursors (and also modified precursors) of the tetracyclines, but none of these compounds has shown an advantage as compared with the tetracyclines introduced. Although a **total synthesis** is possible (Korst et al., 1968; Muxfeldt and Rogalski, 1965), today all tetracyclines are manufactured by **fermentation** and are used in medicine either in the **native form** (tetracycline, oxytetracycline, and chlortetracycline) or after derivatization (rolitetracycline, methacycline, doxycycline, minocycline). The tetracyclines have also been used in very large amounts in animal nutrition for the realization of the nutritive effect, but they should no longer be used today since this gives rise to the spreading of tetracycline-resistant Enterobacteriaceae.

Table 13-6. Tetracyclines Manufactured by Fermentation.

| Name | Formula | | | | Year | Producing agent |
	R_1	R_2	R_3	R_4		(only the first described)
Chlortetracycline	Cl	CH₃	H	OH	1948	*Streptomyces aureofaciens*
Oxytetracycline	H	CH₃	OH	OH	1950	*Streptomyces rimosus*
Tetracycline	H	CH₃	H	OH	1953	Mutants of *Str. aureofaciens*
Demethylchlortetracycline	Cl	H	H	OH	1957	Mutants of *Str. aureofaciens*
Demethyltetracycline	H	H	H	OH	1965	Biotransformation with *Str. aureofaciens* or *Str. rimosus*

Although very much work has been put into the biosynthesis, the formation of derivatives, and the synthesis of the tetracyclines (for a review, see Dürckheimer, 1975), only small advances have been achieved in the direction of **application** in the tetracycline field if this is compared with the β-lactams. Also surprising is the fact that the variation of the tetracyclines in nature is very limited in comparison with the variation in the aminoglycosides or the anthracyclines. Apart from the unusual chelocardin (Oliver et al., 1962; Sinclair et al., 1962; Mitscher et al., 1970a, b), no closely related compounds with a similar action mechanism have been described. The **mode of action** of the tetracyclines has been well studied (see Kaji and Royoji, 1979). The **inhibition of the biosynthesis of protein** in procaryotes by the tetracyclines explains their low toxicity for the cells of warm-blooded animals. Resistance to the tetracyclines is based on a change in the uptake of the tetracyclines and not to an inactivation of the antibiotic or to a changed action site.

The **yields that can be achieved** in tetracycline fermentation are very high at more than 15 g/L. The low water solubility of the products together with their good solubility in organic solvents permits a simple recovery system through a combination of extraction and precipitation (Neidleman, 1978), so that the tetracyclines can be obtained very cheaply. For the manufacture of the tetracyclines as fodder additives it has even been possible to carry out the last stage of the fermentation chain, the production proper, without previous sterilization of the nutrient solution, since with the inoculation material tetracyclines and the polyenes formed simultaneously were already introduced in such large amounts that any infection was suppressed.

Now that it has been possible to expand the action spectrum of the β-lactams into the area of the Gram-negative bacteria and that, today, aminoglycosides which also have a broad action spectrum and are less toxic – in comparison with earlier examples – are available, these antibiotics are penetrating more and more into the fields of application previously reserved to the tetracyclines.

13.5   Macrolide Antibiotics

When Woodward coined the term macrolides in 1957, he covered by it a group of basic and lipophilic antibiotics from actinomycetes acting against Gram-positive bacteria that were characterized by the possession of a large lactone ring. Since large lactone rings are common in microbial metabolites, the group has become greatly expanded and today the classical macrolides form only a subgroup:

a) **Polyoxomacrolides:** erythromycin, spiramycins, oleandomycin, and more than 50 other representatives.

b) **Polyene macrolides:** amphotericin B, nystatin, trichomycin, and more than 50 other representatives.

c) **Macrotetrolides:** nonactin, monactin, dinactin, trinactin, tetranactin, and homologs.

d) **Unusual macrolides:** e.g., chlorothricin, borrelidin, venturicidins, avermectins, zearaleones.

Group a), **polyoxomacrolides,** corresponds to the **classical macrolides,** which are linked not only through the chemical definition – large lactone ring – but also by their action on the Gram-positive bacteria, their action on the biosynthesis of protein in procaryotes at the ribosomal level, their occurrence in actinomycetes, and their inclusion of one or more sugar residues.

Group b), **polyene macrolides,** consists of compounds characterized by the presence of several conjugated double bonds (4 to 7) in the lactone ring and the possession of a similar antifungal action spectrum, while this action can be eliminated by ergosterol or cholesterol (Holz, 1979). However, in addition to this, individual polyene macrolides act against bacteria.

In group c), the **macrotetrolides,** each representative possesses four lactone groups in a large ring system that contains no sugar residues and is active as an ionophore (Bakker, 1979).

In group d) it is possible to include the **unusual macrolides** which cannot be included in groups a)-c). **Borrelidin** inhibits the charging of Thr-t-RNA (Poralla, 1975). **Chlorothricin** is an antagonist of acetyl-CoA (Schindler and Zähner, 1973; Schindler and Scrutton, 1975), and the **avermectins** inhibit, for example, nematodes (Burg et al., 1979; Miller et al., 1979).

The macrolides mentioned hitherto are all products of actinomycetes, but there are also occasionally macrolides in the metabolites of fungi, e.g., curvularin and the zearaleones (Hidy et al., 1977).

Some polyoxomacrolides have found **broad use** in **antibacterial chemotherapy,** but they are under severe competitive pressure from the modern semisynthetic β-lactams. The most important representatives of the polyoxomacrolides are listed in Table 13-7. The whole field of macrolides was described comprehensively by Keller-Schierlein in 1973 and then again by Masamune et al. in 1977.

The polyoxomacrolides are, so far as concerns the macrolide moiety, true polyketides (see Chapter 4, Section 4.6, p. 120) constructed from propionate and acetate units, while in the case of C_{16}-lactones there is also a fragment not constructed directly from acetate (Grisebach, 1978). Even today, the number of polyoxomacrolides is very large, but most strains form a whole gamut of closely related macrolides. The investigations that have been started with the aim of arriving at other, new, macrolides by the protoplast fusion of producing agents of various macrolides promise further expansion, and so do the first attempts that can be recognized to carry out the mutasynthesis and the microbial transformation of the macrolides.

The **manufacture** of the classical macrolides is carried out by the use of strains of actinomycetes in the **batch process,** the macrolides being extracted with organic solvents from the filtrate of the broth. The polyoxomacrolides obtainable on the market all contain an amino

Table 13-7. Some Macrolide Antibiotics (after Keller-Schierlein, 1973; Masamune et al., 1977; and Majer, 1978).

Name	Producing agent	Size of the ring	Sugars	Formula
Erythromycins A, B	*Streptomyces erythreus*	14	desosamine cladinose	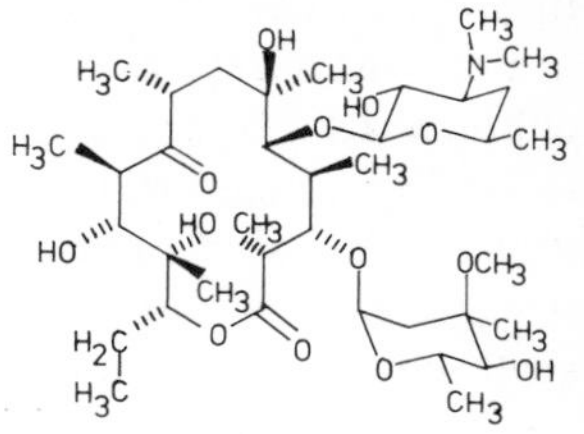 Erythromycin A
Oleandomycin	*Streptomyces antibioticus*	14	desosamine oleandrose	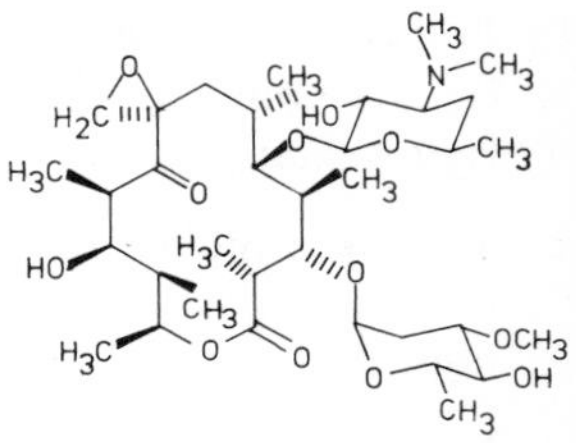
Carbomycins A, B	*Streptomyces halstedii tendae reticuli griseoflavus*	16	mycaminose mycarose	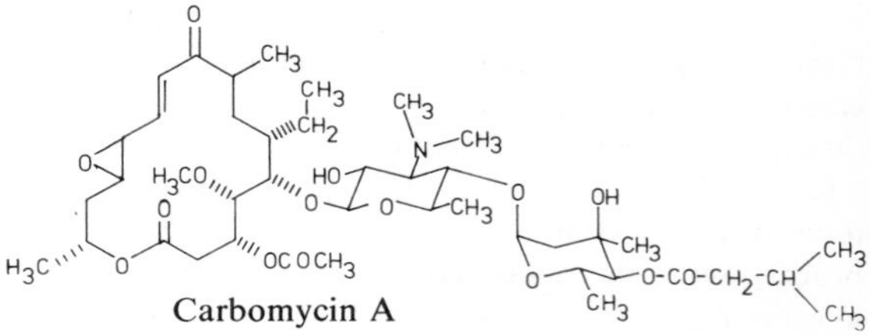 Carbomycin A
Spiramycins I, II, III	*Streptomyces ambofaciens (aureofaciens)*	16	mycaminose mycarose forosamine	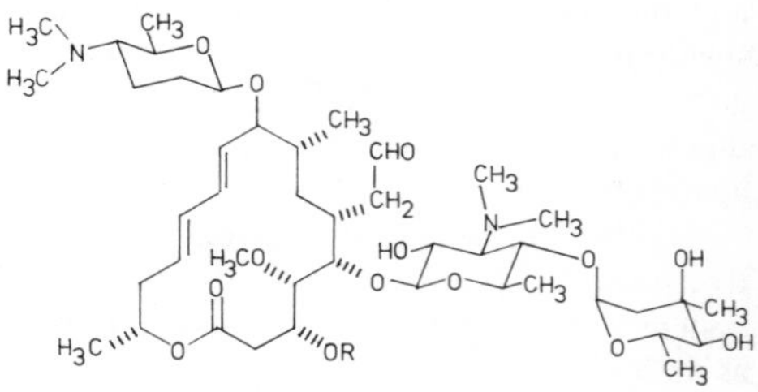

I: R = H
II: R = —COCH₃
III: R = —CO—CH₂—CH₃

Table 13-7. (continued).

Name	Producing agent	Size of the ring	Sugars	Formula
Leucomycins	*Streptomyces reticuli*	16	mycaminose mycarose	
Tylosin–relomycin	*Streptomyces violaceoniger* *Streptomyces hygroscopicus*	16	mycaminose mycarose mycinose	

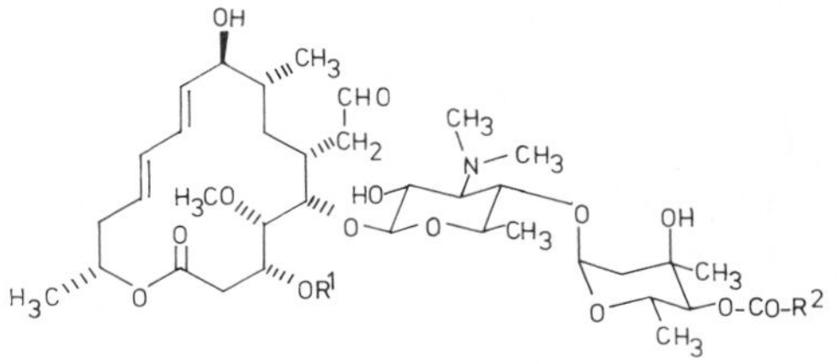

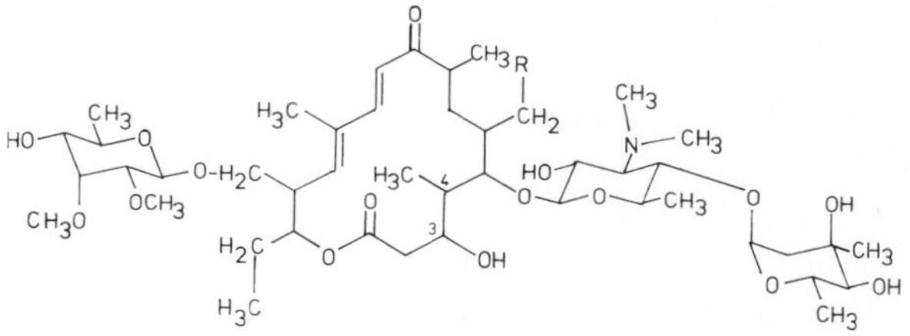

Leucomycin A$_1$
Leucomycin A$_3$
Leucomycin A$_5$
Leucomycin A$_4$
Leucomycin A$_7$
Leucomycin A$_6$
Leucomycin A$_9$
Leucomycin A$_8$

Tylosin: R = —CHO
Relomycin: R = —CH$_2$OH

sugar and consequently show basic behavior which can be utilized for further enrichment (Majer, 1978). In fermentation, care is taken – either by the choice of suitable mutants or by guiding the fermentation in the desired direction – that the therapeutically interesting components are formed preferentially. A **separation** of a **mixture of macrolides** such as certainly occurs in the case of wild strains, is extraordinarily difficult, and modern separating processes such as HPLC, Craig countercurrent distribution, or drop countercurrent distribution (DCCD) must be used.

The high number of possible stereoisomers in the synthesis of polyoxomacrolides represents a challenge in the direction of **stereospecific syntheses** for organic chemistry. Such synthetic investigations are being carried out at the present time in various institutes, but one should probably not envisage the creation of competition to fermentation by a pure synthesis. However, the experience obtained in these investigations may be of great practical importance for making derivatives of polyoxomacrolides. An expansion of the action spectrum in the direction of the Gram-negative bacteria by forming derivatives could recover parts of the lost market for the macrolide.

13.6 Anthracycline Antibiotics

The first anthracycline, **rhodomycin** was described by Brockmann and Bauer in 1950, but the list given by Aszalos and Bérdy (1978) already includes more than 50 representatives, and at the same time it must be considered that a name usually stands for a whole mixture of closely related components. The introduction of **daunorubicin** (= daunomycin) and **adriamycin** into the chemotherapy of tumors has greatly stimulated investigations on anthracyclines (Arcamone, 1978; Carter et al., 1972; Ghione et al., 1975). The two anthracyclines already introduced into therapy still show, in addition to the desired antitumoral action, a considerable general toxicity and, in particular, a very undesirable action on the cardiac activity. In the meantime, anthracyclines have been found which no longer possess this effect, which can easily be recognized on the ECG, or do so only to a highly attenuated degree, e.g., the **carminomycins** and the **aclacinomycins**, but it is still open whether a decrease in the general toxicity is also associated with it. Since the evaluation of antitumoral substances demands substantially more time than that of antibacterial substances, it cannot yet be estimated whether and when new anthracyclines can be placed on the market.

Anthracyclines are O-glycosides consisting of an intensively colored aglycone – an anthracyclinone – and one or more residues of sugars, one of them usually being an amino sugar. In Table 13-8, the most important an-

Daunomycin R=H
Adriamycin R=OH

thracyclinones are grouped around the general parent substance, anthracyclinone (Oki, 1977; Oki and Yoshimoto, 1979). To some extent, further modifications of this basic substance occur. These interrelated anthracyclinones are constructed from one propionate and nine acetate units in the manner typical for the polyketides. Most of the anthracyclines are linked in position 7 to a sugar residue, usually an amino sugar residue. The amino sugar residue may be extended to a short sugar chain, e.g., in the carminomycins and the aclacinomycins, but only sugars not usually involved in the intermediate metabolism are incorporated. Table 13-9 summarizes the sugars that have so far been detected in the anthracyclines. From a combination of the numerous anthracyclinones with one or more sugars which again differ from one another, a very large range of variation can be derived, so that it is not surprising that, of those occurring naturally, alone, more than 200 individual anthracyclines have been described. Through the possibility of mutasynthesis or the protoplast fusion of producing agents of various glycosides (together with the chemical formation of derivatives), the number of accessible anthracyclines will probably rise very greatly in future.

Table 13-8. Structure of the Anthracyclinones.

	R¹	R²

	R^1	R^2
Daunomycinone	Me	COMe
Adriamycinone	Me	COCH$_2$OH
Carminomycinone	H	COMe

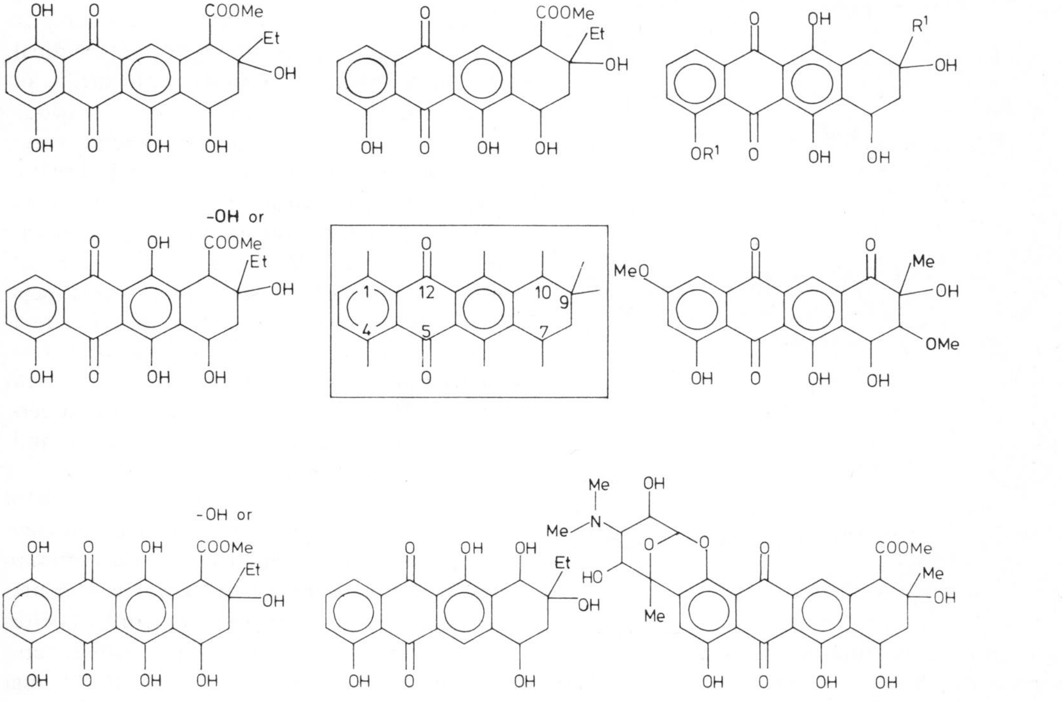

Hitherto, anthracyclines have been found only in actinomycetes. The fermentation **yields achieved** so far are not so high as is the case for other antibiotics manufactured for the market. Most of the wild strains among the anthracycline-producing agents are inhibited by relatively high concentrations of the antibiotic itself in the germination of the spores or, generally, in growth. Some of the anthracyclines are present in the mycelium and can be extracted from it by organic solvents, while the amounts present in the filtrate can likewise be extracted by organic solvents. In the recovery process, acid conditions must be avoided in order to prevent a splitting out of the sugar residues.

The **action** of the anthracyclines is due to their incorporation in the DNA (Neidle, 1978), but it shows some fundamental differences from the action of the actinomycins. This interaction with the DNA, on the one hand, makes their high toxicity understand-

Table 13-9. Sugars from Anthracycline Antibiotics.

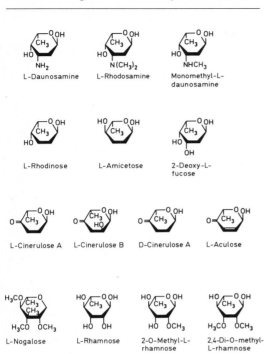

the chemistry of the compounds and says nothing about their mode of action. As can be seen from Table 13-10, the group includes both substances that act on bacteria and not on higher cells and also substances that inhibit eucaryotes. Ansamycins are found in various organisms, and particularly confusing is the occurrence of to some extent identical substances, the **maytansinoids** in Nocardia, an actinomycete, and in the bark of various shrubs. Summarizing accounts of the ansamycins are given by Rinehart and Shield (1976), Wehrli (1977), and Brufani (1977). At the present time, the **rifamycins,** particularly a derivative of rifamycin SV, rifampicin, have found wide use, especially in the fight against tuberculosis. Whether the good antitumoral effect of the maytansinoid representives of the ansamycins can be utilized in practice is an open question. If they can be used, they would certainly be manufactured by fermentation and not isolated from bark.

After practically each name in Table 13-10 there is a whole group of substances, so that the number of representatives is substantially greater than appears at first sight. Here, again, investigations on **biogenesis,** performed with the aid of mutants, are leading to further representatives, e.g., to precursors still having open chains (Knöll et al., 1980; Rinehart et al., 1976; Ghisalba et al., 1978, 1979; Ghisalba and Nüesch, 1978).

The **manufacture** of rifamycin SV, the starting material for the synthesis of rifampicin, is carried out with highly bred strains of *Nocardia mediterranei* in the batch process, efforts being made by the choice of mutants and also by controlling the fermentation to achieve a preferential formation of the SV component. The highly lipophilic nature of the ansamycins facilitates their isolation by extraction processes which, if it is a question of obtaining individual components from a mixture in the pure form must be supplemented by careful chromatography (Ganguly, 1978).

able and, on the other hand, faces the producing cells with the problem of protecting their own DNA from their own antibiotics.

In addition to the anthracyclines, other antitumoral antibiotics are playing an increasing role (Oki and Yoshimoto, 1979; Fuska and Proska, 1978), and special reference should be made to the bleomycins (Hecht, 1979).

13.7 Ansamycins

The ansamycins [the name was proposed by Prelog and Oppolzer (1973)] compose a group of antibiotics each of which consists of a flat aromatic moiety and an aliphatic bridge (see Fig. 13-1). The definition relates exclusively to

Table 13-10. Naturally Occurring Ansamycins.

Name	Year of 1st description	Producing agent	Activity	Literature	Formula (see p. 551)
Rifamycins	1957	*Nocardia mediterranea*	bact, inc. TB reverse transcriptase	Wehrli, 1977; Brufani, 1977	I
Streptovaricins	1957	*Streptomyces spectabilis*	bact, inc. TB reverse transcriptase	Wehrli, 1977; Brufani, 1977; Rinehart and Shield, 1976	III
Halomycins	1967	*Micromonospora halophytica*	bact.	Wehrli 1977; Ganguly et al., 1977	
Naphthomycins	1969	*Streptomyces collinus*	bact, fungi, blocks SH-groups	Wehrli, 1977; Brufani et al., 1979	IV
Geldanamycin	1970	*Streptomyces hygroscopicus*	protozoa, fungi	Sasaki et al., 1970; DeBoer et al., 1970	V
Tolypomycins	1971	*Streptomyces tolypophorus*	bact., inc. TB	Wehrli, 1977; Brufani, 1977	II
Maytansin	1972	*Maytenus ovatus*	antitumor, leukemia	Wehrli, 1977; Brufani, 1977	VI

Table 13-10. (continued).

Name	Year of 1st description	Producing agent	Activity	Literature	Formula (see p. 551)
Maytanbutin	1972	*Maytenus buchananii*	antitumor, leukemia	Wehrli, 1977; Brufani, 1977	
Maytanprin	1972	*Maytenus buchananii*	antitumor, leukemia	Wehrli, 1977; Brufani, 1977	
Colubrinols	1972	*Colubrina texensis*	antitumor, leukemia	Wehrli, 1977; Brufani, 1977	
Herbimycins	1976	*Streptomyces hygroscopicus*	fungi, weeds	Omura et al., 1979; Haneishi et al., 1976; Arai et al., 1976	
Ansamitocins	1977	Nocardia spec.	antitumor, leukemia fungi	Higashide et al., 1977; Asai et al., 1979; Tanida et al., 1980	
Macbecin	1980	Nocardia spec.	antitumor, protozoa	Muroi et al., 1980a, b; Tanida et al., 1980	
Ansatrienin	1981	*Streptomyces collinus*	fungi	Weber et al., 1981	

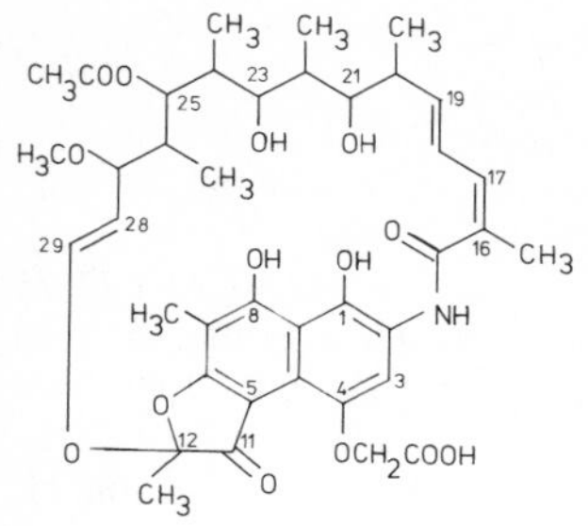

I. Rifamycin B

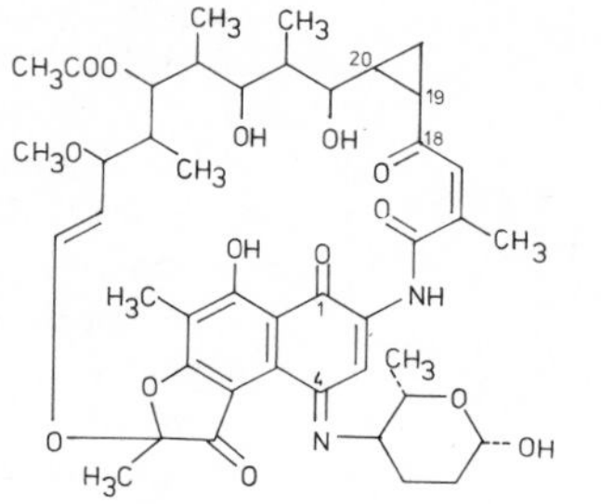

II. Tolypomycin Y

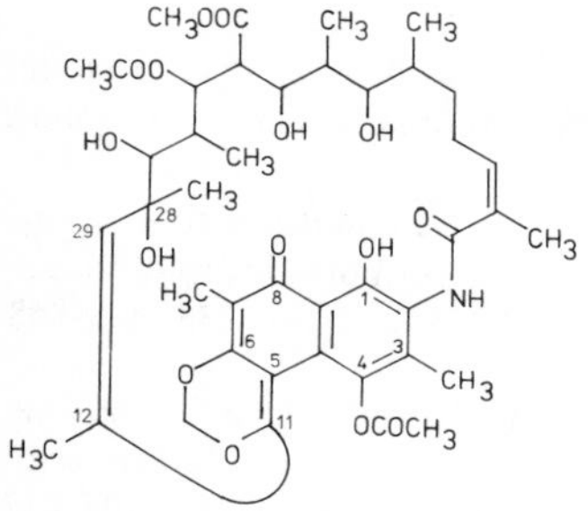

III. Streptovaricin B

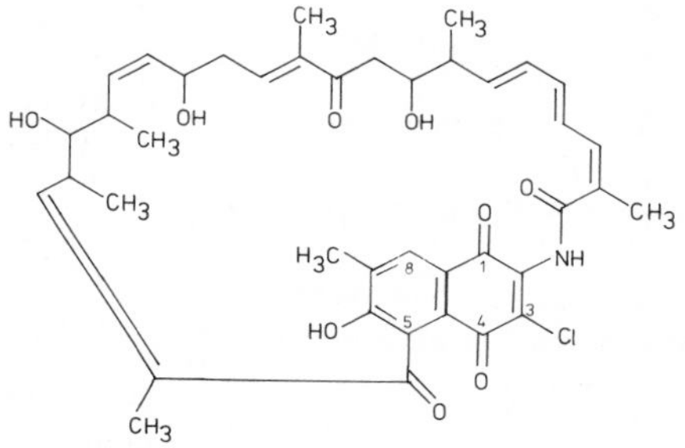

IV. Naphthomycin

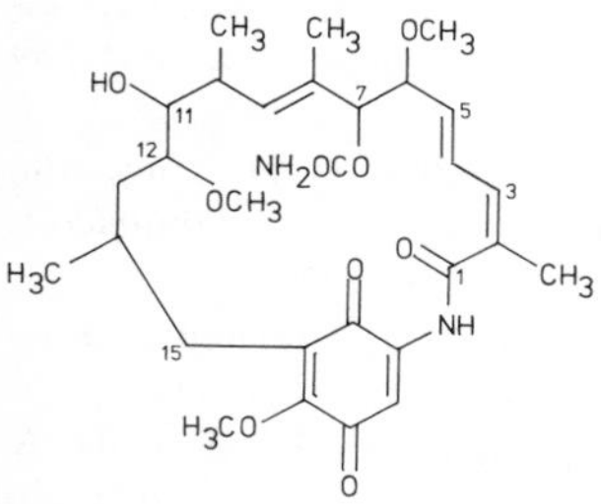

V. Geldanamycin

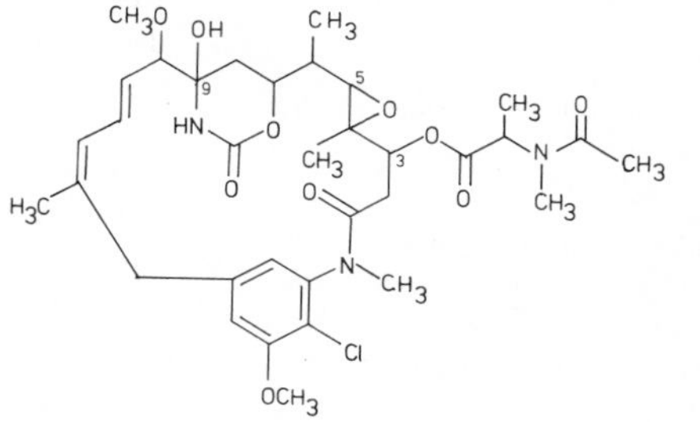

VI. Maytansin

Fig. 13-1. The structures of some representatives of the ansamycins.

13.8   Literature

Some literature references been taken from important handbooks on the subject of "Antibiotics", so that these would have hand to be mentioned repeatedly in the list of literature. They have therefore been given at the beginning and have been numbered.

A   Review Literature

[1] Corcoran, J. W. and Hahn, F. E.: *Antibiotics, III.* Springer Verlag, New York 1975.

[2] Gottlieb, D. and Shaw, P. D.: *Antibiotics, I.* Springer Verlag, New York 1967.

[2] a) Gottlieb, D. and Shaw, P. D.: *Antibiotics, II.* Springer Verlag, New York 1967.

[3] Hahn, F. E.: *Antibiotics, V-1.* Springer Verlag, New York 1979.

[4] Hahn, F. E.: *Antibiotics, V-2.* Springer Verlag, New York 1979.

[5] Hütter, R., Leisinger, T., Nüesch, J. and Wehrli, W.: *Antibiotics and Other Secondary Metabolites.* Academic Press, London 1978.

[6] Perlman, D.: *Structure – Activity Relationships Among the Semisynthetic Antibiotics.* Academic Press, New York 1977.

[7] Weinstein, M. J. and Wagmann, G. H.: *Antibiotics, Isolation, Separation and Purification.* Elsevier Sci. Publ., Amsterdam 1978.

B   Special Literature

The figures placed in square brackets relate to the Review Literature given above.

Abbott, B. J., "Preparation of pharmaceutical compounds by immobilized enzymes and cells", *Adv. Appl. Microbiol.* **20,** 203–257 (1976).

Abraham, E. P.: *Biosynthesis and Enzymatic Hydrolysis of Penicillins and Cephalosporins.* University of Tokyo Press 1975.

Abraham, E. P., "β-Lactam antibiotics and related substances", *Jap. J. of Antibiotics Suppl.* **30,** 1–26 (1977).

Abraham, E. P.: "Developments in the chemistry and biochemistry of β-lactam antibiotics". In: [5], pp. 141–164.

Abraham, E. P., Baker, W., Chain, E. et al., *Nature* **149,** 356 (1942).

Abraham, E. P. and Newton, G. F., "Experiments on the degradation of cephalosporin C", *Biochem. J.* **63,** 628 (1956).

Albers-Schönberg, G., Arison, B. H., Hensen, O. D. et al., "Structure and absolute configuration of thienamycin", *J. Am. Chem. Soc.* **100,** 6491 (1978).

Albers-Schönberg, G., Arison, B. and Smith, H., "New β-lactam antibiotics: structure determination of cephamycin A and B", Tetrahedron Lett. **1972,** 2911.

Ando, K., Murakami, Y. and Nawata, Y., "Tetranactin, a new miticidal antibiotic. II. Structure of tetranactin", *J. Antibiotics* **24,** 418–422 (1971 b).

Ando, K., Oishi, H., Hirano, S. et al., "Tetranactin, a new antimiticidal antibiotic, I.", *J. Antibiotics* **24,** 347–352 (1971 a).

Andreoli, T. E., "The structure and function of amphotericin B – cholesterin pores in lipid bilayer membranes", *Ann. N.Y. Acad. Sci.* **235,** 448–468 (1974).

Aoki, H., Kunugita, K., Hosoda, J. and Imanaka, H., "Screening of new and novel β-lactam antibiotics", *Jap. J. Antibiotics Suppl.* **30,** 207–217 (1977).

Aoki, H., Sakai, H. J., Kohosaka, M. et al., "Nocardicin A, a new monocyclic β-lactam antibiotic. I.", *J. Antibiotics* **29,** 492–500 (1976).

Arai, M., Haneishi, T., Kitahara, N. et al., "Herbicidins A and B, two new antibiotics with herbicidal activity. I.", *J. Antibiotics* **29,** 863–869 (1976).

Arai, M., Ishibashi, K. and Okazaki, H., "Siccanin, a new antifungal antibiotic. I.", *Antimicrob. Agents Chemother.,* 247–252 (1969).

Arcamone, F., "Daunomycin and related antibiotics", *Top. Antibiot. Chem.* **2,** 89–229 (1978).

Arima, K., Imanaka, H., Kousaka, M., Fukuda, A. and Tamura, G., "Studies on pyrrolnitrin, a new antibiotic. I.", *J. Antibiotics* **18,** 201–204 (1965).

Arima, K., Imanaka, H., Kousaka, M. et al., "Pyrrolnitrin", *Agric. Biol. Chem.* **28,** 575 (1964).

Asai, M., Mizuta, E., Izawa, M. et al., "Isolation, chemical characterization and structure of ansamitocin, a new antitumor ansamycin antibiotic", *Tetrahedron* **35,** 1079–1085 (1979).

Asai, M., Muroi, M., Sugita, N. et al., "Enduracidin, a new antibiotic. II.", *J. Antibiotics* **21**, 138–146 (1968).

Aszalos, A. and Bérdy, J., "Cytotoxic and antitumor compounds from fermentation", *Annu. Rep. Ferment. Processes* **2**, 305–333 (1978).

Bakker, E. P.: "Ionophore antibiotics". In: [3] pp. 67–97.

Baldwin, J. E., Christie, M. A., Haber, S. B. and Kruse, L. I., "Stereospecific synthesis of penicillins. Conversion from a peptide precursor", *J. Am. Chem. Soc.* **98**, 3045–3047 (1976).

Ball, C.: "Genetics in the development of the penicillin process". In: [5], pp. 165–176.

Beecham Ltd., D.O.S. 2, 708, 047 (1977).

Benedict, R. G. and Langlykke, G. F., "Antibiotic activity of *Bacillus polymyxa*", *J. Bacteriol.* **54**, 24 (1947).

Bentley, P. H., Berry, P. D., Brooks, G. et al., "Total synthesis of (±)-clavulanic acid", *J. Chem. Soc. Chem. Commun.* **1977**, 748.

Berde, D. and Schild, H. O. (eds.): *Ergot alkaloids and related compounds*. Springer-Verlag, Berlin 1978.

Bérdy, J., "Recent advances in and prospects of antibiotic research", *Process Biochem.* **15**, 28–32 (1980).

Bérdy, J., Aszalos, A., Bostian, M. and McNitt, K. L.: *Handbook of Antibiotic Compounds*, Vol. 1–10. CRC Press 1980–1982.

Berger, J. and Batcho: "Coumarin-glycoside antibiotics". In: [7], pp. 101–158.

Blinov, N. O., Ryabova, I. D., Uspenskaya, T. A. and Khokhlov, A. S., *Antibiotiki Moskow* **7**, 708–713 (1962).

Bodansky, M., Izdebski, J. and Muramatsu, J., "The structure of the peptide antibiotic stendomycin", *J. Am. Chem. Soc.* **91**, 2351 (1969).

Bodansky, M., Muramatsu, I. and Bodansky, A., "Fatty acid constituents of the antifungal antibiotic stendomycin", *J. Antibiotics* **20**, 384–385 (1967).

Bodansky, M., Muramatsu, I., Bodansky, A. et al., "Amino acid constituents of stendomycin", *J. Antibiot.* **21**, 77–78 (1968).

Bodansky, M., Sigler, G. F. and Bodansky, A., "Structure of the peptide antibiotic amphomycin", *J. Am. Chem. Soc.* **95**, 2352 (1973).

Borel, J. F., Feurer, C., Gubler, H. U. and Stähelin, H., *Agents Actions* **6**, 468 (1976).

Boyd, D. B., "Conformational analogy between β-lactam antibiotics and tetrahedrol transition states of a dipeptide", *J. Med. Chem.* **22**, 533–537 (1979).

Brockmann, H. and Bauer, K., "Rhodomycin, ein rotes Antibioticum aus Actinomyces", *Naturwissenschaften* **37**, 492 (1950).

Brockmann, H. and Reschke, T., "Die Konstitution des Resistomycins", *Tetrahedron Lett.* **1968**, 3167.

Brockmann, H. and Schmidt-Kastner, G., "Valinomycin I.", *Chem. Ber.* **88**, 57 (1955).

Brockmann, H. and Schmidt-Kastner, G., "Resistomycin, ein neues Antibioticum aus Actinomyceten", *Naturwissenschaften* **38**, 479 (1951).

Brown, A. G., Butterworth, D., Cole, M. et al., "Naturally occuring β-lactamase inhibitors with antibacterial activity", *J. Antibiot.* **29**, 668–669 (1976a).

Brown, A. G., Corbett, D. F., Eglington, A. J. and Howarth, T. T., "Structures of olivanic acid derivatives MM 4550 and MM 13902. Two new fused β-lactams isolated from *Streptomyces olivaceus*", *J. Chem. Soc. Chem. Commun.* **1977**, 523–525.

Brown, A. G., Howarth, T. T. and Sterling, I., "The formation and X-ray crystal analysis of isoclavulanic acid", *Tetrahedron Lett.* **1976**, 4203–4204 (1976b).

Brufani, M., "The ansamycins", *Top. Antibiot. Chem.* **1**, 91–212 (1977).

Brufani, M., Cellai, L. and Keller-Schierlein, W., "Degradation studies of naphthomycin", *J. Antibiot.* **32**, 167–168 (1979).

Burg, R. W., Miller, B. M., Baker, E. E. et al., "Avermectine, new family of potent antihelmintic agents", *Antimicrob. Agents Chemother.* **15**, 361–367 (1979).

Carter, S. K., DiMarco, A., Ghione, M. et al.: *Adriamycin*. Springer-Verlag, Berlin 1972.

Chaiet, L., Miller, T. W., Goegelman, R. T. et al., "Phosphonomycin: isolation from fermentation sources", *J. Antibiot.* **23**, 336–347 (1970).

Chang, F. N.: "Lincomycin". In: [3], pp. 127–134.

Christensen, B. G., Leanza, W., Beattie, T. R. et al., "Phosphonomycin, structure and synthesis", *Science* **166**, 123 (1969).

Cooper, R. D. G., "New β-Lactam Antibiotics", *Topics in Antibiotic Chem.* **3**, 39-200 (1979).

Corbett, D. F., Eglington, A. J. and Howarth, T. T., "Structure elucidation of MM 17880, a new fused β-lactam antibiotic isolated from *Streptomyces olivaceus*", *J. Chem. Soc. Chem. Commun.* **1977**, 953-954.

Corey, E. J. and Snider, B. B., "A total synthesis of (±)-fumagillin", *J. Am. Chem. Soc.* **94**, 2549 (1972).

Cox, D. A., Richardson, K. and Ross, B. C., "The aminoglycosides", *Top. Antibiot. Chem.* **1**, 1-90 (1977).

Crooy, P. and DeNeys, R., "Virginiamycin: nomenclature", *J. Antibiot.* **25**, 371-372 (1972).

Cundliffe, E.: "Thiostrepton and related antibiotics". In: [3], pp. 329-343.

Daum, S. L. and Lemke, J. R., "Mutational biosynthesis of new antibiotics", *Ann. Rev. Microbiol.* **33**, 241-265 (1979).

Daehne, v. W., Godtfredson, W. O. and Rasmussen, P. R., „Structure-activity relationships in fusidic acid-type antibiotics", *Adv. Appl. Microbiol.* **25**, 95-146 (1979).

DeBoer, C., Meulman, P. A., Wnuk, R. J. and Peterson, D. H., „Geldanamycin, a new antibiotic", *J. Antibiot.* **23**, 442-447 (1970).

Demain, A. L., "Aminoglycosides, genes and regulation", *Jap. J. Antibiotics Suppl.* **32**, 15-20 (1979).

Demain, A. L., Kupka, Y., Shen, Y. Q. and Wolfe, S.: "Microbiological Synthesis of β-lactam Antibiotics". In: *Trends in Antibiotic Research.* Jap. Antibiotic Research Assoc., Tokyo 1982.

Dreyfuss, M., Härri, E., Hofmann, H. et al., "Cyclosporin A and C. New metabolites from *Trichoderma polysporum*", *Eur. J. Appl. Microbiol.* **3**, 125-133 (1976).

Dürckheimer, W.: Tetracycline, "Chemie, Biochemie und Struktur-Wirkungsbeziehungen", *Angew. Chem.* **87**, 751-764 (1975).

Eble, T. E.: "Lincomycin related antibiotics". In: [7], pp. 231-272.

Eble, T. E. and Hanson, F. R., "Fumagillin, an antibiotic from *Aspergillus fumigatus,* H-3", *Antibiot. & Chemother. Washington D.C.* **1**, 54 (1951).

Fleming, A., "On the antibacterial action of cultures of a Penicillium with special reference to their use in the isolation of *B. influenzae*", *Brit. J. Exp. Pathol.* **10**, 226-236 (1929).

Floss, H. G., Mann, P. E., Hamill, R. L. and Mabe, J. A., "Further studies of the biogenesis of pyrrolnitrin from tryptophan by *Pseudomonas*", *Biol. Biochem. Res. Commun.* **45**, 781 (1971).

Flynn, E. H.: *Cephalosporin and Penicillin.* Academic Press, London 1972.

Franck, R. W., "The mitomycin antibiotics", *Progr. Chem. Org. Nat. Prod.* **38**, 1-45 (1979).

Frommer, W., Junge, B., Müller, L. et al., "Neue Enzyminhibitoren aus Mikroorganismen", *Planta Med.* **35**, 195-217 (1979).

Frommer, W., Puls, W., Schäfer, D. and Schmidt, D.: Inhibitoren für Glycosidhydrolasen aus Actinomyceten. D.O.S. 2, 064, 092 (1972).

Fuska, J. and Proksa, B., "Cytotoxic and antitumor antibiotics produced by microorganisms", *Adv. Appl. Microbiol.* **20**, 259-370 (1978).

Ganguly, A.: "Ansamycins". In: [7], pp. 39-68.

Ganguly, A. K., Liu, Y. T., Sarre, O. Z. and Szimelwicz, S., "Structures of halomycin A and C", *J. Antibiot.* **30**, 625-627 (1977).

Gause, G. F.: "Olivomycin, chromomycin and mithramycin". In: [1], pp. 197-202.

Ghione, M., Fetzer, J. and Maier, H.: *Ergebnisse der Adriamycin-Therapie.* Springer-Verlag, Berlin 1975.

Ghisalba, O. and Nüesch, J., "A genetic approach to the biosynthesis of the rifamycin chromophore in *Nocardia mediterranei.* II.", *J. Antibiot.* **31**, 215-225 (1978).

Ghisalba, O., Traxler, P., Fuhrer, H. and Richter, W. J., "Early intermediates in the biosynthesis of ansamycins. II.", *J. Antibiot.* **32**, 1267-1272 (1979).

Ghisalba, O., Traxler, P. and Nüesch, J., "Early intermediates in the biosynthesis of ansamycins. I.", *J. Antibiot.* **31**, 1124-1131 (1978).

Glaxo Ltd., D.O.S. 2,725,690 (1977).

Gosteli, J., "Eine neue Synthese des Antibioticums Pyrrolnitrin", *Helv. Chim. Acta* **55**, 451-460 (1972).

Grisebach, H.: "Biosynthesis of macrolide antibiotics". In: [5], pp. 113-128.

Gröger, D.: "Ergot alkaloids, recent advances in chemistry and biochemistry". In: [5], pp. 201-217.

Grundy, W. E., Sinclai, A. C., Theriault, R. I. et al., "Ristocetin, microbiologic properties", *Antibiot. Annu.*, 687-692 (1956/57).

Haidle, C. W. and Lloyd, R. S.: "Bleomycin". In: [4], pp. 124–154.

Hakenbeck, R., Höltje, J. V. and Labischinski, H. (eds.): *The Target of Penicillin*. Walter de Gruyter-Verlag, Berlin 1983.

Haller, B. and Löffler, W., "Fusidinsäure aus Dermatophyten und andern Pilzen", *Arch. Mikrobiol*. **65**, 181–194 (1969).

Hamill, R. L. and Crandall, L. W.: "Cephalosporin antibiotics". In: [7], pp. 69–100.

Hamill, R. L. and Crandall, L. W.: "Polyether antibiotics". In: [7], pp. 479–520.

Haneishi, T., Terahara, A., Kayamori, H. et al., "Herbimycen A and B, two new antibiotics with herbicidal activity. II.", *J. Antibiot*. **29**, 870–875 (1976).

Harris, T. M., Fehlner, J. R., Raabe, A. B. and Tarbell, D. S., „Oxidative degradation of ristocetin A", *Tetrahedron Lett*. **1975**, 2655.

Harris, C. M., Kibby, J. J. and Harris, T. M., "The biphenyl constituent of ristocetin A", *Tetrahedron Lett*. **1978**, 705.

Harris, C. M., Roberson, J. I. and Harris, T. M., "Biosynthesis of griseofulvin", *J. Am. Chem. Soc*. **98**, 5380 (1976).

Hashimoto, M. and Kamiya, T., "Recent chemical modification of β-lactam antibiotics", *Jap. J. Antibiot. Suppl*. **30**, 218–229 (1977).

Hata, T., Koga, F., Sano, Y. et al., "Carzinophylin, a new tumor inhibitory substance produced by Streptomyces", *J. Antibiot*. **7**, 107–112 (1954).

Hecht, S. M.: *Bleomycin, Chemical, Biochemical and Biological Aspects*. Springer-Verlag, Heidelberg 1979.

Hendlin, D., Stapley, E. O., Jackson, M. et al., "Phosphonomycin, a new antibiotic produced by strains of Streptomyces", *Science* **166**, 122 (1969).

Herrell, W. E.: *Lincomycin*. Modern Sci. Publ., Chicago 1969.

Hickey, R. J., "Bacitracin, its manufacture and uses", *Prog. Ind. Microbiol*. **5**, 93–150 (1964).

Hidy, P. H., Baldwin, R. S., Greasham, R. L. et al., "Zearalenone and some derivatives: Production and biological activities", *Adv. Appl. Microbiol*. **22**, 59–82 (1977).

Higashide, E., Asai, M., Ootsu, K. et al., "Ansamitocin, a group of novel maytansinoid antibiotics with antitumor properties from Nocardia", *Nature* **270**, 721 (1977).

Higashide, E., Hatano, K., Shibata, M. and Nakazawa, K., "Enduracidin, a new antibiotic. I. *Streptomyces fungicidicus* No. B 5477, an enduracidin producing organism", *J. Antibiot*. **21**, 126–137 (1968).

Hirai, K., Nozoe, S., Tsuda, K. et al., "The structure of siccanin", *Tetrahedron Lett*. **1967**, 2177.

Hirai, K., Suzuki, K. T. and Nozoe, S., "The structure and the chemistry of siccanin and related compounds", *Tetrahedron* **27**, 6057 (1971).

Högenauer, G.: "Tiamulin and pleuromutilin". In: [3], pp. 344–360.

Höltje, J. V., "Streptomycin uptake via a inducible polyamine transport system in *Escherichia coli*", *Eur. J. Biochem*. **86**, 345–351 (1978).

Höltje, J. V., "Regulation of polyamine and streptomycin transport during stringent and relaxed control in *Escherichia coli*", *J. Bacteriol*. **137**, 661–663 (1979a).

Höltje, J. V., "Induction of streptomycin uptake in resistent strains of *Escherichia coli*", *Antimicrob. Agents & Chemother*. **15**, 177–181 (1979b).

Holz, R. W., "The effects of the polyene antibiotics nystatin and amphothericin B on the lipid membranes", *Ann. N.Y. Acad. Sci*. **235**, 469–479 (1974).

Holz, R. W.: "Nystatin, amphothericin B and filipin". In: [4], pp. 313–340.

Hopwood, D. A., "Genetics of antibiotic production by Actinomycetes", *J. Nat. Products* **42**, 596–602 (1979).

Horii, S. and Kameda, Y., "Structure of the antibiotic validamycin A", *J. Chem. Soc. Chem. Commun*. **1972**, 747.

Horii, S., Iwasa, T. and Kameda, Y., "Studies on validamycins, new antibiotics. Degradation studies", *J. Antibiot*. **24**, 57–58 (1971a).

Horii, S., Iwasa, T., Mizuta, E. and Kameda, Y., "Studies on validamycins, new antibiotics", *J. Antibiot*. **24**, 59–63 (1971b).

Howarth, T. T., Brown, A. G., Stirling and King, T., *J. Chem. Soc. Chem. Commun*. **1976**, 266–267.

Huber, F. M.: "Griseofulvin". In: [1], pp. 606–613.

Huber, G.: "Moenomycin and related phosphorus-containing antibiotics". In: [3], pp. 135–153.

Hunter, F. E. and Schwartz, L. S.: "Gramicidins". In: [2], pp. 642–648.

Hunter, F. E. and Schwartz, L. S.: "Tyrocidines and gramicidin S". In: [2], pp. 636–641.

Ishibashi, K., "Siccanin, a new antifungal antibiotic produced by *Helminthosporium siccane*", *J. Antibiot.* **15**, 161–167 (1962).

Isono, K. and Suzuki, S., "The polyoxines: pyrimidine nucleoside peptide antibiotics inhibiting fungal cell wall biosynthesis", *Heterocycles* **13**, 333–351 (1979).

Iwasa, T., Higshide, E., Yamamoto, H. and Shibata, M., "Studies on validamycins, new antibiotics. II.", *Antibiot.* **24**, 107–114 (1971a).

Iwasa, T., Kameda, Y., Asai, M. et al., "Studies on validamycins, new antibiotics. IV.", *Antibiot.* **24**, 119–123 (1971b).

Iwasa, T., Yamamoto, H. and Shibata, M., "Studies on validamycins, new antibiotics. I.", *J. Antibiot.* **23**, 595–602 (1970).

Izumiya, N., Kato, T., Aoyagi, H. et al.: *Synthetic Aspects of Biologically Active Cyclic Peptides. Gramicidin S and Tyrocidines.* J. Wiley & Sons, New York 1979.

Jefferys, E. G., "The gibberellin fermentation", *Adv. Appl. Microbiol.* **13**, 283–316 (1970).

Jordan, D. C. and Reynolds, P. E.: "Vancomycin". In: [1], pp. 704–718.

Jung, A. F., Pilgrim, W. R., Poyser, J. P. and Siret, P. J., "The chemistry and antimicrobial activity of new synthetic β-lactam antibiotics", *Top. Antibiot. Chem.* **4**, 1–278 (1980).

Kahan, F. M., Kahan, J. S., Cassidy, P. J. and Kropp, H., "The mechanism of action of fosfomycin", *Ann. N.Y. Acad. Sci.* **235**, 364–386 (1974).

Kahan, J. S., Kahan, F. M., Goegelman, R. et al., "Thienamycin, a new β-lactam antibiotic. Discovery, taxonomy, isolation and physical properties", *J. Antibiot.* **32**, 1–12 (1979).

Kahan, J. S., Kahan, F. M., Stapley, E. O. et al., U.S. Pat. 3, 950, 357 (1976).

Kaji, A. and Royoji, M.: "Tetracycline". In: [3], pp. 304–328.

Kamata, H., Wakagi, S., Fujimoto, Y. et al.: Japan Pat. 8696 (1958a).

Kamata, H., Wakagi, S., Fujimoto, Y. et al., Japan Pat. 5448 (1958b).

Kanzaki, T. and Fujisawa, Y., "Biosynthesis of cephalosporins", *Adv. Appl. Microbiol.* **20**, 159–201 (1976).

Katz, E. and Demain, A. L., "The peptide antibiotics of Bacillus: Chemistry, biogenesis and possible function", *Bacteriol. Rev.* **41**, 449–474 (1977).

Keller-Schierlein, W., "Chemie der Makrolid-Antibiotica", *Fortschr. Chem. Org. Naturst.* **30**, 313–460 (1973).

Keller-Schierlein, W., Prelog, V. and Zähner, H., "Siderochrome (Natürliche Eisen (III)-trihydroxamat-Komplexe)", *Fortschr. Chem. Org. Naturst.* **22**, 279–322 (1964).

Kersten, H. and Kersten, W.: *Inhibitors of Nucleic Acid Synthesis.* Springer-Verlag, Berlin, New York 1974.

Khokhlov, A. S. and Tovarova, I. I.: "Autoregulator from *Streptomyces griseus*". In: Luckner, M. and Schreiber, K. (eds.): *Regulation of Secondary Product and Plant Metabolism.* Pergamon Press, Oxford 1979, pp. 133–145.

Kieslich, K.: *Microbial Transformations of Non-steroid Cyclic Compounds.* Thieme Publ., Stuttgart 1976.

Kitano, K., Nara, K. and Nakao, Y., "Screening for β-lactam antibiotics using a mutant of *Pseudomonas aeruginosa*", *Jap. J. Antibiot. Suppl.* **30**, 239–245 (1977).

Kleiner, E. M., Pliner, S. A., Soifer, V. S. et al., "Structure of A factor, a bioregulator from *Streptomyces griseus*", *Bioorg. Khim.* **2**, 1142–1147 (1976).

Knöll, M. J., Rinehart, K. L., Wiley, P. F. and Li, L. H., "Streptovaricin U, an acyclic ansamycin", *J. Antibiot.* **55**, 249–251 (1980).

Kobel, H. and Sanglier, J. J.: "Formation of ergotoxine alkaloids by fermentation and attempts to control their biosynthesis". In: [5], pp. 233–242.

Kominek, L. A. and Sebek, O. K., "Biosynthesis of novobiocin and related coumarin antibiotics", *Dev. Ind. Microbiol.* **15**, 60–69 (1974).

Kondo, S., Iinuma, K., Naganawa, H. et al., "Structural studies on destomycin A and B", *J. Antibiot.* **28**, 79–82 (1975).

Kondo, S., Sezaki, M., Koike, M. and Akita, E., "Destomycin A. The acid hydrolysis and the partial structure", *J. Antibiot.* **18**, 192–194 (1965b).

Kondo, S., Sezaki, M., Koike, M. et al., "Destomycin A and B, two new antibiotics produced by a streptomycete", *J. Antibiot.* **18**, 38–42 (1965a).

Korst, J. J., Johnston, J. D., Butler, K. et al., "The total synthesis of dl-1-demethyl-6-deoxy-tetracycline", *J. Am. Chem. Soc.* **90**, 439–457 (1968).

Korzybski, T., Kowszyk-Gindifer, Z. and Kurylowicz, W.: *Antibiotics I–III.* Am. Soc. Microbiol., Washington 1978.

Kurita, M., Jomon, K., Komori, T. et al., "Isolation and characterization of nocardicin B", *J. Antibiot.* **29**, 1243–1245 (1976).

Leben, C. and Keitt, G. W., "The effect of an antibiotic substance on apple leaf infection by *Venturia inequalis*", *Phytopathology* **37**, 14 (1947).

Lennon, R. E. and Vezina, C., "Antimycin A, a piscidal antibiotic", *Adv. Appl. Microbiol.* **16**, 56–96 (1973).

Lipinska, E.: "Nisin and its application". In: Woodbine, M. (ed.): *Antibiotics and Antibiosis in Agriculture.* Butterworth, London 1977, pp. 103–130.

McCormick, J. R. D.: "Tetracyclines". In: [2a], pp. 113–122.

Maeda, K., Takahashi, S., Sezaki, M. et al., "Isolation and structure of a β-lactam inhibitor from Streptomyces", *J. Antibiot.* **30**, 770–772 (1977).

Majer, J. P.: "Macrolide antibiotics". In: [7], pp. 273–308.

Malik, V. S., "Chloramphenicol", *Adv. Appl. Microbiol.* **15**, 297–336 (1972).

Mann, R. L. and Bromer, W. W., "The isolation of a second antibiotic from *Streptomyces hygroscopicus*", *J. Am. Chem. Soc.* **80**, 2714 (1958).

Maramatsu, I., Hikawa, B., Hagitani, A. and Miyairi, N., "Quinoline derivatives as degradation products from the antibiotic thiopeptin B", *J. Antibiot.* **25**, 537–538 (1972).

Maramatsu, I., Motoki, Y., Aoyama, M. and Suzuki, H., "Amino acids and derivatives of thiazole-4-carboxylic acid as constituents of thiopeptin B", *J. Antibiot.* **30**, 383–387 (1977).

Marquez, J. A. and Kershner, A.: "2-Deoxystreptamine-containing antibiotics". In: [7], pp. 159–214.

Masamune, S., Bates, G. S. and Corcoran, J. W., "Makrolide, neuere Fortschritte ihrer Chemie und Biochemie", *Angew. Chem.* **89**, 602–624 (1977).

Matsuhashi, M., Ohara, I. and Yoshiyama, Y., "Inhibition of the bacterial cell wall synthesis in vitro by enduracidin, a new polypeptide antibiotic", *Agric. Biol. Chem.* **33**, 134 (1969).

Mattick, A. T. R. and Hirsch, A., "A powerful inhibitory substance produced by group N. streptococci", *Nature,* **154**, 551 (1944).

Mauger, A. and Katz, E.: "Actinomycins". In: [7], pp. 1–38.

Meienhofer, J. and Atherton, E., "Structure-activity relationships in the actinomycins", *Adv. Appl. Microbiol.* **16**, 203–300 (1973).

Merck & Co.: Belg. Pat. 848, 349 (1977).

Miller, A. K., Celozzi, E., Kong, Y. et al., "Cefoxitin, a semisynthetic cephamycin antibiotic: in vivo evaluation", *Antimicrob. Agents & Chemother.* **5**, 33–37 (1974).

Miller, A. K., Celozzi, E., Kong, Y. et al., "Cephamycins, a new family of β-lactam antibiotics. IV.", *Antimicrob. Agents & Chemother.* **2**, 287 (1972a).

Miller, A. K., Celozzi, E., Pelak, B. A. et al., "Cephamycins, a new family of β-lactam antibiotics. III.", *Antimicrob. Agents & Chemother.* **2**, 281 (1972b).

Miller, T. W., Chaiet, L., Cole, D. J. et al., "Avermectins, new family of potent antihelmintic agents", *Antimicrob. Agents & Chemother.* **15**, 368–371 (1979).

Mitscher, L. A., Juvekar, J. V., Rosenbrook, W. et al., "Structure of chelocardin, a novel tetracycline antibiotic", *J. Am. Chem. Soc.* **92**, 6070 (1970).

Mitscher, L. A., Rosenbrook, W., Andres, W. W. et al., "Structure of chelocardin, a novel tetracycline antibiotic", *Antimicrob. Agents & Chemother.*, 38 (1970).

Miyairi, N., Miyoshi, T., Aoki, H. et al., "Studies on thiopeptin antibiotics. I.", *J. Antibiot.* **23**, 113–119 (1970).

Mizuno, K., Asai, M., Horii, S. et al., "Chemistry of enduracidins, new antibiotics", *Antimicrob. Agents & Chemother.* **1970**, 1 (1971).

Mizuno, N. S.: "Streptonigrin". In: [4], pp. 372–384.

Moore, B. A., Jevons, S. and Brammer, K. W., "Peptidoglycan transpeptidase inhibition in *Pseudomonas aeruginosa* and *Escherichia coli* by penicillins and cephalosporins", *Antimicrob. Agents & Chemother.* **15**, 513–517 (1979).

Morin, B. R. and Gorman, M. (eds.): *Chemistry and*

Biology of β-Lactam Antibiotics, Vol. 1–3. Academic Press, London 1982.

Mukherjee, B. B. and Lee, B. K.: "Penicillins and related antibiotics". In: [7], pp. 387–414.

Muroi, M., Haibara, K., Asai, M. and Kishi, T., "The structure of macbecin I and II, new antitumor antibiotics", *Tetrahedron Lett.* **1980,** 309–312 (1980a).

Muroi, M., Izawa, M., Kosai, Y. and Asai, M., "Macbecins I and II, new antitumor antibiotics. II.", *J. Antibiot.* **33,** 205–212 (1980b).

Muxfeldt, H. and Rogalski, W., "A total synthesis of (±)-6-deoxy-6-demethyl-tetracycline", *J. Am. Chem. Soc.* **87,** 933–934 (1965).

Nakano, H., Umio, S., Kariyone, K. et al., "Total syntheses of pyrrolnitrin, a new antibiotic", *Tetrahedron Lett.* **1966,** 737.

Nakatsuka, S., Tanino, H. and Kishi, Y., "Biogenetic-type synthesis of penicillin-cephalosporin antibiotics. I.", *J. Am. Chem. Soc.* **97,** 5008–5010 (1975a).

Nakatsuka, S., Tanino, H. and Kishi, Y., "Biogenetic-type synthesis of penicillin-cephalosporin-antibiotics. II.", *J. Am. Chem. Soc.* **97,** 5010–5012 (1975b).

Nara, T., "Aminoglycoside antibiotics", *Ann. Rep. Ferment. Processes* **1,** 299–326 (1977); *Ann. Rep. Ferment. Processes* **2,** 223–266 (1978).

Neidle, S., "Interactions of daunomycin and related antibiotics with biological receptors", *Top. Antibiot. Chem.* **2,** 230–278 (1978).

Neidleman, S.: "Tetracyclines". In: [7], pp. 715–760.

Neuss, N., Koch, F. K., Molloy, B. B. et al., "Structure of hygromycin B, an antibiotic from *Streptomyces hygroscopicus*", *Helv. Chim. Acta* **53,** 2314–2319 (1970).

Nomoto, S., Teshima, T., Wakamiya, T. and Shiba, T., "The revised structure of capreomycin", *J. Antibiot.* **30,** 955–959 (1977).

Nose, K. and Ende, A., "Mode of action of the antibiotic siccanin on intact cells and mitochondria of *Trichophyton mentagrophytes*", *J. Bacteriol.* **105,** 176 (1971).

Nüesch, J., Hinnen, A., Liersch, M. and Treichler, H. J., "A biochemical and genetical approach to the biosynthesis of cephalosporin C", *Proc. Int. Symp. Genet. Ind. Microorg. 2nd* **1974,** 451–472 (Pub. 1976).

Nüesch, J., "Contribution of genetics to the biosynthesis of antibiotics", *Genet. Ind. Microorg. Proc. Int. Symp.* 3rd **1978,** 77–82 (Pub. 1979).

Okamura, K., Hirata, S., Okamura, Y. et al., "PS-5, a new β-lactam antibiotic from Streptomyces", *J. Antibiot.* **31,** 480–482 (1978).

Oki, T., "New anthracycline antibiotics", *Jap. J. Antibiot. Suppl.* **30,** 70–84 (1977).

Oki, T. and Yoshimoto, A., "Antitumor Antibiotics", *Annu. Rep. Ferment. Processes* **3,** 215–251 (1979).

Oliver, T. J., Prokop, J. F., Bower, R. R. and Otto, R. H., "Chelocardin, a new broad-spectrum antibiotic. I.", *Antimicrob. Agents & Chemother.,* 583 (1962).

Omura, S., Iwai, Y., Takahashi, Y. et al., "Herbimycin, a new antibiotic produced by a strain of Streptomyces", *J. Antibiot.* **32,** 255–261 (1979).

Omura, S., Tanaka, H., Koyama, Y. et al., "Nanaomycins A and B, new antibiotics produced by a strain of Streptomyces", *J. Antibiot.* **27,** 363–365 (1974).

Onda, M., Konda, Y., Noguchi, A. et al., "Revised structure for the naphthalenecarboxylic acid from carcinophylin", *J. Antibiot.* **22,** 42–44 (1969).

Onda, M., Konda, Y., Omura, S. and Hata, T., "A new amino acid and its derivative from carcinophylin", *Chem. Pharm. Bull.* **19,** 2013 (1971).

Onishi, H., Daoust, D. R., Zimmermann, S. et al., "Cefoxitin a semisynthetic cephamycin antibiotic: resistance to β-lactamase inactivation", *Antimicrob. Agents & Chemother.* **5,** 38 (1974).

O'Sullivan, J., Apli, R. T., Stevens, C. M. and Abraham, E. P., „Biosynthesis of a 7-α-methoxycephalosporin. Incorporation of molecular oxygen", *Biochem. J.* **179,** 47–52 (1979c).

O'Sullivan, J., Bleaney, R. C., Huddelston, J. A. and Abraham, E. P., "Incorporation of ^{3}H from δ-(L-α-amino[4,5-^{3}H]adipyl)-L-cysteinyl-D-[4,4-^{3}H]valine into isopenicillin N", *Biochem. J.* **184,** 421–426 (1979a).

O'Sullivan, J., Huddleston, J. A. and Abraham, E. P.: "Biosynthesis of penicillins and cephalosporins in cell-free system". Meeting Royal Soc. 2.–3. May 1979b.

Pan Labs/Sanraku-Ocean., Belg. Pat. 865, 578 (1978).

Paulus, H.: "Polymyxins". In: [2a], pp. 254–267.

Philip, J. E., Schenk, J. R. and Hargie, M. P., "Ristocetin A and B, two new antibiotics, Isolation and properties", *Antibiot. Annu.* **1956/57,** 699.

Pierce, K. E.: "Structure-activity relationships of semisynthetic penicillins". In: [6], pp. 1–86.

Pinkerton, M., Steinrauf, L. K. and Dawkins, P., "The molecular structure and some transport properties of valinomycin", *Biochem. Biophys. Res. Commun.* **35,** 512 (1969).

Poralla, K.: "Borrelidin". In: [1], pp. 365–369.

Prelog, W. and Oppolzer, W., "Ansamycine, eine neuartige Klasse von mikrobiellen Stoffwechsel-produkten", *Helv. Chim. Acta* **56,** 2279–2287 (1973).

Puls, W., Keup, U., Krause, H. P. et al., "Glucosidase inhibition", *Naturwissenschaften* **64,** 536–537 (1977).

Raab, W.: *Natamycin (Pimaricin).* Thieme Verlag, Stuttgart 1972.

Reading, C. and Cole, M., "Clavulanic acid: a β-lactamase inhibiting β-lactam from *Streptomyces clavuligerus*", *Antimicrob. Agents & Chemother.* **11,** 852–864 (1977).

Reden, J. and Dürckheimer, W., "Aminoglycoside antibiotics", *Top. Curr. Chem.* **83,** 105–170 (1979).

Rhodes, A.: Griseofulvin, "Production and biosynthesis", *Prog. Ind. Microbiol.* **4,** 165–188 (1963).

Rinehart, K. L., "Biosynthesis and mutasynthesis of aminocyclitol antibiotics", *Jap. J. Antibiot. Suppl.* **32,** 32–46 (1979).

Rinehart, K. L. and Shield, L. S., "Chemistry of the ansamycin antibiotics", *Prog. Chem. Org. Nat. Prod.* **33,** 231–307 (1976).

Rinehart, K. L. and Stroshane, R. M., "Biosynthesis of aminocyclitol antibiotics", *J. Antibiot.* **29,** 319–353 (1976).

Ryan, M. J.: "Novobiocin and coumermycin". In: [3], pp. 214–234.

Sasaki, K., Rinehart, K. L., Slomp, G. et al., "Geldanamycin. I.", *J. Am. Chem. Soc.* **92,** 7591–7593 (1970).

Sassiver, M. L. and Lewis, A.: "Structure activity relationships among semisynthetic cephalosporins". In: [6], pp. 87–160.

Sawada, Y., Hunt, N. A. and Demain, A. L., "Further studies on microbiological ring-expansion of penicillin", *J. Antibiot.* **32,** 1303–1310 (1979).

Schatz, A., Bugie, E. and Waksman, S. A., "Strepto-mycin, a substance exhibiting antibiotic activity against gram-positive and gram-negative bacteria", *Proc. Soc. Exp. Biol. Med.* **55,** 66 (1944).

Schindler, P. W. and Scrutton, M. C.: Mode of action of the macrolide-type antibiotic chlorothricin. II. Eur. J. Biochem. **55,** 543–553 (1975).

Schindler, P. W. and Zähner, H., "Mode of action of the macrolide-type antibiotic chlorothricin. I.", *Eur. J. Biochem.* **39,** 591–600 (1973).

Schmidt, D. D., Frommer, W., Junge, B. et al., "α-Glucosidase inhibitors", *Naturwissenschaften* **64,** 535–536 (1977).

Sebek, O. K.: "Polymyxins and circulin". In: [2], pp. 142–152.

Sehgal, S. N., Saucier, R. and C. Vezina, "Antimycin. II.", *J. Antibiot.* **29,** 265–274 (1976).

Sheehan, H. C. and Henry-Logan, K. R., "The total and partial general synthesis of the penicillin", *J. Am. Chem. Soc.* **84,** 2983–2990 (1962).

Shemyakin, M. M., Aldanova, N. A., Vinogradova, E. I. and Feigina, M. Yu., "The structure and total synthesis of valinomycin", *Tetrahedron Lett.* **1963,** 1921.

Shiba, T., Nomoto, S., Teshima, T. and Wakamiya, T., "Revised structure and total synthesis of capreomycin", *Tetrahedron Lett.* **1976,** 3907.

Shiba, T., Ukita, T., Mizuno, K. et al., "Total synthesis of L-capreomycidine", *Tetrahedron Lett.* **1977,** 2681.

Sinclair, A. C., Schenck, J. R., Post, G. G. et al., "Chelocardin, a new broad spectrum antibiotic. II.", *Antimicrob. Agents & Chemother.,* 592 (1962).

Sisler, H. D. and Siegel, M. R., "Cycloheximid and other glutarimide antibiotics". In: [2], pp. 283–307.

Smith, C. G. and Hinman, J. W., "Chloramphenicol", *Prog. Ind. Microbiol.* **4,** 137–164 (1963).

Smith, G. A., Smith, K. A. and Williams, D. H., "Structural studies on the antibiotics vancomycin", *J. Chem. Soc. Perkin Trans. I* **1975,** 2108.

Spalla, C. and Marnati, M. P.: "Genetic aspects of the formation of ergot alkaloids". In: [5], pp. 219–232.

Spratt, B. G., "The mechanism of action of penicillin", *Sci. Prog. Oxford* **65,** 101–128 (1978).

Stadtler, P. A. and Stütz, P.: In: Manske, R. H. F. (ed.): *The Alkaloids,* Vol. **15.** Academic Press, New York 1975, pp. 1–40.

Stapley, E. O., Hendlin, D., Mata, J. M. et al., "Phosphonomycin. I.", *Antimicrob. Agents & Chemother.*, 284 (1969).

Stapley, E. O., Jackson, M., Hernandez, S. et al., "Cephamycins, a new familiy of β-lactam antibiotics. I.", *Antimicrob. Agents & Chemother.* **2**, 122 (1972).

Storm, D. R. and Toscano, W. A.: "Bacitracin". In: [3], pp. 1–17.

Suhadolnik, R. J.: *Nucleosides as Biological Probes.* J. Wiley & Sons, New York 1979.

Suhadolnik, R. J., "Naturally occuring nucleoside and nucleotide antibiotics", *Prog. Nucleic Acid Res. Molec. Biol.* **22**, 193–291 (1979).

Suhara, Y., Maeda, K., Umezawa, H. and Ohno, M., "Chemical studies on kasugamycin. V.", *Tetrahedron Lett.* **1966**, 1239–1244.

Suhara, Y., Sasaki, F., Koyama, G. et al., "The total synthesis of kasugamycin", *J. Am. Chem. Soc.* **94**, 6501 (1972).

Suzuki, K., Nawata, Y. and Ando, K., "Tetranactin, a new miticidal antibiotic. V.", *J. Antibiot.* **24**, 675–679 (1971).

Suzuki, S., Nakamura, G., Okuma, K. and Tomyama, Y., "Cellocidin, a new antibiotic", *J. Antibiot.* **11**, 81–83 (1958).

Suzuki, S. and Okuma, K., "The structure of cellocidin", *J. Antibiot.* **11**, 84–86 (1958).

Swartz, R., "The use of economic analysis of penicillin G manufacturing costs in establishing priorities for fermentation process improvement", *Ann. Rep. Ferment. Proc.* **3**, 75–110 (1979).

Takeuchi, S. and Yonehara, H., "Stereochemical characterization of variotin as deduced from the nuclear Overhauser effect in the NMR Spectra", *J. Antibiot.* **22**, 179–180 (1969).

Takhashi, T., Kato, K., Yamazaki, Y., "Synthesis of cephalosporins and penicillins by enzymatic acylation", *Jap. J. Antibiot. Suppl.* **30**, 231–235 (1977).

Tanabe, M. and Seto, S., "Biosynthesis of variotin", *Biochim. Biophys. Acta* **208**, 151 (1970).

Tanaka, N.: "Mikamycin". In: [1], pp. 487–497.

Tanaka, H., Koyama, Y., Awaya, J. et al., "Nanaomycins, new antibiotics produced by a strain of Streptomyces. I.", *J. Antibiot.* **28**, 860–867 (1975a).

Tanaka, H., Koyama, Y., Nagai, T. et al., "Nanaomycins, new antibiotics produced by a strain of Streptomyces. II.", *J. Antibiot.* **28**, 868–875 (1975b).

Tanaka, H., Marumo, H., Nagai, T. et al., "Nanaomycins, new antibiotics produced by a strain of Streptomyces. III.", *J. Antibiot.* **28**, 925–930 (1975c).

Tanaka, N.: "Fusidic acid". In: [1], pp. 436–447.

Tanaka, N.: "Bicyclomycin". In: [3], pp. 18–25.

Tanaka, W., "Development of new bleomycins with potential clinical utility", *Jap. J. Antibiot. Suppl.* **30**, 41–48 (1977).

Tanida, S., Hasegawa, T., Hatano, K. et al., "Ansamitocins, maytansinoid antitumor antibiotics", *J. Antibiot.* **33**, 192–198 (1980).

Tanida, S., Hasegawa, T. and Higashide, E., "Macbecins I and II, new antitumor antibiotics. I.", *J. Antibiot.* **33**, 199–204 (1980).

Tarbell, D. S., Carman, R. M., Chapman, D. D. et al., "The chemistry of fumagillin", *J. Am. Chem. Soc.* **83**, 3096 (1961).

Tarbell, D. S., Carman, R. M., Chapman, D. D. et al., "The structure of fumagillin", *J. Am. Chem. Soc.* **82**, 1005 (1960).

Testa, R. and Tilley, B. C., "Biosynthesis of sisomycin and gentamycin", *Jap. J. Antibiotics Suppl.* **32**, 47–59 (1979).

Thompson, R. Q. and Hughes, M. S., "Stendomycin, a new antifungal antibiotic", *J. Antibiot.* **16**, 187–194 (1963).

Tomasz, A., "The mechanism of the irreversible antimicrobial effects of penicillins: How the β-lactam antibiotics kill and lyse bacteria", *Annu. Rev. Microbiol.* **33**, 113–137 (1979).

Traber, R., Kuhn, M., Loosli, H. R. et al., "Neue Cyclopeptide aus *Trichoderma polysporum*", *Helv. Chim. Acta* **60**, 1568–1578 (1977b).

Traber, R., Kuhn, M., Ruegger, A. et al., "Die Struktur von Cyclosporin C", *Helv. Chim. Acta* **60**, 1247–1255 (1977a).

Treichler, H. J., Liersch, M. and Nüesch, J.: "Genetics and biochemistry of cephalosporin biosynthesis". In: [5], pp. 177–200.

Tripathi, R. K. and Gottlieb, D., "Mechanism of action of the antifungal antibiotic pyrrolnitrin", *J. Bacterial.* **100**, 310 (1969).

Umezawa, H., "Studies on bleomycin. Chemistry and biological action", *Biomedicine* **18**, 459–475 (1973).

Umezawa, H., "Studies on aminoglycoside antibiotics: Enzymic mechanism of resistance and genetics. *Jap. J. Antibiot. Suppl.* **32,** 1–14 (1979).

Umezawa, H., Hamada, M., Suhara, Y. et al., "Kasugamycin, a new antibiotic", *Antimicrob. Agents & Chemother.* **1965a,** 753.

Umezawa, H., Ueda, M., Maeda, K. et al., "Production and isolation of a new antibiotic, kanamycin", *J. Antibiot.* **10,** 181–188 (1957).

Umezawa, H., Okami, Y., Hashimoto, T. et al., "A new antibiotic, Kasugamycin", *J. Antibiot.* **18,** 101–103 (1965b).

Umezawa, H. and Takita, T., "The bleomycins: Antitumor copper binding antibiotics", *Struct. Bonding Berlin* **40** (1980).

Umezawa, S.: The chemistry and conformation of aminoglycoside antibiotics". In: Mitsuhashi, S. (ed.): *Drug Action and Drug Resistance,* Vol. **2.** University Park Press, Tokyo 1975, pp. 3–43.

Umezawa, S., Tanaka, Y., Ooka, M. and Shiotsu, "A new antifungal antibiotic, pentamycin", *J. Antibiot.* **11,** 26–29 (1958a).

Umezawa, S., Nakada, S. and Oonuma, H., "Isolation of 2-methyl-2,4,6,8,10-dodecapentaenedial from oxidative degradation of pentamycin", *J. Antibiot.* **11,** 273–274 (1958b).

Vazquez, D., "Inhibitors of protein biosynthesis", *Mol. Biol. Biochem. Biophys.* **30** (1979).

Vézina, C., Boldoc, C., Kudelski, A. and Sehgal, S. N., "Antimycin A fermentation. I.", *J. Antibiot.* **29,** 248–264 (1976).

Vogler, K. and Studer, R. O., "The chemistry of the polymyxin antibiotics", *Experientia* **22,** 345 (1966).

Wagman, G. H. and Weinstein, M. J.: "Griseofulvin". In: [7], pp. 215–230.

Waksman, S. A.: *Actinomycin, Nature, Formation and Activities.* Interscience Publ., New York 1968.

Waksman, S. A. and Lechevalier, H., "Neomycin, a new antibiotic active against streptomycin-resistent bacteria including tuberculosis organisms", *Science* **109,** 305 (1949).

Weber, J. A. and Ott, J. L.: "Structure activity relationships in the cephalosporins". In: [6], pp. 161–238.

Weber, W., Zähner, H., Damberg, M., Russ, P. and Zeeck, A., "Ansatrienin A u. B", *Zentralbl. Bakteriol. Parasitenk. Infektionskr. Hyg. Abt. 1 Orig.* 122–139, 1981.

Wehrli, W., "Ansamycins, chemistry, biosynthesis and biological activity", *Top. Curr. Chem.* **72,** 21–49 (1977).

Weinstein, M. J., Luedemann, G. M., Oden, E. M. et al., "Gentamycin, a new antibiotic complex from Micromonospora", *J. Med. Chem.* **6,** 463 (1963).

Westley, J. W., "Polyether antibiotics: Versatile carboxylic acid ionophores, produced by Streptomyces", *Adv. Appl. Microbiol.* **22,** 177–223 (1977).

Whiffen, A. J., Bohonos, N. and Emerson, R. I., "The production of an antifungal antibiotic by *Streptomyces griseus*", *J. Bacteriol.* **52,** 610–611 (1946).

Whitefield, G. B., "Biochemical modification of antibiotics", *Proc. Intersec. Congr. of IAMS, Tokyo 1974,* **3,** 472–482.

Williams, D. H. and Kalman, J. R., "Structural and mode of action on the antibiotic vancomycin", *J. Am. Chem. Soc.* **99,** 2768 (1977).

Wipf, H. K., Oliver, A. and Simon, W., "Mechanismus und Selektivität des Alkali-Ionentransportes in Modell-Membranen in Gegenwart des Antibioticums Valinomycin", *Helv. Chim. Acta* **53,** 1605–1608 (1970).

Wipf, K. H. and Simon, W., "Modelle für Kopplungsmechanismus und Träger-induzierten Alkaliionentransport in Mitochondrienmembranen", *Helv. Chim. Acta* **53,** 1732–1740 (1970).

Witteler, F. J., Welzel, P., Duddeck, H. et al., "Zur Struktur des Antibiotikums Moenomycin A", *Tetrahedron Lett.* **1979,** 3493.

Woodward, R. B., "Struktur und Biogenese der Makrolide. Eine neue Klasse von Naturstoffen", *Angew. Chem.* **69,** 50 (1957).

Woodward, R. B., Heusler, K., Gosteli, J. et al., "The total synthesis of cephalosporin C", *J. Am. Chem. Soc.* **88,** 852–853 (1966).

Yonehara, H., Takeuchi, S., Umezawa, H. and Sumiki, Y., "Variotin, a new antifungal antibiotic produced by *Paecilomyces varioti* Bainier var. *antibioticus*.", *J. Antibiot.* **12,** 109–110 (1959).

Chapter 14

Biotransformations

Hans Georg W. Leuenberger and Klaus Kieslich

14.1   Introduction

With the aid of a multiplicity of enzymes, microorganisms are capable of performing a large number of chemical reactions that are necessary for the growth and maintenance of the cell (see Chapters 3 and 4). With their constitutive enzymes or those that can be induced by the substrate, microorganisms can catalyze the individual steps of complex reaction sequences and can thus be used for the catalysis of desired reaction steps on substances supplied.

By **biotransformations** are understood chemical transformations which are catalyzed by microorganisms or their enzymes. Innumerable microbiologically catalyzed reactions of the most diverse types (oxidation, reduction, hydrolysis, C-C linkage, isomerization, introduction of hetero functions) have been described and reviewed in the literature (Capek et al., 1966; Iizuka and Naito, 1967; Fonken and Johnson, 1972; Kieslich, 1976; Sebek and Kieslich, 1977; Kieslich and Sebek, 1980). **Enzymatically** catalyzed reactions may be superior to those catalyzed **chemically** in relation to the following properties:

a) **Reaction specificity:** the catalytic activity of an enzyme is, as a rule, limited to one type of reaction, so that no side reactions take place.

b) **Regiospecificity:** enzyme reactions generally take place specifically in relation to the position of the reaction in the substrate molecule.

c) **Stereospecificity:** enzymes distinguish between the enantiomers of a racemic mixture and therefore, in many cases, transform only one enantiomeric form exclusively or at least preferentially. If in an enzymatic reaction a new center of asymmetry arises, as a rule the product is optically active, i.e., one of the possible enantiomers is formed exclusively or at least preferentially.

d) **Mild reaction conditions:** enzyme reactions take place in aqueous solutions at low temperatures ($<40\,°C$) and at pH values in the neighbourhood of 7.

e) **Lowering of the activation energy:** in the enzyme-substrate complex, the activation energy can be lowered to such an extent that even certain non-activated positions in the substrate molecule are accessible to selective transformation under mild reaction conditions.

Because of these favorable properties, biotransformations are opening up the following operations, given as examples, which are possible by chemical methods only via complicated roundabout pathways or not at all:

- selective functionalization of nonactivated C atoms;

- transformation of one functional group among several groups of similar reactivity;

- resolution of racemates by the selective transformation of one enantiomer; and

- introduction of a center of asymmetry.

14.2   Methods

14.2.1   General

The **working technique** used in biotransformations has recently been described in detail by Perlman (1976). Usually, a microorganism suitable for a desired biotransformation must be sought in a laborious **screening** process. In this process, use is made of pure cultures of microorganisms which have been either isolated from soil samples or have been obtained from public collections (see Appendix, p. 719). The microorganisms are cultivated on a nutrient medium corresponding to their demands by the usual microbiological technique (Perlman, 1976).

Another possibility for **finding microorganisms** with desired enzymatic activity is based on the enrichment of those microorganisms from soil samples which are capable of growing on the substrate to be transformed as the sole source of carbon. After a treatment with mutagenic agents, for example, those mutants are selected by replica plating which can grow on common sources of carbon C but no longer on the substrate to be transformed. In these mutants, the substrate metabolism is blocked. A check is now made as to whether the first steps in the degradation of the substrate still takes place and whether perhaps the desired transformation product is accumulated.

For biotransformation, the substance to be transformed is added either as a pure substance or as a concentrated solution to a solvent with the lowest possible toxicity (water, ethanol, acetone, dimethyl sulfoxide). Various techniques can be used for this purpose: the transformation can be carried out with **growing** or **resting cells** or with **spores**. In special cases, working with isolated enzymes is necessary in order to prevent following reactions due to other enzymes. Finally, the **immobilization** of cells or enzymes makes the repeated use or continuous use of the biocatalyst possible. In each case, after the addition of the substrate, incubation is carried out until the maximum conversion has been achieved. The course of the reaction is followed analytically.

14.2.2 Transformation Techniques

Biotransformation by Growing Cells

The cells are inoculated into a medium permitting the optimum growth and are incubated under suitable conditions (pH, pO_2, temperature). The substrate to be transformed is added during the growth phase. The most favorable moment for the addition of the substrate for the course of the transformation must be determined experimentally. This method is very simple to carry out and is often used in screening for microorganisms with the desired enzymatic activity. It includes the possibility of inducing the desired enzymatic activity by growth in the presence of the substrate. However, good conversions are often achieved only in the stationary phase.

Biotransformation by Stationary Cells

The biomass is cultivated in an optimized growth medium and is harvested by centrifugation or filtration. Then the cells are resuspended in a "**transformation medium**" and the substrate is added. As the transformation medium it is sufficient to use a buffer with the optimum pH. In order to retain viability as long as possible, it is often advantageous to feed certain nutrients, such as glucose, as readily metabolizable sources of energy. In many cases, the desired enzymatic activity can be enhanced by adding small amounts of substrate or related substances to the growth medium even during the initial cultivation. This method has the advantages that growth and biotransformation can take place independently of one another, growth-inhibiting effects of the substrate or product are eliminated, the cell concentration can be adjusted as desired at the beginning of the transformation experiment, the risk of an interfering foreign infection in the transformation medium is greatly reduced, and the isolation of the product from the simple transformation medium is facilitated.

Biotransformation with Spores

Microorganisms capable of sporulation are cultivated under conditions promoting good spore formation. The spores are separated from the mycelium and, in the form of a paste, can be stored in the cooled state for a long time. When required, the biotransformations are carried out by spores in a buffered medium. A comprehensive review of the production of spores and their uses in the field of biotransformations has been given by Vezina et al. (1968). The advantage of the use of spores is their high stability (keepability, repeated use as catalyst).

Biotransformations with Immobilized Cells

An important recent development is the use of microorganisms that are immobilized in an inert **carrier material.** The methods of immobilization and uses have been described in detail in several recent review articles (Abbott, 1978; Chibata et al., 1979; Larsson et al., 1979; Cheetham, 1980). The most frequently used immobilization technique is the inclusion of the microorganisms in a cross-linked polymer permeable to substrate and product, especially **polyacrylamide gel, alginate, κ-carrageenan** or **cellulose.** The fundamental advantage of the use of immobilized cells is the possibility of being easily able to recover and reuse the biocatalyst or even, with the retention of the catalyst in the reaction vessel, to be able to perform continuous biotransformations. In this way, the transformation capacity of the cells is utilized in the optimum manner. Furthermore, as a rule, immobilization considerably enhances the stability of the cells. The highest half-life of an immobilized cell preparation observed so far (aspartase activity of *Escherichia coli* cells immobilized in κ-carrageenan) amounted to almost two years (Sato et al., 1979). On the other hand, however, the enzymatic activity of immobilized cells is usually less than that of the free cells because of a more difficult diffusion situation for substrate and product or because of damage to the cells during immobilization. This **loss of activity** can be compensated by **high cell densities.** Wada et al. (1979) have shown that cells immobilized in κ-carrageenan are capable of proliferation. If the necessary nutrients are added, on the surface of the par-

ticles where the most favorable conditions of growth prevail a thick layer of cells forms which act as efficient biocatalysts for various processes over long periods. The use of immobilized fungal spores for biotransformations has been reported by Johnson and Ciegler (1969).

Biotransformations with Isolated and Immobilized Enzymes

In cases where subsequent or side reactions occur when whole cells are used or where the transport of the substrate is greatly hindered by the membrane barrier, it is necessary to work with isolated enzymes. In the case of reactions that depend on **cofactors,** provision must be made simultaneously for the recycling of the coenzyme. The well-developed technique of enzyme immobilization permits the performance of continuous processes (see Chapter 12).

14.3   Amino Acids

The biotechnical manufacture of amino acids plays an important role, since these structural units of proteins are important as additives to foodstuffs and fodders. Fields of application in medicine, as substances imparting aroma, and in cosmetics are also important.

Today, most natural amino acids can be produced industrially by the **hydrolysis of proteins,** by chemical **synthesis,** or **biosynthetically** by microorganisms. In many cases, a **combination** of chemical synthesis with a biotransformation is advantageous. Various L-amino acids can in fact be prepared from **synthetically available achiral precursors** if the reaction step that is decisive for the introduction of optical activity is brought about by microorganisms or their enzymes. This is done either by the enantioselective hydrolysis of racemic amino acid derivatives,

Table 14-1. Production of L-Amino Acids by the Enantioselective Hydrolysis of Racemic Precursors.

Amino acid	Biotransformation	Microorganism (enzyme)	Concentration of product in g/L (yield)	Process	Literature
Various L-amino acids	Resolution of racemates by enantioselective hydrolysis of DL-acyl amino acids	*Aspergillus oryzae* (L-aminoacylase)	L-Ala.[1]: 6.2 (69.7%) L-Met: 12.0 (80.5%) L-Phe: 14.1 (85.5%) L-Trp: 14.7 (72.0%) L-Val: 9.5 (81.2%)	Continuous flow through a column with L-aminoacylase immobilized on DEAE-Sephadex. ($S^{[2]}$ = 1.2 to 2.8/h)	Chibata et al., 1976
L-Lysine	Enantioselective hydrolysis of DL-α-amino-ε-caprolactam. Racemization of the D form	*Cryptococcus laurentii* (L-α-aminolactam hydrolase) *Achromobacter obae* (D-α-aminolactam racemase)	>100.0 (99.8%)	Batch process using both microorganisms	Fukumura, 1977b
L-Glutamic acid	DL-Hydantoin-5-propionic acid $+ 2\,H_2O \rightarrow$ L-Glu $+ NH_3 + CO_2$	*Bacillus brevis* (hydantoinase)	7.7 (90.0%)	Batch process. Spontaneous racemization of the hydantoin under fermentation conditions	Tsugawa et al., 1966
L-Cysteine	DL-2-aminothiazoline-4-carboxylic acid $+ 2\,H_2O \rightarrow$ L-cysteine $+ NH_3 + CO_2$	*Pseudomonas* sp. (L-hydrolase and D-racemase)	31.4 (95.0%)	Simultaneous hydrolysis of the L-form and racemization of the D-form	Sano et al., 1977b

[1] L-Ala = L-alanine; L-Met = L-methionine; L-Phe = L-phenylalanine; L-Trp = L-tryptophan; L-Val = L-valine.
[2] S = Flow rate: volume of substrate solution per unit volume of immobilized biocatalyst per hour.

by asymmetric synthesis, or by degradation to L-amino acids from suitable precursors (see Tables 14-1, 14-2, and 14-3).

14.3.1 Resolution of Racemates by Enantioselective Hydrolysis

L-Aminoacylase

Immobilized L-aminoacylase (EC 3.5.1.14) from *Aspergillus oryzae* is used for the enantioselective hydrolysis of acyl-DL-amino acids (Tosa et al., 1967). This enzyme selectively hydrolyzes the L-enantiomer of the substrate. The liberated L-amino acid can easily be separated from the acyl-D-amino acid because of their different solubilities. The recovered acyl-D-amino acid can be racemized and the process be repeated (Fig. 14-1).

This process has been used for the industrial manufacture of several amino acids since 1969 and was probably the first technical application of an immobilized enzyme (Chibata et al., 1972). L-Alanine, L-methionine, L-phenylalanine, L-tryptophan, and L-valine can be prepared continuously from the racemic acetyl derivatives in a 1000 L enzyme reactor containing *Aspergillus oryzae* L-aminoacylase immobilized on DEAE-Sephadex (DEAE = diethylaminoethyl) (see Table 14-1) (Chibata et al., 1976). After an operating time of 32 days, in all cases at least 60% of the original activity remains, and by supplying more L-aminoacylase the column can be regenerated repeatedly

to its original activity. The manufacturing costs can be reduced by 40% in comparison with the batch process using the free enzyme.

A comprehensive study on process development and economic aspects of the manufacture of L-amino acids by free or immobilized L-aminoacylase has recently been published by Wandrey and Flaschel (1979). With experimental figures from the resolution of the DL-methionine racemate, these authors show that the continuous manufacture of L-methionine with a soluble enzyme in a membrane reactor is superior from the economic point of view to the column reactor with immobilized aminoacylase.

Recently, a D-aminoacylase from *Streptomyces olivaceus* has also been described (Sugie and Suzuki, 1978).

L-Lysine from DL-α-Amino-ε-caprolactam

With the aid of an α-aminolactam hydrolase (EC 3.5.2) various yeasts are capable of converting DL-α-amino-ε-caprolactam, which is readily available synthetically from cyclohexanone, by selective hydrolysis of the L-enantiomer into L-lysine (Fukumura, 1976a, b). On the other hand, selected bacteria, particularly *Achromobacter obae* are capable of racemizing the remaining D-α-amino-ε-caprolactam (Fukumura, 1977a).

Thus, DL-α-Amino-ε-caprolactam can be converted almost quantitatively into L-lysine in an elegant one-stage process (Fig. 14-2) by the simultaneous action of both microorganisms (Fukumura, 1977b).

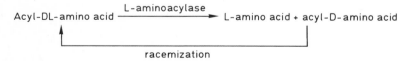

Fig. 14-1. Cleavage of racemates of acyl-DL-amino acids by L-aminoacylase from *Aspergillus oryzae*.

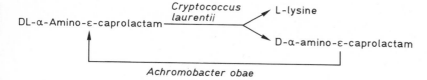

Fig. 14-2. Production of L-lysine from DL-α-amino-ε-caprolactam.

A reaction mixture containing 100 g/L of DL-α-amino-ε-caprolactam and, as biocatalysts, acetone-dried cells of *Cryptococcus laurentii* and lyophilized cells of *Achromobacter obae* yielded L-lysine with a conversion of 99.8%. The L-lysine-HCl isolated from this charge showed an optical purity of 99.5% (Fukumura, 1977b).

neously racemized under the slightly basic fermentation conditions (pH 9; 42 °C) and in this way can also be fed to hydrolysis by the L-specific hydantoinase (Fig. 14-3).

In a similar manner, Sano et al. (1977a) have manufactured L-tryptophan from DL-5-indolyl-methylhydantoin (concentration of the product 7.4 g/L; yield 82%).

Enantioselective Hydrolysis of DL-Hydantoin Compounds

Many microorganisms possess the capacity of liberating L-glutamic acid from DL-hydantoin-5-propionic acid. The highest conversions have been obtained with *Bacillus brevis* (Tsugawa et al., 1966). The hydantoinase is induced by growth in the presence of the substrate. With the aid of this intracellular enantioselective enzyme, *Bacillus brevis* hydrolyzes the L-hydantoin-5-propionic acid exclusively, forming optically pure L-glutamic acid. The D-form of the racemic substrate is sponta-

Enantioselective Hydrolysis of DL-2-Amino-Δ²-thiazoline-4-carboxylic acid

L-Cysteine is formed by many microorganisms from DL-2-amino-Δ²-thiazoline-4-carboxylic acid (DL-ATC). The preferred organism for this biotransformation is a Pseudomonas sp. which, by the simultaneous L-specific hydrolysis and racemization of the D-enantiomer converts DL-ATC almost quantitatively into L-cysteine. In preliminary experiments, with a yield of 95%, up to 31.4 g/L of cysteine was formed (Sano et al., 1977b).

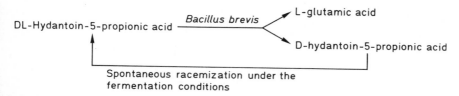

Fig. 14-3. Complete transformation of DL-hydantoin-5-propionic acid into L-glutamic acid by *Bacillus brevis*.

Table 14-2. Formation of L-Amino Acids from Synthetic Precursors.

Amino acid	Biotransformation	Microorganism (enzyme)	Concentration of product, g/L (yield)	Process	Literature
L-Aspartic acid	Fumaric acid + NH_3 → L-Asp.	*Escherichia coli* (aspartase)	179.6 (90%)	Continuous with cells immobilized in x-carrageenan $S^{1)}=1.1/h$	Sato et al., 1979
L-Tyrosine	Phenol + pyruvate + NH_3 → L-Tyr + H_2O	*Erwinia herbicola* (tyrosinase)	60.5 (90%)	Fed batch process	Enei et al., 1973a
	Phenol + DL-serine → L-Tyr + H_2O	*Erwinia herbicola* (tyrosinase)	53.5		Enei et al., 1973b
L-DOPA	Pyrocatechol + pyruvate + NH_3 → L-DOPA + H_2O	*Erwinia herbicola* (tyrosinase)	58.5	Fed batch process	Enei et al., 1973a
	Pyrocatechol + DL-serine → L-DOPA + H_2O		51		Enai et al., 1973b
L-Tryptophan	Indole + pyruvate + NH_3 → L-Trp + H_2O	*Proteus rettgeri* (tryptophanase)	100 (96%)	Batch process	Yamada and Kumagai, 1978
L-Cysteine	β-Chloro-L-alanine + Na_2S → L-cysteine + NaOH + NaCl	*Enterobacter cloacae* (cysteine desulfhydrase)	48 (>80%)	Batch process	Yamada and Kumagai, 1978

[1] S = Flow rate: volume of substrate solution per volume of immobilized biocatalyst per hour.

14.3.2 Formation of L-Amino Acids from Synthetic Precursors

L-Aspartic Acid from Fumaric Acid

A process for the manufacture of L-aspartic acid that is used technically is based on the asymmetric addition of ammonia to fumaric acid with *Escherichia coli* (Fig. 14-4). Strains with high aspartase activities have been selected and immobilized in polyacrylamide gel (Chibata et al., 1974).

The biotransformation can be performed continuously with the aid of columns contain-

L-Tyrosine, L-Tryptophan, L-Cysteine and Related Amino Acids

By α,β-elimination with tyrosinase (EC 4.1.99.2), tryptophanase (EC 4.1.99.1) and cysteine desulfhydrase (EC 4.4.1.1) the corresponding amino acids are degraded in the following way:

a) L-Tyrosine + H_2O → phenol + pyruvate + NH_3

b) L-Tryptophan + H_2O → indole + pyruvate + NH_3

c) L-Cysteine + H_2O → H_2S + pyruvate + NH_3.

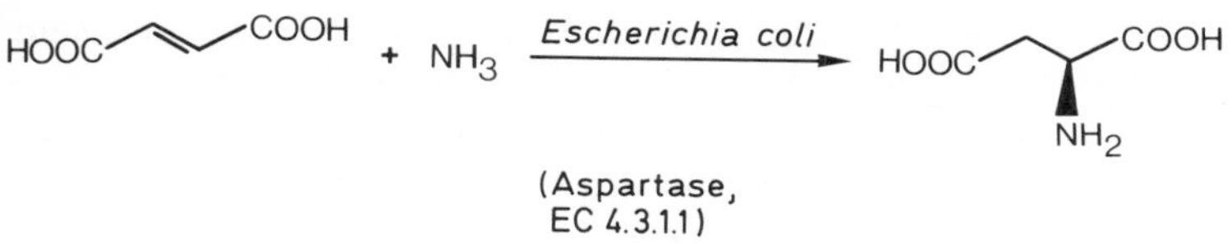

Fig. 14-4. Production of aspartic acid by the asymmetric addition of ammonia to fumaric acid.

ing the immobilized cells. This process for the manufacture of L-aspartic acid has been used industrially since 1973 and possibly forms the first use of immobilized cells on the large technical scale.

It has been possible to increase the stability of the immobilized cells as far as a half-life of 693 days by the use of κ-carrageenan hardened with glutaraldehyde and hexamethylenediamine in place of polyacrylamide gel (Sato et al., 1979).

In an analogous reaction with immobilized cells of *Rhodotorula gracilis* (Nelson, 1976) or with *Sporobolomyces roseus* (Chibata et al., 1978b) L-phenylalanine has been prepared from trans-cinnamic acid and ammonia (NH_3).

The enzymes involved can be used for the synthesis of the corresponding amino acids by the reversal of the α,β-elimination process. In addition they also catalyze β-exchange reactions in which β-substituted alanine derivatives or serine are converted in the presence of phenol into L-tyrosine (tyrosinase), indole is converted into L-tryptophan (tryptophanase), and -SH^- into cysteine (cysteine desulfhydrase) (Yamada and Kumagai 1978).

Related amino acids may arise at very different reaction rates when the corresponding phenol or indole derivatives (Enei et al., 1972) or mercaptans (Kumagai et al., 1974) are used. Processes for the synthesis in this way of L-tyrosine, L-tryptophan, L-cysteine, and related amino acids have been developed with selected microorganisms in which a high suitable enzymatic activity can be induced by cultivation in the presence of the substrates.

The manufacture of **L-tyrosine** is achieved with *Erwinia herbicola* by the reversal of reaction a) in a concentration of 60.5 g/L. If phenol is replaced by pyrocatechol under the same conditions 58.5 g/L of 3,4-dihydroxyphenyl-L-alanine (L-DOPA) is produced (Enei et al., 1973b). With phenol and with pyrocatechol, by β-exchange L-tyrosine and L-DOPA are formed in concentrations of 53.5 g/L and 51 g/L, respectively (Enei et al., 1973a).

L-Tryptophan can be prepared in a concentration of about 100 g/L by the reversal of reaction b) with the aid of *Proteus rettgeri* (Yamada and Kumagai, 1978). If 5-hydroxyindole or 5-methylindole is used in place of indole, the corresponding analogous compound 5-hydroxy- or 5-methyltryptophan is obtained.

High cysteine desulfhydrase activity has been found in *Aerobacter aerogenes* and *Enterobacter cloacae* (Yamada and Kumagai, 1978). **L-Cysteine** is synthesized in an amount of 48 g/L by a β-exchange reaction from β-chloro-L-alanine and sodium sulfide (Na_2S) under the action of *Enterobacter cloacae* (Yamada and Kumagai, 1978). Various S-alkyl-L-cysteines can be synthesized from alkyl mercaptans with *Aerobacter aerogenes* (Kumagai et al., 1974).

The corresponding **hydroxy derivatives** can be obtained by the microbiological hydroxylation of the aromatic L-amino acids. Thus, under the action of *Hydrogenomonas eutropha* L-tyrosine is formed from L-phenylalanine (Friedrich and Schlegel, 1972), and by a subsequent regiospecific hydroxylation with *Aspergillus oryzae* it is converted into L-DOPA (Hanada et al., 1973). On the other hand, *Bacillus subtilis* converts **L-tryptophan** into 5-hydroxy-L-tryptophan (Daum and Kieslich, 1974), the natural precursor of the blood-pressure-controlling and sleep-regulating hormone **serotonin**. However, these hydroxylations take place only at relatively low concentrations of the substrate.

14.3.3 Degradative Biotransformations

L-Alanine from L-Aspartic Acid

Pseudomonas dacunhae has a particularly high L-aspartic β-decarboxylase activity and is thereby capable of producing L-alanine from L-aspartic acid by decarboxylation almost quantitatively in an industrial process (Chibata et al., 1965). An improved process has recently been described in which the decarboxylase activity in *Pseudomonas dacunhae* has been doubled inductively by the addition of L-glutamate during cultivation. In this way, the technical production of L-alanine can be carried out in a supersaturated solution with 1 kg of substrate per liter of fermentation broth. The yield of isolated L-alanine amounts to 93% (Shibatani et al., 1979).

L-Lysine from α,α-Diaminopimelic Acid

The meso isomer of α,α-diaminopimelic acid is transformed into L-lysine by selective decarboxylation with *Bacillus sphaericus*. The DL- form remaining unchanged can easily be epimerized and used again (Gorton et al., 1963).

L-Citrulline from L-Arginine

L-Citrulline is being manufactured continuously from L-arginine by hydrolysis of the Schiff's base with cells of *Pseudomomas pu-*

Table 14-3. L-Amino Acids through Degradative Biotransformations.

Product	Biotransformation	Microorganism (enzyme)	Concentration of the product in g/L (yield)	Process	Literature
L-Alanine	L-Aspartic acid→ L-Ala + CO_2	*Pseudomonas dacunhae* (aspartate β-decarboxylase)	614.0 (93%)	Batch process	Shibatani et al., 1979
L-Lysine	Decarboxylation of meso-α,α-diaminopimelic acid	*Bacillus sphaericus* (decarboxylase)	44.4 (52%)	Batch process	Gorton et al., 1963
L-Citrulline	Hydrolysis of L-arginine	*Pseudomonas putida* (arginine deiminase)	84.1 (96%)	Continuous process with immobilized cells $S^{1)} = 0.19/h$	Yamamoto et al., 1974a
Urocanic acid	L-Histidine→ urocanic acid + NH_3	*Achromobacter liquidum* (L-histidine ammonia lyase)	39.6 (91%)	Continuous process with immobilized cells $S = 0.06/h$	Yamamoto et al., 1974b

[1] S = Flow rate: volume of substrate solution per unit volume of immobilized biocatalyst per hour.

tida immobilized in polyacrylamide gel (Yamamoto et al., 1974a). A 0.5 M solution of arginine-HCl is pumped through the column containing the immobilized cells at a flow rate of 0.19 h^{-1} at 37°C and is 96% transformed into L-citrulline. The stability of the column is very good.

Urocanic Acid from L-Histidine

Urocanic acid is a sunscreening agent and can be produced from L-histidine by the microbiologically catalyzed elimination of ammonia. It is produced by the use of columns containing cells of *Achromobacter liquidum* immobilized on polyacrylamide gel that have previously been subjected to a heat treatment (30 min at 70°C) in order to inactivate the urocanase (Yamamoto et al., 1974b). Jack and Zajic (1977) used *Micrococcus luteus* immobilized with carboxymethylcellulose for the same biotransformation.

14.4   Vitamins

Most vitamins are manufactured industrially by **chemical methods.** The D vitamins are accessible from cheap natural sterols after chemical modification and photochemical opening of the ring B. Vitamin B$_{12}$ and to some extent riboflavin are produced by **biosynthesis** with suitable microorganisms. The technical synthesis of the important vitamin C involves a microbiologically catalyzed reaction step.

L-Ascorbic Acid (Vitamin C)

In the industrial manufacture of L-ascorbic acid, the **classical process of Reichstein and**

Grüssner (1934) starting from D-glucose is still used throughout the world. The D-glucose is reduced catalytically to D-sorbitol. The second reaction step is the regioselective oxidation of D-sorbitol to L-sorbose (Fig. 14-5), which is catalyzed by Acetobacter species, especially *Acetobacter suboxydans,* and, at high substrate concentrations, takes place almost quantitatively (review: Kulhanek, 1970).

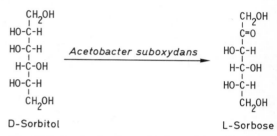

Fig. 14-5. Regioselective oxidation of D-sorbitol.

To protect it against overoxidation, the L-sorbose is acetalated with two molecules of acetone and is now oxidized chemically to diisopropylidene-2-keto-L-gulonic acid which, after the splitting out of the protective groups, is transformed into L-ascorbic acid.

In order to simplify Reichstein's already very cheap synthesis of vitamin C still further, in recent decades several **alternative syntheses** including one or two biotransformations have been developed. The aim was to find a direct approach to the 2-keto-L-gulonic acid, the immediate precursor of L-ascorbic acid. Kulhanek (1970) has given an exhaustive review of the investigations published up to the end of the sixties. Results of more recent literature have been summarized by Crawford and Crawford (1980).

α-Tocopherol (Vitamin E)

Natural α-tocopherol is composed of a chroman ring system and a side chain attached to position 2 of the chroman moiety. The molecule contains three chiral centers with the (2R,4′R,8′R) configuration (Fig. 14-6).

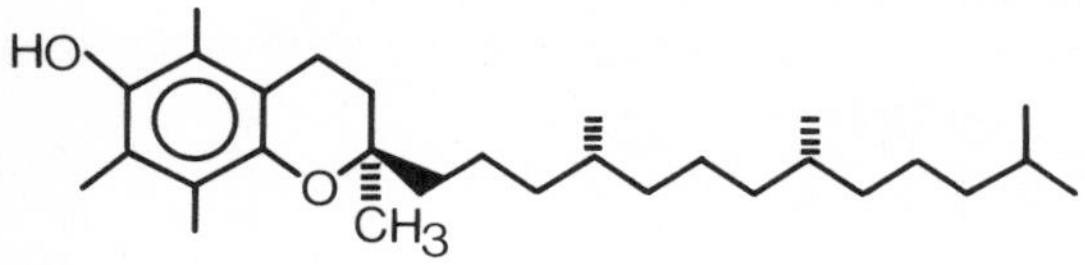

Fig. 14-6. Structure of (2R,4′R,8′R)-α-tocopherol.

Technically, α-tocopherol is manufactured by **chemical synthesis** as the racemate. The first partial synthesis of (2R,4′R,8′R)-α-tocopherol was achieved by the linkage of an optically active chroman aldehyde, readily obtainable by the resolution of the racemate, with an optically active side chain obtained by the degradation of natural phytol (Mayer et al., 1963). Very recently, several total syntheses of natural vitamin E have been made known which also include biotransformations (Fig. 14-7).

To construct the optically active side chain, Cohen et al. (1976) used (S)-β-hydroxyisobutyric acid (2), which was obtained by the microbiological hydroxylation of isobutyric acid (1). A simpler synthetic concept was opened up by the biotransformations that lead to the optically active lactones (4) and (6) (Leuenberger et al., 1979). By the coupling of two molecules of the C₅ lactone (4) (Schmid and Barner, 1979) or (6) (Zell, 1979), after linkage with the achiral C₅ end-piece, (3R,7R)-hexahydrofarnesol was synthesized. In another synthesis, Fuganti and Grasselli (1979) started from fermentation product (8) and, by the ozonolysis of the double bond, liberated a constructional unit for the synthesis of the side chain of α-tocopherol, the optical purity of which, however, was only 74%.

The chiral chroman ring system can be prepared, on the one hand, by the cleavage of a racemate by chemical methods or, on the other hand, by the use of (S)-citramalic acid

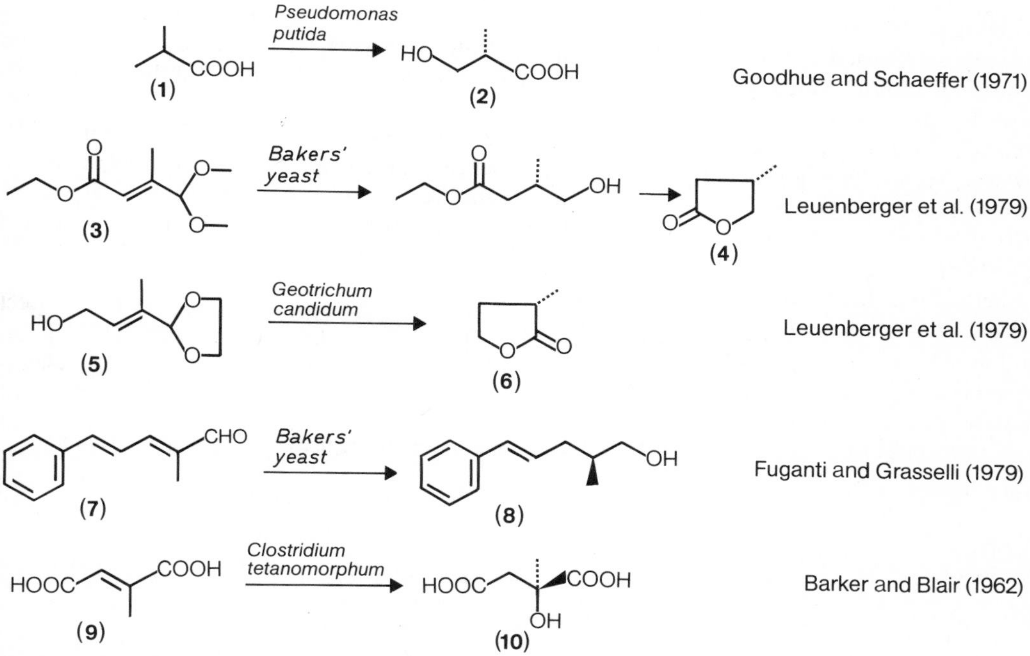

Fig. 14-7. Biotransformations that lead to optically active structural units for the synthesis of (2R,4′R,8′R)-α-tocopherol.

(10), which is available by the enzymatic addition of water to mesaconic acid (Barner and Schmid, 1979).

Vitamin K₁

The C_{15} side chain (3R,7R-hexahydrofarnesol) for α-tocopherol (Schmid and Barner, 1979; Zell, 1979), constructed from the units (S)-3-methyl-γ-butyrolactone (4) and (S)-2-methyl-γ-butyrolactone (6) (Leuenberger et al., 1979) was lengthened by condensation with a trans-C_5-olefin to (7R,11R)-trans-phytol, which was converted by reaction with menadiol monobenzoate into natural vitamin K₁ (7′R,11′R-phylloquinone) (Schmid, 1978, 1982).

Biotin

Goldberg and Sternbach's (1949) chemical total synthesis is used for the industrial manufacture of biotin. Since then, several processes for the microbiological total or partial synthesis of biotin have been described which, however, so far have given only small yields (review: Izumi and Ogata, 1977). However, industrial interest is presented by the microbiological oxidation of the alkyl side chain of the synthetically available precursor DL-cis-tetrahydro-2-oxo-4-n-pentylthieno [3,4-d] imidazoline (DL-TOPTI) by n-paraffin-assimilating corynebacteria, this leading, via the intermediate product DL-biotinol to DL-biotin (Fig. 14-8) (Ogino et al., 1974a, b). However,

when the fermentation time is extended, the DL-biotin is degraded further through β-oxidation. This further degradation of biotin has been reduced to 1/30 by the selection of a mutant which is no longer able to assimilate normal paraffins.

Pantothenic Acid

D-Pantothenic acid, which is active as a vitamin, is composed of the two constructional units β-alanine and D-2,4-dihydroxy-3,3-dimethylbutyric acid (D-pantoic acid) or its lactone (D-2-hydroxy-3,3-dimethyl-γ-butyrolactone = D-pantolactone). Until now, the optically active moiety, namely the D-pantolactone, has been prepared technically by a chemical resolution of the synthetically prepared racemate DL-pantolactone. A microbiological resolution of racemic DL-pantoic acid with microorganisms of the genera Brevibacterium, Corynebacterium, Arthrobacter, and Bacillus has been described in the patent literature (Takahashi and Isono, 1971). The asymmetric reduction of 2-oxopantolactone to D-pantolactone (Fig. 14-9) forms another possibility for the manufacture of this optically active constructional unit of D-pantothenic acid (Lanzilotta et al., 1974).

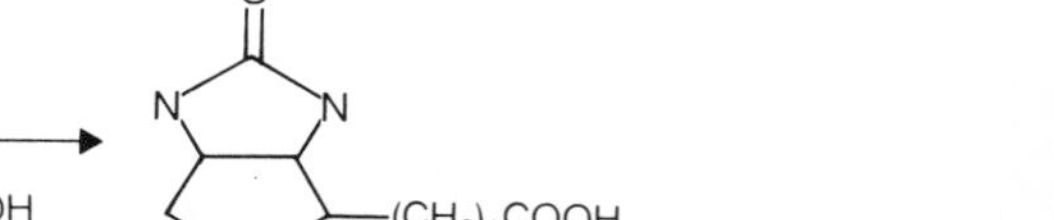

Fig. 14-9. Production of D-pantolactone by the stereoselective reduction of 2-oxopantolactone.

DL-TOPTI   DL-Biotinol   DL-Biotin

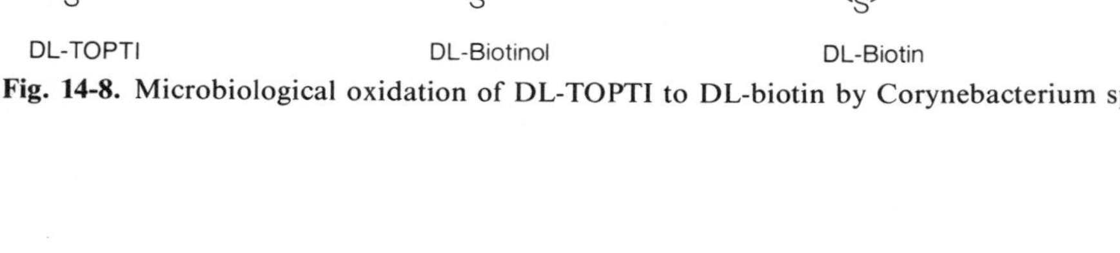

Fig. 14-8. Microbiological oxidation of DL-TOPTI to DL-biotin by Corynebacterium sp.

14.5   Carotenoids and Related Compounds

The carotenoids are among the most wide-spread natural pigments. Of the more than 400 natural carotenoids known, about half possess at least one center of asymmetry and occur in nature in optically active forms (Straub, 1976). In past years, the **chemistry of the carotenoids** has been intensively studied and the **total synthesis** of a large number of carotenoids has been made possible (Mayer and Isler, 1971; Kienzle, 1976; Britton, 1977). However, the total synthesis of optically active hydroxycarotenoids such as, for example, (3R,3′R)-zeaxanthin, (3R)-cryptoxanthin and (3S,3′S)-astaxanthin has only become possible by the use of a microbiological transformation step tak-

ing place enantioselectively (Leuenberger et al., 1976).

The enantioselective reduction of the double bond in oxoisophorone (11), catalyzed by bakers' yeast gives (6R)-2,2,6-trimethylcyclohexane-1,4-dione (12) which, by selective hydrogenation of the C(4) carbonyl group with Raney nickel as catalyst or with triisobutylaluminum (TIBA) as reducing agent can be converted overwhelmingly into (4R,6R)-4-hydroxy-2,2,6-trimethylcyclohexanone (14) (Fig. 14-10).

The trans compound (14) can be separated without difficulty from the cis compound (13) arising as by-product. (4R,6R)-4-hydroxy-2,2,6-trimethylcyclohexanone shows at C4 the absolute configuration corresponding to that of the natural 3-hydroxycarotenoids and therefore represents an ideal key compound for the total synthesis of such hydroxycarot-

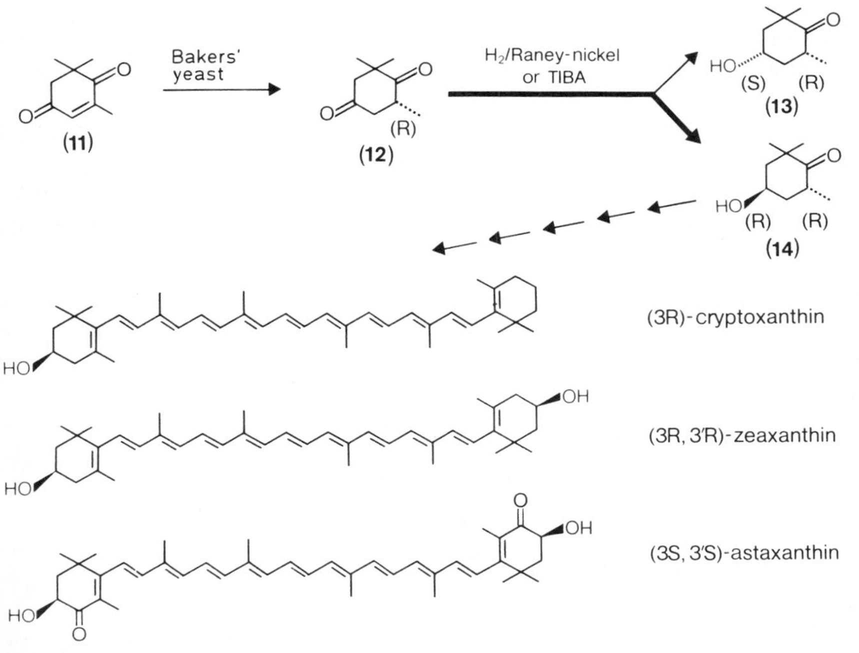

Fig. 14-10. Production of (4R,6R)-4-hydroxy-2,2,6-trimethylcyclohexanone (14) as a constructional unit for the synthesis of natural 3-hydroxycarotenoids and structurally related compounds.

enoids and structurally related natural products.

The enzymatic reduction of oxoisophorone (11) that is decisive for the introduction of the optical activity takes place with bakers' yeast (50 to 100 g/L) as catalyst in a simple sugar solution. Many other microorganisms (yeasts, fungi, and bacteria) are also capable of reducing oxoisophorone (Leuenberger et al., 1976).

Starting from the chiral constructional unit (14), it has been possible to synthesize not only the **natural carotenoids** (3R,3'R)-zeaxanthin, (3R)-cryptoxanthin, and (3S,3'S)-astaxanthin but also many other optically active **xanthophylls** and **apocarotenoids** and also a series of structurally related natural products – namely the plant **growth regulators** (6S)-abscisic acid and (3S,5R,6S)-xanthoxin and the terpenoid **aroma materials** (3S,5R)-loliolide, (5R)-actinidiolide, (5R)-dihydroactinidiolide, (6S,9S)-theaspirone, (6S)-dehydrovomifoliol, (6S,9R)-blumenol A, and picrocrocin (Kienzle et al., 1978; Mayer 1979). In many cases, stereoisomeric forms are accessible simultaneously.

(2S)-Hydroxy-β-ionone is obtained in yields of 60% and 30%, respectively, by the regio- and stereoselective reduction of 2-oxo-β-ionone with bakers' yeast or by the hydroxylation of β-ionone with *Aspergillus niger*. This compound opens up access to the optically active 2-hydroxycarotenoids. (2S)-Hydroxy-β-carotene, the enantiomer of the corresponding natural product, has been synthesized in this way (Ito et al., 1977).

14.6 *Antibiotics*

Enzymatic transformations of antibiotics were first described only as inactivation mechanisms. Only later was it realized that such **transformations on the preparative scale** can

also lead to new types of compounds and that they can be made use of in the following directions:

a) by **microbiological modifications,** transformation products with an improved activity spectrum or properties facilitating application may arise.

b) On the other hand, the knowledge of inactivation pathways can be utilized for the **directed modification** of the sensitive groups responsible for activity in order to prolong the action of the compounds.

c) Microbial degradation products of the active agents may represent starting materials for the chemical resynthesis of modified structures, the **semisynthetic antibiotics.**

Finally, methods have been found for the preparation of new antibiotics which can be regarded as microbiological transformations to only a limited degree. These methods may be based on **changes in the native biosynthesis** and are known as

d) **Directed biosynthesis,** in which inhibitors, promotors, or artificial precursors affect the native routes of antibiotic formation; and

e) biosynthesis modified by **mutation** in which, likewise, modified precursors may be supplied.

These processes give rise to substances which are structurally related to the native products but occasionally exhibit favorable **changes in the action spectrum.**

The multiplicity of examples of the microbiological transformation of antibiotics on the basis of the aims and methods described has been summarized previously in several review articles (Sebek, 1974; Shibata and Uyeda, 1978).

Table 14-4. Types of Reactions in the Biotransformation of Antibiotics with Examples.

Type of reaction	Substrate	Product	Microorganism
Hydrolysis of β-lactams	penicillin	penicillanic acid	*Pseudomonas aeruginosa*
Hydrolysis of peptides	novobiocin	novenamine	*Alcaligenes* sp.
Hydrolysis of lactones	actinomycin	peptides	*Actinoplanes missouriensis*
Hydrolysis of esters	maridomycin	deacetylmaridomycin	*Streptomyces* sp.
Acylation	chloramphenicol	chloroamphenicol-3-acetate	*Streptomyces griseus*
Phosphorylation	kanamycin	kanamycin-3-O-phosphate	*Bacillus circulans*
Formation of nucleotide esters	tobramycin	4-O-adenyltobramycin	*Staph. aureus*
Dehydrogenation	lapachol	dehydro-α-lapachone	*Curvularia lunata*
Oxidation	mycophenolic acid	several oxidation products	various microorganisms
Epoxidation	cis-propenylphosphonic acid	fosfomycin	*Penicillium spinulosum*
Sulfoxidation	lincomycin	lincomycin sulfoxide	*Streptomyces armentosus*
Hydroxylation	josamycin	3''-hydroxyjosamycin	*Streptomyces olivaceus*
Reduction of ketones	daunomycinone	dihydrodaunomycin	*Streptomyces aureofaciens*
Reduction of aldehydes	maridomycin	18-dihydromaridomycin	*Nocardia mexicanus*
Reduction of nitro groups	chloramphenicol	amine	*Streptomyces hemolyticus*
C-Demethylation	griseofulvin	demethylgriseofulvin	*Botrytis alii*
N-Demethylation	clindamycin	N-demethylclindamycin	*Streptomyces punipalus*
Deamination	formycin	formycin B	*Escherichia coli*
Transglycosylation	validoxylamine A	validamycin D	*Rhodotorula* sp.
Isomerization	showdomycin	isoshowdomycin	*Streptomyces* sp.

14.6.1 Microbiological Transformations

Most of the published examples have been carried out with microorganisms which **themselves do not form any antibiotic.** Consequently, these transformations are clearly separated off from possible part-reactions of biosyntheses. The types of reactions found so far are illustrated in Table 14-4 by one example each.

Since these transformations by side reactions or degradative reactions often give only low yields, these processes are generally cost-intensive and uneconomic. Reactions on antibiotics with antitumoral activity provide a possible preparative use (Rosazza, 1978).

As exceptions, the transformation of mannosidostreptomycin into the valuable market product streptomycin (Inamine et al., 1969) and the important hydrolytic cleavage of penicillin G to 6-aminopenicillanic acid (Fig. 14-11) (Huber et al., 1972), the starting material for the production of numerous semisynthetic penicillins (Price, 1977) (see Chapter 4), have gained technical significance.

The **cleavage of penicillin** is carried out by the enzyme penicillin acylase which is widespread in bacteria, fungi, actinomycetes, and yeasts. Two forms of the enzyme differ in their hydrolytic activity with respect to benzylpenicillin and phenoxymethylpenicillin (Cole et al., 1975). Large-scale technical processes are already based on the use of immobilized cells or cell-free enzymes. On the other hand, there is as yet no corresponding microbiological process for a cleavage of cephalosporin in order to obtain 7-aminocephalosporanic acid as the starting point for semisynthetic cephalosporins.

Penicillin acylase can also catalyze the reverse reaction – the formation of various penicillins from 6-aminopenicillanic acid and a suitable acyl residue – which, however, because of satisfactory methods of chemical acylation is not currently being used.

14.6.2 Modified Biosynthesis of Antibiotics

Sometimes, **precursors** offered are incorporated in the biosynthetic process with an increase in yield. In a similar manner, artificial structurally similar precursors can be assimilated with the formation of modified biosynthetic products. However, no examples of new penicillins, echinomycins, pyrrolnitrins, novobiocins, polyoxins, celesticetins, bleomycins, and actinomycins have so far acquired any technical importance.

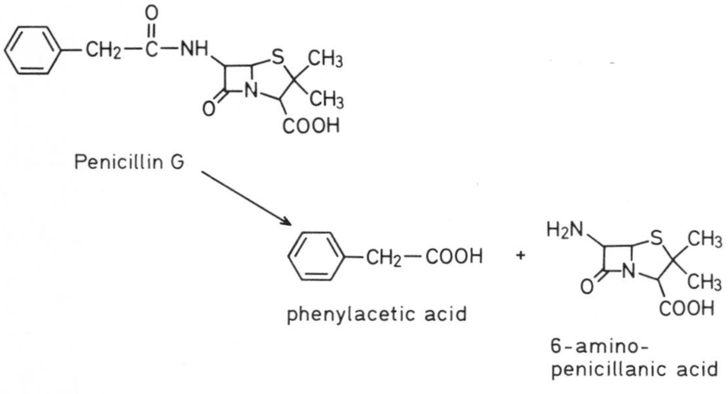

Fig. 14-11. Hydrolytic cleavage of penicillin G.

The **addition of inhibitors** can also lead to new structures by blocking end stages of biosynthesis. Methylation inhibitors give demethyltetracyclines, N-demethylstreptomycin, and N-demethyllincomycin as by-products or main products.

The inhibition of individual biosynthetic stages is also achieved by **mutation of the native strain.** 7-O-Demethylcelesticetin, modified platenomycins, a series of modified cephalosporins, the antitumorally active adriamycin, and accumulated precursors of rifamycin, tetracyclines, and erythromycin have been obtained in this way.

14.6.3   Mutasynthesis

A combination of the use of mutants with additions of precursors was developed ten years ago with aminoglycoside-forming strains of Streptomyces. The formation of 2-deoxystreptamine blocked **by mutation** is replaced by the addition of streptamine or 2-epistreptamine, whereupon, in place of neomycin the new antibiotics hybrimycins A_1, A_2, B_1 and B_2 are produced (Shier et al., 1969). Under similar conditions, this method has led to modified ribostamycins, kanamycins, sisomicins, butirosins, and gentamicins. It has been called **mutational biosynthesis** or **mutasynthesis** and has been described exhaustively by Nara (1977) (see also Chapter 4).

14.7   Steroids

Steroids possess central functions in human metabolism as androgenic (male) and estrogenic (female), progestative (pregnancy) and gluco- and mineralocorticoid **hormones** and, in their natural structures or as derivatives, exhibit antiinflammatory, anabolic, sedative, cytostatic, and contraceptive effects. By chemical modifications, the corresponding antihormonal activities can also be obtained (Applezweig, 1978).

As the **starting materials for the chemical preparation** of the various structures, it is basically the natural product deoxycholic acid (from animal biles), stigmasterol (from soybeans) and diosgenin (see Fig. 14-12) (from the root of the Mexican yam *Dioscorea composita*) that are used.

At first, the compound cortisone, which is highly active against arthritis, could be prepared only from deoxycholic acid via 31 chemical stages. The displacement of the 12α-hydroxy group to form a keto function in position 11 required nine reaction steps. Although this preparation pathway was subsequently optimized to an economic state, a pioneering discovery of the Upjohn company means a decisive simplification of the synthesis of hormones of the adrenal cortex:

In analogy to a hydroxylation of deoxycorticosterone to corticosterone with adrenal cortex, it was possible to introduce a hydroxy group into the 11α position of progesterone (Fig. 14-12) with *Rhizopus arrhizus* or *Rhizopus nigricans* (Peterson and Murray, 1952) in yields of more than 85%. This made available the important corticosteroid hormones with their characteristic oxygen function in position 11 from the cheap natural products **stigmasterol** and **diosgenin**. (Later, hecogenin, which already contains a 12-keto group provided another pathway for the preparation of the corticoids).

Shortly after this, the introduction of a hydroxy group into the 11β position was achieved with *Cunninghamella blakesleeana* (Hanson et al., 1953), by which **hydrocortisone** was obtained directly from Reichstein's compound S.

These trailblazing results made microbiological transformations of steroids a technically important method. The results of the last few years have been summarized in recent reviews (Beukers et al., 1972; Murray, 1976; Kieslich, 1980; Kieslich and Sebek, 1980).

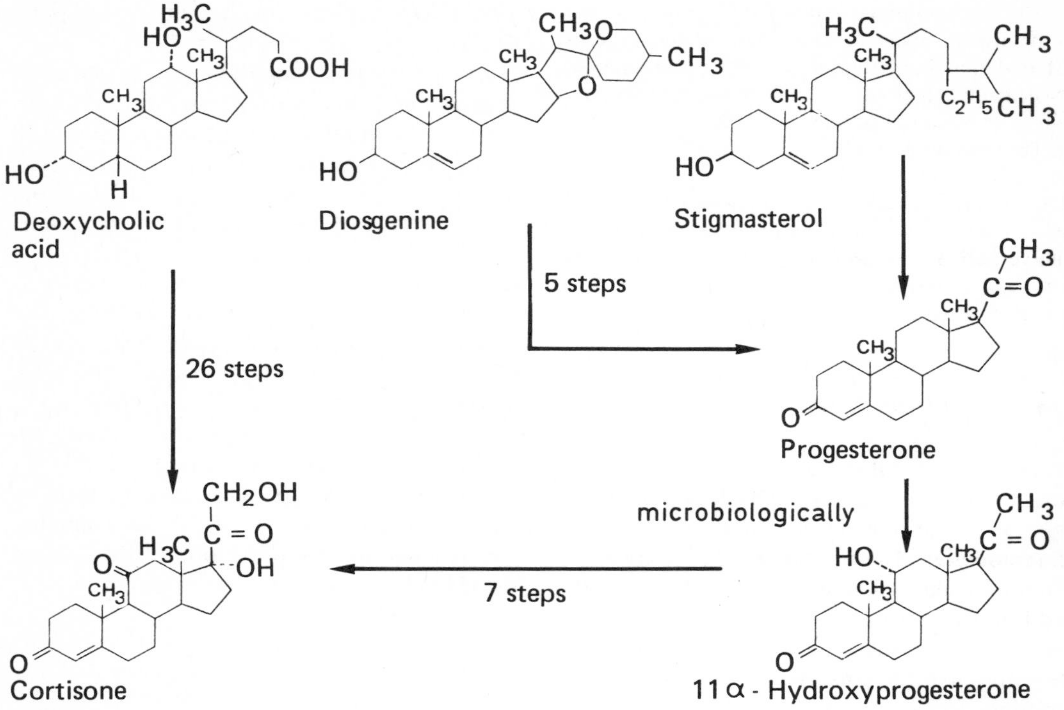

Fig. 14-12. Production of cortisone from natural sterols.

14.7.1   11α-Hydroxylation

Other suitable strains of fungi have been found for the 11α-hydroxylation of **progesterone,** of which *Aspergillus ochraceus* with substrate concentrations of up to 50 g per liter of culture broth and with the formation of only small amounts of the by-product 6β,11α-dihydroxyprogesterone shows particular advantages (Weaver et al., 1960). In addition to progesterone, a number of other steroid structures can be hydroxylated in the 11α position with high regio- and stereospecificities (Kieslich, 1980).

14.7.2   11β-Hydroxylation

On the other hand, the 11β-hydroxylation of **Reichstein's substance S** and its analogs with *Cunningha-*

mella blakesleeana is adversely affected by parallel 6β-hydroxylation and by subsequent oxidation to 11-ketones, which, however, can be partially suppressed by special enzyme inhibition. The fungus *Curvularia lunata,* which is used more frequently, on the other hand, performs unwanted hydroxylations in the 7α, 9α, and 14α positions. These side reactions are excluded by the use of the 17-acetate of Reichstein's substance S (Fig. 14-13), in which the space-filling ester residue protects the rear (α) side of the substrate against undesirable attack without affecting the 11-hydroxylation of the front (β) side (de Fines and v.d. Waard, 1966). Similar screening effects are possible by substituting the 16α position.

In the β-hydroxylation of the D-homo analog of Reichstein's substance S to D-homohydrocortisone, with an antiinflammatory action, the altered ring linkage blocks position 14.

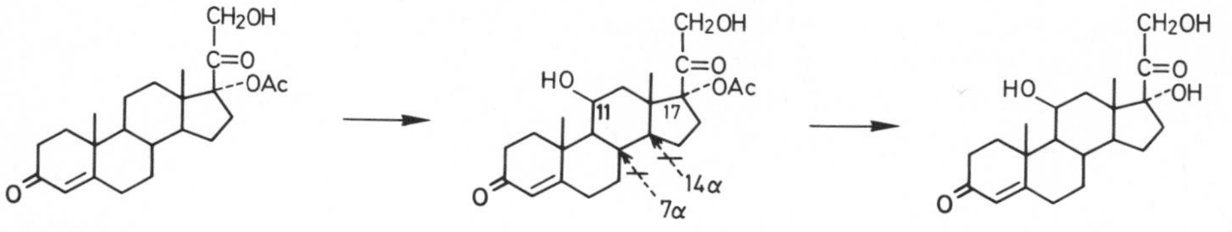

Fig. 14-13. 11β-Hydroxylation of the 17-acetate of Reichstein's substance S by *Curvularia lunata*.

14.7.3 16α-Hydroxylation

In addition to the 11-hydroxylations that are used industrially, the introduction of a 16α-hydroxy group with strains of Streptomyces is acquiring technical importance through the synthesis of the inflammation-inhibiting agent triamcinolone (9α-fluoro-16α-hydroxyprednisolone) (Fig. 14-14).

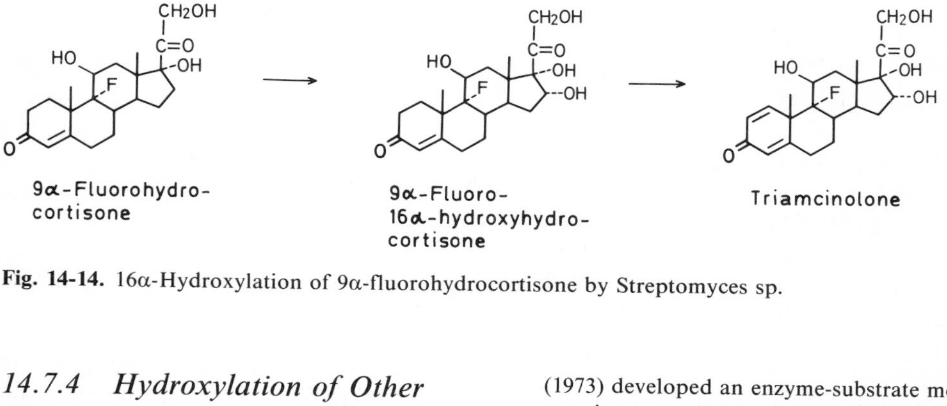

position of a steroid can be hydroxylated, very diverse strains of fungi or, more rarely, species of bacteria being suitable for this purpose.

In the case of nonpolar substrates, there is often a simultaneous introduction of two hydroxy groups, which can likewise be used for preparative purposes (Jones et al., 1971). From broad systematic investigations with representative fungal strains, Jones

Fig. 14-14. 16α-Hydroxylation of 9α-fluorohydrocortisone by Streptomyces sp.

14.7.4 Hydroxylation of Other Positions

Other hydroxylations have found interesting application as useful aids to synthesis in the production of new steroid structures with varied or new types of pharmacological effects (Kieslich, 1980). Since, however, the intermediate or end stages synthesized have acquired no commercial importance, only processes on the semitechnical or laboratory scale have been developed. According to the broad experience available in this field, today basically any

(1973) developed an enzyme-substrate model which permits approximate predictions of the type of attack in mono- and dihydroxylations according to the position of a polar group of the substrate for the enzymatic action process.

14.7.5 1,2-Dehydrogenation

The significant increase in the antiinflammatory action of corticoids brought about by an additional 1,2-double bond has led to the **second microbiological steroid reaction** on the technical scale. For the production of prednisone, prednisolone, triamcinolone, 6-methylprednisolone, dexamethasone, etc., by the dehydrogenation of the corresponding 1,2-saturated structures it is advantageous to use *Bacillus sphaericus, Bacterium cyclooxydans,* and, most frequently, *Arthrobacter (Corynebacterium) simplex* (Nobile et al., 1955). With the last-mentioned bacterium, in a special process, it is possible to convert substrate concentrations up to 500 g of hydrocortisone per liter of culture broth to prednisolone in yields of over 90% in five days. In this process, called **pseudo-crystallofermentation,** the substrate is added in micronized form without a solvent (Kondo and Masuo, 1961). *Arthrobacter simplex* has also been used succesfully for dehydrogenation in immobilized form (Constantinides, 1980).

14.7.6   Ester Saponification and Oxidation of Hydroxy Groups

Since hydrolyzing enzymes are widely distributed in microorganisms, ester saponifications, often coupled with other microbiological reactions in one fermentation step, can be used in practice. In the transformation of a triolone diacetate into Reichstein's compound S with *Flavobacterium dehydrogenans* performed technically (Fig. 14-15), the acetate groups in positions 3 and 21 are hydrolyzed off before the oxidation of the 3β-hydroxy-5-ene system to the 3-keto-4-ene structure takes place. When the pH is carefully kept constant at 6.6, in the corresponding 3β,17α,21-triacetate the 17α-ester group is retained, which leads to the 17-acetate of Reichstein's substance S, an advantageous starting material for a commercial preparation of hydrocortisone (de Flines and v.d. Waard, 1966) (Fig. 14-15).

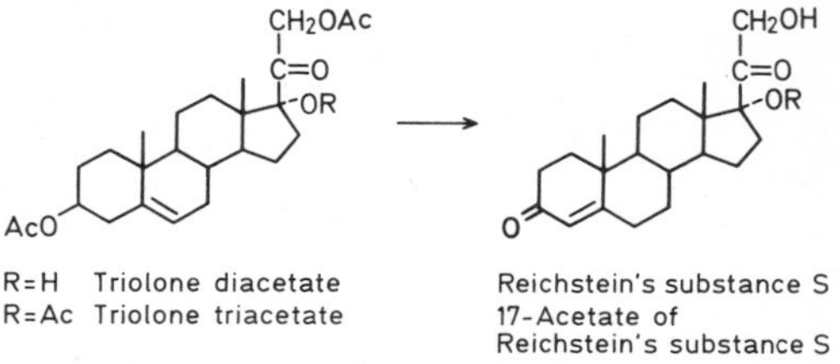

R=H   Triolone diacetate
R=Ac   Triolone triacetate

Reichstein's substance S
17-Acetate of
Reichstein's substance S

Fig. 14-15. Coupled saponification and oxidation of triolone acetates by *Flavobacterium dehydrogenans.*

14.7.7   Reduction of Keto Groups

The reduction of a 17-keto group with yeast was, in 1937, the **first steroid transformation for which a patent was requested** (Schering AG, Schöller, 1937). The process is used technically today only on the small scale for the production of **testosterone** from androst-4-ene-3,17-dione (Fig. 14-16).

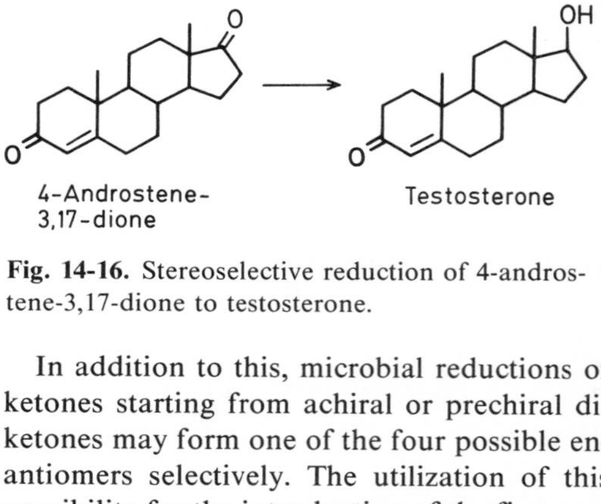

4-Androstene-
3,17-dione

Testosterone

Fig. 14-16. Stereoselective reduction of 4-androstene-3,17-dione to testosterone.

In addition to this, microbial reductions of ketones starting from achiral or prechiral diketones may form one of the four possible enantiomers selectively. The utilization of this possibility for the introduction of the first center of asymmetry by an enzymatic reaction led for the first time to an economic synthesis of steroids. The incorporation of a regio- and stereospecific reduction of one of two equivalent keto groups of a secodione (Bellet et al., 1966) to a secolone (Fig. 14-17) doubled the yield by eliminating the formation of a racemate. The

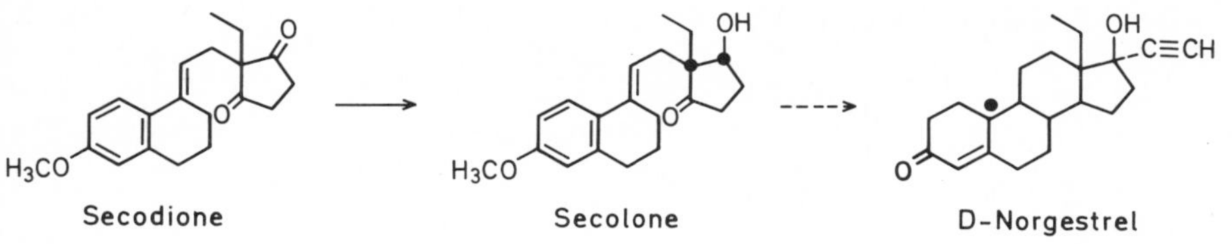

Fig. 14-17. The stereospecific reduction of a seco-dione yields secolone, a constructional unit for the total synthesis of steroids (e.g., D-Norgestrel).

important contraceptive D-norgestrel is largely manufactured in this way (Rufer et al., 1967).

14.7.8 Sterol Side-Chain Degradation

Up to the middle of the fifties, some producers of steroids also used **cholesterol** as the starting material. However, its chemical oxidation to an intermediate product capable of further use gave only low yields.

A **microbial degradation** of the cholesterol side chain has been known basically since 1913. An elucidation of the enzymatic reaction mechanism (Fig. 14-18) (Sih et al., 1967) revealed several possibilities for suppressing the subsequent undesirable degradation of the steroid skeleton.

These methods, which have been treated comprehensively by Martin (1977), are based on the inhibition of the formation of 9α-hydroxyandrosta-1,4-diene-3,17-dione, which is unstable and initiates total degradation (see Fig. 14-18).

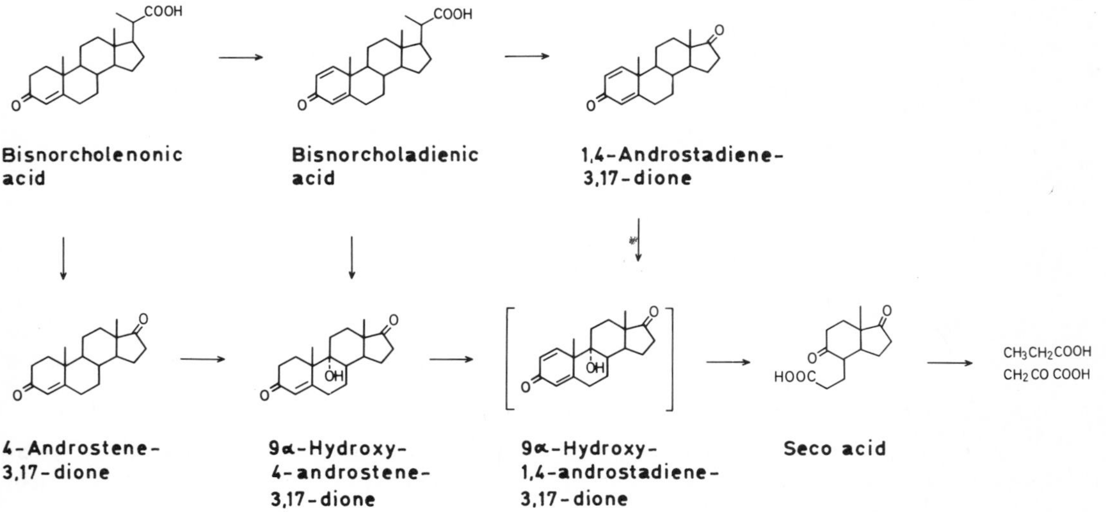

Fig. 14-18. Pathways of enzymatic degradation in steroids.

For the large-scale technical manufacture of androst-4-ene-3,17-dione and androsta-1,4-diene-3,17-dione, the most important compounds at the present time, optimized processes have been developed which are based on special media, additives, and forms of application of the substrate (Martin and Wagner, 1976). At substrate concentrations of several grams per liter, yields of more than 80% of 17-ketosteroids are obtained with the most suitable mycobacteria in fermentation times of three to four days.

In addition to the cholesterol initially destined for this purpose, today **stigmasterol, sitosterol,** and even a **mixture of sterols** containing campesterol, stigmasterol, and sitosterol can be used with equivalent results. Since these products are available cheaply from soybeans and tall oil in large amounts, this has given a new economic starting basis for the production of steroids.

14.7.9 Other Types of Reactions in Microbiological Transformation of Steroids

In addition to the processes used on the large technical scale that have been described, a fairly large number of other types of reactions in microbiological transformations of steroids are known:

Oxidations
- Aromatization of ring A in the dehydrogenation of 19-norsteroids
- Oxidation of pregnan-20-ones to testolactone structures
- Epoxidation of double bonds

Reductions
- Hydrogenation of double bonds
- Dehydroxylation

Hydrolytic Reactions (possibly oxidative)
- Cleavage of phenolic 3-methyl ethers
- Cleavage of glycosides

Glycosidation
- Formation of glucosides at the phenolic 3-hydroxy group
- Formation of glucosides at the 16α-hydroxy group

These reactions have not, however, gone beyond the preparative laboratory scale although basically they possess interest for technical application.

14.8   Prostaglandins

The **pharmaceutical importance of prostaglandins** and analogous compounds (Weeks, 1972; Samuelsson et al., 1975), which, in contrast to steroids, occur in nature only in low concentrations and the isolation of which mainly requires expensive methods of purification, have induced manifold investigations of chemical synthesis for the preparation of these lipoid substances and of derivatives and modified structures (Bindra and Bindra, 1977; Szantay et al., 1978).

Since even the simplest prostaglandins possess three to five centers of chirality (Fig. 14-19), the older total syntheses were generally limited to the production of racemic mixtures. On the other hand, pure chiral structures can be obtained in various ways:

- by **imitating biogenesis** with the incorporation of native constructional units;

- by **chemical synthesis** using an enzymatic – generally microbial – reaction step to introduce the first chirality which directs the subsequent pathway of chemical synthesis to the desired enantiomers; and

- by the **microbial transformation** of native or synthetic prostaglandins to obtain new types of structures with changed action profiles.

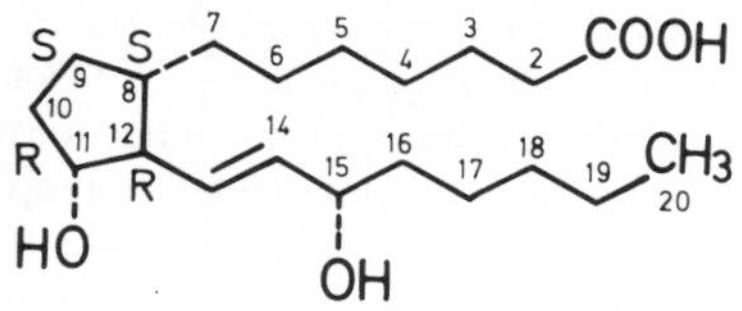

Fig. 14-19. Structures of simple prostaglandins.

zusätzlich	9α-Hydroxy	9-Keto	9-Keto-11-desoxy
—	PGF$_1$α	PGE$_1$	PGA$_1$
cis-Doppelbindung in 5-6-Stellung	PGF$_2$α	PGE$_2$	PGA$_2$
cis-Doppelbindung. in 5-6-und 17-18-Stellung	PEG$_3$α	PGE$_3$	PGA$_3$
Anzahl der Chiralitätszentren	5	4	3

In the last few years, examples of all the pathways mentioned have become known which, on the laboratory scale, form valuable synthetic aids that have not so far led to industrial application. Out of the multiplicity of microbial transformations described in this field (Jiu, 1980), the most important examples have been chosen below.

14.8.1 Imitation of the Biogenesis of Prostaglandins

The **biosynthesis of the prostaglandins** (PGs) is based on essential fatty acids which are cyclized enzymatically with the formation of a cyclopentane ring with α- and ω- side chains. In addition to animal enzyme systems, microorganisms are also capable of transforming unsaturated fatty acids with a 1,4-diene system oxidatively into prostaglandin structures. This possibility has been patented by the Upjohn company with a broad claim to 125 strains of the species Subphylum using polyunsaturated fatty acids as substrates. With the substrate **arachidonic acid** (Fig. 14-20), mixtures of PGE and PGE$_2$ are formed (Beal et al., 1966).

Arachidonic acid can be hydroxylated in position 18 or 19 with *Ophiobolus graminis* and oxidized chemically to the corresponding keto compounds which, on cyclization with animal enzymes, give the corresponding hydroxy- or oxo-PGE structures.

14.8.2 Chemical Synthesis with Supporting Microbiological Reaction Steps

In contrast to **biogenesis, total chemical syntheses** generally start from preformed 5-ring structures. In the course of the synthesis, the 4-hydroxy group of a cyclopentyl derivative becomes the 11-hydroxy function of the prostaglandin system and, with its steric position, can direct the following stereochemistry of the addition of the side chains in positions 8 and 12. The first satisfactory bioorganic total synthesis was based on (+)-4(R)-hydroxycyclopent-2-

ene-1-one. The stereospecific reduction of a 2-(6-methoxycarbonylhexyl)cyclopentane-1,3,4-trione (15) with *Dipodascus uninucleatus* gives a 4(R)- alcohol (16) in 75% yield which can be converted in two subsequent chemical steps into the desired cyclopentyl synthon (17) (Fig. 14-21).

This cyclopentyl synthon (17) can also be obtained more simply in 67% yield by the microbio-

Arachidonic acid

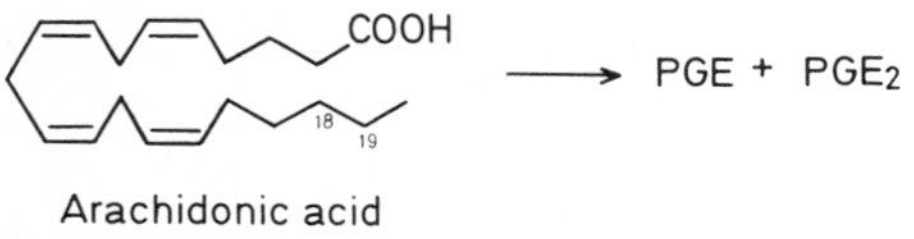

Fig. 14-20. Arachidonic acid as prostaglandin precursor.

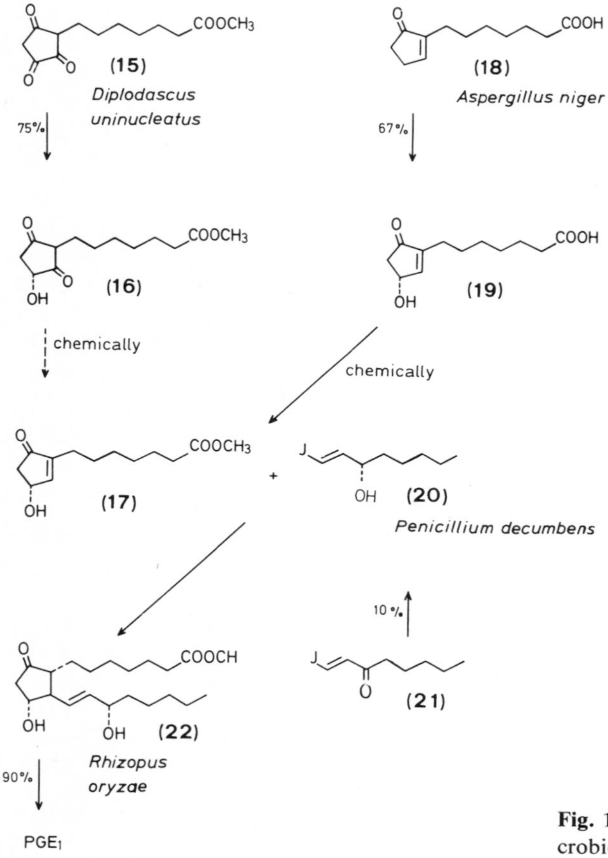

logical hydroxylation of a 2-(6-carboxyhexyl)cyclopent-2-en-1-one (18) with *Aspergillus niger* ATCC 9142 (ATCC = American Type Culture Collection); unfortunately, the product (19) shows a lowered optical purity. To introduce the ω- side chain, the lithium cuprate of a (+)-3(S)-iodooct-1-en-3-ol (20) is used as an octenyl synthon. This chiral alcohol is again obtained by the stereospecific reduction of the corresponding 3-ketone (21) in which, however, *Penicillium decumbens* gives yields of only 10%. The synthetic pathway ends with another microbiological reaction in the form of the saponification of the methyl ester (22) with *Rhizopus oryzae*, giving yields of 90% of free PGE$_1$ (Sih et al., 1973).

PGE$_2$ can be prepared in similar yields in a similar manner to the synthesis of PGE$_1$, starting from

Fig. 14-21. Synthesis of PGE$_1$ with the aid of microbiological reaction steps.

2-(6-methoxycarbonylhex-cis-2-enyl)cyclopentane-1,3,4-trione as the cyclopentyl synthon.

A synthetic pathway developed by Miyano et al. (1975) leads to $\Delta^{8(12)}$-15-keto structures with racemic 11-hydroxy groups (23). Reduction of the 15-keto group takes place in different ways according to the microorganism used. *Flavobacterium sp.* NRRL B-3874 (NRRL = Northern Regional Research Laboratories) gave the trans-diol (24) in 30% yield, *Pseudomonas sp.* NRRL B-3875 formed the trans-diol (25) in 24% yield, and *Rhodotorula glutinis* gave only a d,l-trans-diol, while *Flavobacterium sp.* NRRL B-5641 enabled a mixture of the cis-diols to be obtained.

A specific reduction of an analogous conjugated keto group (Fig. 14-22) with *Kloeckera jensenii* is used preparatively in the synthesis of the active agent sulprostone (26) with the avoidance of the formation of a racemate.

Selective resolutions of racemates are also possible by the saponification of esters of the 11-hydroxy group, an intermediate stage of this synthesis. *Saccharomyces sp.* 1375-143 hydrolyzes the acetate, propionate, or isobutyrate of the R form stereospecifically giving 52% yields of a R- alcohol.

Other regio- and stereoselective hydrolyses have been described for mixtures of cis- and trans-3,5-diacetoxycyclopent-1-ene (27) (Miura et al., 1976).

By the careful control of the saponification with bakers' yeast it has been possible to obtain a maximum of 11.5% of a 3(R)-acetoxy-5(R)-hydroxycyclopent-1-ene (28) (Fig. 14-23), which is also a desirable prostaglandin synthon. The corresponding pure cis-diacetate (29) gives with *Bacillus subtilis* a 56% yield of the 3(S)-acetoxy-5(S)-hydroxy product (30), which is converted chemically into a lactone (31) with the desired absolute configuration (Takano et al., 1976). Unfortunately, the lactone (31) possesses an optical purity of only 35% but is nevertheless an important intermediate in various prostaglandin syntheses (Fried and Sih, 1973).

Microbiological transformation steps have also been used in the **synthesis of artificial prostaglandins,** as in the 15-keto reductions of 9,15-diketo-11-deoxyprostanic acid with *Saccharomyces cerevisae* ATCC 4125 and of 15-dehydroprostaglandins with *Trechispora brinkmanii* CMI 80439 (CMI = Commonwealth Mycological Institute, Kew, England). In addition to the stereospecific keto-reduction, the advantages of mild conditions of enzymatic hydrolysis are frequently made use of in chemical syntheses, using bakers' yeast, *Rhizopus oryzae, Corynespora cassiicola* IMI 56007 (IMI = Imperial Mycological Institute, the former name of the CMI), and various other microorganisms or microbial lipases.

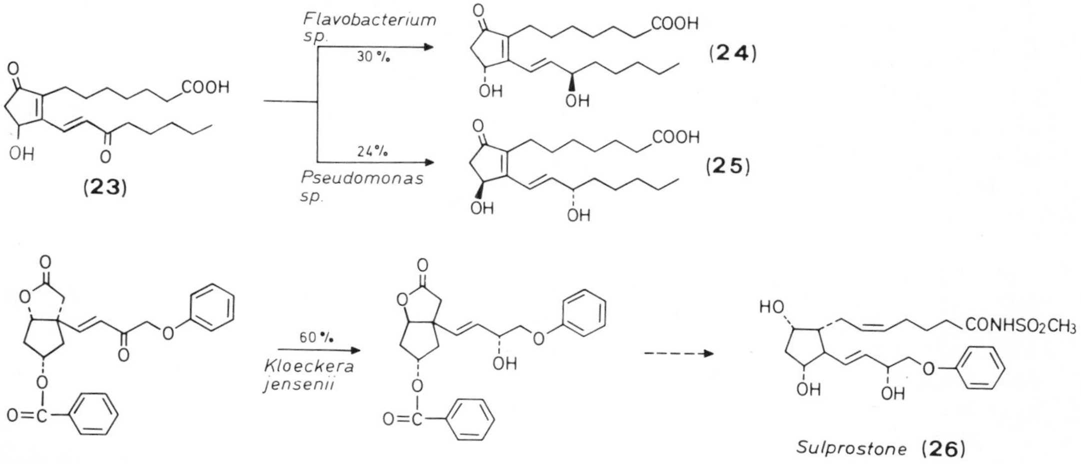

Fig. 14-22. Enantioselective reductions of ketones.

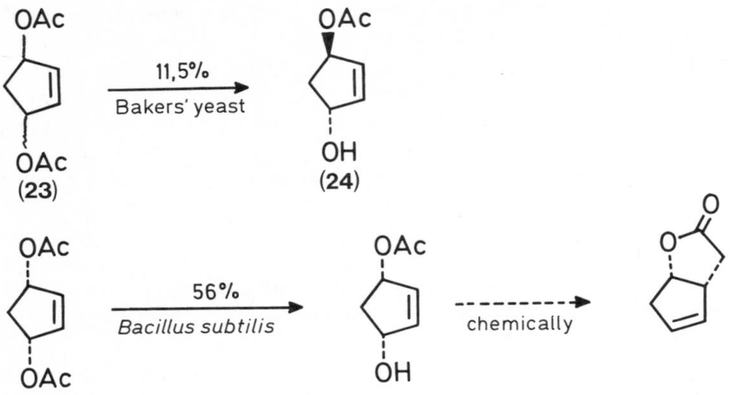

Fig. 14-23. Regio- and stereoselective hydrolysis of 3,5-diacetoxycyclopentenes.

14.8.3 Microbial Transformations of Native and Artificial Prostaglandins

Using bakers' yeast, Schneider and Murray (1973) reduced nat-PGE$_1$ to nat-PGF$_{1\alpha}$, and nat-PGE$_2$ to nat-PGF$_{2\alpha}$, i.e., a 9-keto group was reduced to a 9(S)-OH group without the formation of the 9(R) by-product. When the methyl ester is used in this process, saponification takes place before the keto-reduction.

In the case of racemic PGE$_1$ and PGE$_2$, both enantiomers are reduced to nat-PGF$_{1\alpha}$, nat-PGF$_{2\alpha}$, ent-PGF$_{1\beta}$ and ent-PGF$_{2\beta}$, but with side-reactions and maximum yields of 10%.

The substrate PGA$_2$ (32) is transformed into 15-hydroxy-9-oxoprosta-5,13-dienoic acid (33) by the hydrogenation of the 10,11-double bond with *Cephalosporium sp.* NRRL 5499. *Dactylium dendroides* NRRL 2575 gives as by-product 9,15-dioxaprost-5-enoic acid (34) and 9,15-dioxaprosta-5,8(12)-dienoic acid (35) (Fig. 14-24).

Cunninghamella blakesleena forms, in addition to the 10,11-dihydro compound, an analogous 18-hydroxylated product (36). *Corynespora cassiicola* IMI 56007 can also reduce the 10,11-double bond while hydrolyzing ester groups, and so can Pseudomonas and Streptomyces species in the case of 15-epiprostaglandin A$_2$.

Other **structures of new types** have been obtained by the microbial β-oxidation of natural and synthetic prostaglandins (Hsu et al., 1977). Prostaglandins B$_2$ and A$_2$ have been converted by *Penicillium sp.* M 8904 into tetranor structures, always with attack only on the α- side chain and with the appearance of various by-products. *Mycobacterium rhodochrous* UC 6176 (UC = Upjohn Company, Kalamazoo) can also perform oxidative degradations to tetranor, and also dinor, structures.

Finally, as in steroid transformations, the hydroxylation type of reaction appears useful for the modification of known structures. The transformations described hitherto are summarized in Table 14-5.

14.9 Miscellaneous Products

(1R,2S)-Ephedrine

(1R,2S)-Ephedrine is a natural alkaloid from Ephedra plants with an interesting **pharmaco-**

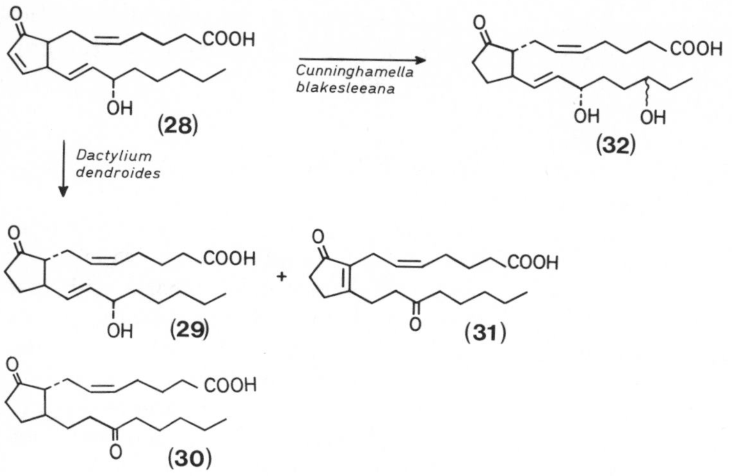

Fig. 14-24. Biotransformations of PGA$_2$ (32).

Table 14-5. Hydroxylation in Prostaglandins

PGF$_{2\alpha}$	Streptomyces UC 5761	18—OH	Sebek et al., 1976
		19—OH	
PGE$_2$	Streptomyces UC 5761	18—OH	Sebek et al., 1976
		19—OH	
PGA$_2$	Streptomyces sp.	17—OH	Marsheck and Miyano, 1975
		18—OH	
		19—OH	
Various prostaglandins	Streptomyces sp.	17—OH	Marx and Doodewaard, 1977
		18—OH	
		19—OH	
		20—OH	
d,l-Prost-13-enoic acid	*Microascus trigonosporus*	18—OH	Lanzilotta, 1977; Lanzilotta et al., 1976
		19—OH	

logical activity. It is used with success particularly in disturbances of the circulation of the blood and in asthma. The racemic ephedrine obtained by chemical synthesis is substantially less active than the natural (1R,2S) enantiomer. Hildebrandt and Klavehn (1934) patented a technical synthesis of (1R,2S)-ephedrine, the first step of which is represented by an asymmetric condensation of benzaldehyde and acetaldehyde brought about by *Saccharomyces cerevisiae.* In a second step the optically active phenyl acetyl carbinol so produced is reduced chemically in the presence of methylamine to (1R,2S)-ephedrine. The center of asymmetry introduced by the biotransformation induces the 2S configuration at the new center of asymmetry arising as a result of the chemical step (Fig. 14-25).

Dihydroxyacetone is used mainly as an active agent in cosmetic preparations for promoting suntan.

L-Malic Acid from Fumaric Acid

L-Malic acid is an important intermediate in the tricarboxylic acid cycle, in which it is formed by fumarase from fumaric acid. It is used for the treatment of liver diseases and as an addition to infusion solutions. In a **continuous industrial process,** L-malic acid is produced by the asymmetric addition of water to fumaric acid with *Brevibacterium ammoniagenes* cells fixed in polyacrylamide gel (Yamamoto et al., 1976, 1977) or *Brevibacterium flavum* cells immobilized in carrageenan (Ta-

Benzaldehyde   Acetaldehyde   (R)-Phenyl acetyl carbinol   (1R,2S)-Ephedrine

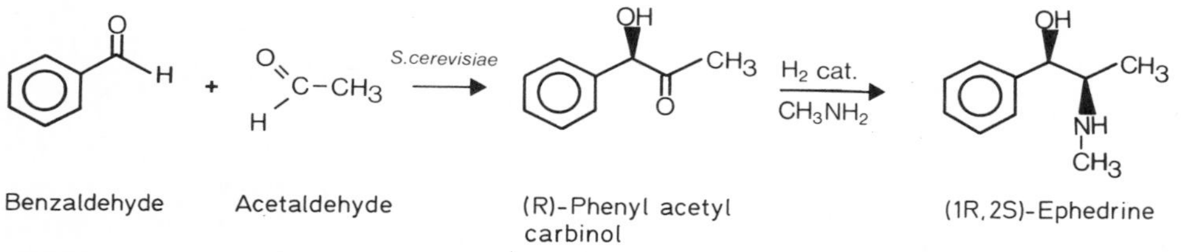

Fig. 14-25. Synthesis of (1R,2S)-ephedrine.

Dihydroxyacetone from Glycerol

Dihydroxyacetone is produced industrially by the regioselective oxidation of glycerol with Acetobacter species, especially *Acetobacter suboxydans* (Green et al., 1961). Under the optimum conditions at a glycerol concentration of 110 g/L an 82% conversion to dihydroxyacetone is observed after 72 h (Green et al., 1961). Flickinger and Perlman (1977) used *Gluconobacter melanogenus* for the same reaction and were able to increase the rate of conversion at least threefold by enriching the aeration flow with pure oxygen.

kata et al., 1980). The formation of the succinic acid that appears as an undesirable by-product is effectively suppressed by treating the immobilized cells with bile extract. The highest fumarase activity and the longest half life (160 days at 37°C) were observed with *Brevibacterium flavum* immobilized in carageenan.

L-Tartaric Acid from Maleic Acid

L-Tartaric acid can be manufactured in an elegant two-stage process from maleic acid. In a first chemical stage, maleic acid is oxidized by hydrogen peroxide (H_2O_2) to cis-epoxysuccinic acid. In a second, microbiological stage, L-tartaric acid is formed almost quantitatively by the asymmetric hydrolysis of the epoxide. The biocatalysts used are *Nocardia tartaricus* (Miura et al., 1976) or *Achromobacter tartarogenes* cells immobilized in polyacrylamide gel (Kawabata and Ichikura, 1976).

Sugar Transformations

A review of the manifold sugar transformations is given by the compilations of Spencer and Gorin (1968) and of Kieslich (1976, pp. 269 to 289). For **technical application,** three processes are of particular importance, namely the isomerization of glucose to fructose by glucose isomerase to increase sweetening power, the hydrolysis of raffinose to sucrose and galactose by α-galactosidase to increase the yields of sucrose from beet sugar molasses, and the hydrolysis of lactose to glucose and galactose by β-galactosidase for the utilization of whey and the production of lactose-free milk products. These processes are carried out industrially on the large scale with the aid of isolated and immobilized enzymes of microbial origin (see Chapter 12). Here we shall mention only processes that have recently been become known that use whole immobilized microorganisms for the same transformations.

Poulsen and Zittan (1976) used a new cell preparation of *Bacillus coagulans* for the **isomerization of glucose.** The cells separated by centrifugation are homogenized, dried, remoistened under standardized conditions, and cross-linked with glutaraldehyde. This immobilized cell preparation is packed into a column and used for the continuous isomerization of glucose. After an operating time of 500 h, 50% of the isomerase activity is still present. It has been possible with 1 kg of catalyst to convert about 1000 kg of glucose into a mixture of 45% of fructose and 55% of glucose.

Chibata et al. (1978a) immobilized *Streptomyces phaeochromogenes* in polyacrylamide and carrageenan and with both polymers obtained a half-life for the glucose isomerase activity of 53 days. It was, however, possible to achieve a considerable further increase in the stability of the cells fixed in carrageenan by hardening with glutaraldehyde and hexamethylenediamine.

Linko et al. (1977) immobilized *Achromobacter missouriensis* on cellulose fibers or beads and studied the isomerization of glucose in a continuous reactor.

The mycelial pellets formed naturally by *Mortierella vinacea* var. *raffinoseutilizer* are rich in α-galactosidase and have been used for the continuous hydrolysis of raffinose. The application of this process in the sugar beet industry has been discussed in detail by Obara et al. (1977).

Whole cells with high β-galactosidase activity, namely *Lactobacillus bulgaricus, Escherichia coli,* and *Kluyveromyces lactis,* have been immobilized in polyacrylamide gel and used for the hydrolysis of the lactose in skim milk (Ohmiya et al., 1977).

Hycanthone and Oxamniquine

The **selective hydroxylation** of an aromatic methyl group has acquired importance with the transformation of the drug lucanthone, which is active against *Schistosoma mansoni* to the more active drug hycanthone with *Aspergillus sclerotiorum* (Rosi et al., 1967). The same reaction is used industrially in the manufacture of the schistosomacide oxamniquine (Fig. 14-26) from the corresponding methyl compound using the same fungus (Richards, 1970).

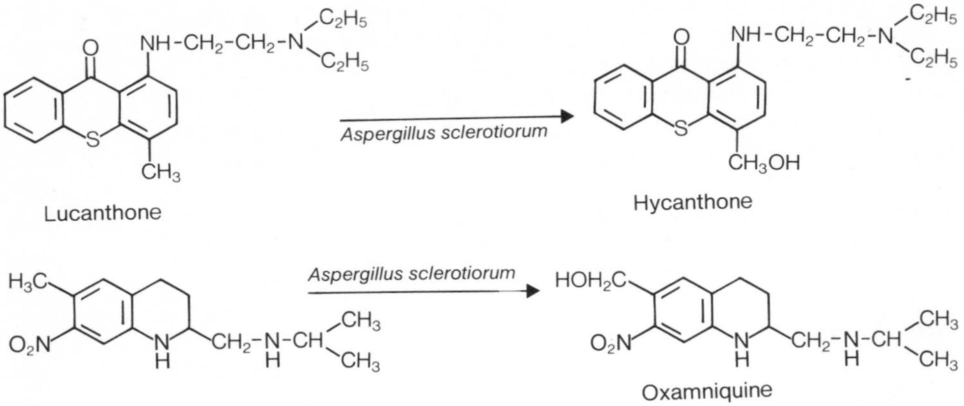

Fig. 14-26. Production of hycanthone and oxaminiquine by the selective hydroxylation of an aromatic methyl group.

Antitumoral Drugs

An exhaustive review of biotransformations applied to various antitumoral drugs has been given by Rosazza (1978) Among the various types of reactions there are reductive cleavages of glycosides, reductions of ketone groups in anthracyclines, hydrolysis of the amine moiety of bleomycin, regioselective hydroxylation in withaferin A and in the aromatic rings of acronycin (acronin) and vinblastine, N-demethylation in D-tetrandrine and vindoline, the formation of ether derivatives and the dimerization of vindoline and the opening of the quinone ring in lapachol. These transformations, and other reactions of the diverse cytostatic drugs have not so far led to compounds with significantly increased activity or reduced toxicity and are therefore not used in practice.

Oxidation of Naphthalene

The first step in the **microbial degradation of aromatic structures** is a double hydroxylation in neighbouring positions. Subsequent oxidations lead via ring cleavages to cis,cis-muconic acid structures. Thus, for example, 2,5-dimethylmuconic acid has been obtained from p-xylene in high yields with *Nocardia corallina* (Hosler and Eltz, 1969).

The first product of the degradation of naphthalene by reductive dihydroxylation is 1,2-dihydroxy-1,2-dihydronaphthalene. The cis isomer is an important precursor of a pesticide and is formed by *Pseudomonas putida* (Cox and Williams, 1980), while the corresponding trans isomer arises under the action of *Nocardia sp.* NRRL 3385 (Wegner, 1973). Subsequent oxidation can lead through several steps to salicylic acid. Even with the most suitable strain, *Corynebacterium renale* ATCC 15070, however, the production of salicylic acid from naphthalene achieved only transient technical significance (Sun Oil Comp., 1965).

14.10   Literature

Abbott, B. J., "Immobilized cells", *Annu. Rep. Ferment. Processes* **2**, 91–123 (1978).

Applezweig, N.: In: Seigler, D. S. (ed.): *Crop Resources*. Academic Press, New York 1978, p. 149.

Barker, H. A. and Blair, A. H., "Enzymatic syntheses of (+)-citramalic acid", *Biochem. Prep.* **9**, 21–29 (1962).

Barner, R. and Schmid, M., "Totalsynthese von natürlichem α-Tocopherol. IV. Aufbau des Chromanringsystems aus Trimethylhydrochinon und einem optisch aktiven C₄- bzw. C₅-Synthon", *Helv. Chim. Acta* **62**, 2384–2399 (1979).

Beal, P. F., Fonken, G. S. and Pike, J. E.: "Microbial conversion of unsaturated fatty acids". US Pat. 3,290,226 (Dec. 6, 1966) (Belg. Pat. 659,983).

Bellet, P., Nomine, G. and Mathieu, J., "Asymmetric reduction by a microbiological route in the total synthesis of steroids", *C. R. Hebd. Séances Acad. Sci. Ser. C* **263**, 88–89 (1966).

Beukers, R., Marx, A. F. and Zuidweg, M. H. J.: "Microbial conversion as a tool in the preparation of drugs". In: Ariens, E. J. (ed.): *Drug Design*, Vol. 3. Academic Press, New York 1972, pp. 1–131.

Bindra, J. S. and Bindra, R.: *Prostaglandin Synthesis*. Academic Press, New York 1977.

Bogoczek, R. (Politechnika Slaska): "2-Oxo-L-gulonic acid by fermentation". Polish Patent 62,547; cited by *C.A.* **76**, 97935p (1972).

Boothroyd, B., Napier, J. E. and Sommerfield, G. A., "The methylation of griseofulvin by fungi", *Biochem. J.* **80**, 34–37 (1961).

Britton, G.: "Carotenoids and polyterpenoids". In: Overton, K. H. (ed.): *Terpenoids and Steroids*, Vol. 7. The Chemical Society, London 1977, pp. 155–175.

Capek, K. A., Hanc, O. and Tadra, M.: *Microbial Transformations of Steroids*. Akademia Press, Prague 1966.

Capek, K. A., Fassitova, O. and Hanc, O., "Progesterone transformations as a diagnostic feature in the genera Alternaria, Stemphylium and Cladosporium", *Folia Microbiol. Prague* **19**, 378–380 (1974).

Capek, K. A., Fassitova, O. and Hanc, O., "Steroid transformations as a biochemical feature of the genus Paecilomyces", *Folia Microbiol. Prague* **21**, 70–72 (1976).

Cargile, N. L. and McChesney, J. D., "Microbiological sterol conversions: utilization of selected mutants", *Appl. Microbiol.* **27**, 991–994 (1974).

Cheetham, P. S. J., "Developments in the immobilisation of microbial cells and their application", *Top. Enzyme Ferment. Biotechnol.* **4**, 189–238 (1980).

Chibata, I., Kakimoto, T. and Kato, J., "Enzymatic production of L-alanine by *Pseudomonas dacunhae*", *Appl. Microbiol.* **13**, 638–645 (1965).

Chibata, I., Tosa, T., Sato, T., Mori, T. and Matsuo, Y., "Preparation and industrial application of immobilized aminoacylase", *Ferment. Technol. Today. Proc. Int. Ferment. Symp.*, 4th **1972**, 383–389.

Chibata, I., Tosa, T. and Sato, T., "Immobilized aspartase-containing microbial cells: Preparation and enzymatic properties", *Appl. Microbiol.* **27**, 878–885 (1974).

Chibata, I., Tosa, T., Sato, T. and Mori, T., "Production of L-amino acids by aminoacylase adsorbed on DEAE-sephadex", *Methods Enzymol.* **44**, 746–759 (1976).

Chibata, I., Tosa, T., Sato, T., Yamamoto, K., Takata, I. and Nishida, Y., "New method for immobilization of microbial cells and its industrial application", *Enzyme Eng.* **4**, 335–337 (1978 a).

Chibata, I., Yamada, S., Nabe, K., Ujimaru, T. and Izumio, N. (Tanabe Seiyaku Co.): "Enzymatic production of L-phenylalanine". Japan. Kokai 7 896 388 (1978 b).

Chibata, I., Tosa, T. and Sato, T., "Use of immobilized cell systems to prepare fine chemicals", *Microb. Technol.* 2nd Ed. **2**, 433–461 (1979).

Cohen, N., Eichel, W. F., Lopresti, R. J., Neukom, C., Saucy, G., "Synthetic studies on (2R,4′R,8′R)-α-tocopherol. An approach utilizing side chain synthons of microbiological origin", *J. Org. Chem.* **41**, 3505–3511 (1976).

Cole, M., Savidge, T., Vanderhaeghe, H.: "Penicillin acylase (assay)", *Methods Enzymol.* **43**, 698 (1975).

Constantinides, A., "Steroid transformation at high substrate concentrations using immobilized *Corynebacterium simplex* cells", *Biotechnol. Bioeng.* **22**, 119–136 (1980).

Cox, D. P. and Williams, A. L., "Biological process for converting naphthalene to cis-1,2-dihydroxy-1,2-dihydronaphthalene", *Appl. Environ. Microbiol.* **39**, 320–326 (1980).

Crawford, T. C. and Crawford, S. A., "Synthesis of L-ascorbic acid", *Adv. Carbohydr. Chem. Biochem.* **37**, 79–155 (1980).

Daum, J. and Kieslich, K., "Darstellung von 5-Hydroxytryptophan durch mikrobiologische Hydroxylierung von L-Tryptophan", *Naturwissenschaften* **61**, 167–168 (1974).

de Flines, J. and v. d. Waard, F.: "11-β-Hydroxysteroids". Dutch Patent Application 66 05 514 (April 4, 1966).

Enei, H., Matsui, H., Okumura, S. and Yamada, H., "Elimination, replacement and isomerization reactions by intact cells containing tyrosine phenol lyase", *Agric. Biol. Chem.* **36**, 1869–1876 (1972).

Enei, H., Matsui, H., Nakazawa, H., Okumura, S. and Yamada, H., "Synthesis of L-tyrosine or 3,4-dihydroxy-L-alanine from DL-serine and phenol or pyrocatechol", *Agric. Biol. Chem.* **37**, 493–499 (1973 a).

Enei, H., Nakazawa, H., Okumura, S. and Yamada, H., "Synthesis of L-tyrosine or 3,4-dihydroxyphenyl-L-alanine from pyruric acid, ammonia and phenol or pyrocatechol", *Agric. Biol. Chem.* **37**, 725–735 (1973 b).

Flickinger, M. C. and Perlman, D., "Application of oxygenenriched aeration in the conversion of glycerol to dihydroxyacetone by *Gluconobacter melanogenus* IFO 3293", *Appl. Environ. Microbiol.* **33**, 706–712 (1977).

Fonken, G. S. and Johnson, R. A.: *Chemical Oxydations with Microorganisms.* Marcel Dekker, New York 1972.

Fried, J. and Sih, J. C., "Total synthesis of prostaglandins. Control of regiospecificity in the alane-epoxide reaction and selective catalytic oxidation of alkynylation products", *Tetrahedron Lett.* **1973**, 3899–3901.

Friedrich, B. and Schlegel, H. G., "Die Hydroxylierung von Phenylalanin durch *Hydrogenomonas eutropha* H 16", *Arch. Mikrobiol.* **83**, 17–31 (1972).

Fuganti, C. and Grasselli, P., "Efficient stereoselective synthesis of natural α-tocopherol", *J. Chem. Soc., Chem. Commun.* **1979**, 995–997.

Fukumura, T., "Screening, classification and distribution of L-α-amino-ε-caprolactam-hydrolyzing yeasts", *Agric. Biol. Chem.* **40**, 1687–1693 (1976 a).

Fukumura, T., "Hydrolysis of L-α-amino-ε-caprolactam by yeasts", *Agric. Biol. Chem.* **40**, 1695–1698 (1976 b).

Fukumura, T., "Bacterial racemization of α-amino-ε-caprolactam", *Agric. Biol. Chem.* **41**, 1321–1325 (1977 a).

Fukumura, T., "Conversion of D- and DL-α-amino-ε-caprolactam into L-lysine using both yeast cells and bacterial cells", *Agric. Biol. Chem.* **41**, 1327–1330 (1977 b).

Goldberg, M. W., Sternbach, L. H. (Hoffmann-La Roche & Co. AG) US Pats. 2,489,232–2,489,238 (1949).

Goodhue, C. T. and Schaeffer, J. R., "Preparation of L(+)-β-hydroxyisobutyric acid by bacterial oxydation of isobutyric acid", *Biotechnol. Bioeng.* **13**, 203–214 (1971).

Gorton, B. S., Coker, J. N., Browder, H. P., Defiebre, C. W., "A process for the production of lysine by chemical and microbiological syntheses", *Ind. Eng. Chem. Prod. Res. Dev.* **2**, 308–314 (1963).

Green, S. R., Whalen, E. A. and Molokie, E., "Dihydroxyacetone: production and uses", *J. Biochem. Microbiol. Technol. Eng.* **3**, 351–355 (1961).

Haneda, K., Watanabe, S. and Takeda, I., "Production of L-3,4-dihydroxy-phenylalanine from L-tyrosine by microorganisms", *J. Ferment. Technol.* **51**, 398–406 (1973).

Hanson, F. R., Mann, K. M., Nielson, E. D., Anderson, H. V., Brunner, M. P., Karnemaat, J., Collingsworth, D. R. and Haines, W. J., "Microbiological transformations of steroids. VIII. Preparation of 17-α-hydroxycorticosterone", *J. Am. Chem. Soc.* **75**, 5369–5370 (1953).

Hildebrandt, G. and Klavehn, W.: US Pat. 1,956,950 (1934).

Hosler, P. and Eltz, R. W.: "Microbial conversion of p-xylene in stirred fermentors". In: Perlman, D. (ed.): *Fermentation Advances.* Academic Press, New York 1969, pp. 789–805.

Hsu, C. F., Jiu, J. and Mizuba, S. S.: 9,15-Dioxo-5-cis-protenoic acid – prepared by fermentation of 15-(S)-hydroxy-9-oxo-5-cis-10,13-transprostatrienoic acid". US Pat. 3,868,412 (Feb. 25, 1975).

Hsu, C. F., Jiu, J. and Mizuba, S., "Microbiol-β-oxidation of prostaglandins", *Dev. Ind. Microbiol.* **18**, 487–497 (1977).

Huber, F. M., Chauvette, R. R. and Jackson, B. G.: In: Flynn, E. H. (ed.): *Cephalosporins and Penicillins.* Academic Press, New York 1972, pp. 27–73.

Iizuka, H., Naito, A.: Microbial transformations of steroids and alkaloids. University of Tokyo Press, Tokyo 1967.

Inamine, E.: In: Perlman, D. (ed.): *Fermentation Advances.* Academic Press, New York 1969, p. 199.

Ito, M., Masahara, R. and Tsukida, K., "Synthesis of (2δ)-β,β-caroten-2-ol", *Tetrahedron Lett.* **1977,** 2767–2770.

Izumi, Y. and Ogata, K., "Some aspects of the microbial production of biotin", *Adv. Appl. Microbiol.* **22,** 145–176 (1977).

Jack, T. R. and Zajic, J. E., "The enzymatic conversion of L-histidine to urocanic acid by whole cells of *Micrococcus luteus* immobilized on carbodiimide activated carboxymethylcellulose", *Biotechnol. Bioeng.* **19,** 631–648 (1977).

Jiu, J., "Microbial Reactions in Prostaglandin Chemistry", *Advances Biochem. Eng.* **17,** 37–62 (1980).

Johnson, D. E. and Ciegler, A., "Substrate conversion by fungal spores entrapped in solid matrices", *Arch. Biochem. Biophys.* **130,** 384–388 (1969).

Jones, E. R. H., Meakins, G. D. and Clegg, A. S.: "Oxidation of Steroids". US Pat. 3,692,629 (April 5, 1971).

Jones, E. R. H., "Microbiological hydroxylation of steroids and related compounds", *Pure Appl. Chem.* **33,** 39–52 (1973).

Kawabata, Y. and Ichikura, S. (Toray Inc., Japan): Japan Kokai 77102496 (1976); CA: **87,** 199200 (1977).

Kienzle, F., "The technical syntheses of carotenoids", *Pure Appl. Chem.* **47,** 183–190 (1976).

Kienzle, F., Mayer, H., Minder, R. E. and Thommen, H., "Synthese von optisch aktiven, natürlichen Carotinoiden und strukturell verwandten Verbindungen. III. Synthese von (+)-Abszisinsäure, (−)-Xanthoxin, (−)-Loliolid, (−)-Actinidiolid und (−)-Dihydroactinidiolid", *Helv. Chim. Acta* **61,** 2616–2627 (1978).

Kieslich, K.: *Microbial Transformation of Non-steroid Cyclic Compounds.* Georg Thieme-Verlag, Stuttgart 1976.

Kieslich, K.: "Steroid conversions". In: Rose, A. H. (ed.): *Economic Microbiology – Microbial Enzymes and Transformations.* Vol. V, 369–465 (1980).

Kieslich, K. and Sebek, O. K., "Microbial transformations of steroids", *Annu. Rep. Ferment. Processes* **3,** 275–304 (1980).

Kondo, E. and Masuo, E., "Pseudo-crystallofermentation of steroid: a new process for preparing prednisolone by a microorganism", *J. Gen. Appl. Microbiol.* **7,** 113–117 (1961).

Koninkl Ned. Gist- en Spiritusfabriek: "Verfahren zur Herstellung von 17α-Acyloxy-21-hydroxysteroiden der Pregnan-Reihe". D.B.P. 1,618,598 (April 24, 1967).

Kuhn, R. and Wieland, T., "Zur Biogenese der Pantothensäure", *Ber. Dtsch. Chem. Ges.* **75B,** 121–123 (1942).

Kulhanek, M., "Fermentation processes employed in vitamin C synthesis", *Adv. Appl. Microbiol.* **12,** 11–33 (1970).

Kumagai, H., Choi, Y., Sejima, S. and Yamada, H., "Synthesis of S-alkyl-L-cysteine from pyruvate, ammonia and alkyl-mercaptan by cysteine desulfhydrase of *Aerobacter aerogenes*", *Biochem. Biophys. Res. Commun.* **59,** 789–795 (1974).

Lanzilotta, R. P., Bradley, D. G. and McDonald, K. M., "Microbial reduction of ketopantoyllactone to pantoyllactone", *Appl. Microbiol.* **27,** 100–134 (1974).

Lanzilotta, R. P., Bradley, D. G., McDonald, K. M. and Tokes, L., "Microbiological hydroxylation of carbon 18 and 19 in 9-oxo-13-(cis and trans)-prostenoic acids", *Appl. Environ. Microbiol.* **32,** 726–728 (1976).

Lanzilotta, R. P.: 18- and 19-Hydroxylated prostaglandins. US Pat. 4,036,876 (July 19, 1977).

Larsson, P. O., Ohlson, S. and Mosbach, K., "Transformation of steroids by immobilized living microorganisms", *Appl. Biochem. Bioeng.* **2,** 291–301 (1979).

Leuenberger, H. G. W., Boguth, W., Widmer, E. and Zell, R., "Synthese von optisch aktiven, natürlichen Carotinoiden und strukturell verwandten Naturprodukten. I. Synthese der chiralen Schlüsselverbindung (4R,6R)-4-Hydroxy-2,2,6-trimethylcyclohexanon", *Helv. Chim. Acta* **59,** 1832–1849 (1976).

Leuenberger, H. G. W., Boguth, W., Barner, R., Schmid, M. and Zell, R., "Totalsynthese von natürlichem α-Tocopherol. I. Herstellung bifunktioneller, optisch aktiver Synthesebausteine für die Seitenkette mit Hilfe mikrobiologischer Umwandlungen", *Helv. Chim. Acta* **62,** 455–463 (1979).

Linko, Y. Y., Pohjola, L. and Linko, P., "Entrapped glucose isomerase for high fructose syrup production", *Process Biochem.* **12** (6), 14–16 (1977).

Marsheck, W. J. and Miyano, M.: "Hydroxylated prostaglandins". US Pat. 3,878,046 (April 15, 1975).

Martin, C. K. A. and Wagner, F., "Microbial transformation of β-sitosterol by *Nocardia sp. M 29*", *Eur. J. Appl. Microbiol.* **2**, 243–255 (1976).

Martin, C. K. A., "Microbial cleavage of sterol side chains", *Adv. Appl. Microbiol.* **22**, 29–58 (1977).

Marx, A. F. and Doodewaard, S.: "Prostaglandin derivatives and their preparation". US Pat. 4,054,595 (Oct. 18, 1977).

Mayer, H., Schudel, P., Rüegg, R. and Isler, O., "Über die Chemie des Vitamins E. III. Die Totalsynthese von (2R,4′R,8′R)- und (2S,4′R,8′R)α-Tocopherol", *Helv. Chim. Acta* **46**, 650–671 (1963).

Mayer, H. and Isler, O.: "Total syntheses". In: Isler, O., Gutmann, H. and Solms, U. (eds.): *Carotenoids*. Birkhäuser, Basel, Stuttgart 1971, pp. 325–575.

Mayer, H., "Synthesis of optically active carotenoids and related compounds", *Pure Appl. Chem.* **51**, 535–564 (1979).

Mitsubishi, Chem. Ind. K. K.: "Microbial oxidation of steroids – to give (17)-hydroxy-androsta-(1,4)-diene-3-one and/or androsta-(1,4)-diene-3,17-dione in presence of fatty acids". Jap. Pat. 5 2070-082 (Dec. 8, 1975).

Miura, S., Kurozomi, T., Toru, T., Tanaka, T., Kobayashi, M., Matsubara, S. and Ishimoto, S., "Prostaglandin chemistry. IV. Microbiological kinetic resolution and asymmetric hydrolysis of 3,5-diacetoxycyclopent-1-ene", *Tetrahedron* **32**, 1893–1898 (1976).

Miura, Y., Yutani, K., Takesue, H., Fujiik, K., Izumi, Y. (Tokuyama Soda Inc. Japan): "L-Tartaric acid". D.O.S. 2,605,921 (1976); *CA:* **86**, 70 103 k (1977).

Miyano, M. and Stealey, M. A., "Prostaglandins. VII. A stereoselective total synthesis of prostaglandin E₁", *J. Org. Chem.* **40**, 1748–1755 (1975).

Murray, H. C.: "Microbiology of Steroids". In: Miller, B. M. and Litzky, W. (eds.): *Industrial Microbiology*. McGraw Hill Book Co., New York 1976, pp. 79–105.

Nara, T.: *Annu. Rep. Ferment. Processes.* **1**, 311–314 (1977).

Nelson, R. P.: US Pat. 3,957,580 (1976).

Nobile, A., Charney, W., Perlman, P., Herzog, H. L., Payne, C. C., Tully, M. E., Jevnick, M. A. and Hershberg, E. B., "Microbiological transformation of steroids. I. Δ¹,⁴-diene-3-ketosteroids", *J. Am. Chem. Soc.* **77**, 4184 (1955).

Obara, J., Hashimoto, S. and Suzuki, H., "Enzyme applications in the sucrose industries", *Sugar Technol. Rev.* **4**, 209–258 (1977).

Ogino, S., Fujimoto, S., Aoki, Y., "Co-oxidation of dl-cis-tetrahydro-2-oxo-4-n-pentyl-thieno-(3,4-d)-imidazoline (dl-TOPTI) by soil isolates of the genus Corynebacterium. *Agric. Biol. Chem.* **38**, 275–278 (1974 a).

Ogino, S., Fujimoto, S., Aoki, Y., "Production of biotin by microbial transformation of dl-cis-tetrahydro-2-oxo-4-n-pentyl-thieno-(3,4-d)-imidazoline (dl-TOPTI)", *Agric. Biol. Chem.* **38**, 707–712 (1974 b).

Ohmiya, K., Ohashi, H., Kobayashi, T. and Shimizu, S., "Hydrolysis of lactose by immobilized microorganisms", *Appl. Environ. Microbiol.* **33**, 137–146 (1977).

Perlman, D.: "Procedures useful in studying microbial transformations of organic compounds". In: Johnes, J. B., Sih, C. J., Perlman, D. (eds.): *Applications of Biochemical Systems in Organic Chemistry*. Part I. John Wiley, New York 1976, pp. 47–68.

Peterson, D. H. and Murray, H. C., "Microbiological oxygenation of steroids at carbon 11", *J. Am. Chem. Soc.* **74**, 1871–1872 (1952).

Poulsen, P. B. and Zittan, L., "Continuous production of high-fructose syrup by cross-linked cell homogenates containing glucose isomerase", *Methods Enzymol.* **44**, 809–821 (1976).

Price, K. E.: In: Perlman, D. (ed.): *Structure-Activity Relationships Among the Semisynthetic Antibiotics*. Academic Press, New York 1977, p. 7.

Reichstein, T. and Grüssner, A., "Eine ergiebige Synthese der L-Ascorbinsäure (Vitamin C)", *Helv. Chim. Acta* **17**, 311–328 (1934).

Richards, H. C. (Pfizer Corp.): "Procédé de préparation de 2-aminoalkyl-tétrahydroquinolines". Swiss Pat. 498,116 (1970).

Rosazza, J. P., "Microbial transformation of natural antitumor agents", *Lloydia* **41**, 297–311 (1978).

Rosi, D., Pertuzotti, G. P., Dennis, E. W., Berberian, D. A., Freele, H., Tullar, B. F. and Archer, S., "Hycanthone a new active metabolite of lucanthone", *J. Med. Chem.* **10**, 867 (1967).

Rufer, C., Kosmol, H., Schröder, E., Kieslich, K. and Gibian, H., "Totalsynthese optisch aktiver Steroide. III. Totalsynthese von optisch aktiven 13-Aethylgonan-Derivaten", *Justus Liebigs Ann. Chem.* **702**, 141–148 (1967).

Samuelsson, R., Granström, E., Green, K., Hamberg, M. and Hammarström, S., "Prostaglandins", *Ann. Rev. Biochem.* **44**, 669–695 (1975).

Sano, K., Yokozeki, K., Eguchi, C., Kagawa, T., Noda, I. and Mitsugi, K., "Enzymatic production of L-tryptophan from L- and DL-5-indolylmethylhydantoin by newly isolated bacterium", *Agric. Biol. Chem.* **41**, 819–825 (1977 a).

Sano, K., Yokozeki, K., Tamura, F., Yasuda, N., Noda, I. and Mitsugi, K., "Microbial conversion of DL-2-amino-Δ^2-thiazoline-4-carboxylic acid to L-cysteine and L-cystine: screening of microorganisms and identification of products", *Appl. Environ. Microbiol.* **34**, 806–810 (1977 b).

Sato, T., Nishida, Y., Tosa, T. and Chibata, I., "Immobilization of *Escherichia coli* cells containing aspartase activity with κ-carrageenan: enzymic properties and application for L-aspartic acid production", *Biochim. Biophys. Acta* **570**, 179–186 (1979).

Schmid, M. (Hoffmann-La Roche & Co. AG): "Verfahren zur Herstellung von trans-Phytol bzw. Vitamin K_1". D.O.S. 2,733,233 (1978).

Schmid, M. and Barner, R., "Totalsynthese von natürlichem α-Tocopherol. II. Aufbau der Seitenkette aus (−)-(S)-3-Methyl-γ-butyrolacton", *Helv. Chim. Acta* **62**, 464–473 (1979).

Schmid, M., Gerber F. and Hirth G., "Stereoselektive Totalsynthese von natürlichem Phytol und Phytolderivaten und deren Verwendung zur Herstellung von natürlichem Vitamin K_1", *Helv. Chim. Acta* **65**, 684–702 (1982).

Schneider, W. P. and Murray, H. C., "Microbiological reduction and resolution of prostaglandins. Synthesis of natural $PGF_{2\alpha}$ and ent-$PGF_{2\beta}$ methyl esters", *J. Org. Chem.* **38**, 397–398 (1973).

Schöller, W.: Manufacture of dihydrofollicle hormones by fermentative reduction. US Pat. 2,184,167 (Feb. 12, 1938), German priority (Feb. 16, 1937).

Sebek, O. K., "Microbial conversion of antibiotics", *Lloydia* **37**, 115–133 (1974).

Sebek, O. K., Lincoln, F. H. and Schneider, W. P., "Conversion of prostaglandins by Streptomycetes and yeasts", *Ferment. Technol. Today, Proc. Int. Ferment. Symp.* 5th, **1976**, 319.

Sebek, O. K. and Kieslich, K., "Microbial transformation of organic compounds", *Annu. Rep. Ferment. Processes* **1**, 267–297 (1977).

Shibata, M. and Uyeda, M., "Microbial transformation of antibiotics", *Annu. Rep. Ferment. Processes* **2**, 267–303 (1978).

Shibatani, T., Kakimoto, T. and Chibata, I., "Stimulation of L-aspartate-β-decarboxylase formation by L-glutamate in *Pseudomonas dacunhae* and improved production of L-alanine", *Appl. Environ. Microbiol.* **38**, 359–364 (1979).

Shier, W. T., Rinehart, K. L. and Gottlieb, D., "Preparation of four new antibiotics from a mutant of *Streptomyces fradiae*", *Proc. Natl. Acad. Sci. USA* **63**, 198–204 (1969).

Sih, C. J., Tai, H. H. and Tsong, Y. Y., "The mechanism of microbial conversion of cholesterol in 17-keto steroids", *J. Am. Chem. Soc.* **89**, 1957–1958 (1967).

Sih, C. J., Heather, J. B., Peruzzotti, G. P., Price, P., Sood, R. and Lee, L. F. H., "Total synthesis of prostaglandins. IV. A completely stereospecific synthesis of prostaglandin E_1", *J. Am. Chem. Soc.* **95**, 1676–1677 (1973).

Spencer, J. F. T. and Gorin, P. A. J., "Microbial transformation of sugars and related compounds", *Prog. Ind. Microbiol.* **7**, 177–220 (1968).

Straub, O.: *Key to Carotenoids: List of Natural Carotenoids*. Birkhäuser, Basel 1976.

Sugie, M. and Suzuki, H., "Purification and properties of D-aminoacylase of *Streptomyces olivaceus*", *Agric. Biol. Chem.* **42**, 107–113 (1978).

Sun Oil Comp.: "Microbial oxydation of polynuclear aromatic hydrocarbons". Brit. Pat. 1,056,729 (1965); cited by *C.A.* **66**, 74955z (1967).

Szantay, C. S. and Novak, L.: *Synthesis of Prostaglandins*. Akadémia Kiadó, Budapest 1978.

Takahashi, T. and Isono, M. (Takeda Ltd.): "Verfahren zur Herstellung von D-Pantoinsäure". D.O.S. 1,643,539 (1971).

Takano, S., Tanigawa, K., Ogasawara, K., "Asymmetric synthesis of a prostaglandin intermediate using microorganisms", *J. Chem. Soc. Chem. Commun.* **1976**, 189–190.

Takata, I., Yamamoto, K., Tosa, T. and Chibata, I., "Immobilization of *Brevibacterium flavum* with carrageenan and its application for continuous production of L-malic acid", *Enzyme Microb. Technol.* **2**, 30–36 (1980).

Tosa, T., Mori, T., Fuse, N. and Chibata, I., "Studies on continuous enzyme reactions. III. Enzymatic properties of the DEAE-cellulose-aminoacylase complex", *Enzymologia* **32**, 153–168 (1967).

Tsugawa, R., Okumura, S., Ito, T. and Katsuya, N., "Production of L-glutamic acid from DL-hydantoin-5-propionic acid by microorganisms. I. Screening of L-glutamic acid-producing microorganisms and some optimal conditions for production of L-glutamic acid", *Agric. Biol. Chem.* **30**, 27–34 (1966).

Vezina, C., Sehgal, S. N. and Singh, K., "Transformation of organic compounds by fungal spores", *Adv. Appl. Microbiol.* **10**, 211–268 (1968).

Wada, M., Kato, J. and Chibata, I., "A new immobilization of microbial cells", *Eur. J. Appl. Microbiol. Biotechnol.* **8**, 241–247 (1979).

Walton, R. B., McDaniell, L. E. and Woodruff, H. B., "Biosynthesis of novobiocin analogues", *Dev. Ind. Microbiol.* **3**, 370–375 (1962).

Wandrey, C. and Flaschel, E., "Process development and economic aspects of enzyme engineering. Acylase L-methionine system", *Adv. Biochem. Eng.* **12**, 147–218 (1979).

Weaver, E. A., Kenney, H. E. and Wall, M. E., "Effect of concentration on the microbiological hydroxylation of progesterone", *Appl. Microbiol.* **8**, 345–349 (1960).

Weeks, R. J., "Prostaglandins", *Annu. Rev. Pharmacol.* **12**, 317–336 (1972).

Wegner, E. H. (Phillips Petroleum Co.): Microbial conversion of naphthalene-base hydrocarbons. US Pat. 3,755,080 (1973); *C.A.* **79**, 113996d (1973).

White, R. F., Birnbaum, J., Meyer, R. T., Ten Broeke, J., Chemerda, J. M. and Demain, A. L., "Microbial epoxidation of cis-propenylphosphonic acid to (−)-cis-1,2-epoxypropylphosphonic acid", *Appl. Microbiol.* **22**, 55–60 (1971).

Wovcha, M. G.: "Verfahren zur Herstellung von 9α-Hydroxyandrostendion". D.O.S. 2,647,895 (Oct. 22, 1976).

Wovcha, M. G. and Biggs, C. D.: "Neue Mikroorganismusmutanten und Verwendung derselben bei der Herstellung von Androst-4-en-3,17-dion". D.O.S. 2,746,383 (Oct. 14, 1977).

Yamada, H. and Kumagai, H., "Microbial and enzymatic processes for amino acid production", *Pure Appl. Chem.* **50**, 1117–1127 (1978).

Yamamoto, K., Sato, T., Tosa, T. and Chibata, I., "Continuous production of L-citrulline by immobilized *Pseudomonas putida* cells", *Biotechnol. Bioeng.* **16**, 1589–1599 (1974a).

Yamamoto, K., Sato, T., Tosa, T. and Chibata, I., "Continuous production of urocanic acid by immobilized *Achromobacter liquidum* cells", *Biotechnol. Bioeng.* **16**, 1601–1610 (1974b).

Yamamoto, K., Tosa, T., Yamashita, K. and Chibata, I., "Continuous production of L-malic acid by immobilized *Brevibacterium ammoniagenes* cells", *Eur. J. Appl. Microbiol.* **3**, 169–183 (1976).

Yamamoto, K., Tosa, T., Yamashita, K. and Chibata, I., "Kinetics and decay of fumarase activity of immobilized *Brevibacterium ammoniagenes* cells for continuous production of L-malic acid", *Biotechnol. Bioeng.* **19**, 1101–1114 (1977).

Zell, R., "Totalsynthese von natürlichem α-Tocopherol. III. Aufbau der Seitenkette mit (−)-(S)-2-Methyl-γ-butyrolacton als zentralem Baustein", *Helv. Chim. Acta* **62**, 474–480 (1979).

Chapter 15

Production of Microbial Biomass

Uwe Faust

15.1 *Definition and Review*

The term **biomass** denotes the **organic cell substance** of plant or animal organisms. It is used both for the total body substance of an organism and as a group term for a biological raw material produced from plants and animals. Correspondingly, by microbial biomass is understood the cell substance of microorganisms that arises during their mass cultivation:

The production of microbial biomass is the technical manufacture of the cell mass of microorganisms from suitable organic raw material.

In technical fermentation processes, in addition to the desired synthesis of a natural substance (e.g., penicillin, citric acid), the multiplication and growth of the culture of microorganisms itself also takes place. As early as the beginning of the twentieth century, it was recognized that this cell mass, or microbial biomass, forms a useful product, so that its production with the substantial exclusion of accompanying processes was made the subject of a new development, the production of **microbial biomass** (Litchfield, 1980).

Chemically, the production of biomass can be formulated in the following manner:

As a **total substance,** biomass is composed of carbohydrates, lipids, proteins, nucleic acids, and special natural products such as vitamins, steroids, isoprenoids, and mineral substances, and it contains structurally bound water (Fig. 15-1).

Here, the main interest is in the **protein component** of the biomass. Consequently, microbial biomass is also called **single-cell protein** (**SCP**) or **bioprotein. The subsidiary components** that it contains can, however, also be utilized, e.g., the lipid fraction (single-cell fat, **SCF**) (Ratledge and Hall, 1979), the nucleic acid, or the vitamin component (particularly the vitamin B complex). In comparison with other biological natural materials this product is produced in relatively large amounts (mass product). Process engineering uses for this purpose on the large technical scale the cheapest possible raw materials and sources of energy that are available in large amounts in simple and low-energy processes.

As an industrial product, microbial biomass competes with biomass products from agriculture, forestry, and fisheries which, although, of course, they are obtained in a different manner, are similar in their basic composition and applicability in view of the universality of biochemistry. It is precisely in these facts that a challenge to biotechnology is seen – namely the production of biomass industrially in a

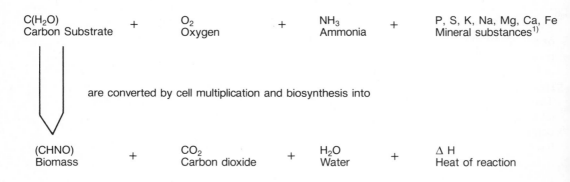

$C(H_2O)$ + O_2 + NH_3 +   P, S, K, Na, Mg, Ca, Fe
Carbon Substrate   Oxygen   Ammonia   Mineral substances[1]

are converted by cell multiplication and biosynthesis into

(CHNO)   + CO_2 + H_2O + ΔH
Biomass   Carbon dioxide   Water   Heat of reaction

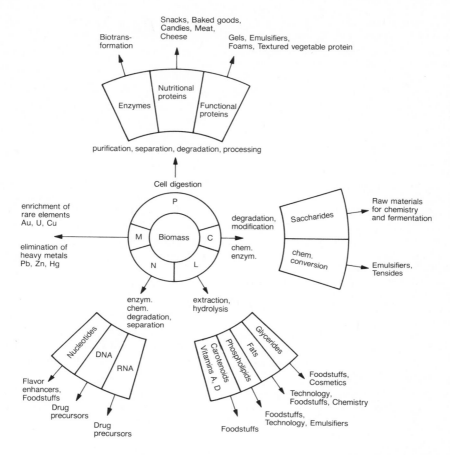

Fig. 15-1. Possibilities of use for components of biomass; – P=proteins; C=carbohydrates; L=lipids; N=nucleic acids, M=minerals.

technically controllable manner independent of soil, climate, and weather. Its development received another impulse when it was discovered that fossil materials can be used as substrates for microorganisms (Söhngen, 1913). Through this new raw material basis, it is possible once again to include the fossil carbon compounds into the life cycle from which they have been excluded for millions of years.

In the meantime, the production of micro-

bial biomass has taken a firm and important place in research, development and technical production and has led to new groups of tasks for microbiology, process engineering, and the development of new bioproducts.

The production of microbial biomass takes place in a **fermentation process.** Here, selected strains of microorganisms are multiplied on suitable raw materials in a technical cultivation process directed to the growth of the culture, and the cell mass so obtained is isolated by separation processes. Process development begins with **microbial screening,** in which suitable production strains are obtained from samples of soil, water, and air or from swabs of inorganic or biological materials (mineral ores, fruit peel) and are subsequently optimized by selection, mutation, or other genetic methods (see Chapter 2). Then the **technical conditions of cultivation** for the optimized strains are worked out and any special metabolic pathways and cell structures are determined (biochemistry, molecular biology). In parallel to these biological investigations, process engineering and apparatus technology adapt the technical performance of the process and the apparatus in which the production of biomass is to be carried out in order to make them ready for use on the large technical scale. Here **economic aspects** (investment, energy, operating costs, scale-up) come to the fore. For the overall profitability of biomass processes, the raw materials, their production and preparation, and the energy demands play the most important role. The various raw materials carriers must be investigated for their applicability from a technical, economic, and biological point of view and be prepared for the special biological process.

The biomass product proper is regarded as a new industrially accessible raw material and requires its own **independent product development** the task of which is, by analyses and biological tests, to determine the properties and composition of the total product and then to find possibilities for utilizing it or its constituents. New **application** are opened up by further processing. These range from the fodder sector through foodstuffs to technical, pharmaceutical, dietetic, and cosmetic products.

Safety demands and questions of environmental protection arise in the production of microbial biomass in relation both to the process and to the product. Finally, safety and the protection of innovation throw up legal and patent aspects, namely operating licenses, product authorizations for particular applications, and the legal protection of new processes and strains of microorganisms.

Thus, the production of microbial biomass includes a complex of technical fields and is becoming an interdisciplinary example of new biotechnology.

15.2   Raw Materials

Carbon-containing substrates (C-substrates) are the main raw material for the production of biomass, since the bulk of the biomass obtained consists of carbon, and then of oxygen and hydrogen, and the energy necessary for the construction of the cell is obtained from the **biocatalytic oxidation** of the C-substrate with oxygen to carbon dioxide and water. Correspondingly, the costs of the C-substrate form the largest item in the costs for the manufacture of biomass. The raw materials (carbon-containing raw materials) used for the production of biomass are summarized in Table 15-1.

The **classical raw materials** are substances containing mono- and disaccharides, since almost all microorganisms can assimilate glucose, related hexose and pentose sugars, and disaccharides. They arise as by-products of agriculture, the foodstuffs industry, and timber processing (whey, molasses, sulfite waste liquor, pressed fruit juices) or are manufactured directly by agrarian means (sugar cane juice, glucose syrup). They are therefore renewable raw materials. This group of materials also finds use in other branches of industry with a high price level which puts the economic aspect of the production of biomass in doubt.

Consequently, the production of biomass employs two other groups of raw materials which cannot be used directly in the area of competition that has been mentioned and are therefore subject to a different evaluation.

15.2.1   Basic Chemical Substances and Intermediates

These include methane (natural gas), methanol, ethanol, acetic acid, and normal paraffins.

Table 15-1. Carbon-containing Raw Materials Used for the Production of Biomass.

Carbon-containing substrates (raw materials)	Source of the substrate (raw material)
C_1 compounds carbon dioxide	air, physiological degradation of carbon-containing substrates, industrial combustion processes, sea water, carbonates;
methane	natural gas, coal, the gasification of wood, digestion processes;
methanol	synthesis gas (carbon monoxide + hydrogen);
C_2 compounds C_2H_5OH, CH_3COOH	ethylene, alcoholic fermentation;
C_5 compounds pentoses	wood sugar, sulfite waste liquor;
C_6 compounds hexoses	sugar cane, sugar beet, glucose syrup, starch;
C_{12} compounds disaccharides	molasses, sugar cane juice, sugar beet juice, whey;
Polysaccharides starch, cellulose	cereals, potatoes, cassava, wood, straw, bagasse;
chitin	wastes from crustacea;
C_{10}–C_{23} compounds normal paraffins	gas-oil.

Methane is one of the primary energy carriers and is available in large amounts both as natural gas and also via the production of synthesis gas from coal or wood. It also arises in the biological digestion of dead organic matter. Large amounts of methane are flared off unused in petroleum production. The favorable availability of methane is counterbalanced by the fact that only a few microorganisms are capable of assimilating methane (methanotrophs) and the technical transformation runs up against process engineering problems. Hitherto, only mixed cultures have been found capable of use for the production of biomass.

Methanol is obtained chemically by partial oxidation from methane or from synthesis gas [carbon monoxide (CO) + hydrogen (H_2)] and is therefore as available as methane. The amount of heat liberated in the partial oxidation can be utilized because of the high temperature level, which is not the case in the direct biological conversion of methane into biomass. Methanol is easy to store and transport without risk and is being developed to form one of the basic raw materials of the chemical industry and as a motor fuel.

From the biological point of view, there is a number of methanolotrophic microorganisms with interesting product properties the production of which offers no technical difficulties. Consequently, methanol is one of the most interesting biomass substrates.

Ethanol can be assimilated by a large number of different microorganisms. Regarded technically, the conversion of ethanol into biomass represents the simplest and neatest variant of the process. However, the raw material is obtained either from carbohydrates by fermentation, so that it is always more expensive than the corresponding substrate, which can also be used directly for the production of biomass, or from ethylene via petrochemical precursors. This basis is not comparable with the methane-methanol line, either, so that for reasons of availability ethanol will probably remain a special substrate for the production of biomass.

Similar points of view apply to **acetic acid,** which is obtained both microbially by the oxidation of ethanol and chemically from ethylene. The conversion of acetic acid into biomass is a simple and readily controllable process.

Normal paraffins with a carbon chain length of C_{10}-C_{23} are present in petroleum and are removed from diesel oil (gas-oil, middle oil) in order to lower its setting point. They are converted by hydrocarbon-degrading microorganisms into biomass. Today, manufacturing processes on the large technical scale are possible. Because they are coupled as a product with gas-oil, however, the availability and evaluation of paraffins are not free.

15.2.2 Complex Organic Compounds

The second group of fermentation substrates comprises complex **organic wastes from the foodstuffs industry, agriculture, forestry, and fisheries.** On the one hand, wastes from these sectors give rise to high disposal costs and, on the other hand, they frequently contain all the constituents necessary for the production of biomass. They can be fed to the production of biomass after a mechanical, thermal, enzymatic, or chemical pretreatment (purification, digestion). Against the low, frequently negative, substrate costs there are the adverse aspects of higher costs of preparation, variability in amount and composition of the wastes, and, frequently, a seasonal supply. The production of biomass – in this case, better upgrading of microbial biomass – often pays only in the case of large tonnages of wastes which are not always achieved in individual factories and therefore do not justify the expense of a fermentation plant.

The following may be mentioned:

- slaughterhouse wastes and blood
- whey
- sulfite waste liquor
- molasses
- fruit pulps
- potato processing wastes
- cereal wastes
- dung from animal rearing
- straw and timber wastes.

A special position is occupied by **carbon dioxide** as a biomass substrate. Carbon dioxide is assimilated directly into biomass by phototrophic and chemolithotrophic microorganisms, and oxyhydrogen bacteria. It is available from industrial combustion processes (thermal power stations), direct from the air, dissolved in sea water, or as carbonate practically free of cost in inexhaustible amounts. The necessary assimilation energy is not, however, as in the case of other raw materials contained in the substrate as bond energy but must be supplied as light in the case of the phototrophic organisms, via reducing substances (hydrogen sulfide, other sulfides, elementary sulfur), or via the oxyhydrogen reaction [hydrogen (H_2) + oxygen (O_2)]. The use of light (e.g., sunlight) makes it necessary to work in **surface culture,** which occupies large areas and is therefore very expensive.

15.2.3 *Sources of Nitrogen*

In addition to the carbon substrates, all biomass processes require nitrogen compounds for the synthesis of proteins and nucleotides. The following compounds are used as sources of nitrogen:

15.2.4 *Other Raw Materials*

Oxygen

All the C-substrates mentioned except carbon dioxide require oxygen for their conversion into biomass, and, because of the intensive mass growth in submerged processes, this is supplied as compressed air or in enriched or pure form. Since oxygen is only slightly soluble in the culture medium (water), it must be introduced continuously into a fermentation system, distributed in the medium, and

Nitrogen (N_2) from the air	for nitrogen-fixing microorganisms, energy-intensive
Ammonia, ammonium salts	cheapest and most common source of nitrogen
Nitrate	can be reduced by many species to ammonia
Urea Amino acids Peptone Proteins }	expensive sources of nitrogen.

The above list shows that, in general, ammonia or ammonium salts of sulfuric acid, hydrochloric acid, or phosphoric acid are the physiologically simplest and cheapest nitrogen compounds for the formation of biomass by microorganisms. The direct fixation of elementary nitrogen (see Chapter 3) is biologically energy-intensive and therefore, in general uneconomic. Moreover, only low rates of growth can be achieved in this way. In the assimilation of ammonium salts, protons are liberated, which lowers the pH of the culture medium (possibility of pH adjustment with ammonia), while when nitrate is used the pH of the culture solution rises and reduction equivalents of the cells (NADH, NADPH) are consumed.

brought into solution before it can be taken up by the microorganisms through diffusion (see Chapter 6). In terms of volume, in biomass processes compressed air is the greatest single component fed. Correspondingly high is the expenditure on the purification, sterilization, compression, and metering of the air or the preparation of pure oxygen. The compressors to be used in a production process are among the largest made.

Mineral Substances

Corresponding to the demand for mineral substances of plants and animals, microorganisms also have a definite requirement for phosphate, sulfate, potassium, sodium, calcium, magnesium, and iron ions, and also for trace elements for the formation of their biomass and the maintenance of their metabolism. These, in the form of an aqueous solution, are mixed in a definite ratio to the biomass to be formed unless they are already present in the process water or in the C-substrate (for example, whey, molasses), and are fed into the process continuously. The dosage of the mineral substances decides the quality of the biomass and the productivity of the process. Incorrectly metered mineral substances lead to deficiency phenomena in the formation of biomass or to the production of metabolites and reserve substances (e.g., polysaccharides, lipids). Moreover, the solution of mineral substances predetermines the osmotic pressure of the culture solution, which must also be kept within tolerable limits for the process to run without problems.

15.2.5   Energy Demand

The industrial production of biomass, unlike the agrarian production of biomass, is not energy-extensive but energy-intensive. Although a comparable consumption of energy per unit biomass produced is to be expected, the nature of the energy used in the two competing production processes differs. In the agrarian field, energy is used mainly for transport, harvesting, and storage and for fuel and heating and cooling agents, as well as for fertilizers and plant protection agents.

In the production of microbial biomass all these items are less important. What is involved here in the way of energy is, in particular, the **energy of compression** for the process oxygen (see the biomass equation) and the energy for removing the heat of fermentation at a low temperature level. While, therefore, in agriculture, forestry, and fisheries it is mobile energy carriers that are used, in the case of a large plant for the production of biomass it is electricity and direct fossil energy carriers (gas, coal via steam).

15.3   Microorganisms

The use of various strains of microorganisms is governed according to the C-substrate available and the desired quality of the biomass obtained. In addition, the choice of a production strain is determined by the technical handling and biological stability of the microorganisms and by safety aspects:

Criteria for the Choice of a Strain for Biomass Production

Given: C-substrate

- genetic stability
- continuous cultivation
- substrate specificity
- substrate yield
- nutrient demands
- submerged process in large fermenters
- separability of the biomass from the culture medium
- quality and composition of the product.

As in the production of other natural microbiological materials, a production strain is isolated by screening in accordance with criteria of choice that have been given and is optimized by selection, mutation, or the directed transmission of hereditary information (see Chapter 2) and by adaption to the technical methods of cultivation. The following classification of the species important for the production of biomass is based on the raw materials.

15.3.1   Methane-assimilating Microorganisms

The oxidative assimilation of C_1 compounds is practised by only a few microorganisms, almost exclusively species of bacteria (see Chapters 2 and 3). It leads from methane via methanol to formaldehyde, which is built up via various metabolic pathways into metabolite structural units. During the assimilation, acetate is formed which inhibits the uptake of the C_1 compound so that, for technical cultivation processes with high cell densities and high growth rates, mixed cultures are used. A methane-oxidizing strain is associated with acetate-assimilating forms which give definite and stable mixed cultures. The following strains have been described (Linton and Stephenson, 1978):

Methylomonas methanooxidans
Methylococcus capsulatus
Pseudomonas sp.

Because of the low water-solubility of methane, these strains have developed large-surface lamella-like internal cell structures which permit a high conversion of low concentrations of dissolved methane or the uptake of gaseous methane. Methane-assimilating microorganisms are found particularly in anaerobic regions of ponds and marshes, in digestion processes in agriculture, and in the utilization of wastes.

15.3.2 Methanol-assimilating Microorganisms

Methanol is miscible with water in all proportions. It arises in nature in fermentation and digestion processes in which methyl groups, e.g., from pectin (fruit peel) are degraded. Methyl groups also arise in dead marine animals, where methylamines form. Correspondingly, methanol-degrading microorganisms are found on rotten fruit and in the neighborhood of anaerobic digestion processes. Both yeasts and bacteria and not only facultative but also obligate methylotrophic organisms are known and can be used for the production of biomass (Cooney and Levine, 1972):

Methanol-assimilating Bacteria

a) Obligate methylotrophs
[Substrates: methane (CH_4), methanol (CH_3OH), acetone (CH_3OCH_3)]
Methylobacter   Methylocystis
Methylococcus   Methylosinus
Methylomonas

b) Facultative methylotrophs
[Substrates: methanol (CH_3OH), carbohydrates, organic acids]
Arthrobacter   Pseudomonas
Bacillus   Rhodopseudomonas
Hyphomicrobium   Streptomyces
Protoaminobacter   Vibrio

Yeasts and Fungi

Facultative methylotrophs
[Substrates: methanol (CH_3OH), carbohydrates, organic acids]
Candida   Pichia
Hansenula   Torulopsis
Kloeckera   Trichoderma

The yeast strains are characterized by a poorer asssimilation of the methanol, a specifically higher oxygen demand, a greater reaction heat, lower fermentation temperature, and a lower protein content in comparison with the methylotrophic bacteria. In addition, they require growth substances. The expenditure on the maintenance of sterility and on the separation of the cells from the culture solution is higher for bacteria. For large-scale technical production, obligate methylotrophic strains assimilating methanol via the hexulose phosphate cycle have been adopted.

15.3.3 Ethanol- and Acetate-assimilating Microorganisms

Ethanol-assimilating strains for the production of biomass are mainly yeasts of the genus *Candida utilis*. Bacterial strains are also known that can assimilate ethanol but the yeasts have become established because they are easier to handle technically and for historic reasons.

Acetate as the central metabolite of the metabolism is assimilated and converted by almost all microorganisms, but for the reasons given under the Raw Materials section, no strains for the production of biomass have yet been obtained by directed development and brought into use.

15.3.4 Carbohydrate-assimilating Microorganisms

The following strains of yeast and fungi are employed to utilize the **pentose-containing raw materials** from wood and wood processing:

Endomyces vernalis
Saccharomyces cerevisiae
Candida utilis.

The various **hexose monosaccharides** and disaccharides are also utilized by many microorganisms. For the production of biomass, not only yeasts but also fungi have been described:

Saccharomyces cerevisiae
Kluyveromyces fragilis
Aspergillus niger.

Fungi are suitable, in particular, for technical processes in which – together with the monomeric hexoses – oligomeric and polymeric carbohydrates from agricultural wastes are used as a mixed substrate and are processed in sim-

ple, robust, nonsterile apparatuses. The separation of fungal mycelium involves only little technical expense.

Polymeric carbohydrates (starch, cellulose, chitin) cannot be assimilated by **yeasts** at adequate rates of conversion. For the production of biomass from these substances, therefore, either **mixed cultures** of yeasts and bacteria are used in which the bacteria perform the step of hydrolysis to oligosaccharides and glucose and the yeasts then assimilate these liberated soluble substrates, or **fungal cultures** such as those mentioned in the case of mono- and disaccharides, are used for simple technical processes:

Cellulomonas alcaligenes
Aspergillus niger
Thermoactinomyces
Trichoderma harzianum, viride
Gliocladium sp.
Endomycopsis fibuligera
Candida utilis
Debaromyces kloeckeri
Sporotrichum pulverulentum
Brevibacterium sp.
Cytophaga sp.

Yeasts of the genus *Candida lipolytica* have come into use for the production of biomass from normal paraffins.

15.3.5 Carbon-dioxide-assimilating Microorganisms

Carbon dioxide is used as a substrate for algal cultures. In technical pilot projects, the following organisms, in particular, are being used:

Scenedesmus sp.
Chlorella
Spirulina maxima
Rhodopseudomonas gelatinosa
Botyococcus braunii.

In the chemolithotrophic assimilation of carbon dioxide, e.g., in the leaching of ores *(Thiobacillus thiooxidans),* however, the formation of biomass has not so far been utilized technically.

The oxyhydrogen bacteria *(Pseudomonas facilis, Alcaligenes eutrophus)* assimilate carbon dioxide in combination with hydrogen and oxygen as substrate. Because of the risk of explosion of the mixture and the lack of availability of cheap hydrogen, however, no interest has been shown in these microorganisms outside research projects.

15.4 Processes and Apparatus

All technical biomass processes follow a common sequence of processes consisting in:

– preparation of the raw material
– fermentation
– mechanical concentration of the biomass
– drying of the product
– final processing of the product.

In the processes based on the chemical raw materials methane, methanol, ethanol, and normal paraffins, the process water separated off during the concentration of the biomass is recycled to fermentation (Topiwala and Khosrovi, 1978). Auxiliary technical steps in the production of biomass are the compression of the air, the cooling of the fermenter, the sterilization of the substrate (facultative), and the provision of drying energy. In large plants, these steps can be included in an interlocking energy system.

15.4.1 Preparation of the Raw Material

The solid raw materials such as mineral salts, cellulose, starch, and sugars are comminuted and dissolved or suspended in water, definite substrate concentrations being established. The cellulose- and starch-containing raw materials are also loosened structurally and partially hydrolyzed by heating and by a pH treatment (alkaline or acid digestion). Depending on the raw material and the production strain, a substantial digestion can be brought about by the addition of cellulases or amylases and glucoamylases (Heynz et al., 1981).

The dissolution or suspension process makes the raw materials mentioned easier to meter out and sterilize in continuous fermentation processes. However, in some cases (see 15.4.2 Fermentation), the production of biomass takes place as a batch process. In these cases (e.g., in rational mini processes), the solid raw materials can be fed with water directly to the fermenter and be treated. The series coupling of the individual process steps in continuous operation becomes a temporal sequence in batch operation, in some cases with the use of a single reactor.

The **liquid raw materials** methanol, ethanol, acetic acid, molasses, glucose syrup, whey, cane sugar juice, normal paraffins, phosphoric acid, and sulfuric acid can, if desired, likewise be mixed with the above-mentioned aqueous nutrient solution to form a complete culture medium or be fed directly to the fermenter from separate storage tanks. In the case of direct dosage, a purification/sterilization step, if necessary, can be achieved by filtration processes.

The gaseous raw materials, air, pure oxygen, methane, ammonia, hydrogen, and carbon dioxide, are sterile-filtered under pressure and likewise metered in directly. They must be free from volatile, aerosol-like, or dust-fine impurities (hydrogen sulfide, hydrocarbons, aromatics, heavy-metal compounds, foreign organisms, lubricating oil). Appropriate purification steps and compressors must be used.

In order to achieve a better distribution in

the fermentation medium, the gaseous media may also be predispersed through blast nozzles.

15.4.2 Fermentation

In accordance with the **empirical equation for biomass,** the production of microbial cell material represents a biological growth process in which the conversion of all the substrates into biomass, carbon dioxide, and water by biosynthesis and cell division takes place with the evolution of heat within the individual microorganism cells added as inoculum that are suspended in a dilute aqueous medium (submerged fermentation).

From the point of view of process engineering, we have a **multiphase contact reaction,** in which the reaction partners are transported to the surface of the cells of all the microorganisms and the by-product carbon dioxide and water are removed. Here it is important that this continuous process operates only when all the reaction partners are present at the surface of the cell in suitable concentrations and further amounts of them are supplied continuously (Faust and Sittig, 1980).

Appropriate contact apparatuses, the fermenters, have been developed on the basis of a knowledge of the construction of chemical apparatus and have been adapted for the different requirements of biological processes (see Chapter 6).

Certain demands are made on a fermenter for the production of biomass (Table 15-2).

For the **production of biomass on the large technical scale,** all substrates and water as the reaction medium are fed in continuously in accurately metered amounts and are kept in uniform admixture with one another in the fermentation reactor, with the simultaneous removal of the heat of the reaction. The physicochemical boundary conditions temperature, pH, partial pressure of oxygen, concen-

Table 15-2. Demands on a Biomass Fermenter.

1. Rapid and uniform distribution of all the reactants over the whole reaction volume
2. Constancy of temperature and pH
3. High substrate yield
4. High oxygen transfer
5. Energy-saving operation
6. Continuous operation
7. Realization on the large technical scale
8. Sterile operation (in some cases).

tration of free substrate, ionic strength, pressure at the head of the reactor, and state of filling are monitored with suitable probes (see Chapter 7) and controlled.

The **inoculation culture** of the production strain required at the **start of the process** is taken from the stock culture in an inoculation chain and added to the presterilized fermenter filled with prepared culture solution and aerated. After a short initial growth phase, continuous flow is switched on. The biomass produced is contained in dilute suspension in the issuing flow.

The carbon substrate (C-substrate) is fed in in such a way that no excess remains in the culture solution, while all the other raw materials (oxygen, source of nitrogen, mineral substances) are present in excess (chemostat principle) (Rehm, 1980).

In **rational mini processes,** the operations are carried out semicontinuously or batchwise. It is true that this lowers productivity of a fermentation plant but permits a simpler and more robust monitoring and control of the process.

The fermenter is filled with water and raw materials, and if necessary it is sterilized and the substrate is digested, and it is then brought to the fermentation temperature, the aeration is switched on, inoculation is carried out, and the process is operated in a closed system. After a desired concentration of biomass has been reached, the fermenter is emptied of the product completely or partially, refilled, and started up again.

In the **cultivation of algae,** submerged cultivation is not used but the operation is carried out in flat trays in which surface cultures are exposed to sunlight and by means of pumps, paddles, or weirs, the material is passed in uniform flow through a closed circuit. To avoid infection and evaporation losses, the system is covered with translucent foil. Thus, the fermentation plant has a flat construction. The cultivation operations follow the day/ night rhythm and, correspondingly, the harvesting of the biomass is carried out not completely continuously but periodically (Tate and Lyle, Annual Report, 1979).

15.4.3 Processing

The working up of the fermented culture solution is based on the fact that only solid biomass and water-containing minerals have to be separated. The bulk of the process water is separated mechanically and returned to fermentation (Topiwala and Khosrovi, 1978).

Fungal mycelium can be filtered off, while **yeast** cultures are thickened to a maximum concentration of solid matter by means of separator centrifuges and decanter centrifuges.

Because of the difficulty of its direct separation, **bacterial biomass** is aggregated by heating, by the addition of ionic or nonionic flocculants, by a change in pH, or in an electric field and it is then, like yeast biomass, thickened in centrifuges (see Chapter 8). The filters and centrifuges that are used (which have been developed for the large-scale technical recovery of biomass) are among the largest unit apparatuses of their type (Gerstenberg et al., 1980).

The concentrated biomass is then heated in order to block the still intact enzyme systems and to break down the biomass (thermolysis).

If the crude biomass is itself the object of the process, this is followed by a drying step. Various large-scale technical drying systems can be employed for this purpose, depending on the intended use of the product (Fig. 15-2).

Apparatuses used for the **drying of the biomass** are also among the largest of their type. The maintenance of the quality of the product and the fully continuous mode of operation of a biomass unit also demand from the drying technique hygienically unobjectionable apparatuses requiring little attention that maintain a narrow temperature profile.

If **individual components** of the biomass are to give the end product, the thickened moist or crude biomass is subjected to a subsequent process of breakdown. Lipids and their individual components, nucleic acids and their monomers, individual protein fractions (soluble, insoluble), vitamins, chromophores, and aroma materials can be recovered by extraction, precipitation, and crystallization, as in the processing of high-value natural materials (see Chapter 8) (Schlingmann and Präve, 1978).

15.5 Process Examples

Most biomass processes developed on the technical scale follow a **general basic scheme** which is divided into the preparation of the raw material, including sterilization of a usually mostly synthetic nutrient solution, in a controlled continuous fermentation that is well supplied with oxygen in airlift loop fermenters, a mechanical separation of the cell mass by centrifuges, including the recycling of the clear phase, and a suitable drying step capable of being performed on the large technical scale – usually spray-drying with combined fluidized-bed granulation (see Fig. 15-2). In the examples given below, therefore, it

Process step	Concentration		Digestion		Drying				
Spec. characteristic	Separators	Decanters	Heaters	Plate evaporators	Spray dryers	Fluidized-bed dryers	Flow dryers	Rotating tube dryers	Flow dryers fluidized bed
	Westfalia: nozzle separator self-cleaning drum g-No. ~8000	Flottweg; Type Z 2L g-No. ~4500	Vessels with double jackets	Holstein und Kappert	Nubilosa: 2-fluid nozzle Niro Atomizer: Centrifugal-atomizer	Niro, Orth, Claudius Peters	Büttner-Schilde-Haas: Rapid circulation dryers	BSH, Lurgi, Krupp	Orth, Convex
Illustration	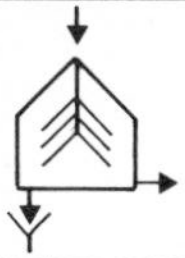	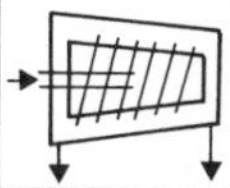	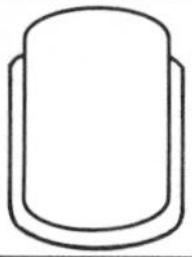	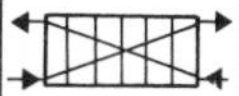	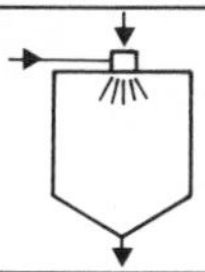	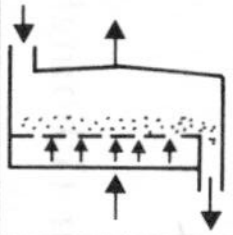	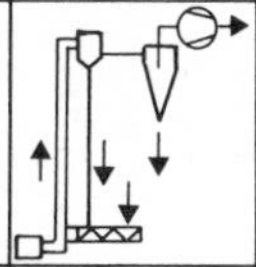	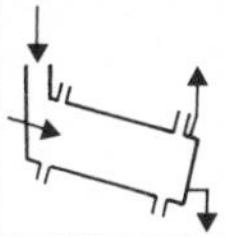	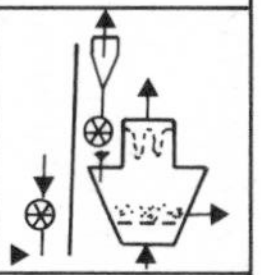
Mode of operation	cont.	cont.	batch and cont.	cont.	cont.		cont. with recycling of dried product	cont. from mixer	cont. from mixer
Mass fraction (%) of cell mass in the feed	2	3–5	15 25–30	~10 (dil. 1:1)	15–18 25–30	35–60 decanter product mixed with spray product	65–70 decanter product mixed with spray product		
Mass fraction (%) of cell mass after the process step	15	25–30	15 25–30	~25	98	95–99	~95	~95	~95
Residence time	500 L/h (nozzle) 8000 L/h (self-cleaning)	680 L/h	5 min 15 min	~3 min	a few seconds	minutes to hours	a few seconds	minutes to hours	minutes to hours
Temperature °C at inlet	10 20	20	90 75	80	Nubilosa: 200 Niro Atomiz.: 290	150	250–380	150	250
Temperature °C of discharge	15 20	20	90 75	50	Nubilosa: 95–100 Niro Atomiz: 110	45–75	100–150	90	75
Remarks on the product after the process step	flowable and pumpable	can be cut	flowable and pumpable	flowable and pumpable	dust-fine bulk density ~0.4 kg	grain size 125–1600 µm	bulk density 0.6–0.7 kg	granulate < 1 mm	granulate < 1 mm

Fig. 15-2. Recovery processes for biomass; – cont. = continuous; dil. = dilution.

is the peculiarities and deviations that are mentioned rather than these basic patterns. For questions of detail, reference may be made to the technical literature cited in each case.

15.5.1 Biomass from Methane

The leading organization in the development of a methane process was the British Shell research organization at Sittingbourne (Kent). In addition to synthetic mixtures, natural gas (93% methane) is used as the raw material. A definite complex mixed culture has been developed as the production culture the main component of which is the methane-assimilating strain *Methylococcus capsulatus*. The subsidiary components Pseudomonas, Nocardia, and Moraxella assimilate metabolites of the main strain and therefore have a stabilizing effect. The operation is carried out with a fully synthetic medium at pH 6.8 in the temperature range of 42 to 45 °C with a computer-controlled mixed gassing with natural gas and air. Equation of the conversion:

3.0 g oxygen + 1.2 g methane → 1 g cells + 1.2 g carbon dioxide + 2.0 g water + 55.3 kJ

The process is operated continuously under semisterile conditions in fermenters with a size of up to the order of 300 L (stirred tanks) at a dilution rate of 0.3 h^{-1}. Cell densities of 25 g/L are achieved. The product is worked up by means of a separator and spray dryer. No analytical or toxicological information about the resulting biomass product is available.

There have been laboratory developments towards a similar process at the Max-Planck Institut für Limnologie at Plön, West Germany.

15.5.2 Biomass from Methanol

As described in the Raw Materials section, **methanol** is the most promising substrate for large-scale technical bioprocesses. For this reason, the production of biomass from methanol is the most developed at the present time. The leaders in this respect are the firm ICI, Billingham, England, who have a production plant with a capacity of about 60 000 tons a year in operation since 1980 (Windass et al., 1980). In addition, Hoechst/Uhde (Faust et al., 1977) (1000 tons per year pilot plant), the Mitsubishi Gas Company (Kuraishi et al., 1979) (Nigata, Japan, 500 tons per year pilot plant), Norprotein (Ebbinghaus et al., 1979) (Sundbyberg, Sweden, 4 m^3 pilot plant), and Phillips Petroleum Provesta (Malik, 1979) (Houston, Texas, pilot plant) have developed their own, similar processes. The production strains used are mostly obligate methylotrophic bacteria of the Methylomonas sp. group. Yeasts, such as *Hansenula polymorpha,* also being worked on for comparison, have a lower protein content and a poorer substrate conversion so that, for economic reasons, they are inferior to bacteria when methanol is used as substrate. The nutrient solutions are fully synthetic. The processes are operated under sterile conditions continuously with the recycling of the clear phase in slender gassed loop reactors. ICI, Hoechst and Mitsubishi Gas Company have carried out technical development of the reactors.

The fermentation of the methanol takes place at pH 6.8 and 37 to 40 °C. For working up, the product is aggregated electrochemically or thermochemically, and the flocculated biomass is then thickened in centrifuges and brought into a storable form in spray-dryers, fluidized-bed dryers, or spin-flash dryers. The Hoechst/Uhde process includes another purification and separation step for taking off the lipids and nucleic acids, so that protein isolates are obtained.

15.5.3   Biomass from Ethanol

The Pure Culture Corp. (formerly: Amoco Corp.) in the USA is operating a fermentation plant for the manufacture of yeast from **ethanol** (capacity 10 000 tons). The course of the process corresponds to the process criteria described at the beginning of this section. Fermentation is carried out in stirred tank fermenters, and the dry product is made up for use in foodstuffs. In addition, a process has been developed in Czechoslovakia (1000 tons/year pilot plant).

15.5.4   Biomass from Normal Paraffins

The **normal paraffin process** was developed between 1965 and 1975 as the first large-scale process generation. Here the British Petroleum Company (BP) carried out the most comprehensive development work and, as well as two fairly large pilot plants (Cape Lavera, France, 20 000 tons/year) it erected a 100 000 tons/year production plant at Sarroch in Sardinia. Since then, the plants have been shut down because of inadequate profitability. However, this work has promoted the development of biomass processes, particularly since here the methods of toxicological and nutritional research necessary for evaluating the product have been worked out and systematized. This has made it possible to show that the microbial biomass manufactured from petrochemical materials is unobjectionable as **animal feed,** being safe and of high nutritional value when the appropriate predetermined biological and technical conditions are maintained. The BP process works with yeasts of the genus *Candida lipolytica* on a sterile continuous basis in stirred tank fermenters in accordance with the transformation formula:

1.12 g paraffin + 2.56 g oxygen + 0.13 g ammonia → 1 g biomass + 1.76 g carbon dioxide + 1.08 g water + 33.5 kJ

Separator centrifuges are used for separating the biomass and spray towers for drying it. Fermentation is carried out at 30°C and a pH of 4.5 (Watts, 1976).

Comparable processes have been developed as far as the pilot scale and tested by Dainippon (Ohiwa, 1975), by Kanegafuchi (Takata, 1969), by Hoechst/Uhde (Knecht et al., 1977), and by Petrochemie Schwedt (Bauch et al., 1978). In some cases, unpurified gas-oil containing normal paraffins is used, and after fermentation it is separated in three-phase separators. The end product is freed from residual hydrocarbons by extraction with isopropanol (BP, Schwedt). In addition to BP, the firm Liquichimica S.A. in Italy has erected production plants using the Kanegafuchi process, and Roniprot in Romania one using the Dainippon process (60 000 tons per year). In the Soviet Union, such plants with an output of more than 100 000 tons/year of biomass are in operation (Bauch et al., 1978).

15.5.5   Biomass from Carbohydrate-containing Raw Materials

The production of biomass from various **carbohydrate-containing substrates** has an old tradition when one thinks of the yeast fermentation of molasses, whey, and sulfite waste liquor from the production of cellulose. The processes carried out technically today have now arrived at plants of medium size producing from a few hundred to a few thousand tons of biomass per year and are adapted individually to the local raw materials situation. The technology usually involves a **combined utilization of wastes,** as, for example, in the case of whey, sulfite waste liquor, molasses, and wastes from the foodstuffs industry or agriculture. Here we shall give details of two processes, as examples:

The **Pekilo process** of the firm of Tampella, Finland (Romantschuk and Lektomäki, 1978) is based on **pentose-containing sulfite waste liquors from wood processing.** The sulfite is driven off by heating and the solution is then fermented continuously with the fungus *Paecilomyces varioti* at pH 4.5, 30°C, and a dilution rate $D = 0.2$ h^{-1}. A plant with a productivity of 10000 tons per year of biomass from 100 m^3/hr of sulfite waste liquor is in operation at Jämsänkoski, Finland. It uses a 360 m^3 stirred tank fermenter under sterile conditions. Ammonia, potassium chloride, and phosphoric acid are added as nutrient salts. The fungal mycelium produced is separated by means of filter presses and dried on a belt dryer to form a flaky product.

The firm of Tate and Lyle, Reading, England has developed a **rational mini technology** by which, on the small scale, the **fruit** of a tree growing in arid zones *(Ceratonia siliqua)* is converted by fermentation with the fungus *Aspergillus niger* (Imrie and Vlitos, 1973). The fruit is extracted with hot water which yields a 7% sugar solution to which ammonium sulfate and dihydrogen phosphate are added. This solution is fermented batchwise at 36°C in a 3000-liter stirred tank for 24 hr with 45% yield, which gives a cell density of more than 30 g/L. The protein content is 35%. The culture solution is thickened in rotary vacuum filters, and is dewatered in a ring dryer to give a keepable powder.

A similar process has been developed by Hoechst/Uhde as a mobile unit which can supply various animal farms with protein feedstuffs obtained from certain agrarian wastes (Schneider, 1980).

15.5.6 Biomass from Carbon Dioxide

In addition to yeasts, bacteria, and fungi, **phototrophic microorganisms** have been used for the production of biomass. Here a technology is employed which has been adapted to the demand for light. Microalgae or phototrophic bacteria of the genera Spirulina, Scenedesmus, Rhodopseudomonas, and Chlorella are cultivated in flat trays turned toward the sunlight, the culture solution being treated with additional nutrients and being circulated by pumps. This technique is area-intensive, particularly since only low concentrations of biomass are reached before the absorption of light by the cells becomes the limiting factor.

During the night, no growth can take place, so that the generation times are important (about 24 h). The corresponding plants are therefore designed more particularly for small biomass capacities (50-500 tons/year) and preferably for equatorial zones with a high intensity of light.

A variant of the process is the **mixed cultivation of algae** on **liquid organic wastes,** when it is less the production of biomass and more the **elimination of effluents** that is in the foreground. Neither of these developments has yet gone beyond the research stage. Thus, for example, the firm Tate and Lyle have operated an experimental station in the form of terraces at the University of Liège (Tate and Lyle, Annual Report, 1979) in order to manufacture **fish food** for the breeding of fish with the multicellular filamentous alga Hydrodictyon. The waste water from the breeding of the fish is recirculated to the algal unit.

A Canadian process from the University of Sherbrook using *Spirulina maxima* has achieved a biomass productivity of 0.05 g/L·h, which is about 1% of the level achieved with yeast and bacteria (Leduy and Therien, 1979). The area yield is 12 g of biomass per m^2 per day, i.e., 20 tons per hectare per year. Thus, the yield is no higher than for conventional cultural products.

In a German/Indian project, plastic trays with a volume of 10000 L each were covered with translucent sheets (Becker, 1979). The culture solution, harvested daily, was processed by means of separator centrifuges or textile filters and was dried on roller dryers on 120°C.

15.5.7 Biomass Products and Economic Aspects

The bioproducts made in the processes described form **unconventional sources of protein** the use of which as fodder or foodstuffs components must be shown to be safe by careful analytical, microbiological, toxicological, and nutritional testing. For this purpose, recommendations of IUPAC and of the Protein Advisory group (see Appendix) that give a recommended minimum set of limits have been generally adopted. In addition to this, other special investigations are indicated that depend on the intended use and also on the raw material and the manufacturing technique. These measures are required particularly with the use of **petrochemical substrates** such as gas-oil, coal gas, and normal paraffins, and also methanol. For this reason, the products from the processes described are among the best-described and best-studied fodders and foodstuffs of all. For all the processes tested on the relatively large scale (BP, ICI, Kanegafuchi, Hoechst) it has been possible to demonstrate the **toxicological safety** and the **biological value** of the products (see the cited literature). This has formed the first step to the introduction of the marketing of new biomass products. However, before their use becomes established, further stagewise testings of the technology, profitability, and possible applications will follow. Table 15-3 gives a typical review of some analytical characteristics of selected bioproteins. Table 15-4 shows the most important tests for safety and nutritive aspects.

When the **economic aspects** of the technical manufacture of biomass are considered (Sittig

et al., 1978), it can be seen that 50 to 70% of the manufacturing costs are for the raw materials. Consequently, the profitability of a process is decided by the costs either of substrates coupled to agricultural products or by the rise in the price of petrochemical feedstocks and energy carriers. From this, it may be expected that biomass products can become profitable and therefore can become a meaningful supplementation of existing sources of protein the greater the extent to which they are purified, show high-value properties, and can open up **new fields of application.** Here, their use as fodder components for the mass rearing of animals can be only a first stage in development. Some other aspects of profitability are dealt with in Chapter 18. So far, single-cell proteins have shown the following **possibilities of application**

in animal nutrition:
– fattening calves
– fattening poultry
– feed for laying hens
– fish breeding
– fattening pigs
– feed for domestic animals;

in the foodstuffs area:
– as aroma carriers
– as vitamin carriers
– as emulsifying aids
– to improve the nutritive value of baked products
– in soups
– in ready-to-serve meals
– in diet recipes;

in the technical field:
– in paper processing
– in leather processing
– as foam stabilizers.

In addition to the production of microbial biomass that has been described, it may be

Table 15-3. Comparative Analyses of Various Biomass Products.

Biomass products	Bacteria/ methanol	Yeasts/ paraffin	Yeasts/ carbohydrates	Fungi/ carbohydrates	Algae/ carbon dioxide
Crude protein (%)	80	55–60	45–50	35–45	40–60
Nucleic acids (%)	10–15	5–8	5	10	6
Fat (%)	8	9	8	2–5	5–9
Mineral substances (%)	7–8	8	7	5–10	10–15
Amino acids (g/16 g nitrogen):					
Isoleucine (Ileu)	4.5	3	4.5	5	5–6
Alanine (Ala)	7	6	6	6.5	
Leucine (Leu)	7	5.5	6.5	7	8–9
Glycine (Gly)	5.5	3	5	5	
Lysine (Lys)	6	6.5	6.5	6.5	4–5
Phenylalanine (Phe)	3.5	2.5	3.5	4	4–5
Methionine (Met)	2.5	2	1.5	2	2–3
Proline (Pro)	3.5	2.5	3.5	4	
Threonine (Thr)	4.5	3.5	5.5	4	5
Aspartic acid (Asp)	9	8	8	9	
Tryptophan (Trp)	1	0.5	1	1	1
Glutamic acid (Glu)	10	9	10	2	–
Valine (Val)	5	3.5	5	5	6–7
Tyrosine (Tyr)	3	3	3.5	3.5	5
Arginine (Arg)	4.5	3.5	4.5	5	9–10
Histidine (His)	2.5	2	3	2	1.8
Serine (Ser)	3.5	3	3.5	4	–

The Table shows various biomass products that are produced by a given group of organisms when growing on a given carbon substrate, e.g., bacteria growing on methanol (bacteria/methanol).

Table 15-4. Animal Experiments and other Investigations Recommended for Testing the Quality of Biomass as Animal Fodder.

Safety	**Nutritive aspects**
Acute and chronic toxicity	Biological protein value
Carcinogenicity	Biological digestibility
Teratogenicity	Availability of the amino acids and mineral components
Mutagenicity	Metabolizable energy
	Stability on storage, mixing stability
	Effect on animal tissues that may be used as foodstuffs
	Compatibility with conventional fodders.

mentioned, finally, that the production of bakers', brewers', and wine yeasts, of starter cultures, of definite strains for research and therapy, and of humus cultures for soil inoculations, and also cultures of edible fungi, must be included in the production of microbial biomass. These techniques are operated on similar principles to those described but form **special areas,** which are discussed more fully to some extent in Chapter 9.

15.6   Economic Aspects

The industrial manufacture of microbial biomass is greatly affected from the economic point of view by the C-substrate used. While in the case of locally available highly diversified waste substrate no general consideration of profitability is possible, more accurate calculation can be made for the synthetic raw materials methane, methanol, normal paraffins, and ethanol.

Figure 15-3 gives a rough **cost distribution** for the substrates mentioned. The actual cost factors depend greatly on the local conditions. The main variables can be discussed in the following way:

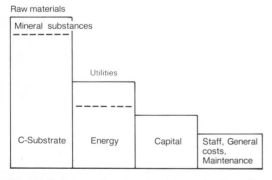

Fig. 15-3. Key to the costs for the production of biomass with synthetic raw materials.

15.6.1   Variables Resulting form the Process

Substrate Costs

In every case, the substrate costs form the largest single cost factor. A variation in these costs therefore means the greatest possibility of affecting the total manufacturing costs. The raw materials costs can be minimized, on the one hand, by choosing a site for the production of biomass where the raw materials are available cheaply. Costs can be saved by simplifying the manufacture and purification of the raw material, e.g., in the case of methanol or ethanol. Moreover, the manufacture of raw materials is more economical in larger plants for producing them. Finally, the substrate yield (referred to biomass) affects the raw materials costs.

Factors involved in the raw materials costs are, then

- site
- raw material production process
- capacity of the plant
- substrate yield
- product concentration/quality of the biomass.

Utilities

The energy for compressing air, cooling, sterilizing, and drying forms the next most important cost factor. Sites with cheaply available thermal, electrical, fossil, or process-derived energy are to be preferred. The biomass manufacturing process can then be adapted to the particular form of energy. If the main energy base is natural gas (e.g., in combination with a methane- or methanol-producing plant), both the production of compressed air and of electricity and also of sterilization and drying can be provided through natural gas (gas turbine with waste heat utilization).

Available steam can also be used correspondingly.

A considerable amount of energy can be saved by interconnecting the individual process steps and by coupling with another industrial plant (power station, methanol synthesis plant, sugar factory).

In particular, savings in air compression are possible if a substantial utilization of the oxygen of the fermenter air is ensured by the appropriate construction of the fermenter. The substrates mentioned have different, specific, oxygen demands, and demands for cooling in the following sequence:

- methane
- paraffins
- methanol
- ethanol
- carbohydrates.

Capital load

The capital-dependent costs are determined, on the one hand, by the **cost of the apparatus** for the process, the capacity of a plant, and the **capacity conditions.** The main variable here is the **size of the plant.** Small plants can be profitable only if they include simplifications of processes and material to a considerable degree:

- nonsterile working
- cheap apparatus materials
- high fermenter productivity
- simple separation technique (sedimentation, filtration)
- renouncement of the drying of the product.

The greater expenditure on apparatus in processes with cheap, simple, and unpurified raw materials (natural gas, gas-oil, cellulose wastes) usually does not pay in comparison with more expensive pure substrates with simpler technology.

The distribution of costs for **fermentation, mechanical concentration,** and **thermal drying** is approximately in equal parts. High productivities and biomass concentrations in fermentation (small fermenters) are compensated by the greater expenditure on energy to achieve these productivities, so that optimum productivities can be determined. Furthermore, high productivities run in parallel with a high nucleic acid content and a low protein content, so that they are important only for producing nucleic acids.

The other process-specific cost factors play only a subordinate role in comparison with the main parameters that have been mentioned.

15.6.2   Product-Specific Variables

The process costs arising are covered only by the product produced. The **absolute value of the product** is governed by the amount of product referred to the costs involved (yield, continuity of the manufacturing process) and by the quality of the product.

The **quality of the product** is poorer for a low-value unpurified product of a rational mini process with varying composition or one including numerous subsidiary components than for upgraded products. The upgrading of the product may consist of a purification and separation into the components of the biomass or the imparting of functional properties to the end product such as taste, aroma, bite, emulsifiability, foaming, complex-formation, extrudability, elasticity, water-binding capacity, and water solubility (Schlingmann and Präve, 1978).

Because of genetic variability, the possibilities of technical control in manufacture, and the simplicity of the process, microbial biomass is more suitable for such special products than biomass from the plant or animal kingdom.

Correspondingly, the use of bioprotein (single-cell protein, SCP) for animal nutrition may be only a first step of development in this direction, since because of the quantitative conversion loss, animal feed must always be cheaper than enriched end products.

15.7 Literature

Bauch, J. et al., „Verfahren zur Gewinnung von Fermosin-Futterhefe aus Erdöldestillaten", *Chem. Tech. Leipzig* **30** (6), 284 (1978).

Becker, E. W.: *Manual on Cultivation and Processing of Algae as Source of SCP*. Inst. f. chem. Pflanzenphysiologie, 7400 Tübingen.

Cooney, C. L., Levine, D. W., *Adv. Appl. Microbiol.* **15**, 337 (1972).

Ebbinghaus, L., Eriksson, M., Lindblom, M., "Mikrobiell protein from methanol", *Kem. Kemi* **6**, 311 (1979).

Faust, U., Präve, P., Sukatsch, D. A., "Continuous biomass production from methanol", *J. Ferment. Technol.* **55** (6), 609 (1977).

Faust, U., Sittig, W., "Methanol as carbon source for biomass production", *Adv. Biochem. Eng.* **17**, 63 (1980).

Gerstenberg, H., Sittig, W., Zepf, K., „Aufarbeitung von Fermentationsprodukten", *Chem. Ing. Tech.* **52**, 1, 19 (1980).

Heisel, M., „Verfahrenstechnik, Biologie und Wirtschaftlichkeit eines neuen Verfahrens zur Biosynthese von Eiweiß", *Linde Ber. Tech. Wiss.* **45**, 84 (1979).

Heynz, F. K., Reinefeld, F., Thielecke, K.: „Technologie der Kohlenhydrate". In: Winnacker-Küchler: *Chemische Technologie*. Hansa-Verlag, München 1981.

Imrie, F. K. L., Vlitos, A. J.: "Production of fungal protein from carob". 2nd International SCP Symposium. M.I.T. Boston, USA, May 1973.

Knecht, R. et al., "Microbiology and biotechnology of SCP produced from n-paraffin", *Process Biochem.* **12** (4/9), 25 (1977).

Kuraishi, M. et al., "Microbiology applied to biotechnology", *DECHEMA Monogr.* **83**, 111 (1979).

Leduy, A., Therien, N., "Cultivation of *Spirulina maxima*", *Can. J. Chem. Eng.* **57**, 489 (1979).

Linton, J. D., Buckee, J. C., "Interactions in a methane utilizing mixed bacterial culture in a chemostat", *J. Gen. Microbiol.* **101**, 219 (1977).

Linton, J. D., Stephenson, R. J., "Preliminary study of growth yields", *FEMS Microbiol. Lett.* **3**, 95–98 (1978).

Litchfield, J. H., "Microbial cells on your meal", *CHEMTECH*, April 1980, S. 218.

Malik, E.: Brochure of Fa. Phillips Provesta, Bartlesville, Oklahoma 74003 (1979).

Ohiwa, J., "Outlines of hydrocarbon yeasts", SCP-Symposium 1975, Philadelphia. ACS National Meeting.

Ratledge, C., Hall, M. S., "Accumulation of lipid by *Rhodotorula glutinis* in continuous culture", *Biotechnol. Lett.* **1** (3), 155 (1979).

Rehm, H. J.: *Industrielle Mikrobiologie,* 2nd Ed. Springer-Verlag, Berlin, Heidelberg, New York 1980, p. 138.

Romantschuk, H., Lektomäki, M., "Operation experience of first full scale Pekilo SCP-Mill Application", *Process Biochem.* **13**, 3 (1978).

Schlingmann, M., Präve, P., "Single Cell Proteine mit reduz. Nukleinsäure- und Fettgehalt", *Fette-Seifen-Anstrichm.* **80**, 283 (1978).

Schneider, E.: „Einfachverfahren zur Herstellung von Hefeprotein". 2. Symposium Mikrobielle Proteingewinnung 1981, GBF-Braunschweig. Verlag Chemie, Weinheim.

Sittig, W., Faust, U., Präve, P., Scholderer, J., „Technologische und wirtschaftliche Aspekte der Einzellerproteingewinnung", *Chem. Ind.* **30**, 713 (1978).

Söhngen, N. L., „Benzin, Petroleum und Paraffin als Kohlenstoff- und Energiequelle für Mikroben", *Zentralbl. Bakteriol. Parasitenk. Infektionskr. Abt. 2* **37**, 595 (1913).

Takata, T., "From n-paraffins to proteins", *Hydrocarbon Process.* **48**, 99 (1969).

Tate & Lyle, Annual Report 1979, Reading, England.

Topiwala, H. H., Khosrovi, B., "Waterrecycle in biomass production process", *Biotechnol. Bioeng.* **20**, 73–78 (1978).

Watts, H., "Single cell protein", *Chem. Ind. London* **1976**, 537.

Windass, D. J., et al., "Improved conversion of methanol to SCP", *Nature* **287**, 396 (1980).

Chapter 16

Environmental Biotechnology

Klaus Mudrack, Hermann Sahm, and
Wolfgang Sittig

Purification of Effluents with Aerobic Processes

16.1   Historical Development

In order to be able to evaluate the present state of sewage treating processes correctly, the steps in development will be given in a few words (Imhoff, 1979).

Until the 19th century, excrements were stored above or below ground in the neighborhood of dwellings and, when necessary, transported to the fields or poured into open waters (Dunbar, 1907). With the introduction of the water closet in the 19th century, this method of disposing of excrements was no longer adequate. The excrement was rinsed from the collecting pits onto the streets and collected in the open gutters provided for taking off rainwater. The consequence was intolerable states of hygiene and epidemics. Only by the construction of underground sewers for transporting the wastewater from the populated area, i.e., with the introduction of **flushing drainage** was it possible to eliminate the nuisance. At this stage of development, therefore, only purely constructional measures were necessary and for this reason, naturally, the problem of disposing of sewage was exclusively in the hands of engineers and builders. Hygienists were involved in the development only to the extent that they recognized wastewater as causes of sickness and encouraged the building of sewers. Chemists and biologists were not concerned with the problems at this period.

With the rapid development of industry and the increase in the density of population in the industrial areas, it was found that the problem had not been solved but the nuisance had merely been displaced from the areas of population into the water bodies. The disastrous situation in rivers overloaded with sewage, the receiving bodies, made a **purification of the sewage** urgently necessary. In this situation, it was logical that the sewage purification stations, which were regarded as the final stage of the sewerage system were likewise constructed by building engineers, hygienists and chemists being involved in the development of the "biological processes." A "technical microbiology" that could actively cooperate in the development of sewage purification processes did not yet exist at this period. Finally, the small degree of representation of microbiology in the field of sewage purification which has lasted to the present time can be understood from this development situation.

16.2   Wastewater

Wastewater as a substrate for the organisms present in the "reactor clarification unit" can be defined precisely only in the rarest cases. In broad terms, it is possible to distinguish **communal sewage,** the various types of **industrial effluents** and **mixed sewage.**

Apart from industrial effluents with extremely one-sided composition, it is impossible to characterize qualitative and quantitative compositions of sewage adequately by individual parameters (e.g., fat, sugars, chlorides). Attempts have therefore been made to determine the sum of the organic pollutants present in sewage directly by oxidizing it under definite conditions and determining the amount of oxidizing agent necessary for this purpose. In the case of the **"biochemical oxygen demand" (BOD$_5$),** the amount of oxygen (mg O_2/L) consumed by microorganisms in 5 days during the biological transformation of the pollutants is given. In the determination of the **"chemical oxygen demand" (COD)** with the aid of chemical oxidation by potassium dichromate or potassium permanganate, either the amount of oxidizing agent consumed (e.g., mg $KMnO_4$/L) or the equivalent amount of oxygen calculated from it (mg O_2/ L) is given.

None of the methods can determine the amount of soil (pollution) "absolutely correctly," i.e., the results must be interpreted in each case in the light of the analytical method used.

16.2.1 Communal Sewage

By communal sewage is understood the wastewater arising in households, communal establishments (schools, hospitals), and small-scale industry (slaughterhouses, laundries, hotels) within a community. According to Imhoff (1979), the **amount of sewage** per inhabitant

shows characteristic fluctuations over 24 hours (Fig. 16-1). Likewise, the **composition** and **concentration** of the pollutants fluctuate in the course of a single day. If the soil load that is to be treated in the clarification plant is calculated (e.g., as kg BOD_5/h) from the amount of sewage and its concentration, the figures during the daily peak may amount to a multiple of the night minimum values (Fig. 16-2). On an average, one can calculate with the amounts of soil, referred to an inhabitant (or per m^3 of sewage) given in Table 16-1.

If the community includes industrial enterprises, the composition and amount of the "mixed sewage" will be affected by these additional input contributors according to the nature and size of the enterprise.

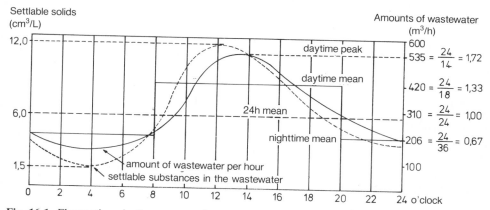

Fig. 16-1. Fluctuations in the amount of wastewater and the settlable solids contents from a town of 50 000 inhabitants in the course of 24 h (after Imhoff, 1979).

Table 16-1. Amounts of Wastes per Head of the Population (H) or per 1 m^3 of Sewage (Imhoff, 1979).

	Mineral (in g/H·d)	Organic	Total	BOD_5	Mineral (in g/m^3)	Organic	Total	BOD_5
Settlable solids	10	30	40	20	50	150	200	100
Nonsettlable solids	5	10	15	10 } 40	25	50	75	50 } 200
Dissolved matter	75	50	125	30	375	250	625	150
Total	90	90	180	60	450	450	900	300

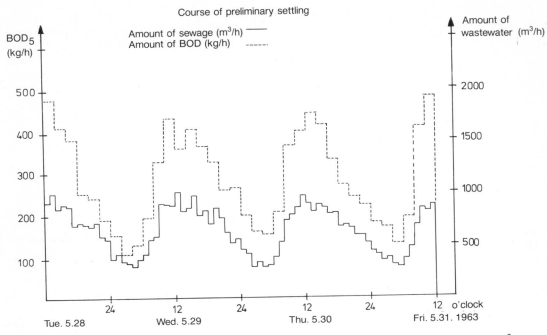

Fig. 16-2. Fluctuations in the amount of wastewater and the BOD$_5$ load in the mixed wastewater of a German town (about 180000 population equivalents).

16.2.2 Industrial Effluents

The term industrial effluents denotes the effluents that arise in industrial and manufacturing enterprises in connection with the production processes. The amount and composition are therefore determined by the **nature of the crude products** and the **treatment processes.** The reader is referred to the relevant literature (Meinck et al., 1968; Sierp, 1967; Imhoff, 1979).

In principle, those effluents are accessible to biological purification that arise from all factories processing **plant** or **animal** materials such as, for example, foodstuffs industries, distilleries, paper mills, tanneries, and wool-scouring plants. But organically polluted effluents from the **chemical** industry can also be purified by biological treatment. While pre-

viously the view was held that concentrated industrial effluents must be "diluted" with communal sewage before biological purification, experience has shown that it is often more economic to subject concentrated industrial effluents to a partial purification (50 to 70% degradation) in highly loaded aerobic or anaerobic stages and to carry out the final purification together with other wastewater or alone in subsequent weakly loaded stages.

In order to be able to relate the effluent load of a factory to that of a communal or other industrial enterprise, use is made of the term **"population equivalent."** This is the BOD$_5$ load of the factory referred to the mean daily amount of BOD$_5$ of an inhabitant (60 g BOD$_5$/d).

While the processes for the aerobic biological purification of communal sewage have

Table 16-2. "Population equivalents" of Some Industrial Enterprises.

Enterprise	Processing	Population equivalents*⁾
Brewery	1000 L of beer	150–350
Dairy (without cheese section)	1000 L of milk	25–70
Starch factory	1 ton of maize or wheat	500–900
Wool-scouring plant	1 ton of wool	2000–4500
Papermill	1 ton of paper	200–900

* 1 population equivalent $= 60$ g BOD_5/d

largely been developed to a mature state, industrial effluents still offer problems in the identification of constituents difficult to degrade and in the optimization of economic efficiency and safety in operation.

16.2.3 Properties of the Substrate "Wastewater"

When, in biotechnology, it is desired to transfer proven processes to the practice of the purification of communal and industrial effluents, the following properties of the wastewater, which differ from those of ordinary substrates, must be taken into account:

– Wastewater changes in amount and composition according to the time of day (day-night), the day of the week (working day-holiday), the season of the year (seasonal operation, holiday period), and the operating situation in trade and industry. Consequently, no uniform supply of substrate, either qualitatively or quantitatively, is possible.

– The amount of substrate supplied may undergo a brief manifold increase owing to uncontrollable and unforeseeable events (e.g., "technical hitches" in factories, storm waters after a long dry period) (load surges).

– As a rule, because of its large amount, wastewater cannot be treated under sterile conditions, i.e., the use of pure cultures is impossible. With certain industrial effluents, the working-in phase can be shortened by inoculation with adapted bacterial cultures.

– Apart from a few highly concentrated types of industrial effluents, the concentration of the substrate in the wastewater is so low that in a flow-through reactor the rate at which the organisms are washed out is always greater than their rate of growth. The processes must therefore include possibilities for retaining and recycling biomass.

16.3 Aims and Limitations of the Aerobic Biological Processing of Wastewater Purification

The loading of water bodies by wastewater discharges consists mainly in the **disturbance of the oxygen economy** by oxygen-consuming organic substances and ammonium compounds. Biological clarification plants were therefore developed with the aim of eliminating these substances from the sewage. Consequently, the **efficiency of a clarification plant** is measured by the decrease in the BOD_5 concentration and by the oxidation of ammonium (nitrification). In the course of time, it has been possible to develop empirical assessment parameters with the aid of which purification plants are being erected which achieve a high degree of elimination of BOD_5 and nitrification.

In the last few years, however, yet other demands have been made on the quality of the biologically purified sewage which cannot be completely satisfied by mechanical-biological purification processes. When biologically purified sewage is discharged into lakes or reservoirs, the phosphorus and nitrogen compounds that they still contain promote the **eutrophication** of the water. The additional elimination of these organic nutrients in the purification plant can be carried out biologically in the case of **nitrogen** (nitrification-denitrification). As a rule, **phosphates** are eliminated by chemical methods (precipitation, flocculation by means of iron, aluminum, and calcium compounds). **Biological processes** have been developed in the last few years. They are based on an incorporation of the phosphate either into the organisms of the activated sludge (Barnard, 1976 and 1980; Levin et al., 1975) or into algae (Sekoulov, 1978).

These **processes for the elimination of phosphorus and nitrogen** are therefore termed "further purification" or **"the tertiary purification stage."** The necessity for using surface waters as drinking water and as water for industrial purposes has directed attention to the **refractory substances** difficult or impossible to degrade biologically that are introduced with the sewage (Bernhardt, 1980). Attempts have therefore been made by varying the aerobic biological processes for sewage purification to go beyond the original aim and eliminate these substances as well. The use of two- or multistage biological processes has given some success. In these, in the first step the easily degradable oxygen-consuming substances are assimilated by the microorganisms, and in the following stages biocenoses can then develop which can even metabolize "difficultly degradable substances" as nutrients. If this biological method is impossible, additional physicochemical methods must be used such as, for example, precipitation, flocculation, adsorption, and ion exchange.

16.4   Trickling Filter Process

In 1894, Corbett at Salford (England) brought the trickling filter process to technical maturity. In principle, the trickling filter corresponds to a fixed-bed reactor in which the biomass ("trickling filter film") has settled on broken material or shaped plastic bodies.

The **trickling filter film** (biomass) is a living community of **bacteria, fungi, protozoa, entomostracans,** and **insect larvae** (Liebmann, 1960). Additionally **blue and green algae** can develop on illuminated surfaces. Corresponding to the decreasing supply of nutrients from the surface to the bottom of the trickling filter a vertical stratification of the biocenosis can be observed. Likewise, there are differences in the living community between weakly loaded and highly loaded trickling filters. The elimination of the pollution present mainly in dissolved and colloidal form is carried out essentially by the bacteria, fungi and protozoa. The higher forms (worms, insects, larvae) act to prevent blockage of the packing of the trickling filter by a mechanical loosening or reduction of the film of biomass. When the trickling filter cools down greatly in the winter, the number of higher organisms and the purifying effect fall off.

Oxygen is supplied through the air circulating in the void volume. The wastewater is distributed as evenly as possible over the surface with the aid of rotating spargers and trickles over the films on the trickling filters. The undisturbed operation of the system requires the rate of growth of the biomass, which is limited by the supply of nutrients (BOD_5 loading, kg of $BOD_5/m^3 \cdot d$), to be in equilibrium with the rinsing effect that depends on the supply of wastewater to the surface of the trickling filter (m^3 of wastewater/m^2 of surface $\cdot$ h = m/h). Consequently, in 1936 Halvarson developed the high-rate trickling filter in which by recycling purified wastewater the washing effect is increased to such an extent that even the growth of biomass due to higher

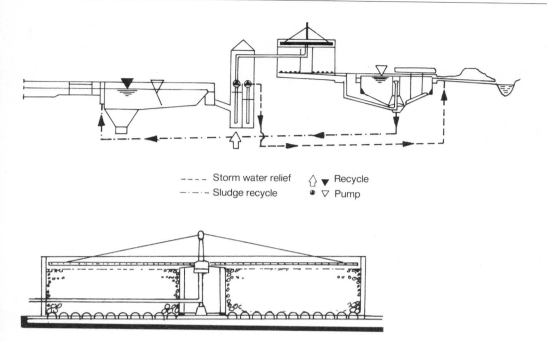

---- Storm water relief	⇧ ▼	Recycle
-·-·- Sludge recycle	◉ ▽	Pump

Fig. 16-3. Flow sheet of a trickling filter plant and cross sections through a trickling filter.

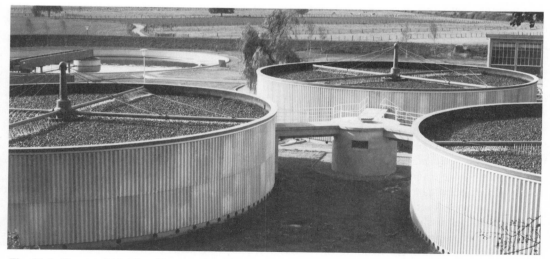

Fig. 16-4. Group of trickling filters at the Fröndenberg clarification plant (photograph: Archiv Ruhrverband).

loading is washed of. This prevents a blockage of the trickling filter and, accordingly, the trickling filter is released from the task of bringing about a "mineralization" of the biomass, in addition to purifying the wastewater.

In general, a purification plant using the trickling filter process consists of the following structures:

A **mechanical purification stage** (rakes, sand trap, settling tanks) must precede the trickling filter in order to prevent a blockage of the filter bed by the sludge materials present in the wastewater.

The **trickling filter** itself (Figs. 16-3 and 16-4) consists of a cylinder about 2.80 to 4.20 m high the diameter of which is determined by the amount of sewage and the BOD_5 load and the desired space loading. About 0.5 m above the base of the filter there is a grid of prefabricated concrete parts or the like upon which filter packing material is placed. The side walls of the hollow base are provided with openings through which a circulation of air through the trickling filter is possible. The wastewater that has percolated through the filter together with the parts of the biological film that have been rinsed off collects on the bottom of the hollow base and flows to the final settling tank.

The **packing material** consists of lumps of lava tuff, slag, or weather-resistant brick. With a grain size of 40 to 80 mm both a large specific surface (90 to 96 m^2/m^3) and also a sufficiently large void fraction (40 to 60%) are achieved, which makes a good purification efficiency with good aeration possible. Recently, shaped plastic inserts have also been developed which permit larger surfaces (up to 250 m/m^3) and void fractions (up to 95%).

The particles of sludge rinsed out are separated from the purified wastewater in a **final settling tank** following the trickling filter and, as a rule, are recycled to the preliminary settling section for joint treatment.

In a **weakly loaded trickling filter** the rinsing effect is slight, so that the trickling filter film is rinsed out from the filter very slowly. The specific BOD_5 loading must therefore be so small that a blockage of the trickling filter by a too vigorous growth of the biological film is avoided. In these trickling filters, in addition to a very substantial elimination of the BOD, a nitrification of the ammonium compounds also generally takes place. The organic parts of the sludge having largely been eliminated in the trickling filter, the amount of sludge rinsed out is diminished. It exhibits a fairly low water content and is hardly digestible.

In the case of **highly loaded trickling filters,** the rinsing effect is kept so high by the recycling of purified wastewater that excess biomass is immediately washed out (high-rate trickling filter). In this case, the trickling filter serves only for wastewater purification and no longer has the task of sludge treatment, so that the BOD_5 loading can be higher. The washed out sludge is still capable of being digested and has a high water content.

Recently, very highly loaded plastic trickling filters have been used for the **partial purification** of concentrated wastewater as the first stage of a multistage plant. In this case, the loading may be made so high that, for example, only 50% of the BOD_5 input is eliminated.

The **aeration** of trickling filters takes place naturally as a result of the temperature difference between the internal and external air. The air in the trickling filter adopts the temperature of the wastewater, i.e., it is colder than the external air in summer and warmer in winter. There is a resulting upward or downward flow of the air through the filter. A prerequisite for good aeration is a sufficient void volume throughout the filter. In special cases, the trickling filter may be covered and be artificially aerated, which may be necessary, for example, to protect neighboring residential areas against odor nuisance and filter flies.

In contrast to the classical trickling filter in which the biomass is fixed and the wastewater moves, there are processes in which the biomass is moved through the sewage. Thus, for example, in the **immersing disk process** circular disks are fixed at a small distance apart from one another on a horizontal shaft. These disks are half immersed in a trough through which wastewater is flowing. By slow rotation of the disks the attached biomass is alternatively immersed in water and exposed to the air, giving an alternating supply of the organisms with substrate and oxygen.

In other solutions to the problem, **hollow rollers** rotating on a shaft are filled with pieces of plastic or covered by a plastic sheath which serves as a surface for the organisms to settle upon and these likewise by slow rotation bring about alternating contact with sewage and atmospheric oxygen. The supply of oxygen can be increased by a special design of the parts. When additional bacterial flocs form in the sewage, a **combination of trickling filter and activated sludge processes** is obtained. A more detailed description of the various process combinations available on the market must be renounced within the framework of this account.

Exhaustive descriptions of the theoretical principles and practical application of trickling filters and immersing disk devices can be found in the Lehr- und Handbuch der Abwassertechnik, Bd. II [Textbook and Handbook of Sewage Technique, Vol. II] (1975) and in the ATV-Arbeitsblatt (Association of Sewage Technicians, Worksheet) A 135 (1982).

16.5 Activated Sludge Process

The activated sludge process was developed by Ardern and Lockett in Manchester in 1913. They recognized that the flocs of sludge arising when sewage was aerated in a bottle were responsible for the purification process and called them "activated sludge." As a matter of process engineering this led to the task of enriching this biomass in the reaction tank and supplying it with the necessary oxygen in a continuous purification process. As a rule, the concentration of nutrients in wastewater is so low that in a flow-through reactor the washing out the biomass is greater than its rate of growth. Consequently, the activated sludge must be separated from the purified sewage in a subsequent settling tank and be returned to the activated sludge tank. **Activated sludge tank** and **final settling tank** therefore form a unit the functioning of which is only ensured when the settling properties of the flocs of activated sludge permit their separation and concentration in the final settling tank.

As a rule, an **activated sludge plant** consists of a preliminary settling tank, activated sludge tank, and final settling tank (Figs. 16-5 and 16-6). However, the preliminary settling step is not absolutely necessary – as it is in the case of the trickling filter process – i.e., even crude wastewater can be treated in an activated sludge tank, e.g., in the oxidation ditch.

In the **activated sludge tank,** the organic pollutants are converted by microbes into inorganic end products (carbon dioxide, water, salts) or they are incorporated into the activated sludge. Consequently, a close contact is necessary between wastewater, flocs of activated sludge, and oxygen by means of an adequate circulation in the tank. Aeration is carried out either with compressed air or by means of surface aerators, a distinction being made between brush aerators and centrifugal aerators. They simultaneously bring about the necessary circulation. In more recent developments, the units for aeration and circulation are separate. In the last few years, another path has been followed for the better utilization of the atmospheric oxygen introduced by the development of high **bubble-column-like reactors** with a 20 to 120 m depth of water.

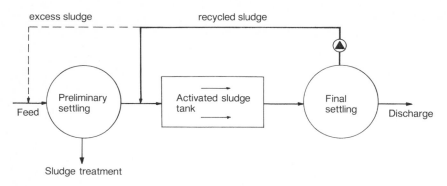

Fig. 16-5. Flow sheet of an activated sludge plant.

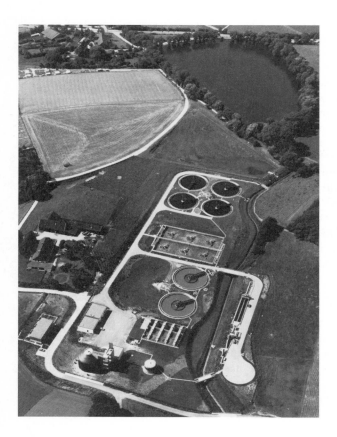

Fig. 16-6. Aerial photograph of the Abtsküche clarification plant (released by Regierungspräsidium Düsseldorf, No. 08 K 14, Archiv Ruhrverband).

Because of the pressure-proportional increase in the solubility of oxygen with increasing depths of water, there is a decrease in the amount of waste air and a better supply of the flocs of activated sludge with oxygen. Since, as a rule, activated sludge with good settling and thickening properties develops under the given conditions, the reactors can be operated with higher concentrations of sludge. Taken all together, this leads to conditions which permit a higher specific load (see Chapter 6). So far, the following processes have been used in practice:

– The "deep-shaft" process, an airlift reactor created in a well-drilling process with a 70 to 120 m depth of water (Hines, 1979).

– The Turmbiologie® activated sludge process, a bubble-column reactor 30 m high which is gassed at the base by two-phase injectors (Diesterweg et al., 1978).

– The Biohoch® process, a reactor with internal air lift circulation upon which a bubble-column section is set (Müller and Sell, 1979).

In the last few years, instead of air, technically pure oxygen has also been used for the gassing of the wastewater (Rinke, 1980). **Oxygen gassing** offers advantages particularly in the case of odor-intensive effluents (slaughterhouse operations, fish processing) because of the small gas throughput (Bischofsberger, 1980).

Depending on the nature of the supply and the design of the activated sludge tank (Fig. 16-7), a distinction is made between the **completely mixed tank** with uniform loading of the activated sludge and the "classical" **longitudinal-flow basin,** in which, however, a more uniform loading can also be achieved by distributed supply of the wastewater (stepwise loading). In the **cascade basin,** on the other

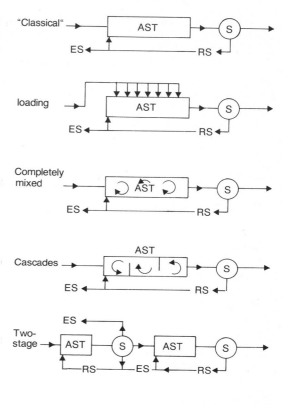

AST = activated sludge tank   RS = recycled sludge
S   = settling tank   ES = excess sludge

Fig. 16-7. Some possibilities for performing the activated sludge process.

hand, an alternation between high loading in the first stage and weak loading in the following ones is brought about deliberately. As other variants, the two-stage activated sludge plants with separate sludge circuits must be mentioned, while combinations between the trickling filter and the activated sludge processes are possible.

Elongated basins, circular basins, and Dortmund basins are used as **final settling stages.** The fastest possible return of the settled sludge is important in order to keep the anaerobic phase for the sludge organisms short.

The **purification efficiency** of an activated sludge plant is determined by the BOD_5-sludge load (kg BOD_5/kg DS · d; DS = dry solids), i.e., by the ratio between the amount of pollutant and the amount of activated sludge, or the specific supply of nutrients for the activated sludge organisms. The concentration of sludge (kg DS/m^3) gives the BOD_5 load (kg BOD_5/m^3 · d) and therefore the size of the activated sludge tank (Imhoff K., and Imhoff K. R., 1979; ATV, 1975).

In order to keep a constant concentration of sludge in the activated sludge tank, an amount of activated sludge corresponding to its daily growth must be taken off as **"excess sludge."** As a rule, the excess sludge is still capable of being digested and is therefore fed to the sludge-treatment unit.

In plants with **joint aerobic sludge stabilization** (e.g., oxidation ditches, activated sludge ditches, compact plants), the BOD_5-sludge load is made so low that the excess sludge is no longer capable of being digested. Since, as a rule, a preliminary settling stage for sludge substances is no longer provided, no unit for sludge digestion is necessary.

The **"activated sludge,"** i.e., the biomass in the activated sludge tanks, consists essentially of **bacterial flocs** which are mainly responsible for the elimination of the pollution. Investigations hitherto on the species composition of the bacterial flocs have shown that it consists mainly of Gram-negative non-spore-forming species that must be assigned to the genera Achromobacter, Flavobacterium, Alcaligenes, and Pseudomonas. Small amounts of Gram-positive species have been found that belong to the family of the Micrococcaceae. A list of the most important genera of bacteria that have so far been found in activated sludge is contained in ATV (1975).

In addition to the flocs of bacteria, the pattern of the activated sludge is determined by occurrence of typical Protozoa and occasionally Rotifera and Nematoda. They are of sub-ordinate importance for the purification effect, but as "filterers" contribute to reducing the turbidity of the purified wastewater. More important is their "indicator function," since, depending on the load, the supply of oxygen, turbulence, and other factors they set up definite **living communities** which can be used to judge the functioning of the biological sewage treating stage (Scherb, 1968; Buck, 1968).

Because of the multiplicity of species in the mixed biocenosis of the activated sludge, the system can adapt well to seasonal changes in temperatures, the influence of toxic substances (e.g., phenols, cyanides), pH values deviating from neutral (between about pH 6 and pH 9), salt concentrations, anaerobic phases (e.g., in the final settling tank), and changes in the composition of the wastewater.

An important phenomenon for clarification plant operation which is very interesting from the scientific point of view is the **bulking sludge problem.** It has already been mentioned that the separation and thickening of the activated sludge in the final settling step is an indispensible prerequisite for the functioning of the activated sludge process. Disturbances occur when microorganisms growing in the form of threads develop in the activated sludge; these have a decisively adverse effect on the settling process. The growth of these organisms can be triggered off both by the composition of the wastewater (e.g., carbohydrates, organic acids, sulfides) and also by factors determined by the operation of the plant (e.g., sludge loading, transport of the recycled sludge) (Matsché, 1977). Although the symptoms of the development of bulking sludge have long been known in practice and considerable operating difficulties are caused by them, our knowledge of the organisms concerned is still inadequate. Eikelboom (1979) has worked out a method of determination which permits an identification of the various organisms. Work is being performed in various institutes on the environmental demands and metabolic physiology of the organisms. For combating the organisms and improving the settling properties of the sludge, iron salts, chlorine, and changes in the operating conditions are used in practice (Matsché, 1977; ATV, 1975).

16.6   Lagoon Processes

Lagoons have long been used for the purification of effluents. A comprehensive review of the present situation has been drawn up, by the ATV working group "Abwasserteiche" ("Wastewater Lagoons") (1979). In general the biological or biochemical purification effect is to be ascribed mainly to the metabolic activities of various microorganisms and even macroorganisms that are suspended in the water or settled in the bottom mud. In the treatment of crude wastewater, sedimentation processes for settlable materials also play a fundamental role.

In comparison to the trickling-filter and activated-sludge processes, in which heterotrophic organisms play an exclusive role, **autotrophic organisms** also play a part in the purification process in lagoons. The biocenoses are therefore richer in species and, in the case of low loading, correspond in numerous respects to those of a receiving body. For this reason, even inorganic fertilizers such as nitrates and phosphates can be partially eliminated with the other pollutants. Furthermore, the autotrophic organisms also contribute to the supply of oxygen to the wastewater lagoon to an extent depending on the illumination. In order to ensure a supply of oxygen independent of the season of the year and time of day even in highly loaded lagoons, they may also be aerated by technical means.

The following types of wastewater lagoons can be distinguished on the basis of their application:

– **Settling lagoons** are used mainly for the separation of settlable materials from the crude effluent. Dimensional criteria are residence time, amount of sludge produced, and frequency of discharge. Because of the high loadings normally prevailing, such lagoons are predominantly anaerobic. For this rea-

son, they will not be discussed further at this point (see Sections 16.11.1 and 16.11.2).

– **Unaerated wastewater lagoons** are reservoirs, artificially constructed or naturally present, which serve for the biological treatment of wastewater. Oxygen is supplied to unaerated wastewater lagoons naturally through the surface of the water (water/air boundary) and by photosynthesis (biogenic aeration). Depending on the relationship between the supply and consumption of oxygen, and aerobic milieu becomes established in the top layer of the water in the lagoon, while in the deeper layers anaerobic conditions may prevail – depending on the load.

– **Aerated wastewater lagoons** achieve an intensification of the purification process through additional technical aeration and forced circulation. Of particular importance for degradation is the contact zone between water and bottom sludge and the biologically active growth on the wetted surfaces of the lagoon if a good mass transfer and an adequate supply of oxygen are ensured there by the aeration-circulating unit. In addition, flocs of bacteria that develop in the free water contribute to the purification process. Since, however, they reach concentrations of only about 0.05 g DM/L, their effect is low in comparison with activated sludge (3 to 5 kg DM/L). A post-clarification zone (usually an unaerated lagoon) is necessary to separate off the suspended matter.

– **Polishing lagoons** – in contrast to the wastewater lagoons, which are fed with unclarified or only mechanically treated wastewater – are used for further purification after, for example, a trickling filter or activated sludge unit (see Section 16.6). In the case of receiving bodies of low capacity or of particularly high demands on the quality of the waters, polishing lagoons are a simple and reliable process for improving the effluent from a biological clarification plant.

Wastewater lagoons are used mainly by relatively small communities. On the other hand, they have come into use for the treatment of effluents from foodstuffs and chemical industries. In various cases, lagoon processes provide the possibility of autoadaptation to the specific requirements of the individual types of industrial effluents. For example, peak loads in seasonal operations of the foodstuffs industry can be accepted, or difficultly degradable substances can be treated in following lagoons with long residence times.

16.7 Sewage Treatment Processes as Special Forms of Biotechnology

Basically, the biological processes for purifying effluents must be included in biotechnology. In each case, an initial substrate (crude wastewater) is converted by microorganisms (activated sludge, trickling filter film) into end products (purified effluent, excess sludge, water, and carbon dioxide). However, in various points the prerequisites and operating conditions differ basically from those of the usual processes of biotechnology. They will therefore be pointed out briefly here.

The initial substrate "wastewater" is neither quantitatively nor qualitatively constant or capable of being deliberately modified. In spite of these great fluctuations, the processes must yield an end product (purified wastewater with limiting concentrations) as uniform as possible.

In order to achieve low final "nutrient" concentrations (final BOD_5) the substrate concentrations in the reactor must be very low. Under these conditions, only very low rates of growth are possible for the organisms.

It is possible to affect the biocenosis by, for example, constant reaction temperatures, pH values, composition of the nutrients, etc., to a limited extent only in exceptional cases. It is impossible to work with pure cultures under sterile conditions.

16.8 Column Wastewater Reactors

In the last ten years, activated sludge processes have been developed for treating highly loaded industrial effluents which take place in high reactors similar to bubble columns. Because of the increasing solubility of oxygen in the water, which is proportional to the pressure at any depth of water, increased oxygen turnover can be achieved and the residence time of the wastewater to be treated in the activated sludge plant can be shortened (see section 16.5). The "**deep shaft**" system (Hines, 1979), which uses an airlift reactor with a depth of water of 70 to 120 m constructed in a well-drilling operation belongs to these processes. Aeration takes place at a depth of 30 m in the downstream compartment. The total lowering of the density in the upstream compartment is sufficient to entrain the injected fresh air downwards against its natural tendency to rise.

Mann (1980) has reported on a Turmbiologie® ("tower biology") activated sludge process which is carried out in a bubble column reactor 30 m high gassed with the aid of two-phase nozzles, while Müller and Sell (1979) use a Biohoch-Reaktor® provided with internal airlift circulation and surmounted by a bubble-column section (Fig. 16-8). In addition to the small volume of the plant, the reduced amount of waste air and the substantially reduced demand for constructional area of these processes are emphasized. A further possibility is opened up by the addition of finely ground activated carbon upon which the microorganisms settle. This makes the retention of the sludge simpler (see page 631) and simultaneously the activated carbon is able to adsorb harmful substances which could not otherwise be degraded and feed them gradually to the degradation process.

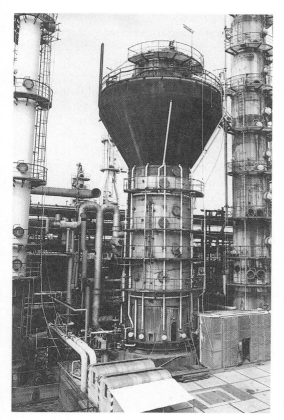

Fig. 16-8a. Biohoch-Reaktor (Hoechst AG).

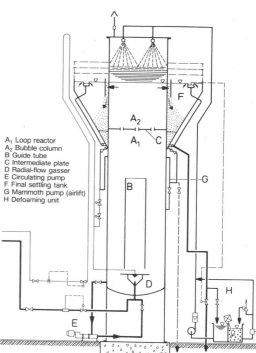

A₁ Loop reactor
A₂ Bubble column
B Guide tube
C Intermediate plate
D Radial-flow gasser
E Circulating pump
F Final settling tank
G Mammoth pump (airlift)
H Defoaming unit

Fig. 16-8b. Biohoch-Reaktor (sketch).

Purification of Effluents by Anaerobic Processes

16.9   General

Wherever, in nature, organic material is degraded microbially under anaerobic conditions and in the absence of sulfate and nitrate, methane is produced. Thus, as early as 1776 the Italian physicist A. Volta discovered the occurrence of a combustible gas over marshes and ponds (Hoppe-Seyler, 1886). The well-known "will o' the wisps" in marshes and bogs arise through the combustion of methane (marsh gas), although even today it is still not clear how the ignition of this gas comes about. The **microbial formation of methane** takes place, however, not only in inland-water and seawater sediments, in tundras, and flooded rice fields, but also in the rumen of ruminant animals. Investigations have shown that in the stomach of a cow about 8 to 10% of the fodder is converted into 100 to 200 L of methane per day (Hungate, 1966; Wolfe, 1971). It is estimated that on the Earth about $1000 \times 10^9 \ m^3$ of methane is formed by microorganisms and passed into the atmosphere each year (Ehhalt, 1976). This means that about 5% of the carbon assimilated by photosynthesis is converted into methane by anaerobic microorganisms (Vogels, 1979). This demonstrates the importance of this process for the carbon cycle in nature under anaerobic conditions.

The capacity of anaerobic bacteria for degrading organic substances to methane and carbon dioxide (biogas) has been utilized on the large technical scale since 1911 to stabilize the sludge arising in various sections of effluent purification processes (Hobson et al., 1974; McCarty, 1964). Since this **anaerobic sludge digestion process** is frequently being carried on today according to the state of bio-

logical knowledge of the fifties, the rates of conversion and the stability of the process are sometimes not very great. However, it is beginning to be realized more and more that the bad name that has been attached to methane fermentation for this reason for years is not justified. An extented and more profound knowledge about this process has shown that the residence times can be substantially shortened and that many experiments that previously failed in sludge digestion can be carried out successfully today. Because of increasing energy costs **methane fermentation** has recently attracted great interest in the purification of effluents with high loads of organic matter (Lettinga et al., 1980; Sahm, 1984). In this chapter, therefore, a summarizing account of the biology and technical application of the formation of methane will be given.

16.10   Biology of the Formation of Methane

While it was assumed for a long time that in the anaerobic conversion of organic substances into methane and carbon dioxide only two different groups of bacteria are involved (Barker, 1956), it has been possible to show in the last few years that there are at least three different groups (Bryant, 1979). As can be seen from Fig. 16-9, in the degradational or nutritional chain the various organic compounds are degraded to acids, alcohols, hydrogen, and carbon dioxide by one group of microorganisms in a first step. The second group of bacteria then converts these alcohols, acids, etc., into acetic acid, hydrogen, and carbon dioxide, which are then used as substrates by the last group, the methane bacteria, and are converted into methane and carbon dioxide.

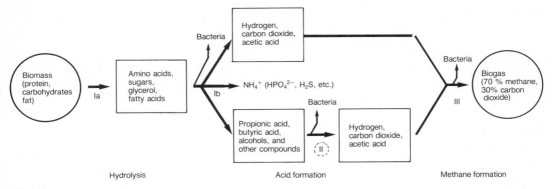

Fig. 16-9. Scheme of the fermentation of organic substances to biogas by three different groups of bacteria.

16.10.1 Hydrolytic and Acid-forming (Fermentative) Bacteria

The first group of bacteria is very heterogeneous; thus, in addition to obligate anaerobic strains such as, for example, Bacteroides, Clostridia, Bifidobacteria, facultative anaerobic Enterobacteria and Streptococci (Hobson et al., 1974; Crowther and Harkness, 1975) also occur. These organisms, which occur in digestion sludge in numbers of about 10^6 to 10^8 cells/mL, first hydrolyze the macromolecular compounds such as polysaccharides, proteins, and fats with the aid of extracellular enzymes (hydrolases). While most biopolymers can be split relatively easily and rapidly, lignocellulose-containing materials are degraded only slowly and incompletely, since the lignin, which cannot be cleaved anaerobically, has a very pronounced inhibiting effect (Hackett et al., 1977). With the exception of the fatty acids, the hydrolysis products are then fermented by the well-known metabolic pathways predominantly to hydrogen, carbon dioxide, acetic acid, propionic acid, butyric acid, lactic acid, valeric acid, ethanol, ammonia, and hydrogen sulfide (Thauer et al., 1977; Gottschalk, 1979). The partial pressure of hydrogen (pH_2) has a certain influence on the formation of the various fermentation products. Thus, at a high pH_2 more propionic and butyric acids and less acetic acid, hydrogen, and carbon dioxide are formed than at a low pH_2 (Bryant, 1979; Hungate, 1966; Thauer et al., 1977).

16.10.2 Bacteria Forming Acetic Acid and Hydrogen (Acetogenic Bacteria)

While it was believed for a long time that the methane bacteria are capable of utilizing the fermentation products of the first group of bacteria (Barker, 1956), only recently the group of microorganisms has been discovered that forms a link between the acid-forming bacteria and the methane bacteria. This group degrades propionic acid and butyric acid and the longer-chain fatty acids, alcohols, aromatics, other organic acids, etc., to acetic acid, hydrogen, and carbon dioxide. So far, only a few strains are known, since these organisms can grow in pure culture only at a very low pH_2, as can be seen from the following example. Bryant et al. (1967) have shown that a culture of *Methanobacillus omelianskii* which was capable of forming methane from ethanol in accordance with the following equation:

$$2\,CH_3CH_2OH + CO_2 \rightarrow 2\,CH_3COOH + CH_4 \quad (1)$$
$$\Delta G = -132,6 \text{ kJ}$$

is a **synergistic mixed culture** of two different species of bacteria. One bacterium is the S-organism forming acetic acid and hydrogen from ethanol:

$$CH_3CH_2OH + H_2O \rightarrow CH_3COOH + 2\,H_2 \quad (2)$$
$$\Delta G = 6,2 \text{ kJ}$$

The other bacterium is *Methanobacterium bryantii,* which assimilates the hydrogen liberated and forms methane:

$$4\,H_2 + CO_2 \rightarrow CH_4 + 2\,H_2O \quad (3)$$
$$\Delta G = -138,9 \text{ kJ}$$

Since the conversion of ethanol into acetate at pH 7.0 is, as can be seen from Eq. (2), endergonic, this reaction can take place only when it is "drawn along" by an exergonic one. As can be seen from Fig. 16-10, with decreasing partial pressure of hy-

drogen ($pH_2 < 0.5$ bar) the assimilation of ethanol becomes exergonic. This is achieved in the mixed culture by the fact that the bacterium degrading ethanol lives in a close syntrophic association with the hydrogen-consuming methane bacterium (Fig. 16-11). As Eq. (1) shows, the overall conversion of the two organisms together is an exergonic process.

This example of the conversion of ethanol also applies, mutatis mutandis, for the degradation of propionic acid, butyric acid, long-chain fatty acids, aromatic aldehydes, etc., and quite generally for substances which are degraded under anaerobic conditions to acetic acid, hydrogen, and carbon dioxide and the free enthalpy of which is positive under standard conditions (McInerney et al., 1979; Ferry and Wolfe, 1976; Bryant, 1979; Mah et al., 1977). Since very low pH_2 values ($< 2 \times 10^{-3}$ bar and $< 9 \times 10^{-5}$ bar, respectively) are necessary for the anaerobic degradation of butyric acid and propionic acid, the hydrogen produced must be consumed immediately at the position where it arises. An intimate contact between the cells of the **acetogenic** and **methanogenic bacteria** is necessary to meet this requirement, since this low pH_2 value can-

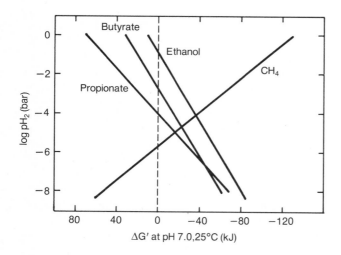

Fig. 16-10. Influence of the partial pressure of hydrogen (pH_2) on the free energy ($\Delta G'$) for the degradation of 1 mmol of ethanol, propionate, or butyrate and for the formation of methane from hydrogen and carbon dioxide (after Thauer et al., 1977).

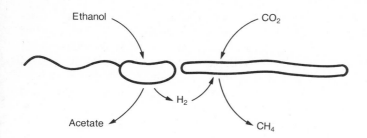

Fig. 16-11. Interspecies hydrogen transfer. Transfer of hydrogen from acetogenic to methanogenic bacteria.

not be maintained by the diffusion of the hydrogen alone. For fermentation practice, the existence of such cell associates means that particular attention must be devoted to their limited stability in relation to physical effects, such as those due to turbulences and shearing forces. This applies particularly to the starting-up phases of methane fermentation while the concentrations of bacteria are still relatively low. When the concentration of sulfate in the medium is low, sulfate-reducing bacteria such as, for example, strains of Desulfovibrio, can convert ethanol or lactic acid into acetic acid, hydrogen, and carbon dioxide if the methane bacteria assimilate the hydrogen (Bryant et al., 1977; Widdel and Pfennig, 1977). There are indications that this transfer of hydrogen from the acetogenic to the methanogenic bacteria is frequently a limiting factor in the microbial generation of methane.

16.10.3 Methane-forming (Methanogenic) Bacteria

This group of bacteria are among the **most oxygen-sensitive organisms** known today. They require for growth a redox potential of about −300 mV and some are very rapidly killed by oxygen (Paynter and Hungate, 1968). In order to be able to isolate these strictly obligate anaerobic bacteria in pure culture and to grow them in the laboratory, special techniques had to be developed (Hungate, 1950; Bryant,

1972). Today, more than 20 different methane-forming bacterial species, which are morphologically very diverse, have been isolated in pure culture. There are bacilli, spirilla, cocci, and sarcinas (Wolfe, 1971; Zeikus, 1977; Balch et al., 1979). As can be seen from Table 16-3, the methanogenic bacteria, as the last group in the chain of anaerobic degradation, have a very **limited substrate spectrum.** Most species so far isolated are capable of assimilating hydrogen as the sole source of energy. The conversion of hydrogen into methane is highly exergonic, so that the equilibrium lies on the side of the formation of methane (see Eq. (3)). The affinity of the methane bacteria is very high. Thus, Hungate (1967) found, for example, that the K_m value for the conversion of hydrogen into methane in the rumen is 10^{-6} mol/L. Many of the methane-forming bacteria can also consume formic acid as substrate:

$$4\,HCOOH \rightarrow CH_4 + 3\,CO_2 + 2\,H_2O \qquad (4)$$
$$\Delta G = 111 \text{ kJ}$$

Although about 70% of the methane that is formed in nature arises from acetic acid, so far only a few **methane bacteria assimilating acetic acid** are known (Smith et al., 1980). Thus, Methanosarcinas are capable of growing not only on hydrogen + carbon dioxide, methanol, methylamine, dimethylamine, and trimethylamine, but also on acetic acid (Stadtman and Barker, 1951; Hippe et al., 1979; Smith et al., 1980; Scherer and Sahm, 1979):

$$4\,CH_3OH \rightarrow 3\,CH_4 + CO_2 + 2\,H_2O \qquad (5)$$
$$\Delta G = -106 \text{ kJ}$$

$$4\,CH_3NH_2 + 2\,H_2O \rightarrow 3\,CH_4 + CO_2 \qquad (6)$$
$$+ 4\,NH_3 \qquad \Delta G = -77 \text{ kJ}$$

$$CH_3COOH \rightarrow CH_4 + CO_2 \qquad (7)$$
$$\Delta G = -32 \text{ kJ}$$

Recently, some other rod-forming methane bacteria have been isolated which are likewise capable of converting acetic acid into methane and carbon dioxide (Cappenberg 1975; van den Berg et al., 1976; Zehnder et al., 1980). Since in the conversion of acetic acid into methane and carbon dioxide only a relatively small amount of energy is liberated ($\Delta G = 32$ kJ), the growth of the methane-forming bacteria on this substrate is very slow. The idea that was held for a relatively long time that the methane bacteria are capable of converting into methane not only hydrogen, for-

Table 16-3. Characteristics of Methanogenic Species in Pure Culture.

Species	Morphology	Substrates	Cell wall composition
Methanobacterium	long rods	H_2, formate	pseudomurein
formicium	to	H_2	
bryantii	filaments	H_2	
thermoautotrophicum			
Methanobrevibacter	lancet-shaped	H_2, formate	pseudomurein
ruminantium	cocci	H_2, formate	
smithii	short rods	H_2	
arboriphilus			
Methanococcus	motile irregular	H_2, formate	polypeptide
vannielii	small	H_2, formate	subunits
voltae	cocci	H_2, formate	
thermolithotrophicus	pseudosarcina	H_2, methanol,	
mazei		methylamines,	
		acetate	
Methanomicrobium	motile short	H_2, formate	polypeptide
mobile	rods		subunits
Methanobacterium	motile irregular	H_2, formate	polypeptide
cariaci	small cocci	H_2, formate	subunits
marisnigri			
Methanospirillum	motile regular	H_2, formate	polypeptide
hungatei	curved rods		
Methanosarcina	irregular cocci	H_2, acetate	heteropoly-
barkeri	as single cells	methanol	saccharide
	packets, pseudo-	methylamines	
	parenchyma		
Methanothrix	rods to	acetate	no muramic
soehngenii	long filaments		acid
Methanothermus	non-motile	H_2	pseudomurein
fervidus	rods		

mate, and acetate but also longer-chain fatty acids such as butyric acid, valeric acid, and caproic acid (Barker, 1956) appears not to be supported by the evidence, since the species so far isolated in pure culture are incapable of doing this. The earlier findings that even higher fatty acids can be converted into methane probably resulted from the use of mixed populations.

As a series of biochemical and molecular-biological investigations in the last few years has shown, the methane-forming bacteria exhibit a number of peculiarities in comparison with most other bacteria (Balch et al., 1979; Thauer and Fuchs, 1979):

a) the cell wall of these bacteria contains no murein, which is a typical cell wall component of almost all bacteria;

b) the cytoplasmic membrane is constructed of isoprenoid lipids instead of the fatty acid esters of glycerol that are usually found;

c) these bacteria contain coenzymes which have not so far been found in any other organism such as, for example, coenzyme M (2-mercaptoethanesulfonic acid) and coenzyme F_{420}, a deazariboflavin derivative which fluoresces and therefore makes it possible to identify methane bacteria specifically in the fluorescence microscope;

d) comparisons of the base sequences of ribosomal RNAs have shown that the methanogenic bacteria are only distantly related to most other bacteria. It is assumed that this group of bacteria diverged from the other species of bacteria very early in evolution. Therefore the methanogenic bacteria belong to the Archaebacteria which is an ancient group phylogenetically distinct from the typical procaryotes.

The reduction of carbon dioxide to methane takes place in stages with the intermediates formate, formaldehyde, and methanol, occurring not in the free state but bound to carriers (Fig. 16-12). An important carrier here is **coenzyme M,** which has recently been isolated by Wolfe et al. (Balch et al., 1979). It has been shown that this coenzyme M plays an important role as methyl carrier in the synthesis of methane. In which way the synthesis of ATP is coupled with the exergonic process of methane formation is largely obscure. It is assumed that this takes place via a chemiosmotic mechanism. Labelling data and enzymatic studies indicate that these bacteria synthesize their cell material when growing on hydrogen and carbon dioxide as the sole source of carbon not via the Calvin cycle but via acetyl-CoA, pyruvate, oxalacetate and α-ketoglutarate (Fuchs et al., 1982).

16.11 Technical Processes

16.11.1 Sludge Digestion

For **stabilizing sewage sludges,** which arise in large amounts (40×10^6 m^3/year in West Germany) in the aerobic purification of effluents in wastewater treatment plants an anaerobic sludge treatment (sludge digestion process) has been carried out for many years. Here more than 50% of the organic constituents in the sewage sludge are converted into methane and carbon dioxide, which results in a residual sludge that is substantially odorless, is

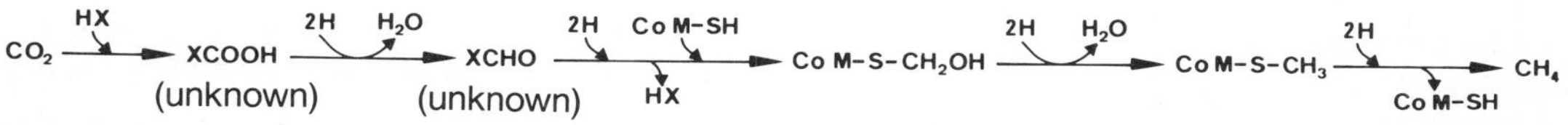

$$CO_2 \xrightarrow[\text{HX}]{} XCOOH \xrightarrow[\text{2H}]{\text{H}_2\text{O}} XCHO \xrightarrow[\text{2H} \quad \text{HX}]{} CoM\text{-}S\text{-}CH_2OH \xrightarrow[\text{2H}]{\text{H}_2\text{O}} CoM\text{-}S\text{-}CH_3 \xrightarrow[\text{2H} \quad CoM\text{-}SH]{} CH_4$$
(unknown)   (unknown)

Fig. 16-12. Reduction of carbon dioxide to methane via carrier-bound intermediates (after Balch et al., 1979).

easy to dewater, and, because of the minerals and humic acids that it contains, can be used as a **valuable fertilizer.**

The **first sludge digestion plants,** which were built about the turn of the century and some of which are still used today in smaller domestic clarification units, consist of simple digesting pits. A further development consist of a two-storied unit (Emscher tank) in which the sludge sinks directly into the digestion chamber, where microbial degradation takes place under anaerobic conditions (Fig. 16-13) (Roediger, 1967). Since the sludge is brought to a uniform temperature to a certain extent by the effluent flowing over it, under favorable conditions the formation of methane may take place in the digestion chamber. Depending on the conditions, however, the residence times here amount to between three months and one year.

most favorable conditions for the very **sensitive methane bacteria,** in the last few years the following measures have proved to be desirable for operating the digestion towers: preheating, inoculation, and good mixing of the fresh sludge during charging, substantially constant operating temperatures (32 to 37 °C), prevention of the formation of covering floating layers, and removal of indigestible floating matter, together with good circulation and degassing of the contents of the digestion chamber. In this way, it has been possible to shorten the **residence times** of the sludge in the digestion towers from 30 to 40 days to about 15 to 20 days and to raise the volume-related load from 1 to 4 kg of dry organic solids/m^3 of digester volume per day. With a degree of degradation of 60% of the organic substances in the sludge, the amount of biogas formed per day then averages 2 to 2.5 m^3/m^3 of diges-

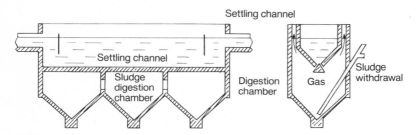

Fig. 16-13. Sketch of two-storied settling and digestion kit. This type is known as the "Emscher tank".

In order to achieve a more reliable and faster anaerobic treatment of sludge, since 1925 sludge settling tanks, as a rule, separate from the sludge digestion chamber have been installed. These sludge digestion vessels may, as can be seen from Fig. 16-14, be compared basically with the reactor vessels of other biotechnological processes. As a rule, they are egg-shaped or cylindrical and have an average size of 500 to 10 000 m^3. In order to create the

tion chamber. Since about 60 to 70 vol% of this biogas consists of methane, with a calorific value of 23 100 kJ/m^3, it can be used directly for heating purposes inside or outside the wastewater treatment plant (Roediger, 1974). Very recently, there have also been attempts to carry out this process of sludge digestion in two stages, which is said to achieve an increase in the stability and in the conversion yield (Ghosh and Klass, 1978).

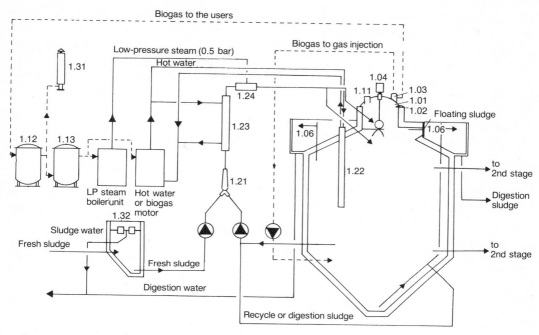

Fig. 16-14. Flow sheet of a digestion plant with three heating systems that can be used alternatively or in combination. (With the kind permission of the Roediger Anlagenbau-Gesellschaften, D-6450 Hanau, CH-4142 München stein/Basel.)

1.01 Gas cap
1.02 observation window
1.03 gas takeoff dome
1.11 device preventing gas over- and underpressure
1.04 floating layer preventer
1.06 takeoff device for digestion water
1.05 floating sludge port
1.12 gravel filter

1.13 ceramic filter
1.21 inoculum mixer
1.22 immersion heating unit
1.23 tube jacket heat exchanger
1.24 low-pressure steam nozzle
1.31 gas flaring unit
1.32 takeoff device for sludge water

16.11.2 Degradation of Wastewater Highly Loaded with Organic Matter

Since sewage sludge is, in principle, an effluent enriched with organic and inorganic contaminants, the application of this anaerobic process directly to the treatment of industrial effluents highly loaded with organic matter (e.g., from the foodstuffs industry or agriculture) was obvious (Baader et al., 1978). In fact, in comparison with the aerobic processes, it has the following advantages:

– The energy demand is much lower, since no aeration but only a slight mixing of the contents of the digestion chamber is necessary.

– More than 90% of the organic substances are converted into methane and carbon dioxide, so that only very small amounts of bacterial biomass (degraded sludge) are formed.

– The anaerobic transformation takes place in closed vessels, so that no odor nuisance arises.

– The wastewater may have a very high solids content (up to 15%).

– The biogas produced can be used for heating purposes.

In addition to the classical digestion tower, which, as a rule, is operated as a semicontinuous flow-through reactor, the following variants of the process have been developed in the last few years for the anaerobic purification of effluents with high loads of organic matter:

Contact Digestion

In this process, which was developed specially for the anaerobic treatment of wastewater, in analogy to the aerobic activated sludge process, part of the bacterial biomass of the outflow is separated from the liquid phase and returned to the reactor (Fig. 16-15) (Steffen and Bedker, 1961). In this way, the wastewater can pass through the reactor at a higher rate of flow than the rate of growth of the microorganism would permit, since the recycling procedure controls and prevents the wash-out of the bacterial biomass. The main problem here is, however, an effective and reliable **separation of the microorganisms** from the liquid phase, since, because of their low specific gravity difference and the bubbles of gas still attached to them the bacteria sediment only very poorly (van den Berg and Lentz, 1979). Attempts have been made to achieve better sedimentation with the aid of vacuum degassing, flocculating agents, centrifugation, lowering the temperature, etc. (Lettinga et al., 1980).

In the **Anamet process,** which works according to the principle of the contact process and has been used successfully on the large technical scale for some years in the purification of

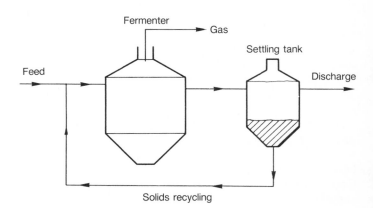

Fig. 16-15. Contact process.

sugar factory effluents, the recycling of the sludge takes place via a **lamellar separator** (Hoffmann-Walbeck and Pellegrini, 1978). Here, at a mean residence time of nine days and a sludge content in the reactor of 5 kg/m^3, about 80% of the BOD load (5.6 kg/m^3) in the wastewater is degraded. In a subsequent aerobic purification stage there is another decrease in BOD to about 25 g/m^3. Similar figures have also been achieved for the anaerobic degradation of yeast factory effluents, but in this case it was possible to shorten the residence time to 5 to 7 days (Köhler, 1973). Since the turnover rates are substantially affected by the concentration of active microorganisms in the reactor, the efficiency of this process depends decisively on the separation and return of the sludge.

Anaerobic Filters

In analogy to the aerobic trickling filter process, **anaerobic fixed-bed reactors,** i.e. anaerobic filters, have also been developed. Here the washing out of the microorganisms is prevented by an inert supporting material upon which the microorganisms grow, so that no external separation and recycling of the sludge is necessary (Coulter et al., 1957; Young and McCarty, 1969). The **filling materials** used are gravel, packed plastic plates provided with profiles of the most diverse types, or Raschig rings. As can be seen from Fig. 16-16, the wastewater is passed through the reactor from the bottom upwards, during this process, on contact with the microorganisms, the organic material is degraded to methane and carbon dioxide. While the biogas is taken off at the top of the reactor, the particles of mud and the excess of biomass can be removed at the bottom of the reactor. This process is particularly suitable for wastewater containing no or only very few solid particles, since these would block the anaerobic filter.

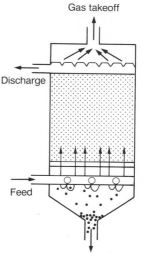

Fig. 16-16. Anaerobic fixed-bed reactor system (anaerobic filter).

As laboratory and pilot experiments have shown, this process can be used to purify potato starch effluent, with a high load of organic matter, and also effluents from the pharmaceutical industry with turnover rates of 10 kg COD/m^3 per day (Lettinga et al., 1980; Jennett and Dennis, 1975). In spite of this very good efficiency, the anaerobic filter has not yet come into wide use. A reason for this could be that, in contrast to the aerobic fixed-bed reactors, in the anaerobic filters the packing elements serve less as surfaces of attachment for the bacteria than as coalescing aids for the bubbles of gas from the microorganisms. This has the consequence that the microorganisms agglomerate into larger flocs of sludge which are then no longer distributed uniformly in the reactor but mainly settle at the bottom (Lettinga et al., 1980). This could be prevented, for example, by immobilizing the bacteria which are still very active even in the support-fixed state, as has recently been shown (Karube et al., 1980).

Column Reactors

A further development of the anaerobic filter is the **UASB process** (upflow anaerobic sludge blanket process) which has been developed by Lettinga et al. in Holland during the last few years (Lettinga et al., 1980). As can be seen from Fig. 16-16 and 16-17 here a **simple column reactor** without additional packing material is used. Under suitable conditions, the microorganisms agglomerate to form dense-packed particles which sediment very well. A high concentration of bacteria develops in the bottom part of the column, and the concentration falls off towards the top. Since the wastewater is pumped through the reactor from the bottom upwards, it is mainly the bacterial particles in the bottom of the column which converts the organic substances into biogas, some of which remains adhering to the particles and draws them upward. In the top part of the column a **gas separator** ensures that the bubbles

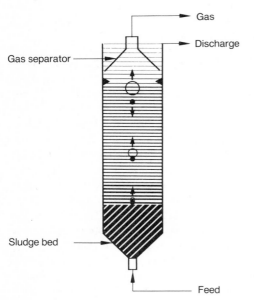

Fig. 16-17. Sketch of an aerobic column reactor (UASB).

of gas are separated from the particles. Hence there is no appreciable wash-out of the sludge. The gas-free particles then sink to the bottom again and the same process is repeated. This leads to a thorough mixing of the whole reactor without any mechanical stirring being necessary.

With sugar factory effluents, this gives hydraulic retention times of 3 to 6 hours, a methane productivity of 2.5 to 3.5 m^3 per m^3 of reactor per day, and a reduction of the COD in the effluent of more than 95% at a load of 15 to 30 kg of COD/m^3 per day. These high rates of conversion can be achieved because, on the one hand, very high concentrations of bacteria (up to 150 kg/m^3) with a specific activity of 1 kg of COD reduction per kg per day are present in the bottom part of the column reactor and, in the second place, thorough mixing is achieved because of the very pronounced formation of gas. As has been shown, a 200 m^3 plant in a sugar factory can, when necessary, be shut down for several months without long waiting times having to be accepted in return when it is started up again. By means of this process, wastewater containing solids can also be purified, in a two-stage installation (Pipyn and Verstraete, 1979). Thus, distillery effluents with a COD of 10 kg/m^3 were fermented in the first stage mainly to acids, and these were then converted into biogas in a secondary column reactor, a reduction in the COD of 85% being achieved at a residence time of 14 hours.

16.12   Process Conditions

Since the growth and metabolic activities of the anaerobic microorganisms producing biogas are substantially affected by the composition of the wastewater, the temperature and the pH, these factors will be considered briefly below.

16.12.1 Composition of the Wastewater

Since the composition of the wastewater is very heterogeneous, depending on its origin, as a rule **the sum of the organic pollutants present in the wastewater** is determined, in terms of the biological and chemical oxygen demands (see p. 625). Wastewater with a COD of 1 to 100 kg/m³ is suitable for an anaerobic treatment (Fig. 16-18) since in the case of wastewater with a lower COD problems arise in the retention of the biomass (Frostell, 1979). A series of investigations has shown that anaerobic microorganisms can degrade a **multiplicity of different organic compounds** to methane and carbon dioxide (Buswell and Mueller, 1952). The few substances which apparently cannot, or can only very slowly, be anaerobically converted include hydrocarbons, lignin, organic ethers, and certain plastics, although, from a thermodynamic point of view, all organic carbon compounds can be degraded to methane and carbon dioxide (Schoberth, 1978). Theoretically, the maximum achievable proportion of methane in the biogas can be determined for almost all organic compounds by means of the following disproportion equation:

$$C_nH_aO_b + \left(n - \frac{a}{b} - \frac{b}{2}\right)H_2O$$

$$\rightarrow \left(\frac{n}{2} - \frac{a}{8} + \frac{b}{4}\right)CO_2 + \left(\frac{n}{2} + \frac{a}{8} - \frac{b}{4}\right)CH_4$$

(Buswell and Mueller, 1952).

The more reduced an organic compound, the higher is the proportion of methane in the biogas formed by its anaerobic decomposition; in the case of alcohol, for example, it is 75% while for carbohydrates it is only 50% (Fig. 16-19). In these figures, the solubility of carbon dioxide as a function of the pH has not been taken into account.

The various organic substances are metabolized at different rates by the microorganisms. Thus, carbohydrate- and protein-assimilating anaerobic bacteria, for example, grow very rapidly (generation time <1 day) and also ferment these substances very rapidly (O'Rourke, 1968). On the other hand, the degradation of fatty acids is very slow, and organisms grow only with very long generation times (about 5 days). Frequently, therefore, in the methane fermentation the degradation of the fatty acids is also the rate-limiting step (O'Rourke, 1968). In the case of cellulose-containing materials Pfeffer and Liebman (1976)

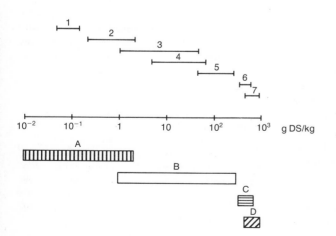

Fig. 16-18. Various processes for the treatment of effluents and residues with different solids contents. 1: Communal wastewater; 2: effluent from the pulp industry; 3: effluent from the foodstuffs industry; 4: sewage sludge; 5: liquid manure; 6: garbage; 7: plant residues. A: Aerobic treatment; B: anaerobic treatment; C: composting; D: combustion.

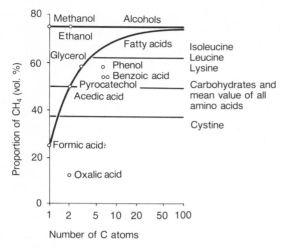

Fig. 16-19. Amounts of methane in the biogas in the anaerobic conversion of various organic substances (after Schoberth, 1978).

have shown that the hydrolysis of the cellulose in this overall process may be rate-determining.

For the microorganisms to be able to grow, however, they require not only organic substances as sources of carbon and energy but also a number of **nutrient salts.** Altogether, all the elements necessary for cell mass synthesis must be available in assimilable compounds (see Chapter 3). While such substances are normally present in sufficient amounts in communal wastewater, in the case of certain industrial effluents it may be necessary to add phosphate, ammonium, or some trace salts, such as sulfides. Since the amount of bacterial biomass formed, referred to the COD degraded ($< 10\%$) is considerably less in the anaerobic than in the aerobic process, the demand for nutrient salts here is correspondingly lower.

Several substances which may also occur in effluents at times inhibit the metabolic activities of the anaerobic bacteria and, in the extreme case, render an aerobic purification of the wastewater impossible. Thus, **chlorinated hydrocarbons** such as, for example, chloroform and carbon tetrachloride have an inhibiting effect on the methane bacteria even in very low concentrations (1 to 2 mg/L). **Cyanides** are also toxic for the methanogenic bacteria, even in concentration of 0.5 to 1 mg/L, although not for the acid-forming bacteria (Thiel, 1969). The inhibiting influence of heavy metals on the formation of methane depends very greatly on the concentration of sulfide (Lawrence and McCarty, 1965).

16.12.2 Temperature

The temperatures used most frequently today in the anaerobic treatment of sludge and wastewater lie between 32 and 37°C (mesophilic range). A **relatively strictly constant temperature** must be maintained, since deviations by only a few degrees soon lead to a drastic fall in the rates of conversion and therefore of gas production. It has recently been shown that in thermophilic sludge digestion processes residence times of 10 days at 35°C could be reduced to 4 days at 60°C, the gas yield being raised by 70% (Pfeffer, 1974).

Since very little experience with large technical thermophilic plants is yet available, it is still impossible to foresee whether the shorter residence times and the higher yields of gas will justify the higher heating costs, particularly under European climatic conditions. If, however, the pasteurization of the digested sludge is made a legal requirement, this will give a positive balance for the thermophilic process since in this case, in contrast to the mesophilic process, no additional costs will arise. The use of thermophilic anaerobic processes can therefore represent an economically advantageous further development of the mesophilic anaerobic sludge stabilization processes used hitherto. Very little is yet known about the anaerobic thermophilic degradation of effluents with high loads of organic matter.

16.12.3 pH

The **pH optimum** in methane fermentation lies between pH 6.7 and 7.4. If, because of a disturbance of the equilibrium between the acid-producing and the acid-consuming bacteria, an **overproduction of acid** and, therefore, a fall in the pH in the medium to below 6 take place, the activity of the methane bacteria is greatly inhibited. Moreover, a pronounced **production of ammonia** in the degradation of proteins can lead to an inhibition of methane formation if the pH rises above 8 (McCarty, 1964). Normally, with the formation of only slightly fluctuating amounts of acid and ammonia, the pH is kept constant because of the buffer action of the carbon dioxide or carbonate that arises during the fermentation. Thus, falling pH, increasing amount of volatile acids, increasing amount of carbon dioxide in the gas, and decreasing production of gas show that the methane bacteria are no longer working in the optimum manner and that a regulating intervention into the process must be made in order to prevent overacidification ("unbalancing").

Conclusion

Summarizing, it can be stated that the anaerobic microbial conversion of organic residues into methane and carbon dioxide, which has been carried out in the stabilization of sewage sludge on the large technical scale for more than 50 years (sludge digestion) has also become of great interest for the purification of effluents in recent years because of the continuously increasing cost of energy. As can be seen from Table 16-4, in the case of certain effluents highly loaded with organic matter from the foodstuffs industry, the composition and concentration of which fluctuate only slightly, degrees of purification and rates of turnover can be achieved with some newly developed anaerobic processes that are comparable with those of aerobic processes. To what extent this energy-saving process can be applied to the purification of communal sewage and chemical effluents has yet to be shown by further intensive research in the fields of microbiology, process engineering, and biotechnology.

Table 16-4. Characteristics of Anaerobic Treatment Processes.

Parameter	High rate digester	Contact process	Anaerobic filter/fluidized bed process	UASB process
Suitable wastes and wastewaters	sludge, manure solid wastes	wastewaters from food industry	wastewaters from food industry	sugar industry wastewaters
Suitable COD-concentration (mg L^{-1})	>20000	2000–20000	500–10000 (40000)	1000–50000
Treatment temperature (°C)	a) 30–40 b) 55–60	30–40	20–35	7–35
Organic load COD (kg m^{-3} d^{-1})	1–8	1–5	1–15	3–15
Sludge load (kg COD per kg sludge)	–	0.2–0.5	–	0.8–1.0
Waste sludge production (kg sludge per kg COD degraded)	–	0.03–0.10	0.03–0.10	0.04
Solids retention time (d)	a) 10–30 b) 5–15	>20	>100	>100
Hydraulic retention time (d)	a) 10–30 b) 5–15	0.5–25	0.2–3	0.2–3
Effiency (% COD)	30–70	60–90	70–95	80–90
Methane content of gas (% v v^{-1})	50–75	50–90	50–90	80–90

Biological Purification of Waste Air and Degradation of Solid Wastes

16.13 Processes for the Biological Purification of Waste Air

Biological processes for the purification of waste air have been used only for a few years. They are based essentially on the principle of absorbing the harmful and odorous substances on solid or aqueous phases and degrading them further by means of microorganisms (Jager and Schildknecht, 1974). The advantage of biological purification resides in the fact that, in contrast to absorption alone, which works only at relatively high capacities of the absorbent for the odorous substances, the microorganisms keep their concentration in the medium low through their metabolism. Biofilters, beds of packing bodies through which liquid is trickling, biowashers, i.e., spray towers, or bubble columns are used. Table 16-5 (after Steinmüller et al., 1979) gives examples of the **elimination of odor** by microorganisms, and Table 16-6 shows the degradation pathways of various microorganisms in the degradation of odor-causing materials. A calculation and description of biofilters is given by Gust, Grochowski, and Schirz (1979) and one for biowashers by Gust, Sporenberg, and Schippert (1979).

The waste air from **garbage composting plants** (Helmer, 1974), from **carcass processing facilities** (Körbitz and Brocke, 1968), from **agricultural enterprises** (Dratwa, 1968), of **sewage plants** (Carlson and Leiser, 1966), and even from **industrial plants** such as foundries (Reither, 1977) have also now been purified successfully by biological processes. Biological processes are also used for **fermentation plants** (Carlson and Gumerman, 1966). In the near future the purification of sulfur-containing power plant waste gases must be considered, as must the binding of malodorous substances from the waste air of chemical plants with the aid of biosynthesis.

16.14 Processes for the Biological Degradation of Solid Wastes

The **putrefaction of solid substances** and their destruction by the attack of microorganisms is an undesirable event in many cases: the corrosion of metals caused by microorganisms, which may be ascribed to the secretion of acids, the rotting of wood and, not least, the spoilage of stored foodstuffs are continuously causing great losses. On the other hand, the putrefaction of solid wastes to form soluble substances capable of being incorporated in the food chain again is a process which must be deliberately promoted (Finstein and Morris, 1975).

Table 16-7 gives examples of what groups of **organisms** are capable, according to present experience, of degrading what substances. The most prominent are aerobic fungi (up to 63 °C) and, in addition, thermophilic bacteria (up to 70 °C and even 78 °C) (Lacey, 1973).

Composting processes range from simple controlled landfills with semianaerobic condi-

Table 16-5. Biological Degradation of Malodorous Substances from Mixtures of Complex Composition.

Source	Main constituents	Microorganisms identified	System
Pig feces	lower fatty acids	*Streptomyces griseus* *S. antibioticus*	surface culture
Culture of *Anabaena circinalis*	geosmin	*Bacillus cereus* *B. subtilis,* Sarcina sp., Mima sp.	submerged culture
Atmosphere	carbon monoxide, ethylene, acetylene	aerobic soil bacteria	earth columns
Actinomycetes in water reservoirs	–	*Bacillus cereus*	submerged culture
Industrial waste	phenol	*Bacillus cereus*	sand filter
Foundry waste air	phenols, formalde-hyde, amines, ketones, aldehydes	adapted activated sludge	biowasher
Meat processing	lower fatty acids	Nocardia sp. *Microthrix parvicella*	activated sludge process

tions through the comminution of solid wastes and mixing with sewage sludge up to continuous composting in towers or drums, i.e., true aerated reactors. By mixing with liquid manure followed by composting, cellulose-containing dry wastes such as straw, paper, sawdust, can be prepared for soil improvement (Schuchardt, 1978). The composting of horse dung to give a suitable substrate for the growing of edible fungi has acquired economic importance (Grabbe, 1978, see Chapter 9).

Because of the high resistance to natural putrefaction of a number of **modern plastics,** which has led to considerable pollution of the environment as the result of the use of no-return packages, compositions have been de-veloped the plasticisers, lubricants, stabilizers, fillers, or residual monomers in which are subject to appropriate enzymatic or microbial degradation (Pirt, 1980).

Finally, reference must be made to the fermentation of solids which can also be used for certain wastes (Cannel and Moo-Young, 1980) and which is linked with the deliberate **use of wastes in the energy cycle** because of consideration imposed by the increasing expense of energy (Bruin, 1980). The methanization of wastes in controlled dumps, which are regarded as fermentation reactors, has been described by Rees (1980) who particularly emphasizes the importance of an adequate moisture content of the dumped masses.

Table 16-6. Microbial Degradation of Substances with Intense Odors.

Substrate	Degradation products	Degradation pathway	Microorganisms
Methanol Formaldehyde	carbon dioxide, water	assimilation via the serine transhydroxy-methylase pathway	*Pseudomonas AM 1*
Lower alcohols and fatty acids	acetyl-CoA	β-oxidation	many bacteria and fungi
Methyl ketones		subterminal attack by monooxygenases	*Pseudomonas multivorans*
Dimethylamine	methylamine and formaldehyde	hydroxylase	*Pseudomonas aminovorans*
n-Propylamine	propionate	amine dehydrogenase	*Mycobacterium convolutum*
Phenol	acetaldehyde and pyruvate	meta-cleavage	*Pseudomonas putida*
Phenol	acetyl-CoA and succinate	ortho-cleavage	*Trichosporon cutaneum*
p-Cresol	protocatechuic acid	ortho-cleavage	*Pseudomonas fluorescens*
m-Cresol	fumarate and pyruvate	gentisic acid pathway	Pseudomonas sp.
Benzaldehyde	benzyl alcohol and benzoic acid	dismutation	*Acetobacter ascendens*
Aniline	2-hydroxyacetanilide, 4-hydroxyaniline		*Aspergillus ochraceous*
Aniline	pyrocatechol	dioxygenation	Nocardia sp.
Pyridine, 4-methylpyridine			Pseudomonas sp.
Indole	pyrocatechol		*Chromobacterium violaceum*
Indole	tryptophan		*Neurospora crassa*
Camphor	lactonic acid		*Pseudomonas putida*

Table 16-6. (continued).

Substrate	Degradation products	Degradation pathway	Microorganisms
3-Fluorophenol, 4-fluorophenol, and 4-chlorophenol	acetyl-CoA, succinate and HF or HCl	ortho-cleavage	Bacterium NCIB 8250
Methyl mercaptan			Pseudomonas, Bacillus, Nocardia, Flavobacterium, Micrococcus
Methyl mercaptan, dimethyl sulfide, dimethyl disulfide			Thiobacillus
4-Methylthio-phenol	4-methylsulfinyl-phenol	oxidation	Nocardia calcarea
4-Methylsulfinyl-phenol	2-hydroxy-5-methyl-sulfinylmuconic acid semialdehyde	meta-cleavage	Nocardia calcarea

Table 16-7. Degradation of Solids by Microorganisms.

Cellulose	Trichoderma, Mucor
Cotton	Aspergillus species, Mucor
Animal fibers	B. mesentericus
Gum rubber	S. lipmanii, Nocardia, Thiobacilli
Vulcanized rubber	Acremonium charticola
Polyurethane	Cladosporium resinae, Penicillium citrinum, Asp. niger
Poly(vinyl alcohol)	Pseudomonas
Fats, oils	Pseudomonas, Bacillus, Xanthomonas, Aspergillus, Fusarium
Water-based paints	P. aeruginosa

Table 16-7. (continued).

Linseed oil paints	Flavobacterium, *Pullularia pullulans*
Calcimines	*Cladosporium herbarum*
Oil paints	*Alternaria dianthicola, Aureobasidium pullulans*
Arsenic oxide	*Mucor mucedo, Aspergillus glaucus*
Kerosine	*Claudosporium resinae*
Trinitrotoluene	*Pseudomonas aeruginosa*
Picric acid	Corynebacteria
Leather	*Penicillium aculeatum, Scopulariopsis brevicaulis, Fusiarium oxysporum*
Concrete	Thiobacillus
Glass	Aspergillus, Penicillium, Scopulariopsis, Desulfovibrio, Thiobacillus
Cyanides	*Thiobacillus denitrificans, B. stearothermophilus, Rhizoctonia solani*
Detergents	Pseudomonas
Wood	fungi

16.15   Literature

ATV: *Lehr- und Handbuch der Abwassertechnik,* Vol. 2, 2nd Ed. Verlag W. Ernst und Sohn, Berlin 1975.

ATV, "Abwasserteiche für kommunales Abwasser", *Korrespondenz Abwasser* **26**, 403–415 (1979).

ATV: *Arbeitsblatt A 135: Grundsätze für die Bemessung von Tropfkörpern und Scheibentauchkörpern in einstufigen biologischen Kläranlagen,* 1982.

Baader, W., Dohne, E. and Brenndörfer, M.: "Biogas in Theorie und Praxis", *KTBL-Schrift* **229** (1978).

Balch, W. E., Fox, G. E., Magrum, L. J., Woese, C. R. and Wolfe, R. S., "Methanogens: Reevaluation of a unique biological group", *Microbiol. Rev.* **43**, 260–296 (1979).

Barker, H. A.: *Bacterial Fermentations.* John Wiley and Sons, Inc., New York 1956.

Barnard, J. L., "A review of biological phosphorus removal in the activated sludge process", *Water SA* **2**, 136–144 (1976).

Barnard, J. L., "Biologische Phosphor- und Stickstoffbeseitigung", *Gewässerschutz – Wasser – Abwasser* **42**, 803–834 (1980).

Bernhardt, H., "Anforderungen an die Elimination schwer abbaubarer Stoffe aus der Sicht der Trinkwasseraufbereiter", *Gewässerschutz – Wasser – Abwasser* **42,** 157–199 (1980).

Bischofsberger, W., "Belebungsanlagen mit Sauerstoffbegasung für industrielle Abwässer in Deutschland", *Gewässerschutz – Wasser – Abwasser* **42,** 609–633 (1980).

Bruin, S., "Biomass as a source of energy", *Biotechnol. Lett.* **2** (5), 231–238 (1980).

Bryant, M. P., Wolin, E. A., Wolin, M. J. and Wolfe, R. S., "*Methanobacterium omelianskii,* a symbiotic association of two species of bacteria", *Arch. Mikrobiol.* **59,** 20–31 (1967).

Bryant, M. P., "Commentary on the Hungate technique for culture of anaerobic bacteria", *Am. J. Clin. Nutr.* **25,** 1324–1328 (1972).

Bryant, M. P., Campbell, L. L., Reddy, C. A. and Crabill, M. R., "Growth of Desulfovibrio in lactate or ethanol media low in sulfate in association with H_2-utilizing methanogenic bacteria", *Appl. Environ. Microbiol.* **33,** 1162–1169 (1977).

Bryant, M. P., "Microbial methane production – theoretical aspects", *J. Anim. Sci.* **48,** 193–201 (1979).

Buck, H., "Die Ciliaten des Belebtschlammes in ihrer Abhängigkeit vom Klärverfahren", *Münch. Beitr. Abwasser, Fischerei, Flußbiol.* **5,** 206–222 (1968).

Buswell, A. and Mueller, H. F., "Mechanism of methane fermentation", *Ind. Eng. Chem.* **44,** 550–552 (1952).

Cannel, E. and Moo-Young, M., "Solid-state fermentation systems", *Proc. Biochem.* **8,** 24–28 (1980).

Cappenberg, Th. E., "A study of mixed continuous cultures of sulfate-reducing and methane-producing bacteria", *Microb. Ecol.* **2,** 60–72 (1975).

Carlson, D. A. and Gumerman, R. C., "Hydrogen sulfide and methyl mercaptan removals with soil columns", *Eng. Ext. Ser. Purdue Univ.* **121,** 172–191 (1966).

Carlson, D. A. and Leiser, C. P., "Soil beds for the control of sewage odours", *J. Water Pollut. Control Fed.* **38,** 829–840 (1966).

Coulter, J. B., Soneda, S. and Ettinger, M. B., "Anaerobic contact process for sewage disposal", *Sewage Ind. Wastes* **29,** 468–477 (1957).

Crowther, R. F. and Harkness, N.: "Anaerobic Bacteria". In: Curds, C. R. and Hawkes, H. A. (eds.):

Ecological Aspects of Used-water Treatment. Academic Press, Inc., New York 1975, pp. 65–91.

Diesterweg, G., Fuhr, H. and Reher, P., "Die Bayer-Turmbiologie", *Industrieabwässer,* June **1978,** 7–13.

Dratwa, H., "Das Biofilter, ein Verfahren zur Geruchsbeseitigung", *Staub-Reinh. Luft* **28,** 516–520 (1968).

Dunbar, W. Ph.: *Leitfaden für die Abwasserreinigungsfrage,* 3rd Ed. München 1954.

Ehhalt, D. H.: "The atmospheric cycle of methane". In: Schlegel, H. G., Gottschalk, G. and Pfennig, N. (eds.): *Microbial Production and Utilization of Gases.* E. Goltze-Verlag, Göttingen 1976.

Eikelboom, D. H., "Leitfaden für die Bestimmung fadenförmiger Mikroorganismen in Belebtschlamm", IMG-TNO-Bericht Nr. A 93, Juli 1979.

Ferry, J. G. and Wolfe, R. S., "Anaerobic degradation of benzoate to methane by microbial consortium", *Arch. Microbiol.* **107,** 33–40 (1976).

Finstein, M. S. and Morris, M. L., *Adv. Appl. Microbiol.* **19,** 113–151 (1975).

Frostell, B.: "Anaerobic waste-water treatment with emphasis on sludge retention". PhD thesis, Stockholm 1979.

Fuchs, G. et al., Zentralbl. Bakteriol. Parasitenk. Infektionskr. Hyg. Abt. I Orig. C **3,** 277 (1982).

Ghosh, S. and Klass, D. L., "Two-phase anaerobic digestion", *Proc. Biochem.* **13,** 15–24 (1978).

Gottschalk, G.: *Bacterial metabolism.* Springer-Verlag, Heidelberg 1979.

Grabbe, K., *Grundl. Landtech.* **28,** 64–69 (1978).

Gust, M., Grochowski, H. and Schirz, S., *Staub-Reinh. Luft* **39** (11), 397–402 (1979).

Gust, M., Sporenberg, F. and Schipper, E., *Staub-Reinh. Luft* **39** (9), 308–314 (1979).

Hackett, W. F., Connors, W. J., Kirk, J. K. and Zeikus, J. G., "Microbial decomposition of synthetic 14C-labelled lignins in nature", *App. Environ. Microbiol.* **33,** 43–51 (1977).

Helmer, R., "Abluftreinigung in Müllkompostwerken mit Hilfe der Bodenfiltration", *Beitr. Müll Abfall* **5,** 140–146 (1974).

Hines, D. A., "The use of deep-shaft process in uprating and extending sewage treatment works", *Ind. Water Poll. Contr.,* London (1979).

Hippe, H., Caspari, D., Fiebig, K. and Gottschalk, G., "Utilization of trimethylamine and other N-methyl compounds for growth and methane formation by *Methanosarcina barkeri*", *Proc. Natl. Acad. Sci. USA* **76**, 494–498 (1979).

Hobson, P. N., Bousfield, S. and Summers, R., "Anaerobic digestion of organic matter", *CRC Crit. Rev. Environ. Control* **4**, 131–191 (1974).

Hoffmann-Walbeck, H. P. and Pellegrini, A., "Fortschritte bei der Aufbereitung von Zuckerfabrikabwässern", *Zuckerindustrie Berlin* **103**, 841–847 (1978).

Hoppe-Seyler, F., "Über die Gärung der Cellulose mit Bildung von Methan und Kohlensäure. I. Über das Vorkommen der Entwicklung von Methan und Kohlensäure in wasserhaltigem Erdboden", *Z. Physiol. Chem.* **10**, 201–217 (1886).

Hungate, R. E., "The anaerobic mesophilic celluloytic bacteria", *Bacteriol. Rev.* **14**, 1–49 (1950).

Hungate, R. E.: *The Rumen and its Microbes.* Academic Press Inc., New York 1966.

Hungate, R. E., "Hydrogen as an intermediate in the rumen fermentation", *Arch. Microbiol.* **59**, 158–164 (1967).

Imhoff, K. R., "Die Entwicklung der Abwasserreinigung und des Gewässerschutzes seit 1868", *GWF Wasser Abwasser* **120**, 563–576 (1979).

Imhoff, K. and Imhoff, K. R.: *Taschenbuch der Stadtentwässerung,* 25th Ed. Oldenbourg-Verlag, München, Wien 1979.

Jager, J. and Schildknecht, H., *Beitr. Müll Abfall* **5**, 145–148 (1974).

Jennett, J. C. and Dennis, N. D., "Anaerobic filter treatment of pharmaceutical waste", *J. Water Pollut. Control Fed.* **47**, 104–121 (1975).

Karube, I., Kuriyama, S., Matsunaga, T. and Suzuki, S., "Methane production from wastewaters by immobilized methanogenic bacteria", *Biotechnol. Bioeng.* **22**, 847–857 (1980).

Köhler, R., "Anaerober Abbau von Hefefabrikabwasser", *Wasser, Luft Betr.* **17**, 342–346 (1973).

Körbitz, H. G. and Brocke, W., "Geruchsquellen bei Tierkörperverwertungsanstalten und technische Maßnahmen zur Vermeidung von Nachbarschaftsbelästigung", *Schriftenr. LIB Landesanst. Immissions-Bodennutzungsschutz des Landes Nordrhein-Westfalen* **19**, 16–20 (1968).

Lacey, J.: In: Sykes, G., Skinner, F. A. (eds.): *Actinomycetales.* Academic Press, London, New York 1973, pp. 231–251.

Lawrence, A. W. and McCarty, P. L., "The role of sulfide in preventing heavy metal toxicity in anaerobic treatment", *J. Water Pollut. Control Fed.* **37**, 392–406 (1965).

Lettinga, G., van Velsen, A. F. M., Hobma, S. W., De Leeuw, W. and Klapwijk, A., "Use of the upflow sludge blanket (USB) reactor concept for biological wastewater treatment, especially for anaerobic treatment", *Biotechnol. Bioeng.* **22**, 699–734 (1980).

Levin, G. V., Topol, G. J. and Tarnay, A. G., "Operation of full-scale biological phosphorus removal plant", *J. Water Pollut. Control Fed.* **47**, 577–590 (1975).

Liebmann, H.: *Handbuch der Frischwasser- und Abwasserbiologie,* Vol. 2. München, Wien 1960.

Mah, R. A., Ward, D. M., Baresi, L. and Glass, T. L., "Biogenesis of methane", *Annu. Rev. Microbiol.* **31**, 309–341 (1977).

Mann, Th.: *Bayer-Turmbiologie.* Lecture at DECHEMA-Meeting 1980.

Matsché, N., "Blähschlamm-Ursachen und Bekämpfung", *Wien. Mitt. Wasser Abwasser Gewässer* **22**, M1–M28 (1977).

McCarty, P. L., "Anaerob waste treatment fundamentals. I. Chemistry and microbiology", *Public Works* **94**, 107–112 (1964).

McInerney, M. J., Bryant, M. P. and Pfennig, N., "Anaerobic bacterium that degrades fatty acids in syntrophic association with methanogenes", *Arch. Microbiol.* **122**, 129–135 (1979).

Meinck, F., Stoof, H., Kohlschütter, H.: *Industrie-Abwässer.* Gustav Fischer-Verlag, Stuttgart 1968.

Müller, G. and Sell, G., "Der Biohoch-Reaktor, eine platz- und energieeinsparende Abwasserreinigungsanlage", *DECHEMA Monogr.* **86**, 589–596 (1979).

O'Rourke, J. T.: "Kinetics of anaerobic treatment of reduced temperatures". Ph. D. Thesis, Stanford University 1968.

Paynter, M. J. B. and Hungate, R. E., "Characterization of *Methanobacterium molilis* sp.n. isolated from the bovine rumen", *J. Bacteriol.* **95**, 1943–1951 (1968).

Pfeffer, J. T., "Temperature effects on anaerobic fermentation of domestic refuse", *Biotechnol. Bioeng.* **16**, 771–787 (1974).

Pfeffer, J. T. and Liebman, J. C., "Energy from refuse by bioconversion, fermentation and residue disposal process", *Resour. Recovery Conserv.* **1**, 295 (1976).

Pipyn, P. and Verstraete, W., "A pilot scale anaerobic upflow reactor treating distillery wastewaters", *Biotechnol. Lett.* **1**, 495–500 (1979).

Pirt, S. J., "Microbial degradation of synthetic polymers", *J. Chem. Technol. Biotechnol.* **30**, 176–179 (1980).

Rees, J. F., *J. Chem. Technol. Biotechnol.* **30**, 161–175 (1980).

Reither, K., "Gießereiabluft kann sauberer sein", *TL-Umweltschutztechnik* **30**, 5 (1977).

Rinke, G., "Anwendungs- und Planungsbeispiele für Belebungsanlagen mit Sauerstoffbegasung in der BRD", *Gewässerschutz – Wasser – Abwasser* **42**, 635–661 (1980).

Roediger, H.: *Die anaerobe alkalische Schlammfaulung.* Verlag R. Oldenbourg, München 1967.

Roediger, H.: Bau und Betrieb von Schlammfaulungsanlagen. *Münch. Beitr. Abwasser Fisch Flußbiol.* **24**, 1–16 (1974).

Sahm, H., "Anaerobic wastewater treatment", *Adv. Biochem. Eng. Biotechnol.* **29**, 83–115 (1984).

Scherb, K., "Zur Biologie des belebten Schlammes", *Münchner Beiträge* **5**, 158–205 (1968).

Scherer, P. and Sahm, H., "Züchtung von *Methanosarcina barkeri* auf Methanol oder Acetat in einem definierten Medium", 4th Symposium on Technical Microbiology, Berlin, 281–290 (1979).

Schoberth, S.: "Mikrobielle Methanisierung von Klärschlamm". In: *Biologische Abfallbehandlung.* BMFT 1978, pp. 87–135.

Schuchardt, F., *Grundl. Landtech.* **28**, 69–75 (1978).

Sekoulov, J., "Nachreinigung von Abwässern durch Belebt-Algenverfahren", *Gewässerschutz – Wasser – Abwasser* **25**, 365–278 (1978).

Sierp, F.: *Die gewerblichen und industriellen Abwässer.* Berlin 1967.

Smith, M. R., Zinder, S. H. and Mah, R. A., "Microbial methanogenesis from acetate", *Proc. Biochem.* **15**, 34–39 (1980).

Stadtman, T. C. and Barker, H. A., "Studies on the methane fermentation. IX. The origin of methane in the acetate and methanol fermentations by Methanosarcina", *J. Bacteriol.* **61**, 81–86 (1951).

Steffen, A. J. and Bedker, M., "Operation of full-scale anaerobic contact treatment plant for meat packing wastes", *Eng. Ext. Ser. Purdue Univ.* **109**, 423–437 (1961).

Steinmüller, W., Claus, G. and Kutzner, H. J., "Mikrobiologischer Abbau von luftverunreinigenden Stoffen", *Staub-Reinh. Luft* **39** (5), 149–153 (1979).

Thauer, R. K., Jungermann, K. and Decker, K., "Energy conservation in chemotrophic anaerobic bacteria", *Bacteriol. Rev.* **41**, 100–180 (1977).

Thauer, R. K. and Fuchs G., "Methanogene Bakterien", *Naturwissenschaften* **66**, 89–94 (1979).

Thiel, P. G., "The effect of methane analogues on methanogenesis in anaerobic digestion", *Water Res.* **3**, 215–223 (1969).

Van den Berg, L., Patel, G. B., Clar, D. S. and Lentz, C. P., "Factors affecting rate of methane formation from acetic acid by enriched methanogenic cultures", *Can. J. Microbiol.* **22**, 1312–1319 (1976).

Van den Berg, L. and Lentz, C. P., "Factors affecting sedimentation in the anaerobic contact fermentation using food processing waste", *Ann. Arbor Science* **1979**, 185–193.

Vogels, G. D., "The global cycle of methane", *Antonic van Leeuwenhoek J. Microbiol. Ser.* **45**, 347–352 (1979).

Widdel, F. and Pfennig, N., "A new anaerobic, sporing, acetate-oxidizing, sulfate-reducing bacterium, *Desulfotomaculum* (emend.) *acetoxidans*", *Arch. Microbiol.* **112**, 119–122 (1977).

Wolfe, R. S., "Microbial formation of methane", *Adv. Microb. Physiol.* **6**, 107–146 (1971).

Young, J. C. and McCarty, P. L., "The anaerobic filter for waste treatment", *J. Water Pollut. Control Fed.* **41**, R 160–R 173 (1969).

Zehnder, A. J. B., Huser, B. A., Brock, Th. D. and Wuhrmann, K., "Characterization of an acetate-decarboxylating non-hydrogen oxidizing methane bacterium", *Arch. Microbiol.* **124**, 1–11 (1980).

Zeikus, J. G., "The biology of methanogenic bacteria", *Bacteriol. Rev.* **41**, 514–541 (1977).

Zeikus, J. G., Fuchs, G., Kenealy, W. and Thauer, R. K., "Oxidoreductases involved in cell carbon synthesis of *Methanobacterium thermoautotrophicum*", *J. Bacteriol.* **132**, 604–613 (1977).

Chapter 17

Microbial Leaching

Klaus Bosecker

17.1   Introduction

The increasing shortage of nonregenerable raw materials to be expected for the future makes it necessary to intensify endeavors to develop new sources of raw materials and to utilize known deposits with the aid of improved or new technology.

The introduction of **microbial leaching processes** which may achieve importance for the future supply of metallic raw materials offers new possibilities. Bacterial leaching, i.e., the winning of metals with the aid of bacteria, is based on the capacity of certain bacteria of the genus Thiobacillus to convert sparingly soluble metal compounds by biochemical reaction mechanisms into **water-soluble metal sulfates.** It is now possible with the aid of microbiological leaching processes to make profitable use of ores no longer worth being processed by conventional methods, so-called **low-grade ores,** and **metal-containing industrial residues.** Technically, the bacterial leaching of ores is used today mainly for recovering metal from copper and uranium ores.

17.2   Microorganisms

17.2.1   Thiobacilli

A fundamental role in microbial leaching is played by bacteria of the genus Thiobacillus. They are Gram-negative, non-spore-forming rods about 0.5 μm thick and 1.3 μm long, which, with two exceptions, are provided with flagella at the poles. Most thiobacilli are strictly **chemolithoautotrophic** and grow under aerobic conditions. They obtain their energy by the oxidation of elementary sulfur and of **reduced sulfur compounds** and use the carbon

dioxide of the air as the sole source of carbon. The end product of the oxidation of sulfur is sulfate (Vishniac and Santer, 1957; Trudinger, 1967).

Bacterial leaching is carried out in acid solutions at pH values between 2.0 and 3.0 at which metal ions remain in solution. For this reason the species *T. thiooxidans* and *T. ferrooxidans* living exclusively in acid media are of particular importance. Other thiobacilli are also capable of oxidizing sulfur and sulfides, but they grow only at higher pH values at which, because of hydrolysis, metal ions cannot normally be brought into solution.

Thiobacillus thiooxidans

T. thiooxidans was isolated in 1922 by Waksman and Joffe. The rods, with a length of 1 to 2 μm, occur individually and, more rarely, in pairs or short chains. They oxidize elementary sulfur and thiosulfate to sulfuric acid and sulfate, the pH in the medium falling to 1.5 to 1. In extreme cases values of less than 1 can actually be reached. The intensive production of acid leads to a rapid decomposition of the rock so that acid-soluble metal compounds can pass into solution as sulfates. Sulfides are not oxidized.

Thiobacillus ferrooxidans

However, there is no doubt that the more important role in bacterial leaching processes is played by *T. ferrooxidans*. This bacterium was first isolated in 1947 by Colmer and Hinkle from coal pit waters containing sulfuric acid. Morphologically they are identical with *T. thiooxidans,* but they differ from the latter by the very much slower course of the oxidation of elementary sulfur. *T. ferrooxidans* is distinguished from all other thiobacilli by the fact that, in addition to sulfur and reduced sulfur compounds, it also oxidizes bivalent iron.

In addition to *T. ferrooxidans,* two other chemoautotrophic bacteria have been described which likewise use bivalent iron as a source of energy: *Ferrobacillus ferrooxidans* (Leathen et al., 1956) and *Ferrobacillus sulfooxidans* (Kinsel, 1960). These species cannot be distinguished morphologically but only on the basis of their capacities for using inorganic sulfur compounds as oxidizable substrates. According to this classification, *T. ferrooxidans* oxidizes bivalent iron, sulfur, sulfides, and thiosulfate, while *F. ferrooxidans* uses only bivalent iron as the energy-providing substrate and *F. sulfooxidans* grows with bivalent iron and sulfur. Detailed investigations by Kelly and Tuovinen (1972) have shown, however, that all three species oxidize sulfur and thiosulfate, as well as bivalent iron, so that there is no longer any justification for a taxonomic differentiation. The terms *F. ferrooxidans* and *F. sulfooxidans* now serve merely as synonyms for *T. ferrooxidans.*

17.2.2 Thermophilic Microorganisms

In the meantime, thermophilic chemoautotrophic bacteria were described (Brierley and Brierley, 1973) which oxidize bivalent iron, elementary sulfur, and sulfides and leach molybdenite and chalcopyrite (Brierley and Murr, 1973).

The bacteria grow at a temperature of 45 to 70°C. The pH optimum is 2. Physiologically and morphologically, these acido-thermophilic bacteria now belong to the genus Sulfolobus (*S. brierleyi,* Zillig et al., 1980) which was first described by Brock et al. (1972).

Other facultative thermophiles, Thiobacillus-like bacteria, oxidize pyrite, pentlandite, and chalcopyrite at 50°C (Brierley and Le Roux, 1977). Thermophilic Thiobacillus-like organisms have been isolated from leaching dumps. They use bivalent iron as a source of energy but grow only in the presence of yeast extract (Brierley, 1978).

The thermophilic microorganisms are still too little studied to permit their use for technical leaching processes. However, they will be advantageous in those processes (dump leaching, in situ leaching), in which because of higher temperatures, the mesophilic species *T. thiooxidans* and *T. ferrooxidans* are no longer viable.

17.3 Reaction Mechanisms

At the present time, microbial leaching processes are based exclusively on the activity of *T. ferrooxidans* and *T. thiooxidans,* which convert sparingly soluble metal compounds via biochemical oxidation reactions into water-soluble metal sulfates. The most important reaction steps are summarized in simplified form in the equations 17-1 to 17-7 given below.

In general, in microbial leaching two reaction mechanisms can be distinguished: direct and indirect bacterial leaching (Silverman and Ehrlich, 1964).

17.3.1 Direct Bacterial Leaching

In direct bacterial leaching, a physical contact exists between bacteria and sulfide mineral, and oxidation to sulfate takes place through several enzymatically catalyzed intermediate steps. In this process, pyrite is oxidized to iron(III) sulfate (Silverman, 1967):

$$2\,FeS_2 + 7\,O_2 \xrightarrow{\ T.\ ferrooxidans\ } 2\,FeSO_4$$
$$+\,2\,H_2O \qquad\qquad +\,2\,H_2SO_4$$
$$(17\text{-}1)$$

$$4\,FeSO_4 + O_2 \xrightarrow{\ T.\ ferrooxidans\ } 2\,Fe_2(SO_4)_3$$
$$+\,2\,H_2SO_4 \qquad\qquad +\,2\,H_2O$$
$$(17\text{-}2)$$

Very recent investigations have shown that the following noniron metallic compounds can be oxidized by *T. ferrooxidans* directly (Torma, 1977):

Covellite (CuS)   Molybdenite (MoS₂)
Chalcocite (Cu₂S) Stibnite   (Sb₂S₃)
Sphalerite (ZnS)   Cobalt sulfide (CoS)
Galena   (PbS)   Millerite   (NiS)

For direct sulfide leaching, therefore equation 17-3 can be formulated:

$$MeS + 2 O_2 \xrightarrow{\text{T. ferrooxidans}} MeSO_4 \qquad (17\text{-}3)$$

17.3.2 Indirect Bacterial Leaching

The indirect mechanism covers processes in which the leaching agent is merely produced or regenerated by microorganisms.

For example, sulfide minerals can be oxidized by Fe^{3+} ions and leached by an exclusively geochemical mechanism without the interaction of bacteria (Dutrizac, 1974):

$$MeS + Fe_2(SO_4)_3 \rightarrow MeSO_4 + 2 FeSO_4 + S \quad (17\text{-}4)$$

The bivalent iron arising in this reaction can be reoxidized to iron(III) ions by *T. ferrooxidans* in accordance with equation 17-2 and as such can take part in the oxidation process again. In this leaching process, the bacteria have only a **catalytic** function because they accelerate the oxidation of iron(II) ions which takes place only very slowly under normal conditions, i.e., in the absence of bacteria. According to investigations by Lacey and Lawson (1970), in the pH range between 2 and 3 the rate of the bacterial oxidation of iron(II) ions is about 10^5 to 10^6 times higher than that of the chemical oxidation of iron(II) ions.

The sulfur arising simultaneously (equation 17-4) is likewise oxidized to sulfuric acid by *T. ferrooxidans*, but this takes place much fas-

ter under the action of *T. thiooxidans*, which frequently occurs together with *T. ferrooxidans*.

$$2 S + 3 O_2 + 2 H_2O \xrightarrow{\text{T. thiooxidans}} 2 H_2SO_4 \quad (17\text{-}5)$$

The role of *T. thiooxidans* in microbial leaching obviously consists in creating favorable conditions for the growth of *T. ferrooxidans* and for the oxidation of iron because of its good **production of acid.**

As an example of the **indirect reaction mechanism** we may mention the bacterial leaching of uranium ores.

The tetravalent form of uranium that is usually present in the ore is insoluble in the leaching liquid. On the other hand, the hexavalent uranium compounds are water-soluble. The oxidation to hexavalent uranium can take place with iron(III) ions in accordance with the following equation:

$$UO_2 + Fe_2(SO_4)_3 \rightarrow UO_2SO_4 + 2 FeSO_4 \quad (17\text{-}6)$$

The oxidation potential necessary for the oxidation of uranium(IV) to uranium(VI) can be provided by *T. ferrooxidans* through the oxidation of iron(II) compounds (e.g., the pyrite that is widely distributed in uranium ores) to trivalent iron-compounds in accordance with the following equation obtained by summing equations 17-1 and 17-2:

$$\begin{aligned} 2 FeS_2 + H_2O \ &\xrightarrow{\text{T. ferrooxidans}} \ Fe_2(SO_4)_3 \quad (17\text{-}7) \\ + 7\tfrac{1}{2} O_2 \qquad & \qquad\qquad + H_2SO_4 \end{aligned}$$

In the leaching of uranium, iron(III) ions form the oxidant, which is then continuously regenerated by the *T. ferrooxidans*.

On the whole, microbial leaching is based on interlocking biochemical and chemical oxidations in which particular importance must be attributed to the cycle between iron(II) ions and iron(III) ions. It is not always easy to distinguish between direct and indirect leaching mechanisms. In technical leaching processes, this distinction is pointless, anyway, since because of the complex composition of the ores the two leaching mechanisms are frequently superposed upon one another.

17.4 Modification of the Bacterial Activity

The effectiveness and profitability of microbial leaching processes are largely dependent on the **activity of the bacteria** and on the **chemical** and **mineralogical composition** of the ore to be leached. The maximum yields of metal can be achieved only when the leaching conditions correspond to the optimum conditions of growth of the bacteria.

17.4.1 Nutrients

As chemoautotrophic organisms, the thiobacilli are relatively undemanding and require only a few mineral nutrients which, in general, are obtained from the surrounding rock. Apart from the energy-yielding iron and sulfur compounds, ammonium and magnesium salts, together with phosphate and sulfate, are the most important essential mineral components. Details on concentrations concerned are given by Tuovinen et al. (1971) and Tuovinen and Kelly (1972). In the laboratory, *T. ferrooxidans* is usually cultivated in Silverman and Lundgren's 9 K medium (1959) or in the culture medium of Leathen et al. (1951). For *T. thiooxidans*, Starkey's nutrient solution (1925), with the addition of elementary sulfur, is usually used (Table 17-1).

It is impossible to give exact concentration figures for leaching processes with respect to

Table 17-1. Nutrient Media for the Cultivation of *T. ferrooxidans* and *T. thiooxidans*.

	T. ferrooxidans		*T. thiooxidans*
Constituents	Leathen et al. (1951)	9 K Medium Silverman and Lundgren (1959)	Starkey (1925)
$(NH_4)_2SO_4$	0.15 g	3.0 g	0.3 g
KH_2PO_4	—	—	3.5 g
K_2HPO_4	0.05 g	0.5 g	—
$MgSO_4 \cdot 7 H_2O$	0.5 g	0.5 g	0.5 g
$CaCl_2 \cdot 2 H_2O$	—	—	0.25 g
$Ca(NO_3)_2$	0.01 g	0.01 g	—
KCl	0.05 g	0.10 g	—
$Fe_2(SO_4)_3 \cdot 9 H_2O$	—	—	0.01 g
Flowers of sulfur	—	—	10 g
aqua dest.	1000 mL	700 mL	1000 mL
$10 N H_2SO_4$	—	1.0 mL	—
$FeSO_4 \cdot 7 H_2O$	10 mL of a 10% solution (wt./vol.)	300 mL of a 14.74% solution (wt./vol.)	—
pH	3.5	3.0–3.5	3.5

the **demand for mineral salts.** Some inorganic nutrients pass into solution during the leaching process while others may be sorbed on the surface of the material to be leached or deposit as precipitates from the leaching liquid. The addition of pyrite can accelerate indirect leaching, while too high iron(III) ion concentrations inhibit the bacterial oxidation of iron(II) ions competitively (Kelly and Jones, 1978).

An adequate **supply of oxygen** can be achieved in the laboratory by aeration, stirring, or shaking. In the case of leaching on the technical scale, particularly in the case of dump leaching, difficulties may occur in relation to the optimum rates of aeration. The advantages of microbial leaching can be utilized to the maximum extent only when the factors for the transfer of oxygen into the leaching liquid are adequately known and taken into account (Torma, 1977).

Additional gassing with **carbon dioxide** stimulates the growth of *T. ferrooxidans* (Nielson and Beck, 1972) and promotes the leaching of metal sulfides (Bruynesteyn and Duncan, 1971; Torma et al., 1972). Figures for carbon dioxide concentrations range from 0.1 to 2% (Torma, 1977). According to more recent investigations by Kelly and Jones (1977), however, an optimum supply of carbon dioxide is not necessary in technical leaching processes, since even nongrowing bacteria are active for a relatively long time, and the oxidation of iron is independent of growth.

17.4.2   pH and Eh

The adjustment of the **correct pH** is a necessary condition for the growth of the thiobacilli active in leaching and is decisive for the solubility behavior of the metal compounds. The influence of the pH on the activity of *T. ferrooxidans* has been studied in detail (Silverman and Ehrlich, 1964). Figures between 2.0

and 2.5 have been found as the pH optimum for the bacterial oxidation of iron(II) ions and sulfide (Bodo and Lundgren, 1974; Sakaguchi et al., 1976). At pH values below 2, a considerable inhibition of the activity of *T. ferrooxidans* can be observed, but Tuovinen and Kelly (1973) succeeded in adapting *T. ferrooxidans* to pH values of down to 1.3 by increasing additions of acid.

As an aerobic bacterium, *T. ferrooxidans* requires redox systems with positive redox potentials. Starting from 300 mV, towards the end of the logarithmic growth phase *Eh* (standard oxidation-reduction potential) levels of about 600 mV are reached as a consequence of the oxidation of iron(II) ions (Dugan and Lundgren, 1964).

17.4.3   Temperature

The temperature optimum for the oxidation of iron(II) ions and sulfide by *T. ferrooxidans* is between 28 and 30°C (Silverman and Lundgren, 1959; Razzell and Trussell, 1963a; Torma et al., 1970). At low temperatures, because of a recession in the bacterial activity a decrease in the rates of extraction of metal is also to be expected. At higher temperatures (50 to 80°C), thermophilic microorganisms can be used for leaching purposes (Brierley and Murr, 1973; Brierley and Le Roux, 1977).

17.4.4   Chemistry and Mineralogy of the Leaching Material

The **chemical and mineralogical composition** of the material to be leached is of primary importance. When the carbonate content is high, the pH level in the leaching liquid rises, which leads to a pronounced inhibition or complete suppression of the bacterial activity. The low pH values necessary for the growth of the thiobacilli can be achieved in such cases by the external addition of acid, but this may place the profitability of a microbial process in doubt (Bosecker et al., 1978). Only in rare cases the mineral composition corresponds to simple stoichiometry, and chemically identical minerals occur in different crystal forms (e.g., iron and zinc sulfides) which usually exhibit different leaching properties (Silvermann et al., 1961; Khalid and Ralph, 1977).

17.4.5 Grain Size and Concentration of the Substrate

According to investigations by Razzell and Trussell (1963b) and Duncan et al. (1966a), the rate of leaching depends on the **surface** of the substrate leached. A decrease in the grain size means an increase in the particle-specific surface and in the total surface, so that higher yields of metal can be obtained with no change in the total mass of the particles. A grain size of about 42 µm is regarded as the optimum (Torma, 1977, summarizing literature). However, these figures were obtained on sulfide concentrates and cannot be transferred to the leaching of low-grade ores. A decrease in the grain size leads not only to an enlargement of the surface of the sulfides but simultaneously to an enlargement of the surface of the gangue material, which, in the case of low-grade ores leads to a "dilution" of the sulfide component.

A greater total particle surface can also be achieved by raising the pulp density, in which case the total mass of the particles likewise increases. An increase in the pulp density may result in an increased dissolution of certain compounds which have an inhibiting or even toxic effect on the growth of the thiobacilli. In practice, therefore, the optimum value for the particle size and for the substrate concentration must be determined beforehand for each substrate to be leached.

17.4.6 Surface-active Agents and Organic Extractants

In contrast to older publications (Duncan et al., 1964), according to which surface-active agents accelerate the leaching process and stimulate the growth of the thiobacilli, more recent investigations by Torma et al. (1976) have shown that after the addition of surface-active agents, because of a decrease in the surface tension, the mass transport of oxygen is greatly reduced and the growth of the bacteria is increasingly inhibited.

The organic extractants used in solvent extraction obviously have a similar effect (Torma and Itzkovitch, 1976). In recent years, solvent extraction processes have acquired technical importance for the selective extraction of certain metals from the leaching liquids and for increasing the concentration of metal ions in highly diluted aqueous solutions by back-extraction from the organic phase.

When bacterial leaching and solvent extraction are coupled, after the separation of the phases it is desirable to return the aqueous phase to the leaching process in order to save costs. Depending on the solubility of the solvent and extractant used, the recycled solution may contain different amounts of organic components which may affect the activity of the thiobacilli.

17.4.7 Heavy Metals

The choice of bacterial strains tolerant of heavy metals is of particular importance. Many heavy metals in low concentrations are necessary constituents of the nutrient medium as trace elements, but in higher concentrations they have a toxic effect. In general, thiobacilli have a high tolerance to heavy metals (Marchlewitz et al., 1961). Duncan and Bruynesteyn (1971) observed strains that were active in uranium mines even at concentrations as high as 10 g of uranium/L. High tolerance limits have also been found for copper (55 g/L), nickel (50 g/L), and zinc (112 g/L) (Sakaguchi et al., 1976; Bosecker, 1977; Torma et al., 1972). Different strains of the same species may show completely different sensitivities to heavy metals (Marchlewitz et al., 1961; Ebner and Schwartz, 1974; Bosecker, 1977). It is often possible to adapt individual strains to higher concentrations of metals or to specific substrates by gradually increasing the concentration of metals or substrates.

17.4.8   Light

Finally, reference may be made to the light-sensitivity of thiobacilli (Bryner et al., 1954). Investigations by Le Roux and Marshall (1977) have shown that it is particularly the **short-wave region** of visible light that is active. Inhibition by UV irradiation can be reversed by visible light. At the present time, nothing is known about the influence of light on biohydrometallurgical processes nor is there any information on the relative distribution of bacteria in the dump and the oxidation or collecting tank. Photoinactivation certainly has no effect on bacteria below the surface of the dump.

Only in laboratory experiments with weakly inoculated cultures may difficulties due to the action of light occur, but these can be avoided if the initial phase of growth is arranged during the night. Under normal conditions with a high density of inoculation there are no difficulties due to the particle effect.

17.5   Microbial Leaching Processes

17.5.1   Laboratory Investigations

Microbial leaching is now used industrially to recover copper and uranium, in particular, from low-grade ores and residues of conventional mining. The profitability of biohydrometallurgical processes depends fundamentally on the chemical and mineralogical characteristics of the ore to be leached, so that processes tested on individual types of ores cannot be transferred to other ores. Hence, before preparations are made for microbial leaching on the large technical scale, the leaching characteristics of the ore concerned must be thoroughly studied. In the first place, it must be decided whether the material is suitable for microbial leaching, in general. Then follow investigations to optimize the leaching conditions. Various processes are available in the laboratory for this purpose.

Percolator Leaching

The first experiments on the bacterial leaching of sulfide ores were carried out in air-driven percolators (Bryner et al., 1954) and in stationary leaching vessels (Razzell and Trussell, 1963b). In the simplest case, the percolator (Fig. 17-1) consists of a glass tube provided in its bottom part with a sieve plate and filled with comminuted samples of ore. The ore packing is irrigated or flooded with a nutrient that has been inoculated with thiobacilli, and the leaching liquid flowing from the packing is pumped back on to the sample material with a sterile stream of air which simultaneously takes care of the aeration of the system. This recycling is necessary, since in contrast to other microbiological transformations,

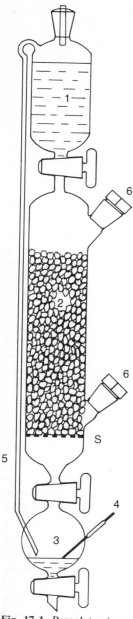

Fig. 17-1. Percolator (according to Wagner and Schwartz, 1967). – 1 = Reservoir of the circulating liquid; 2 = reaction vessel filled with ore and sieve plate (S); 3 = receiver with rise tube (5); 4 = tube for introducing compressed air; 6 = filling nozzles.

the bacterial oxidation of sulfides takes place relatively slowly.

There are no hard and fast rules concerning the design and size of the percolators. The dimensions are obviously governed by the amount of material available and by any special questions that are to be answered. The percolators developed by Wagner and Schwartz (1967) have a diameter of 30 to 60 mm. The reaction vessel contains 200 to 600 g of ore, depending on the type of ore and the size of the percolator. The total volume of the circulating leaching liquid amounts to a maximum of 200 mL. Because of the sometimes very long experimental phases, evaporation losses frequently take place which are made up by the addition of sterile distilled water. To monitor the course of the leaching process, samples are taken at intervals from the collecting vessel and the state of the leaching process is determined on the basis of pH measurements, microbiological investigation, and chemical analysis of the metals that have passed into solution.

Suspension Leaching in Shake Flasks

Because of the often inadequate supply of oxygen and the unfavorable surface ratio, percolator leaching is fairly lengthy, and series of experiments lasting 100 to 300 days are no rarity (Razzell and Trussell, 1963b). Furthermore the rates of extraction of metal are often very low (Bryner et al., 1954). In the laboratory, therefore, percolator leaching has been substantially displaced by suspension leaching in shake flasks. In **suspension** or **submerged leaching,** fine-grained material (grain size < 100 μm) is suspended in the leaching liquid and is kept in motion on the shaking table or by means of a stirrer (Duncan and Trussell, 1964). As compared with percolator leaching, the ratio of the surface of the ore to the amount of ore added is multiplied, so that a substantially larger reaction surface is available to the biological and chemical agents. Higher rates of aeration and a more accurate monitoring and control of the various parameters favor the growth and the activity of the bacteria, so that the reaction times are considerably shortened and the yields of metal are substantially raised. Thus, for example, in the leaching of copper schist in a percolator, less than 1% of the copper was leached in 100 days, while in shaking experiments 80 to 85% of the copper was extracted in 20 days (Bosecker et al., 1978).

Suspension leaching has proved to be outstanding in the laboratory, both when it is a question of investigating variables and elucidating the actual mechanisms and also when it is a question of determining whether a certain material is suitable for microbial leaching. To clear the last point, the fine-milled sample material is leached under the optimum conditions of growth: in this way, it can be decided after only a few weeks – in contrast to percolator leaching – under what conditions the microbial leaching process can be performed. Preferably, the fine-grained sample material is suspended in nutrient solution (usually 9 K medium) and, where necessary, is acidified with sulfuric acid with stirring or shaking until the pH remains constant between 2.0 and 2.5. Even during this phase, the first information is obtained on the consumption of acid and the solubility of various mineral components in acids. After this, massive inoculation with bacteria is carried out. Samples are taken at definite intervals and the metal contents of the leaching liquid are determined. For sterile controls, a 2% alcoholic solution of thymol is added instead of the bacterial suspension (Torma and Subramanian, 1974). Other authors add mercury nitrate (100 ppm) in order to inhibit any growth (Razzell and Trussell, 1963b). A heat sterilization of the ore (Bryner et al., 1954) should be renounced until it has been shown that no chemical and mineralogical changes take place in the substrate material during sterilization.

When only a small amount of metal or none at all passes into solution during such a test experiment or when the consumption of acid is extremely high, it appears unrealistic to expect appreciable yields of metal from a large-scale technical plant. When, however, significant concentrations of metal are measured in the leaching liquid, metal yields and rates of extraction can be determined. On the basis of these results it can then be decided whether microbiological leaching processes can be used (Figures 17-2 and 17-3).

Bruynesteyn and Duncan (1977) have developed a two-phase test process in order to check the realizability of a planned leaching project. In the first phase, preliminary experiments are performed in shake flasks. These are followed by a series of column tests from which important information for a practical, commercial application can be derived.

Column Leaching

Column leaching operates on the principle of percolator leaching and can be regarded as a **model for a heap or dump leaching process.** As in the percolator, in column leaching there are no hard and fast general rules in relation to dimensioning. Depending on their size, the columns may be made of glass, plastic, lined cement pipes, or steel. Their capacity ranges from several kilograms to a few tons. The columns used by Bruynesteyn and Duncan (1977) are about 2.50 m high with a capacity of 1 to 2 tons. Probably the largest test columns have been installed at the New Mexico Institute of Mining and Technology in Socorro, USA (Murr and Brierley, 1977) (Fig. 17-4). Approximately 200 tons of ore are leached microbially in steel vessels 12 to 30 m high with an internal diameter of 3.10 m.

Almost all column systems have, at various distances from the head of the column, devices for taking samples and for the installa-

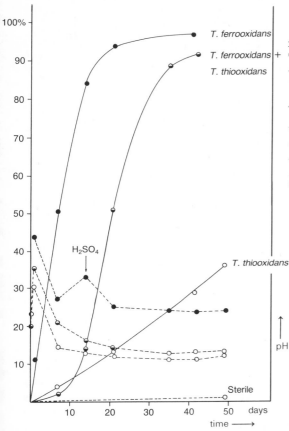

Fig. 17-2. Bacterial leaching of uranium ore in shake flasks. Change in pH and extraction of uranium on leaching with *T. ferrooxidans, T. thiooxidans,* and a mixed culture of the two strains [grain size <600 μm; pulp density 5% (wt./vol.)].

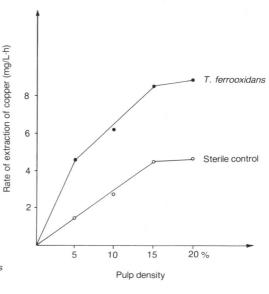

Fig. 17-3. Leaching of copper schist with *T. ferrooxidans*. Rate of extraction of copper as a function of pulp density.

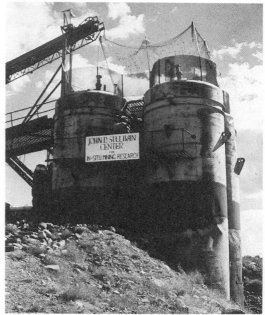

Fig. 17-4. Column leaching. Pilot plant at the J. D. Sullivan Center for in situ Mining Research, New Mexico Institute of Mining and Technology, Socorro, New Mexico, USA.

tion of special measuring instruments (temperature, humidity, oxygen, carbon dioxide), or additional gassing devices. In this way, both the changes in the leaching liquid during its passage through the column and also the leaching conditions in the charge material and changes in these conditions during the leaching process can be investigated. This gives important information on the variables to be expected in dump or heap leaching, together with indications on how the **leaching conditions can be optimized.** A number of particularly important parameters have been summarized by Bruynesteyn and Duncan (1977) and will be given briefly here. These are:

- supply of oxygen and carbon dioxide
- humidity conditions
- pH gradient
- temperature gradient
- precipitation of iron(III) salts
- particle size
- particle breakdown and particle migration
- appearance of impermeable layers.

Many of these variables can be studied meaningfully only on the semitechnical scale. For more detailed investigations, reference may be made to the publications of Bruynesteyn and Duncan (1977) and of Murr and Brierley (1978).

17.5.2 Technical Leaching Processes

The technical performance of microbial leaching consists, in the simplest manner, of piling up ore-containing rock, irrigating it in a suitable manner with a bacteria-containing suspension, collecting the leaching liquid flowing from the pile and extracting the metals dissolved in it (Fig. 17-5). Since the bacterial oxidation of sulfide takes place very slowly in comparison with other biotechnological processes, it is desirable to work in a **circulating**

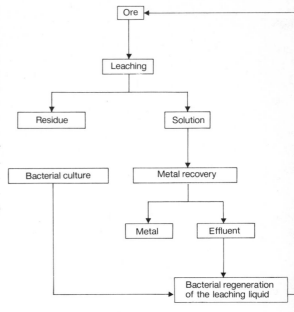

Fig. 17-5. Flow sheet of a bacterial leaching process.

system and to pump the leaching liquid over the ore continuously. In practice, essentially three processes are used: dump leaching, heap leaching, and in situ leaching.

Dump Leaching

The oldest process is dump leaching. Although the construction of dumps and the technology of leaching may differ very greatly from plant to plant, nevertheless they practically all work on the same principle (Corrans et al., 1972; Fletcher, 1970; Karavaiko et al., 1977; Malouf, 1972; Zajic, 1969). Overburden material and ores with a low content of metal, so-called low-grade ores, which are not suitable for conventional processes because of excessive transport and production costs, are, depending on the features of the land, deposited in dumps or tipped onto the slopes of mountains, or smaller steep-sided valleys are filled with them. Tipping on a slope and filling small valleys have the advantage that, because of the natural gradient, the problems of irrigation and drainage are simpler to handle. A prerequisite is that a seeping of the leaching liquid into the subsoil can be excluded on the basis of the geological conditions. Otherwise it is necessary to seal the soil in some way or other, whether by asphalting, cementing, or the application of a thick layer of clay, or by laying down a fixed layer of plastic.

The size of the dumps may vary considerably. Old dumps may be up to 200 m high and contain 50000 to 100000 tons of ore. The "finger dumps" constructed recently are several hundred meters long and about 40 m broad, and only 10 to 20 m high (Robinson, 1972). The development of this type of dump has, as the result of more favorable surface ratios, led to a considerable improvement in the aeration situation in the dump, and simultaneously the danger of an excessive rise of the temperature in the interior of the dump has been substantially decreased.

The leaching liquid is pumped onto the dump and percolates through the material of the dump. Various processes are used for irrigating the dumps. The cheapest, but also the least effective method consists in constructing dams and the continuous or alternating flooding of the dammed areas. Substantially more efficient is the irrigation of the surface of the dump with the aid of perforated hoses or the spraying of the leaching liquid with sprinkler systems. The last method has the advantage that the leaching liquid is enriched with oxygen during spraying. A disadvantage is the high rate of evaporation in dry areas and the high energy costs for pumping. Frequently, in order to achieve a better aeration of the dump, after the dump has been made, its surface, which has been compacted by the heavy large-capacity machines, is loosened. In addition,

special aeration boreholes may be made (Robinson, 1972).

The **leaching liquid** flowing out from the foot of the dump is collected and, after **extraction of the valuable metals,** it is pumped back to the dump. Frequently, before being pumped back, the leaching solution is passed into a so-called **oxidation tank** in which the bacteria and iron(III) ions are regenerated. Since iron(III) ions very readily undergo hydrolysis reactions and then precipitate from the leaching liquid as hydroxide compounds, in some plants the leaching suspension is acidified to pH 2.0 by the addition of sulfuric acid before being pumped back to the dump. This simultaneously means that at least part of the iron precipitated on the mineral surface is redissolved so that the oxidation of the sulfides is not blocked (Fig. 17-6).

Heap Leaching

Dump leaching and heap leaching are two processes which – apart from different size relationships – are distinguished by the fact that, because of their smaller amount of material, the heaps are constructed substantially from the aspect of the most favorable leaching conditions. Heap leaching is applied predominantly to finely divided oxide-sulfide ores which are not suitable for concentration by flotation. Leaching is carried out in concrete-lined basins or tanks that are provided with double bottoms so that the leaching liquid can percolate through the layer of ore. The basins have a capacity of up to 12000 tons and are usually arranged on the countercurrent principle (Torma, 1977).

In Situ Leaching

In situ leaching is, essentially, carried out in old, shutdown, underground mines. In some

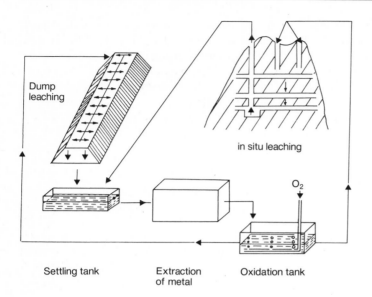

Dump
leaching

in situ leaching

O₂

Settling tank   Extraction   Oxidation tank
                       of metal

Fig. 17-6. Flow sheet of a dump and in situ leaching process (after Karavaiko et al., 1977).

cases, galleries and tunnels are flooded, and in other cases ore present but no longer worth digging out and ore-containing underground rubbish is sprayed or washed under pressure. The outflowing liquid is collected in lower galleries and pits and is pumped to the surface to the preparation plant (Fisher, 1966; Mac Gregor, 1966). The best-known example of this type of leaching, which is also called **underground leaching** is the uranium leaching operation of Stanrock Uranium Mines Ltd. at Stanrock, Ontario, Canada (see Section 17.6.2).

Deposits, which because of a low content of valuable metals or small extent cannot be profitably worked by conventional methods, can be extracted in situ by forcing the bacteria-containing leaching suspension through boreholes into the ore bodies previously fractured in place and, after a certain reaction time, pumping it up again through neighboring boreholes or horizontal collecting tunnels driven previously (Karavaiko et al., 1977). A precondition is an adequate permeability of the ore body and a sufficiently high imper-

meability of the surrounding gangue rock so that any seepage of the leaching liquid is prevented.

Stirred-tank Process

Because of the high metal yields in suspension leaching, a transition from shake flasks to bioreactors by analogy with other biotechnological processes was tested very early (Bruynesteyn and Duncan, 1971). At the present time, the stirred tank process is still in the development stage and, in view of the capacity of the reaction vessels in current use (up to 50 L), one can speak only of a **semitechnical** scale.

With the optimum control of the important leaching parameters, depending on the pulp density in the bacterial leaching of zinc sulfide concentrates, zinc yields of more than 80% have been achieved, with zinc extraction rates of 640 mg/L·h and a zinc concentration of 120 g/L in the leaching liquid (Torma et al., 1972). The bacterial leaching of chalcopyrite concentrates, a material very difficult to leach, gave extraction rates of 500 to 700 mg of copper/L·h in the batch process and led to copper concentrations of 25 to 28 g/L in the leaching suspension (Bruynesteyn and Duncan, 1971). In the meantime, a continuous stirred-tank process has been developed which with the same extraction rate of 400 mg copper/L·h has led to copper concentrations of 35 to 50 g/L in the leaching liquid (McElroy and Bruynesteyn, 1978).

On the basis of these results, the use of a microbial tank leaching process for the extraction of sulfide ore concentrates appears thoroughly realistic. Thus, flow sheets have been developed, cost plans have been drawn up, and patent applications have already been filed on the leaching of sulfide copper, zinc, cobalt, nickel, and lead concentrates on the basis of material turnovers of 100 to 200 tons/day (Bruynesteyn and Duncan, 1971; McElroy and Bruynesteyn, 1978; Torma, 1973; Torma, 1978a and Torma, 1978b).

17.6 Technical Applications

17.6.1 Leaching of Copper Ores

Intensive attempts to elucidate the bases of microbial leaching have led to the situation that biohydrometallurgical processes are now being used on the large technical scale for extracting copper and uranium from low-grade ores and residues of conventional mining.

We must first mention the dump leaching of low-grade copper ores carried out mainly in the USA but also in Canada, Mexico, South Africa, Australia, Portugal, Spain, Yugoslavia, the USSR, and some other countries (Table 17-2). A total of about 5% of the annual world production of copper is obtained by bacterial leaching (Malouf, 1971). In the USA alone,

the amounts of copper obtained annually by dump leaching are estimated at more than 227000 tons (Fletcher, 1970).

The largest plant for microbial leaching is that for dump leaching of the **Kennecott Copper Corporation at Bingham Canyon,** Utah, USA. The contents of the dumps stored there are estimated at more than $3.6 \cdot 10^9$ tons. Another 25000 tons of overburden material arises every day, and this is tipped onto the slopes of the mountains or is piled into dumps. The irrigation of the dumps is carried out through a system of pipes more than 12 km long. About 150 m^3 of leaching liquid is sprayed per minute. The leaching of the dumps and the recovery of the metal are combined to form a circulating system. The copper-free leaching liquid leaving the cementation plant is acidified with sulfuric acid to pH values between 1.9 and 2.4 before it is returned to the dump in order to keep iron in solution and to ensure favorable conditions for the growth of the bacteria. At Bingham, about 200 tons of copper are recovered every day by the leaching of the dumps.

At the **Chino Mine in New Mexico,** USA, which also belongs to the Kennecott Corporation, about 10000 tons of copper ore are mined per day. The rich ore with copper contents of 0.8 to 2.5% is sent directly for smelting, while low-grade ore and rubbish material is piled into dumps each of which contains approximately 1.5 million tons of ore. The average copper content of the dumps amounts to 0.27%. About 80 m^3 of water/min is consumed for irrigation, which is carried out partly by discontinuous flooding of the head of the dump and partly through sprinkler systems (Figs. 17-7 and 17-8). Because of the high pyrite content of this type of ore, no acid is added. The copper content of the leaching liquid leaving the dump amounts to about 0.5 g/L. In the Chino Mine, approximately 30% of the production of copper is obtained by microbial leaching.

In the **Miami Mine in Arizona,** USA, an in situ process is used in order to extract copper from low-content residues of a deposit which has previously been mined by conventional methods. In this process, the residual ore bodies are irrigated from the surface. The area to be leached amounts to about 0.5 km^2. The leaching liquid passes through the layer of ore, which is about 180 m thick, in 3 to 4

Table 17-2. Examples of the Large Technical Scale Dump Leaching of Low-Grade Copper Ores (after Corrans et al., 1972).

Locality	Dump material copper content (%)	Production of copper (tons/year)	Year
Arizona			
Bagdad Copper Co.	0.5	7800	1965
Esperanza	0.3	2000	1965
Inspiration Co.		3800	1965
Miami Co.		13000	1965
Ray (Kennecott)	0.24	9000	1965
Silver Bell		2400	1965
New Mexico			
Chino (Kennecott)	0.25	27000	1965
Utah			
Bingham (Kennecott)		70000	1965
Mexico			
Cia Minerva de Cananea	0.3	3300	1965
Spain			
Rio Tinto		18000	1945
Australia			
Rum Jungle		375	1967
Tasmania			
Mt. Lyell		100	1970

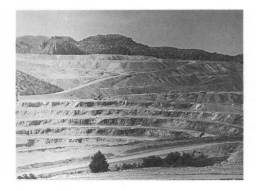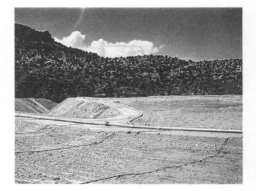

Fig. 17-7. Dumps for the bacterial leaching of low-grade copper ores (Chino Mine, New Mexico, USA).

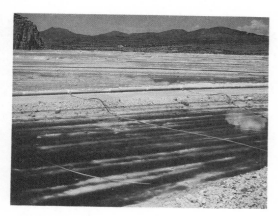

Fig. 17-8. Dump leaching of low-grade copper ores by discontinuous flooding of the surface of the dumps (Chino Mine, New Mexico, USA).

weeks and is collected in the old pits below. The extraction of copper is improved by discontinuous irrigation with a dry phase of about 3 months. The copper content of the leaching liquid amounts to 2 g of copper/L. By cementation 25 tons of copper are produced per day (Fletcher, 1970).

In practice, all dump leaching processes take place by the same principle (see Section 17.5.2). However, there is a considerable heterogeneity in relation to the technical details (construction of the dump, size of dump, method of irrigation, metal recovery) – due to the type of ore, the deposit, and the topographic features – which cannot be discussed here in detail. Further information on plants now in operation is given by Karavaiko et al. (1977).

17.6.2 Leaching of Uranium Ores

The microbial leaching of uranium is operated essentially as in situ leaching in conventional uranium mines that have been shut down.

A classic example is the leaching of uranium at the **Stanrock Mine in the Elliot Lake region** of On-

tario, Canada. A fall in the uranium content of the ore led to a marked rise in production costs, so that in 1964 a change was made to a bacterial process (MacGregor, 1966). Walls, roofs, and floors of the former mining galleries, and rubbish material present in side tunnels are washed under high pressure.

The washing process is carried out in two six-man shifts per day, each man dealing with an area of about 500 m² per shift. After three months in each case, the washing process is repeated.

In the meantime, several changes take place in the ore which indicate that the leaching process is proceeding. In the first place, the oxidation of the sulfide to sulfates leads to a dark, almost chocolate-brown discoloration of walls and floors. With increasing oxidation of the uranium, bright yellow efflorescences are visible through the brown coating, the color of which corresponds to that of the "yellow cake." Under the powerful jet of the next washing process, the uranium passes into solution and the surface of the ore is liberated for further oxidation processes. The washwater is collected in lower passages and shafts and is pumped into the processing plant. The water used for the washing process has a pH of 5.0, and after the washing process the leaching water has a pH of 2.3. The annual production of uranium is about 50 000 kg of triuranium octaoxide (U_3O_8). Attempts to raise the yields of uranium by the addition of salts of the 9 K medium gave no appreciable success (MacGregor, 1969).

A similar process is used in the **Milliken Mine** of the Rio Algom Mines Ltd. at Elliot Lake, Canada. Initially, the galleries were lightly sprayed and not washed under pressure. This showed that washing by a spray process was not sufficient to remove the basic iron deposits and to liberate the soluble uranium. More successful was washing under pressure, as practised at Stanrock. In contrast to Stanrock, however, after the addition of the nutrient salts of the 9 K medium the intermediate phase could be shortened to 4 to 5 weeks. The yields of uranium rose simultaneously. During a year, about 60 000 kg of uranium is extracted by bacterial leaching (Fisher, 1966).

A **vat leaching process,** i.e., leaching in large tanks, or heap leaching has been proposed for the leaching of carbonate-rich uranium ores (Flöter et al., 1979).

17.7   Future Aspects

Two microbial leaching processes, the dump leaching process and the in situ leaching process, are already being used commercially to recover copper and uranium from ores of relatively low value that can no longer be processed profitably by conventional methods.

Although, particularly in the dump leaching process, enormous areas with sometimes millions of tons of rubbish material are leached and considerable yields of metal are obtained, most plants operate only as **auxiliary hydrometallurgical operations** in which the phenomenon of the bacterial leaching of metals is in fact used, but not deliberately. Thus, in dump leaching there is no doubt that substantially higher yields of metal are achieved if, when new dumps are set up, the results obtained in model experiments are taken into greater account to optimize the most important leaching parameters (grain size, irrigation of the dumps, aeration of the dumps, control of the pH). In the case of older dumps, a corresponding optimization can be achieved by restructuring the dump.

At the present time, the use of microbial leaching processes is still limited essentially to the extraction of copper and uranium. For the future, however, it must be considered that these processes will play a primary role in metal extraction, so that in addition to copper and uranium other metals, such as zinc, nickel, cobalt, and molybdenum, will be leached bacterially (Table 17-3). As compared with the conventional pyro- and hydrometallurgical processes, microbial leaching processes involve only low capital and process costs. The plants can be erected in the immediate neighborhood of the deposits so that no high transport costs arise. The performance of the process is simple and easy to control and requires no wide technical knowledge. There is much to indicate that this biotechnology will probably be of great interest for obtaining raw materials in developing countries, in particular.

The development of **suspension leaching** has opened up new prospects for the use of microorganisms in the extraction and recovery of valuable metals. **Tank leaching** is being seriously considered for the extraction of metals from ore concentrates (Torma, 1978a; McElroy and Bruynesteyn, 1978). For conventional ore concentrates, the suspension leaching process is hardly competitive with the classical smelting processes. However, it will always be advantageous for **finely disperse concentrates** that cannot be, or can be only inadequately, processed by conventional metallurgical processes, or when, because of remote or only small ore deposits, the erection of a classical processing plant does not appear to be justified. Moreover, suspension leaching is remarkably harmless to the environment and, unlike pyrometallurgical roasting processes, leads to no pollution of the atmosphere.

Besides the metal sulfates that have passed into solution, the sparingly soluble metals, such as gold, silver, and lead, enriched in the residue are attracting increasing interest. From low-value **lead sulfide concentrates,** after the extraction of soluble interfering accompanying metals (zinc, cadmium, and copper), high-value residual ores can be obtained from which the lead is then obtained in conventional smelting plants (Torma, 1978a). A corresponding process has been envisaged for recovering **gold,** which occurs in finely divided form together with iron, arsenic, copper, and zinc sulfides (Pinches, 1971).

In addition, the use of tank leaching for the **recovery** of metals from fine-grained **industrial mineral residues** is being considered (Duncan et al., 1966b), by which, in addition to possibilities for ensuring the supply of raw material, solutions to problems of environmental protection could be found. Thus, for example, from zinc electrolysis residues almost 70% of the copper content and 50% of the zinc con-

Table 17-3. Range of Application for Microbial Leaching According to: Duncan et al. (1966b), Karavaiko et al. (1977), Torma (1977), Schwartz (1973), and Zajic (1969).

I. Thiobacilli

Iron:
Pyrite	FeS_2	
Marcasite	FeS_2	
Pyrrhotite	FeS	
Arsenopyrite	FeAsS	

Copper:
Bornite	Cu_5FeS_4
Covellite	CuS
Chalcocite	Cu_2S
Chalcopyrite	$CuFeS_2$
Enargite	$CuAsS_4$
Tetrahedrite	$Cu_8Sb_2S_7$

Zinc:
Sphalerite	ZnS
Marmatite	ZnS

Nickel:
Millerite	NiS
Pentlandite	$(Ni, Fe)_9S_8$
Violarite	$(Ni, Fe)_3S_4$
Bravoite	$(Ni, Fe)S_2$

Molybdenum:
Molybdenite	MoS_2

Lead:
Galena	PbS

Antimony:
Antimonite	Sb_2S_3

Cobalt:
Cobaltite	CoAsS

Tin:
Stannite	Cu_2FeSnS_4

Arsenic:
Orpiment	As_2S_3

Uranium:
Uranium oxide	(indirect)

II. Heterotrophic bacteria and fungi

Copper oxide	Gold
Copper carbonates	Platinum metals
Manganese oxide	
Uranium ores	

tent have been extracted with thiobacilli. 35% of the copper and almost 95% of the zinc have been brought into solution from sulfide-containing dusts arising in the smelting of copper (Ebner, 1978).

At the present time, microbial leaching is carried out on the technical scale exclusively with *T. ferrooxidans*. In the case of industrial mineral residues, these bacteria may fail, since in the case of fly ash and filter ash and, particularly, slags, it is mainly metal oxide compounds that occur rather than metal sulfides. However, metal oxides can be brought into solution through the biological production of sulfuric acid with *T. thiooxidans*, although in many cases chemical acid leaching will be simpler. Microbial leaching with *T. thiooxidans* may be advantageous when in chemical leaching high costs would arise for the transport of the acid and, on the other hand, sufficient sulfur for a bacterial production of acid is available cheaply as a waste product. Another advantage of microbial leaching consists in the fact that as a consequence of the growth of *T. thiooxidans* the pH falls only gradually, so that the metals pass into solution at different rates corresponding to their solubilities and can be separated from the leaching suspension selectively (Sullivan et al., 1979).

In the case of oxide, carbonate, and silicate ores, again, limits are set to the use of thiobacilli. In these cases, the employment of **heterotrophic bacteria and fungi** with which a mobilization of heavy metals through the formation of salts with organic acids or through chelate formation with organic components from the culture medium can take place is being considered (Schwartz, 1973; Silverman and Munoz, 1970). The mobilization of **gold** by various species of Bacillus and Pseudomonas has been described several times (summary in Karavaiko et al., 1977), although so far gold contents not exceeding 1.5 mg/L have been achieved.

Uranium and copper can be brought into solution by leaching with heterotrophic microorganisms (Berthelin et al., 1977; Kiel, 1977; Wenberg et al., 1971). **Manganese oxides** are leached enzymatically by a multiplicity of bacteria (particularly bacilli and pseudomonads) and nonenzymatically by fungi through reducing organic acids (Ehrlich, 1979).

The use of heterotrophic microorganisms for recovering **valuable metals** is still in its initial stage, and much development work is still necessary before its technical realization. Whether this will also lead to a commercial application will be decided in the final account by the supply of raw material and its costs.

17.8   Literature

Berthelin, J., Belgy, G. and Magne, R.: "Some aspects of the mechanism of solubilization and insolubilization of uranium from granites by heterotrophic microorganisms". In: Schwartz, W. (ed.): *Conference Bacterial Leaching*. Verlag Chemie, Weinheim 1977, pp. 251–260.

Bodo, C. and Lundgren, D. G., "Iron oxidation by cell envelopes of *Thiobacillus ferrooxidans*", *Can. J. Microbiol.* **20**, 1647–1652 (1974).

Bosecker, K.: "Studies in the bacterial leaching of nickel ores". In: Schwartz, W. (ed.): *Conference Bacterial Leaching*. Verlag Chemie, Weinheim 1977, pp. 139–144.

Bosecker, K., Neuschütz, D. and Scheffler, U.: "Microbiological leaching of carbonate-rich German copper shale". In: Murr, L. E., Torma, A. E. and Brierley, J. A. (eds.): *Metallurgical Applications of Bacterial Leaching and Related Microbiological Phenomena*. Academic Press, New York 1978, pp. 389–401.

Brierley, J. A., "Thermophilic iron-oxidizing bacteria found in copper leaching dumps", *Appl. Environ. Microbiol.* **36**, 523–525 (1978).

Brierley, J. A. and Brierley, C. L., "A chemoautotrophic microorganism isolated from an acid hot spring", *Can. J. Microbiol.* **19**, 183–188 (1973).

Brierley, J. A. and Le Roux, N. W.: "A facultative thermophilic Thiobacillus-like bacterium: oxidation of iron and pyrite". In: Schwartz, W. (ed.): *Conference Bacterial Leaching*. Verlag Chemie, Weinheim 1977, pp. 55–66.

Brierley, C. L. and Murr, L. E., "Leaching: use of a thermophilic and chemoautotrophic microbe", *Science* **179**, 488–490 (1973).

Brock, T. D., Brock, K. M., Belly, R. T. and Weiss, R. L., "Sulfolobus: a new genus of sulfur-oxidizing bacteria living at low pH and high temperature", *Arch. Mikrobiol.* **84**, 54–68 (1972).

Bruynesteyn, A. and Duncan, D. W., "Microbiological leaching of sulphide concentrates", *Can. Metall. Q.* **10**, 57–63 (1971).

Bruynesteyn, A. and Duncan, D. W.: "The practical aspects of laboratory leaching studies". In: Schwartz, W. (ed.): *Conference Bacterial Leaching*. Verlag Chemie, Weinheim 1977, pp. 129–137.

Bryner, L. C., Beck, J. V., Davis, D. B. and Wilson, D. G., "Microorganisms in leaching sulfide minerals", *Ind. Eng. Chem.* **46**, 2587–2592 (1954).

Colmer, A. R. and Hinkle, M. E., "The role of microorganisms in acid mine drainage; a preliminary report", *Science* **106**, 253–256 (1947).

Corrans, I. J., Harris, B. and Ralph, B. J., "Bacterial leaching: an introduction to its application and theory and a study on its mechanism of operation", *J. S. A. Inst. Min. Metall.* **72**, 221–230 (1972).

Dugan, P. R. and Lundgren, D. G., "Model mechanism of iron oxidation by the chemoautotroph *Ferrobacillus ferrooxidans*", *Bacteriol. Proc.* **92** (1964).

Duncan, D. W. and Bruynesteyn, A., "Enhancing bacterial activity in a uranium mine", *CIM Bull.* **64**, 32–36 (1971).

Duncan, D. W. and Trussell, P. C., "Advances in the microbiological leaching of sulfide ores", *Can. Metall. Q.* **3**, 43–55 (1964).

Duncan, D. W., Trussell, P. C. and Walden, C. C., "Leaching of chalcopyrite with *Thiobacillus ferrooxidans:* effect of surfactants and shaking", *Appl. Microbiol.* **12**, 122–126 (1964).

Duncan, D. W., Walden, C. C. and Trussell, P. C., "Biological leaching of mill products", *CIM Bull.* **59**, 1075–1079 (1966a).

Duncan, D. W., Walden, C. C. and Trussell, P. C., "Biological leaching of mill products", *Trans. Can. Inst. Min. Metall. Min. Soc. N. S.* **69**, 329–333 (1966b).

Dutrizac, J. E. and MacDonald, R. J. C., "Ferric iron as a leaching medium", *Miner. Sci. Eng.* **6** (2), 59–100 (1974).

Ebner, H. G.: "Metal recovery and environmental protection by bacterial leaching of inorganic waste materials". In: Murr, L. E., Torma, A. E. and Brierley, J. A. (eds.): *Metallurgical Applications of Bacterial Leaching and Related Microbiological Phenomena*. Academic Press, New York 1978, pp. 195–206.

Ebner, H. G. and Schwartz, W., "Mikrobiologische Untersuchungen XII. Verhalten von Mikroorganismen auf uranhaltigen Gesteinen", *Z. Allg. Mikrobiol.* **14**, 93–102 (1974).

Ehrlich, H. L.: "Bacterial leaching of manganese ores". In: Trudinger, P. A., Walter, M. R., Ralph, B. J. (eds.): *Biogeochemistry of Ancient and Modern Environments*. Australian Academy of Science, Canberra 1980, pp. 609–614.

Fisher, J. R., "Bacterial leaching of Elliot Lake uranium ore", *Trans. Can. Inst. Min. Metall. Min. Soc. N. S.* **69**, 167–171 (1966).

Fletcher, A. W., "Metal winning from low-grade ore by bacterial leaching", *Trans. Can. Inst. Min. Metall. Min. Soc. N. S.* **79**, 247–252 (1970).

Flöter, W., Sadowski, R. and Wirth, G., "Mikrobielle Laugung", *Metall Berlin* **33** (1), 56–58 (1979).

Karavaiko, G. I., Kuznetsov, S. I. and Golonizik, A. I.: *"The Bacterial Leaching of Metals from Ores"* (Engl. translation by W. Burns). Technology Ltd., Stonehouse, England 1977.

Kelly, D. P. and Jones, C. A.: "Factors affecting metabolism and ferric iron oxidation in suspensions and batch cultures of *Thiobacillus ferrooxidans:* Relevance to ferric iron leach suspension regeneration". In: Murr, L. E., Torma, A. E. and Brierley, J. A. (eds.): *Metallurgical Applications of Bacterial Leaching and Related Microbiological Phenomena*. Academic Press, New York 1978, pp. 19–44.

Kelly, D. P. and Tuovinen, O. H., "Recommendation that the names *Ferrobacillus ferrooxidans* Leathen and Braley and *Ferrobacillus sulfooxidans* Kinsel be recognized as synonyms of *Thiobacillus ferrooxidans* Temple and Colmer", *Int. J. Syst. Bacteriol.* **22**, 170–172 (1972).

Khalid, A. M. and Ralph, B. J.: "The leaching behaviour of various zinc sulphide minerals with three *Thiobacillus species*". In: Schwartz, W. (ed.): *Conference Bacterial Leaching*. Verlag Chemie, Weinheim 1977, pp. 165–173.

Kiel, H.: "Laugung von Kupferkarbonat- und Kupfersilikat-Erzen mit heterotrophen Mikroorganismen". In: Schwartz, W. (ed.): *Conference Bacterial Leaching*. Verlag Chemie, Weinheim 1977, pp. 261–270.

Kinsel, N. A., "New sulfur oxidizing iron bacterium: *Ferrobacillus sulfooxidans* sp. n.", *J. Bacteriol.* **80**, 628–632 (1960).

Lacey, D. T. and Lawson, F., "Kinetics of the liquid-phase oxidation of acid ferrous sulfate by the bacterium *Thiobacillus ferrooxidans*", *Biotechnol. Bioeng.* **12**, 29–50 (1970).

Leathen, W. W., McIntyre, L. D. and Braley, S. A., "A medium for the study of the bacterial oxidation of ferrous iron", *Science* **114**, 280–281 (1951).

Leathen, W. W., Kinsel, N. A. and Braley, S. A., "*Ferrobacillus ferrooxidans,* a chemosynthetic autotrophic bacterium", *J. Bacteriol.* **72**, 700–704 (1956).

Le Roux, N. W. and Marshall, V. M.: "Effect of light on Thiobacilli". In: Schwartz, W. (ed.): *Conference Bacterial Leaching*. Verlag Chemie, Weinheim 1977, pp. 21–35.

McElroy, R. O. and Bruynesteyn, A.: "Continuous biological leaching of chalcopyrite concentrates: demonstration and economic analysis". In: Murr, L. E., Torma, A. E. and Brierley, J. A. (eds.): *Metallurgical Applications of Bacterial Leaching and Related Microbiological Phenomena*. Academic Press, New York 1978, pp. 441–462.

MacGregor, R. A., "Recovery of U_3O_8 by underground leaching", *Trans. Can. Inst. Min. Metall. Min. Soc. N. S.* **69**, 162–166 (1966).

MacGregor, R. A., "Uranium dividends from bacterial leaching", *Min. Eng. Littleton, Colo.* **21** (3), 54–55 (1969).

Malouf, E. E., "The role of microorganisms in chemical mining", *Min. Eng. Littleton, Colo.* **23** (11), 43–46 (1971).

Malouf, E. E., "Current copper leaching practices", *Min. Eng. Littleton, Colo.* **24** (8), 58–60 (1972).

Marchlewitz, B., Hasche, D. and Schwartz, W.: "Untersuchungen über das Verhalten von Thiobakterien gegenüber Schwermetallen", *Z. Allg. Mikrobiol.* **1**, 179–191 (1961).

Murr, L. E. and Brierley, J. A.: "The use of large-scale test facilities in studies of the role of microorganisms in commercial leaching operations". In: Murr, L. E., Torma, A. E. and Brierley, J. A. (eds.): *Metallurgical Applications of Bacterial Leaching and Related Microbiological Phenomena*. Academic Press, New York 1978, pp. 491–520.

Nielson, A. M. and Beck, J. V., "Chalcocite oxidation and coupled carbon dioxide fixation by *Thiobacillus ferrooxidans*", *Science* **175**, 1124–1126 (1972).

Pinches, A., "Bacterial leaching of sulphide minerals", *Min. Miner. Eng.* **7** (9), 14–16 (1971).

Razzell, W. E. and Trussell, P. C., "Isolation and properties of an iron-oxidizing Thiobacillus", *J. Bacteriol.* **85**, 595–603 (1963a).

Razzell, W. E. and Trussell, P. C., "Microbiological leaching of metallic sulfides", *Appl. Microbiol.* **11**, 105–110 (1963b).

Robinson, W. J., "Finger dump preliminaries promise improved copper leaching at Butte", *Min. Eng. Littleton, Colo.* **24** (9), 47–49 (1972).

Schwartz, W., "Verwendung von Mikroorganismen zu Leaching-Prozessen", *Metall Berlin* **27** (12), 1202–1206 (1973).

Silverman, M. P., "Mechanism of bacterial pyrite oxidation", *J. Bacteriol.* **94**, 1046–1051 (1967).

Silverman, M. P. and Ehrlich, H. L., "Microbial formation and degradation of minerals", *Adv. Appl. Microbiol.* **6**, 153–206 (1964).

Silverman, M. P. and Lundgren, D. G., "Studies on the chemoautotrophic iron bacterium *Ferrobacillus ferrooxidans*. I. An improved medium and a harvesting procedure for securing high cell yields", *J. Bacteriol.* **77**, 642–647 (1959).

Silverman, M. P. and Munoz, E. F., "Fungal attack on rock: solubilization and altered infrared spectra", *Science* **169**, 985–987 (1970).

Silverman, M. P., Rogoff, M. H. and Wender, I., "Bacterial oxidation of pyritic materials in coal", *Appl. Microbiol.* **9**, 491–496 (1961).

Starkey, R. L., "Concerning the physiology of *Thiobacillus thiooxidans*, an autotrophic bacterium oxidizing sulfur under acid conditions", *J. Bacteriol.* **10**, 135–162 (1925).

Sullivan, E. A., Zajic, I. E. and Jack, T. R.: "Comparison of biological and chemical leaching: heap leaching using Thiobacillus thiooxidans", In: Trudinger, P. A., Walter, M. R., Ralph, B. J. (eds.): *Biogeochemistry of Ancient and Modern Environments*. Australian Academy of Science, Canberra 1980, pp. 557–562.

Torma, A. E.: "Verfahren zum biohydrometallurgischen Extrahieren von Kobalt und Nickel aus sulfidischen Erzen, Konzentraten und synthetischen Sulfiden". D.O.S. 2,303,388 (1973).

Torma, A. E., "The role of *Thiobacillus ferrooxidans* in hydrometallurgical processes", *Adv. Biochem. Eng.* **6**, 1–37 (1977).

Torma, A. E.: "Complex lead sulfide concentrate leaching by microorganisms". In: Murr, L. E., Torma, A. E. and Brierley, J. A. (eds.): *Metallurgical Applications of Bacterial Leaching and Related Microbiological Phenomena*. Academic Press, New York 1978a, pp. 375–388.

Torma, A. E.: "Selective bacterial cyclic leaching process". Can. Pat. 1,023,947 (1978b).

Torma, A. E. and Itzkovitch, I. J., "Influence of organic solvents on chalcopyrite oxidation ability of *Thiobacillus ferrooxidans*", *Appl. Environ. Microbiol.* **32**, 102–107 (1976).

Torma, A. E. and Subramanian, K. N., "Selective bacterial leaching of a lead sulfide concentrate", *Int. J. Miner. Process* **1**, 125–134 (1974).

Torma, A. E., Gabra, G. G., Guay, R. and Silver, M., "Effects of surface active agents on the oxidation of chalcopyrite by *Thiobacillus ferrooxidans*", *Hydrometallurgy* **1**, 301–309 (1976).

Torma, A. E., Walden, C. C. and Branion, R. M. R., "Microbiological leaching of a zinc sulfide concentrate", *Biotechnol. Bioeng.* **12**, 501–517 (1970).

Torma, A. E., Walden, C. C., Duncan, D. W. and Branion, R. M. R., "The effect of carbon dioxide and particle surface area on the microbiological leaching of zinc sulfide concentrate", *Biotechnol. Bioeng.* **14**, 777–786 (1972).

Trudinger, P. A., "The metabolism of inorganic sulphur compounds by Thiobacilli", *Rev. Pure Appl. Chem.* **17**, 3–4 (1967).

Tuovinen, O. H. and Kelly, D. P., "Biology of *Thiobacillus ferrooxidans* in relation to the microbiological leaching of sulfide ores", *Z. Allg. Mikrobiol.* **12**, 311–346 (1972).

Tuovinen, O. H. and Kelly, D. P., "Studies on the growth of *Thiobacillus ferrooxidans* I. Use of membrane filters and ferrous iron agar to determine viable numbers, and comparison with $^{14}CO_2$-fixation and iron oxidation as measures of growth", *Arch. Mikrobiol.* **88**, 285–298 (1973).

Tuovinen, O. H., Niemela, S. I. and Gyllenberg, H. G., "Effect of mineral nutrients and organic substances on the development of *Thiobacillus ferrooxidans*", *Biotechnol. Bioeng.* **13**, 517–527 (1971).

Vishniac, W. and Santer, M., "The Thiobacilli", *Bacteriol. Rev.* **21**, 195–213 (1957).

Wagner, M. and Schwartz, W., "Geomikrobiologische Untersuchung VIII. Über das Verhalten von Bakterien auf der Oberfläche von Gesteinen und Mineralien und ihre Rolle bei der Verwitterung", *Z. Allg. Mikrobiol.* **7**, 33–52 (1967).

Waksman, S. A. and Joffe, I. S., "Micro-organisms concerned with the oxidation of sulphur in soil. II. *Thiobacillus thiooxidans,* a new sulphur oxidizing organism isolated from the soil", *J. Bacteriol.* **7**, 239–256 (1922).

Wenberg, G. M., Erbisch, F. H. and Volin, M. E., "Leaching of copper by fungi", *Min. Eng. Littleton, Colo.* **23** (11), 74 (1971).

Zajic, J. E.: *Microbial Biogeochemistry.* Academic Press, New York 1969.

Zillig, W., Stetter, K. O., Wunderl, S., Schulz, W., Priess, H., Scholz, J., "The Sulfolobus-"Caldariella" group: Taxonomy on the basis of the structure of DNA-dependent RNA polymerases", *Arch. Microbiol.* **125**, 259–269 (1980).

Chapter 18

Economic Aspects of Fermentation Processes

Leo Hepner and Celia Male

18.1 Introduction

The **profitability** of an industrial process determines its technical realization and its successful use. This applies particularly to biotechnological processes, which, with continuously improving technology, have had a very variable history. An example of this is the manufacture of **butanol and acetone** which existed even before the first world war:

The shortage of natural rubber and the successful polymerization of isoprene and butadiene, as well as the high demand for explosives, led to the setting up of a series of plants for the fermentation manufacture of butanol and acetone. Many of these were closed in the post-war period but were restarted with the development of the automobile industry. Until the advent of the large-scale production of an-

tibiotics, butanol-acetone fermentation occupied second place in economic importance amongst microbiological processes, after the production of alcohol. However, the cheapness and high availability of petroleum after the second world war suppressed this industry almost completely, and only in a few centrally-planned economies, in South Africa as well as Egypt and Brazil, are such plants still in operation. In view of the new evaluation of petroleum as a basic material, on the one hand, and further developments in biotechnological development, on the other hand, a revival of this technology in various regions of the world is conceivable.

The profitability of biotechnological processes is related to the sometimes lenghty and **intensive expenditure on research and development** which must be invested in this field today before any particular laboratory process is suitable for application on a large technical scale (Fig. 18-1).

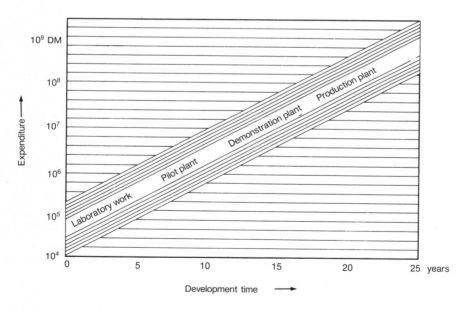

Fig. 18-1. Development costs and time for new technology.

This expenditure of time, research work, and capital for an interdisciplinary development is in general higher than for chemical synthesis. In relation to the market possibilities it may be prohibited, particularly if the costs for **toxicological investigations** of the new product sometimes necessary are included. There is hardly one discipline that has recently shown as many possibilities as biotechnology. Nevertheless, there are only a limited number of fermentation products with a market comparable with chemical products.

These include, in the first place **fermentation products** with **pharmaceutical applications** (Chapter 13), of high chemical complexity and high value (e.g., antibiotics). In addition, a series of **food-related** components (Chapter 9 and 10), whose importance is not so much due to chemical structure, but rather the specific aroma, taste, or physical properties (bakers' yeast, alcoholic beverages, vinegar, fermented spices, cheese) belong to these bioproducts. Furthermore, processes have become significant where large amounts of material to be processed are converted with relatively low concentrations of active substrate as, for example, the **leaching of ores** (Chapter 17), and **biological wastewater processes** (Chapter 16).

The field of **industrial enzymes** (Chapter 12) is only now beginning to develop in a profitable manner. In contrast to this, one group of chemically defined relatively simple compounds is in continuous competition with chemically synthesized products, and here it is less the technology than the costs of the substrate that decide profitability. Finally, the same applies to the **biotechnological manufacture of biomass** (Chapter 15) as feed and food compared with biomass obtained by agricultural means. In developing products for the food sector, the price fluctuations of conventional food components make difficult any reliable economic forecasts. Below we classify the factors that affect the profitability of a bioprocess, illustrated by examples.

18.2   Main Factors of Profitability

The success of a product depends on its **quality,** production technology, and toxicological safety as well as feasibility of production at prices that can be born by the market. The **price** at which a bioproduct is put on the market is composed of various factors. Depending on the sector, economic area, legal requirements, and the structure of the manufacturer, these must be evaluated in different manners. So far as plant and national economic considerations, such as duties, taxes, advertising costs, general operating costs, and profits are concerned, reference may be made to the relevant economic textbooks. The **manufacturing costs** must be regarded as specifically product-linked and can be divided into **fixed** and **variable** costs. Even if an individual cost can be considered under various circumstances both as component of the fixed cost or as part of the variable cost, according to whether the cost component is assumed as a long-term one and is written off over a fixed period or whether it is subject to short-term changes. In the following section, for clarity, we shall adhere to a conventional classification of the types of costs.

Fixed Costs

Fixed costs contain expenditure for the acquisition of the **production facilities,** the **buildings** and **utilities,** including installation and start-up, together with general factory and administrative costs. Usually, the management of the **business and of the plant** are included under the fixed costs, and so is a contribution for **safety, insurance, quality control, research costs,** and the **calculated maintenance costs.**

Variable Costs

Variable costs include the cost of **raw materials, fuel, energy, production personnel,** and other **variable services.** These costs differ from plant to plant and are determined by the management. Thus, for example, in the production of a range of fermentation products in one plant, the fixed costs may be apportioned to the profitable products alone, while only the variable costs may be charged to the products that do not yield a profit. In this way, a more flexible and broader production is possible than where everything is equally apportioned. The **capital charge** for the installed production plant is highly dependent on the financial conditions of the company and the site. Although fermentation plants are capital-intensive, service charges on the capital are not the main factor of the manufacturing cost in most bioprocesses. The following analysis therefore deals with the variable costs that are specific to bioprocesses.

18.2.1   Energy

Fermentation processes are carried out at ambient temperatures and pressures in an aqueous medium. These compare favorably with the operational conditions in chemical processes. Furthermore, no corrosive solvents, acids, or alkalis with extreme demands on material are used. In comparison with the agricultural production of natural products, substantially higher yields are achieved. Nevertheless, biotechnological processes also make special demands on the form and consumption of energy.

The primary, even if not the most important in all cases, input of energy in fermentation processes is required for the **mixing** and **maintenance in the mixed state** of all reactants, including the microorganisms, enzymes or fixed systems, in a homogenized multiphase system which, if left to itself, could undergo phase separation. In most fermentations, this requirement is taken care of by **mechanical mixing energy** in combination with aeration of the reaction mixture. In these aerobic processes, air represents the most important substrate, with a correspondingly high compression energy. Therefore, technological improvements in the energy-saving for mixing and compression demand attention.

The second form of energy in biotechnological processes appears in the **recovery** and **isolation** (Chapter 8) of the product. The active ingredient is generally present at low concentration in the aqueous solution. The necessary cost of separation is considerable, regardless of whether it is carried out by mechanical means (centrifugation, filtration, extraction, chromatography) or by thermal means (distillation, drying). In addition to these two areas of energy, there are other process-specific energy requirements:

In many biological processes, **thermal sterilization** of the vessels and media with steam is necessary. In addition to this, higher reaction temperatures are unfavorable in relation to cooling; depending on the process, this may become an item consuming much energy (Table 18-1).

Evaluating the different forms of energy, including indirect energy such as, for example, manual labor and the consumption of energy in the manufacture of the process equipment, has been standardized. This has acquired importance just for biotechnological processes, as compared with competing processes. In the fermentation production of solvents and fuel such as acetone/butanol and ethanol, and also in the production of biogas, the energy input of the production process is compared with the energy content of the product obtained. Here, biological processes are comparable with petrochemical processes. In the production of nutrients, similar comparisons have been made by the energy input of agricultural,

Table 18-1. Consumption of Energy in Biotechnological Processes.

Process step	Process
Micro- and macromixing in fermentation	stirring, pumping, shaking, gassing
Aeration	compression, air separation
Cooling	water and vacuum cooling
Product separation	centrifugation, filtration, chromatography, distillation, drying, extraction, crystallization
Sterilization	steam sterilization, electrical sterilization, sterilization with energy-rich rays

forestry, and fishery products, and here again, biotechnological processes can be validly compared. It can be seen from these examples that the advantages and disadvantages of bio-processes, from the view-point of energy, can hold the balance, but that the principle energy factors are different from those for chemical and agricultural processes.

18.2.2 Fermentation Substrates

Apart from biological waste treatment processes and leaching of ores, **substrate costs** form the most important individual elements of the production cost. Organic carbon compounds are used as substrates and as **sources of biological energy** for maintenance metabolism and nutrient metabolism of the microorganisms used. Nitrogen compounds are sources of nitrogen and minerals, and also in individual cases, growth factors, precursors, and trace elements. In general, the **sources of carbon** make up by far the greatest proportion, both in quantity and cost. Even though fermentation processes based **on hydrocarbons or methanol,** i.e., petrochemical compounds, are known, most bioprocesses use **carbohy-**

drates and **fats** as the main substrates. Consequently, these processes are at least indirectly dependent on the market situation of agricultural products, which is traditionally variable and unstable. **Sugar-** and **starch-containing**

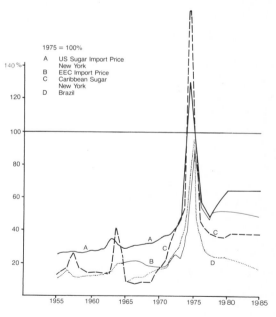

Fig. 18-2. Index of the price of sugar.

raw materials have for long been the most important fermentation substrates in the manufacture of antibiotics, the production of bakers' yeast, the ethanol fermentation, the manufacture of citric acid, and the production of enzymes. Fig. 18-2 shows the change in the price of sugar during 1955 to 1984. The world market price of the raw materials is extraordinarily sensitive to temporary shortages, and price rises by a factor of 2 to 3 are possible. Figures 18-3 and 18-4 show the corresponding changes in the price of molasses and maize.

This price situation is complicated by regional **price characteristics,** since only 2% of the production reaches international markets in the case of sugar and molasses. Most output is consumed nationally and part of it regionally, without the need to sell on open markets. A large part of the balance has already been contracted for at fixed prices before its production. Only the remainder is traded at the so-called world price. Furthermore, in Europe, because of the high threshold price of the EEC for cereals and cereal starch, maize is two to three times dearer than in the USA.

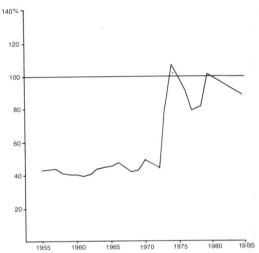

Fig. 18-4. Index of the price of maize.

For the reasons mentioned, many fermentation plants are endeavoring to develop new substrates from agricultural wastes, cellulose or, as already mentioned, from fossil energy sources, which have more stable prices, in order to avoid this dependence on prices. These considerations may lead to locating bioprocess plants in regions with cheap agricultural excesses or with fossil raw materials.

18.2.3 Working Materials

Apart from **electricity, steam,** and **fuel gas** for the production of the necessary mechanical and thermal process energy and compressed air, the only materials required are **process** and **cooling water** of various grades. The direct costs of these, including disposal, are negligi-

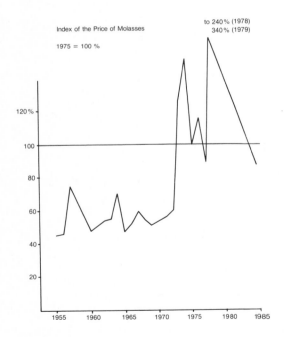

Fig. 18-3. Index of the price of molasses.

ble in comparison with the energy demands and will not therefore be mentioned further.

18.2.4 Environmental Protection

However, fermentation plants produce considerable amounts of gaseous and liquid effluents, some of which require a treatment to inactivate them. This applies to waste gases from fermenters and spray towers, which may sometimes lead to odor problems if they are not treated. In the case of highly active bioproducts such as pharmaceuticals and enzymes, a careful **purification of the waste gases and effluents** is necessary. Since, in general, this involves handling large amounts of medium with a low concentration of material, purification is particularly expensive. In some cases, the active microbial biomass also represents a problem requiring treatment.

Nevertheless, the environmental demands of fermentation plants are different from chemical and agricultural plants. Generally, biological treatment and possibly further use or recycling of the wastes is possible.

18.2.5 Capital Costs

Microbiological transformations in bioprocesses are based on similar process concepts. With small differences in detail, they are similar from process to process and therefore capital costs can be determined as well.

Basically, a fermentation process can be divided into the **preparation of the raw materials,** the **microbiological reaction step,** and the **recovery** and, if necessary, **purification of the products. Auxiliary items** that must be mentioned are: stores for raw materials and products, preparation of energy and working materials, management and staff rooms, maintenance shops, culture preparation laboratories, and the treatment of effluents and wastes. In addition to this classification of technical processes, the construction operations can be divided into plant and equipment, piping, measuring and control technique, electrical equipment, buildings and steel construction, engineering operations, and start up. Each of these individual operations makes an individual contribution to the capital costs; however, in general, the fermenter unit with its specific supply of energy and cooling water and measuring and control equipment coupled to the fermenter usually make up more than half the capital cost. An exception is ethanol, where distillation is roughly twice as capital-intensive as fermentation. This indicates that a purely thermal process stage is more expensive than equipment used for biological processes. On the other hand, for biotechnological processes larger plants are needed in relation to the yield. This fact is due to the use of simple large fermentation vessels and dilute culture media. This is undergoing a change in the new processes where fixed cell systems or immobilized enzymes are used. The bioreactors are smaller and achieve higher space/time yields but are more expensive in construction and in relation to the carrier material for the enzymes.

In view of the wide range of different fermentation processes, in addition to this general introductory discussion of the main cost factors – substrate, energy, capital load – the profitability of biotechnological processes is illustrated based on a few selected examples.

18.3 Examples of Products

18.3.1 Manufacturing Costs for *Penicillin G*

The manufacture of penicillin is divided into the important sterilization of the plant and medium, propagation of the microbial culture, fermentation, and recovery of the product from the culture solution. Since early antibiotic days up to modern processes, a series of improvements that are of economic significance have been developed.

The decisive breakthrough for **large-scale commercial production** was brought about by a **change from surface cultivation to submerged cultivation,** for which strains and nutrients had to be adapted. It was possible to raise the **concentration of products** in the fermented broth from less than 100 mg per liter to more than 25 g/L. This increased the productivity of production plant, shortened fermentation cycles and downtime, additional sterilization of the medium was carried out continuously. **Productivity** affects the capital costs relating to equipment. Furthermore, the yield of product has been increased by due and better appreciation of process conditions including dosed metering of individual substances in combination with an optimized control of temperature and pH and of the stirrer speed and rate of aeration. In view of the high component of the cost represented by substrate, this likewise means a significant saving.

Table 18-2. Capital Costs of a Penicillin Production.

Cost factor	Costs
Equipment of the plant	18%
Steel structure	4%
Insulation	1%
Measuring and control technique	2%
Piping	9%
Electrical installation	12%
Buildings	9%
Working material devices	16%
Land	2%
Laboratories	3%
Spare parts	0.5%
Engineering operations	7%
Installation	5%
Stocks, operating capital, maintenance apparatus, vehicles, management buildings and miscellaneous	9%

For a modern production (Europe, 1984), the individual costs are summarized in Tables 18-2 and 18-3.

Table 18-3. Operating Costs of a Penicillin Production Unit.

Cost factor	Fermentation costs		Recovery costs
Raw materials	46%		3%
Staff	5%		6%
Maintenance	12%		3%
Laboratories		0.3%	
Working materials			
steam	2%		3%
electricity	13%		2%
water		0.3%	
effluent elimination		2%	
Miscellaneous		2%	

In view of the importance of the influence of the **fermentation raw materials,** these are classified further (Table 18-4).

Table 18-4. Costs of Raw Materials.

Raw material	Costs
Glucose	47%
Sodium phenylacetate	40%
Corn steep liquor	4%
Ammonium sulfate	2%
Potassium phosphate	2%
Miscellaneous	5%

The ratio of the fixed and variable costs can be seen from Table 18-5:

Table 18-5. Total Manufacturing Costs.

Type of costs	Fermentation costs	Recovery costs
Variable costs	51%	12%
Fixed costs	21%	5%
Overhead costs		8%

The figures given, which are representative of a series of more expensive fermentation processes, show the main items of the costs and therefore the points of attack for further improvements in profitability.

The sales price for crude penicillin in the Federal Republic of Germany in 1985 was 80 DM/kg, and the variable costs for this area alone are given as 50 DM/kg. The bulk of production is, however, marketed not as crude material but in the form of finished drugs, for which the price is 140 to 160 DM/kg. This commercial form represents higher added value and improved profit margins are achieved which are not primarily related to material and energy costs but include considerable proportion of costs for quality control, advertising, packaging, and sales operations.

18.3.2 Manufacturing Costs for Penicillin Amidase

Penicillin amidase has been selected as an example of the **manufacture of an enzyme.** This enzyme catalyzes the splitting off of the side chain of penicillin to form 6-aminopenicillanic acid (6-APA), the starting material for a series of semisynthetic antibiotics. It is obtained as an exoenzyme by aerobic fermentation from cultivated mutants of the bacterium *Escherichia coli* with the addition of the inductor phenylacetic acid. Table 18-6 contains the variable costs of the production of the enzyme for a 10 m^3 fermenter.

Table 18-6. Variable Costs of the Production of Penicillin Amidase (1985; 10 m^3 reactor, for yield see text).

Cost factor	Costs
Fermentation and extraction	800 DM
Labor	2800 DM
Services	455 DM
	4075 DM

The yield of a 10 m^3 reactor would permit the production of 410 kg of penicillin G. The variable costs are therefore given by the cost of 1.65 kg penicillin G at DM 130 plus the enzymatic transformation, 16 DM, thus making DM 146. The corresponding market price of 6-APA is 165 DM/kg (1985).

18.3.3 Manufacturing Costs of Citric Acid

Citric acid by fermentation has replaced citric acid extracted from citrus fruit. In the aerobic batch fermentation of *Aspergillus niger,* apart from mineral substances carefully metered in, various forms of molasses can be used as the main substrate. The pH- and temperature-controlled fermentation lasts about five days, and the labor costs are minimized by computer control. The critical cost factors in the manufacture of citric acid are therefore the main substrate, the consumption of energy, including cooling, and the capital costs in relation to the low space/time yields.

Technically, about 800 kg of citric acid can be obtained from a ton of sugar. The variable costs of a batch fermentation process are given in Table 18-7.

From one batch is obtained 9 tons of citric acid, corresponding to variable costs of about 2.20 DM/kg. The sales price for citric acid (Federal Republic of Germany, 1985) is about 3.50 DM/kg.

Table 18-7. Variable Costs of the Manufacture of Citric Acid (Figures for a 9-ton batch, 1985).

Cost factor	Costs	
Raw materials		
molasses	6 500 DM	
others	1 280 DM	24%
extraction	1 450 DM	7%
Total raw materials	9 230 DM	40%
Services and working materials	11 400 DM	50%
Labor	2 000 DM	10%

18.3.4 Manufacturing Costs of Fuel Alcohol

In addition to the traditional beverage alcohol industry, in some regions of the globe the manufacture of **industrial alcohol** by fermentation from agrarian raw materials and wastes has successfully competed against the synthetic production of ethanol from ethylene, particularly where the appropriate raw materials are available cheaply and in large

Table 18-8. Manufacturing Costs for Industrial Ethanol (Brazil, 1979).

Cost factor	Basis			
	Cassava		Sugar cane	
Investments	17 M US-$		15.5 M US-$	
Main substrate	228 $/m³	60%	204 $/m³	57%
Enzymes, chemicals, working materials	60 $/m³	16%	6 $/m³	4%
Staff	13 $/m³	3%	15 $/m³	4%
Maintenance, insurance, management	18 $/m³	5%	25 $/m³	7%
Taxes	15 $/m³	4%	24 $/m³	7%
Depreciation	32 $/m³	8%	49 $/m³	14%
Net proceeds	29 $/m³	8%	50 $/m³	14%
Determined sales price fob	379 $/m³	100%	358 $/m³	100%

amounts, while petrochemical substrates have to be imported. An example of an aerobic process for the manufacture of a basic chemical is given in Table 18-8, summarizing the manufacturing costs of a conventional ethanol fermentation for Brazil (1979).

Table 18-9 gives a statement of the expenditure of energy in ethanol fermentation (based on crude sugar juice from beets) for an energy-optimized continuous ethanol process in Europe:

Table 18-9. Consumption of Energy in the Manufacture of Ethanol.

Process step	Energy (kWh/L of ethanol)
Cultivation of the raw material	2
Transport of the raw material	1
Preparation of the raw material	1
Fermentation	–
Distillation	1
Treatment of effluent (utilization of biogas)	– 1
Calorific value of the ethanol	8.5

It can be seen that even under the unfavorable European conditions, where there is no utilization of bagasse for the production of energy, analysis of the energy utilization shows that a significant net gain in energy can be achieved by careful management. This becomes important when it is borne in mind that the energy input may convert domestic solid fuel (coal) to a high-value liquid fuel.

18.3.5 Manufacturing Costs of Bioprotein from Methanol

The production of microbial biomass from synthetic organic chemicals, particularly methanol, for use as feed and in specified form as food ingredient, has achieved importance. A percentage distribution of manufacturing costs is shown in Table 18-10 (plant capacity 100000 tons/a):

Table 18-10. Cost Factors in the Manufacture of Bioprotein from Ethanol.

Cost factor	Costs
Energy	17%
Personnel, maintenance, general costs	9%
Capital load	28%
Material costs	46%
including methanol	35%
ammonia	4%
phosphoric acid	5%

This process is an example of a capital-intensive large-scale process with non-agriculture raw material. Depending on the site conditions and the price situation for raw materials, the methanol component may vary between about 25 and 50%.

18.4 Economic Data for Various Manufacturers and Product Capacities of Bioproducts

For a better understanding of the market potential of various fermentation products, below we list companies and production capacities in several tables (Tables 18-11 to 18-16).

Table 18-11. West European Antibiotics Manufacturers (1985).

Firm	Country	Type
Fermenta/ Pierrel/ISF	Sweden, Italy	P, T, O
Biochemie	Austria	P
RIT (SKF)	Belgium	O
Novo	Denmark	P
Rhône-Poulenc	France	P, O
Roussel-Uclaf	France	T, O
Bayer	Germany	P, O
Hoechst	Germany	P, T, O
Dow	Italy	T
Ciba-Geigy	Italy	O
Cyanamid	Italy/United Kingdom	T, O
Farmitalia/Lark	Italy	T, O
Pierrel	Italy	O
Proter	Italy/Ireland	T, O
SPA	Italy	T
Squibb	Italy	P, O
Gist Brocades	Netherlands, Portugal	P
Apothekernes	Norway	O
CIPAN	Portugal	T, O
Antibioticos	Spain	P, O
Cepa	Spain	O
Beecham	United Kingdom	P
Lilly	United Kingdom	O
Glaxo	United Kingdom	P, T, O
Pfizer	United Kingdom/ France/Spain	T, O

P = penicillin
T = tetracycline
O = other antibiotics

Table 18-12. Manufacturers of Organic Acids in Western Europe (1985).

Firm	Country	Acid
Jungbunzlauer	Austria	C
Citrique Belge	Belgium	C
Finnish Sugar	Finland	G
Lesaffre	France	C
Rhône-Poulenc	France	I, L
Roquette	France	G
Benckiser	Germany	C, G
Biacor	Italy	C
Akzo	Netherlands	G
Chemie Combinatie	Netherlands	L
Ayuso	Spain	L
Ebro	Spain	C
Sika	Switzerland	G
Croda	United Kingdom	L
Pfizer	United Kingdom/ Ireland	C, G, I
Sturge	United Kingdom	C

C = citric acid; G = gluconic acid; I = itaconic acid; L = lactic acid.

Table 18-13. Manufacturers of Enzymes in Western Europe.

Firm	Country
Category A – Bulk products:	
– Grinstet	Denmark
– Novo	Denmark/Switzerland
– Miles-Kali	Germany
– Röhm	Germany
– Gist Brocades	Netherlands/France
– ABM	United Kingdom
– Glaxo	United Kingdom
Category B – Specialities:	
– Boehringer Mannheim	Germany
– E. Merck	Germany
– Genzyme	United Kingdom

Table 18-14. Amino Acid Manufacturers in Western Europe (1985).

Firm	Country	Type
Eurolysine/Orsan	France	L & MSG
Carvazerre	Italy	MSG
Peniberica	Spain	MSG

MSG = monosodium glutamate; L = lysine.

Table 18-15. Manufacturers of Other Fermentation Products in Western Europe (1985).

Firm	Country	Product
Fromageries Bel	France	SCP
Rhône-Poulenc	France	B_{12}, X
Roussel-Uclaf	France	B_{12}
Farmitalia	Italy	E
Poli	Italy	E
Attisholz	Switzerland	SCP
Biochemie	Austria	E
Fisons	United Kingdom	D
Glaxo	United Kingdom	B_{12}
ICI	United Kingdom	SCP
Pfeifer & Langen	Germany	D

B_{12} = vitamin B_{12}; D = dextran; E = ergot alkaloid; G = gibberellic acid; SCP = single cell protein; X = xanthan gum.

Table 18-16. Amounts of Fermentation Products (1985).

Category of fermentation product	Western Europe, tons	World, tons
Antibiotics		
(human + veterinary)		
Penicillin	6000 – 7000	10000
Tetracycline	2000 – 3000	3000 – 4000
Other antibiotics	1500 – 2000	4000 – 5000
Organic acids		
Citric acid	140000–150000	350000
Gluconic acid		
Itaconic acid	30000 – 40000	50000 – 60000
Lactic acid		
Miscellaneous products		
Vitamin B_{12}	5	10
Ergot alkaloids	10	10
SCP	50000–100000	300000–400000
Dextrans	1000	2000
Xanthan gum	4000	15000
Amino acids	60000	270000

Appendix

Appendix I
Journals, Periodicals, Reviews

Acta Biochemica et Biophysica,
Hungary.

Acta Microbiologica,
Hungary.

Acta Microbiologica Polonica,
Poland.

Acta Microbiologica Sinica,
People's Republic of China.

Advances in Applied Microbiology,
USA.

Advances in Biochemical Engineering,
Federal Republic of Germany.

Agricultural and Biological Chemistry Journal,
Japan.

American Society for Microbiology News,
USA.

Angewandte Chemie,
Federal Republic of Germany.

Annales de Microbiologie,
France.

Annual Reports on Fermentation Processes,
USA.

Antibiotics and Chemotherapy,
USA.

Antimicrobial Agents and Chemotherapy,
USA.

Antonie van Leeuwenhoek Journal of Microbiology and Serology,
The Netherlands.

Applied and Environmental Microbiology,
USA.

Applied Biochemistry and Microbiology,
USA.

Applied Microbiology,
USA.

Archiv für Genetik,
Switzerland.

Archiv für Mikrobiologie,
Federal Republic of Germany.

Ascatopics,
USA.

ATCC-Quarterly Newsletter,
USA.

Bacteriological Reviews,
USA.

Biochemische Zeitschrift,
Federal Republic of Germany.

Biochimica et Biophysica Acta,
The Netherlands.

Biologie in unserer Zeit,
Federal Republic of Germany.

Biotechnology,
United Kingdom.

Biotechnology and Bioengineering,
USA.

Biotechnology Letters,
United Kingdom.

Biotechnology Newswatch,
USA.

Brauwelt,
Federal Republic of Germany.

Canadian Journal of Genetics and Cytology/
Journal Canadien de Genétique et de Cytologie,
Canada.

Canadian Journal of Microbiology,
Canada.

Central Patents Index,
United Kingdom.

Chemical Engineering,
USA.

Chemical Engineering Science,
USA.

Chemie Ingenieur Technik,
Federal Republic of Germany.

Chemie, Technik,
Federal Republic of Germany.

CRC – Critical Reviews in Biochemistry,
USA.

CRC – Critical Reviews in Food Technology,
USA.

CRC – Critical Reviews in Microbiology,
USA.

Current Genetics,
Federal Republic of Germany.

Current Microbiology,
USA.

Dechema-Monographie: Biotechnologie,
Federal Republic of Germany.

Derwent Biotechnology Abstracts,
United Kingdom.

Die Pharmazie,
German Democratic Republic.

Enzyme and Microbial Technology,
United Kingdom.

Enzyme Technology Digest,
USA.

European Chemical News,
United Kingdom.

European Journal of Applied Microbiology,
USA.

European Journal of Applied Microbiology
and Biotechnology,
Federal Republic of Germany.

FEMS Microbiology Letters,
USA.

Fermentation Research Institute Report,
Japan.

Fleischwirtschaft,
Federal Republic of Germany.

Folia Microbiologica,
United Kingdom.

Forum Mikrobiologie,
Federal Republic of Germany.

Food Technology,
USA.

Genetics,
USA.

Genetic Technology, News,
USA.

Giornale di Microbiologia,
Italy.

Immunological Communications,
USA.

Immunology,
United Kingdom.

Indian Journal of Microbiology,
India.

Indian Journal of Mycology and Plant Patho-
logy,
India.

Interdisciplinary Science Reviews,
United Kingdom.

International Journal of Biochemistry,
United Kingdom.

International Journal of Systematic Bacteriology,
USA.

Japanese Journal of Microbiology,
Japan.

Journal of Agriculture and Food Chemistry,
USA.

Journal of Antibiotics,
Japan.

Journal of Applied Bacteriology,
United Kingdom.

Journal of Applied Biochemistry,
USA.

Journal of Applied Chemistry and Biotechnology,
United Kingdom.

Journal of Bacteriology,
USA.

Journal of Carbohydrates-Nucleosides-
Nucleotides,
USA.

Journal of Chemical Technology and
Biotechnology,
United Kingdom.

Journal of Chromatography,
The Netherlands.

Journal of Chromatography Biomedical
Applications,
The Netherlands.

Journal of Fermentation Technology,
Japan.

Journal of General and Applied
Microbiology,
Japan.

Journal of Microbiological Methods,
The Netherlands.

Journal of General Microbiology,
United Kingdom.

Journal of the American Chemical Society,
USA.

Microbiologica,
Italy.

Microbiological Reviews,
USA.

Microbiology,
USSR.

Microbiology Abstracts Section B.
Bacteriology,
USA.

Microbiology and Immunology,
Japan.

Mikrokosmos,
Federal Republic of Germany.

Nature,
United Kingdom.

Naturwissenschaften,
Federal Republic of Germany.

Naturwissenschaftliche Rundschau,
Federal Republic of Germany.

Pharmazie in unserer Zeit,
Federal Republic of Germany.

Process Biochemistry,
United Kingdom.

Ringdoc Literature Documentation,
United Kingdom.

Science,
USA.

Spektrum der Wissenschaft,
Federal Republic of Germany.

Swiss Chemical Industry,
Switzerland.

Tetrahedron Letters,
United Kingdom.

Trends in Biochemical Science,
The Netherlands.

Trends in Biotechnology,
The Netherlands.

Umschau in Wissenschaft und Technik,
Federal Republic of Germany.

Verfahrenstechnik,
Federal Republic of Germany.

VDI-Nachrichten,
Federal Republic of Germany.

Zentralblatt für Bakteriologie, Parasiten-
kunde, Infektionskrankheiten und Hygiene,
Federal Republic of Germany.

Zeitschrift für Allgemeine Mikrobiologie,
Federal Republic of Germany.

Zeitschrift für Naturforschung, Ausgabe C:
Biosciences,
Federal Republic of Germany.

Appendix II

Biotechnological Abbreviations, Formulas, and Symbols

Biotechnology, as an interdisciplinary barrier, makes use of technical terms, basic units, formulas, and abbreviations from various fields, so that it is impossible, especially in the case of abbreviations and symbols, to use unitary terms.

The following collection therefore contains a list of the most common terms arranged according to their fields of application. They have been compiled with the aim and hope of promoting understanding and dialogue in the developing field of biotechnology and hence of being of general use for biotechnologists.

A II.1   Fermentation Terms

Term	Abbreviation	Unit
Amount of inoculum	*IO*	%, L
Biological oxygen demand	*BOD*$_5$	$gO_2 \cdot (L \cdot 5d)^{-1}$ (specific consumption of oxygen in 5 days)
Biomass	*X*	$g \cdot L^{-1}$
Bubble diameter (gas)	d_B	mm
Cell concentration	*X*	$g \cdot L^{-1}$
Cell multiplication rate	v	h^{-1}
Cell weight, dry	DW	$g \cdot L^{-1}$
Chemical oxygen demand	*COD*	$gO_2 \cdot L^{-1}$
Concentration of carbon dioxide in the waste gas	$CO_2\uparrow$	vol.%
Concentration of oxygen	c_{O_2}	
– in the culture solution	$\bar{c}_{O_2}$	$mg \cdot L^{-1}$
– in the waste gas	$O_2\uparrow$	vol.%
– of saturation	$c^*_{O_2}$	$mg \cdot L^{-1}$
Concentration of product	c_{PR}	$g \cdot L^{-1}$
Concentration of substrate		
– in the feed of medium	S_o	$g \cdot L^{-1}$
– in the fermenter	*S*	$g \cdot L^{-1}$
Conversion	*U*	%
Critical dilution rate (wash out)	D_{crit}	h^{-1}
Cycle time	t_c	s
Dextrose equivalent	*DE*	% molar reduction equivalents in the substrate referred to glucose $= 100$
Dilution rate (F/V)	*D*	h^{-1}
Doubling time	t_D	h

Term	Abbreviation	Unit
Flow rate of the medium	F	$L \cdot h^{-1}$
Maintenance coefficient	m	g/g of substrate converted per dry biomass per hour during maintenance metabolism only
Maximum growth rate	μ_{max}	h^{-1}
Michaelis-Menten constant	K_m	$g \cdot L^{-1}$
Microorganisms	MO	—
Monod constant	K_m, K_s	$g \cdot L^{-1}$
Mortality constant	K_d	s^{-1}, h^{-1}
Oxygen transfer rate	OTR	$mmol \cdot L^{-1} \cdot h^{-1}$
Oxygen uptake	Q_{O_2}	$mmol \cdot L^{-1}$
Oxygen uptake rate	OUR	$mmol \cdot L^{-1} \cdot h^{-1}$
Partial pressure (gas)	p	mbar
Partial pressure of carbon dioxide	p_{CO_2}	mbar
Partial pressure of oxygen	p_{O_2}	mbar
P/O ratio	P/O	$\dfrac{\text{mol of esterified phosphate}}{\text{mol of oxygen converted}}$
Production of carbon dioxide	Q_{CO_2}	$mol \cdot L^{-1}$
Productivity	PR	$g \cdot L^{-1} \cdot h^{-1}$
Rate of gassing	Q_G	$m^3 \cdot m^{-3} \cdot h^{-1}$ (volumes of gas throughput per volume of liquid per minute)
Redox potential	E_h	mV
Reflux rate	F_R	$L \cdot h^{-1}$
Respiratory coefficient	RQ	$\dfrac{\text{mol } CO_2}{\text{mol } O_2}$
Saturation constant	K_s	$g \cdot L^{-1}$
Total carbon content	TC	%
Total inorganic carbon content	TIC	%
Total organic carbon content	TOC	%
Yield factors		
– referred to the substrate	YX/S	$\dfrac{\text{g dry biomass formed}}{\text{g substrate converted}}$
– referred to ATP	Y_{ATP}	$\dfrac{\text{g dry biomass formed}}{\text{mol ATP converted}}$
– referred to oxygen	Y_0	$\dfrac{\text{g dry biomass formed}}{\text{mol of oxygen consumed}}$
– referred to substrate electrons	Y_{ave-}	$\dfrac{\text{g dry biomass formed}}{\text{number reactive substrate electrons}}$

A II.2   Biotechnological Formulas

Rate of growth (Monod equation):

$$\mu = \frac{1}{X}\frac{dX}{dt} = \frac{\mu_{max} S}{K_s + S}$$

Oxygen transfer rate:

$$OTR = k_L \cdot a (c_{O_2}^* - \bar{c}_{O_2})$$

Doubling time:

$$t_D = \frac{\ln 2}{\mu}$$

Productivity:

$$PR = D \cdot X = \frac{dX}{dt}$$

Reaction rate (Michaelis-Menten equation):

$$v = \frac{v_{max} S}{K_m + S}$$

Respiratory quotient:

$$RQ = \frac{mol\, CO_2\, produced}{mol\, O_2\, consumed}$$

A II.3   Biochemical Compounds and Abbreviations

Abbreviation	Name
A	Adenosine, a nucleoside, a constituent of nucleic acids
AA	Amino acids
ADH	Alcohol dehydrogenase, oxidizes alcohol to aldehyde
Acetyl-CoA	Acetyl(coenzyme A), coenzyme that activates acetyl groups for transfers
Ala	Amino acid alanine
Arg	Amino acid arginine
Asp	Amino acid aspartic acid
ATP	Adenosine 5'-triphosphate, energy-rich mononucleotide
C	Cytidine, a nucleoside, a constituent of nucleic acids
Cys	Amino acid cysteine (comprising a SH group)
DNAs	Deoxyribonucleic acids
dRib	Deoxyribose, a pentose sugar
EC	Enzyme Commission
FAD	Flavine adenine dinucleotide
FMN	Flavine mononucleotide (riboflavine 5'-phosphate)
Fru	Fructose, a hexose sugar
G	Guanosine, a nucleoside, a constituent of nucleic acids
Gal	Galactose, a hexose sugar
Glc	Glucose, a hexose sugar
GlcN	Glucosamine, a constituent of bacterial cell walls
GlcNAc	N-Acetylglucosamine, a constituent of bacterial cell walls
GlcUA	Gluconic acid, a constituent of bacterial cell walls

Glu	Amino acid glutamic acid
Gly	Amino acid glycine
Hb	Hemoglobin, an oxygen-binding blood pigment
HbO_2	Oxyhemoglobin, an oxygen-bound blood pigment
His	Amino acid histidine
I	Inosine, a nucleoside that arises on the deamination of adenosine
Ile	Amino acid isoleucine
kat	katal, international unit of enzyme activity
Leu	Amino acid leucine
Lys	Amino acid lysine
Man	Mannose, a hexose sugar
Met	Amino acid methionine, containing sulfur
MNAc	N-Acetylmuramic acid, carbohydrate, a cell wall constituent
NAD	Nicotinamide adenine dinucleotide, oxidized form
NADP	Nicotinamide adenine dinucleotide phosphate, oxidized form
Phe	Amino acid phenylalanine
Pro	Amino acid proline
Rib	Pentose sugar ribose, a constituent of RNA
RNAs	Ribonucleic acids, polynucleotides as sequence transmitters in the biosynthesis of proteins
mRNAs	Messenger RNAs, transfer the genetic code from DNAs to the site of protein biosynthesis
tRNAs	Transfer RNAs with specific binding for individual amino acids, activate and transfer one amino acid in each case to the site of protein biosynthesis
S	Substrate
Ser	Amino acid serine
T	Thymidine, a nucleoside, a constituent of nucleic acids
U	Uridine, a nucleoside, constituent of nucleic acids
Val	Amino acid valine

A II.4 Genetic Engineering Terms (according to Gassen, Kontakte 1/81)

Clones:	Identical daughter cell derived from a single mother cell by multiplication
DNA ligases:	Enzymes which bind DNA fragments together
Insertion:	Incorporation of a newly synthesized or isolated short DNA sequence into a plasmid or chromosome
Introns:	Sequences in DNAs which are in fact transcribed into mRNAs but are subsequently split out and therefore form no permanent constituents of the mRNAs (only in eucaryotes)
Ligation:	Direct linkage of nucleic acid fragments
Operator:	Regulatory section in a nucleic acid with binding capacity for a repressor protein for blocking the synthesis of mRNAs

Plasmid:	Annular nucleic acid in cells outside the central chromosome with a lower molecular weight than the central chromosome; bearer of nonessential additional information, e.g., sex factors (F factors) and resistance factors (R factors)
	Plasmids and viral nucleic acids with known functions such as resistance or sequences are denoted by trivial abbreviations derived from their function or origin, e.g., SV 40 for simian virus, pBR322 for a plasmid imparting resistance to antibiotics
Promotor:	Regulatory section in a nucleic acid with the capacity for binding RNA polymerase
Repressor:	Regulatory protein with binding capacity for operators
Restriction endonucleases:	Enzymes which specifically cleave DNAs at a definite information-bearing sequence of nucleotides and thereby permit an insertion of foreign sequences.
	Restriction endonucleases are named in genetic engineering by trivial abbreviations that are derived from the name of the originating cell, e.g., EcoRI from *Escherichia coli* RY13, HindII from *Haemophilus influenza,* HpaII from *Haemophilus parainfluenza,* or PstI from *Providencia stuartii*
Transduction:	Introduction of foreign genetic material into a cell by means of a virus or, in the case of bacteria, by means of phages
Transformation:	Uptake of free nucleic acids or plasmids into a cell
Transcription:	Conversion of a DNA (gene) information sequence into a mRNA sequence
Translation:	Synthesis of proteins on mRNAs
Vector:	Plasmid or virus that after ligation with a foreign DNA is used to introduce new information into the cell.

A II.5   Selection of Antibiotics (Names and Formulas)

(These antibiotics are described in more detail in Chapter 13)

I Chloramphenicol   II Griseofulvin   III Chlortetracycline

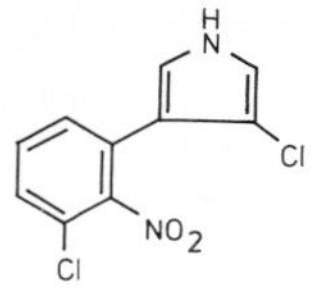

IV Pyrrolnitrin

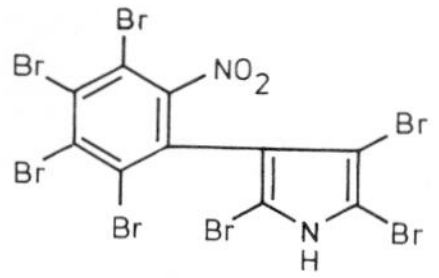

IX Borrelidin

XIII Isonitrin A

V Bromonitrin

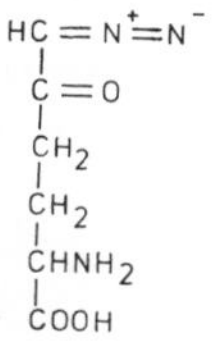

X Toyocamycin

XIV Ferrioxamine B

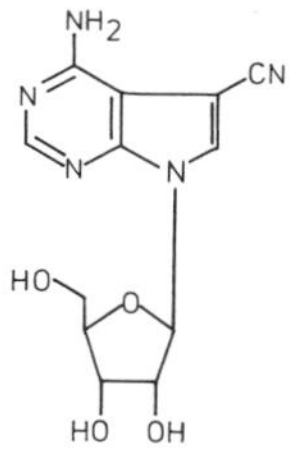

VI DON

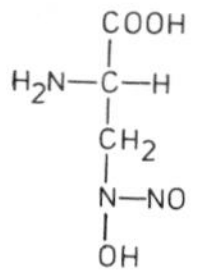

XI Alanosine

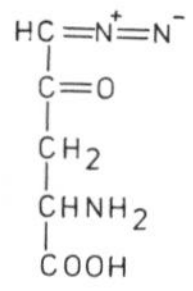

VII Azaserine

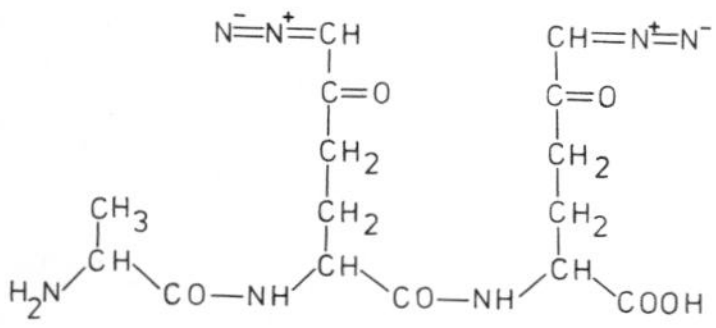

VIII Alazopeptin

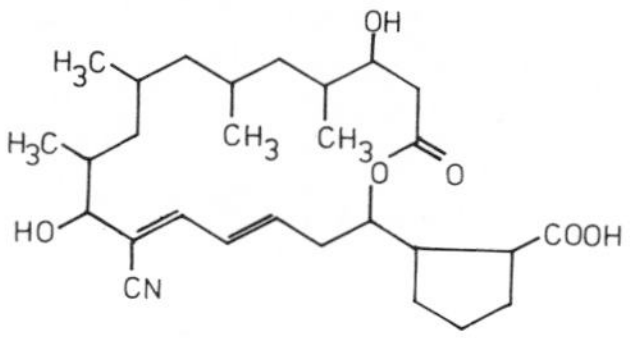

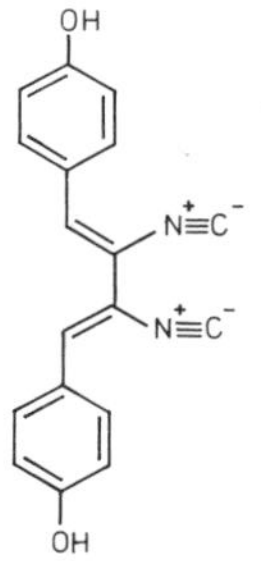

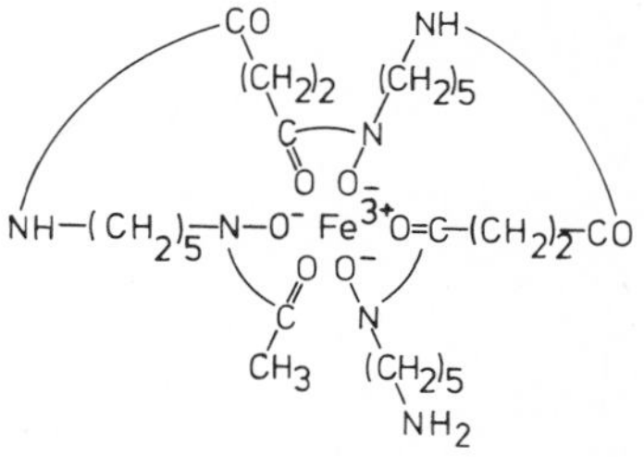

XII Xanthocillin

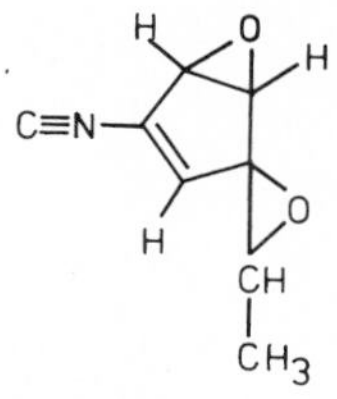

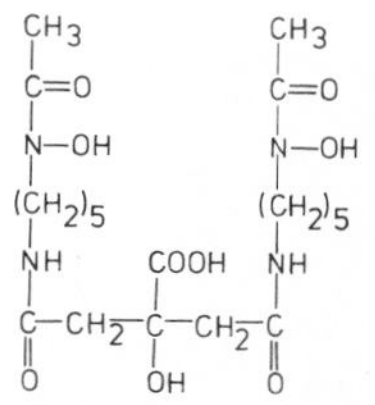

XV Arthrobactin

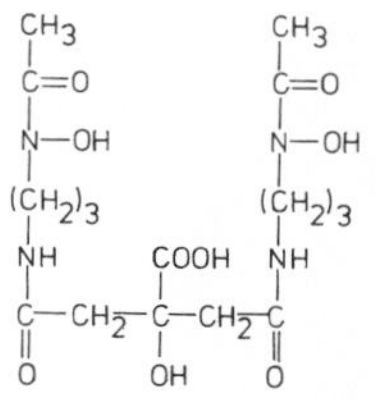

XVI Schizokinen

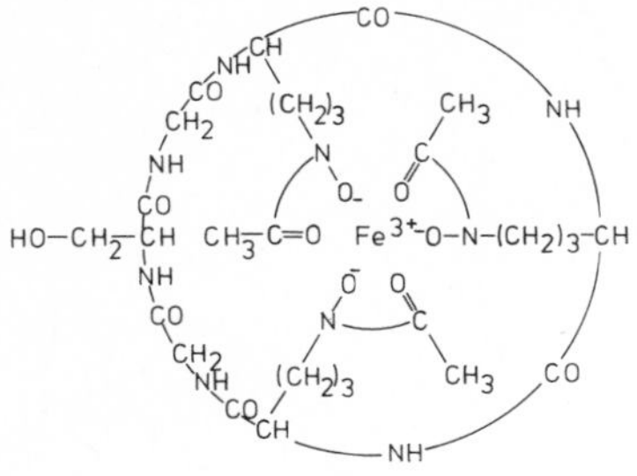

XVII Ferricrocin

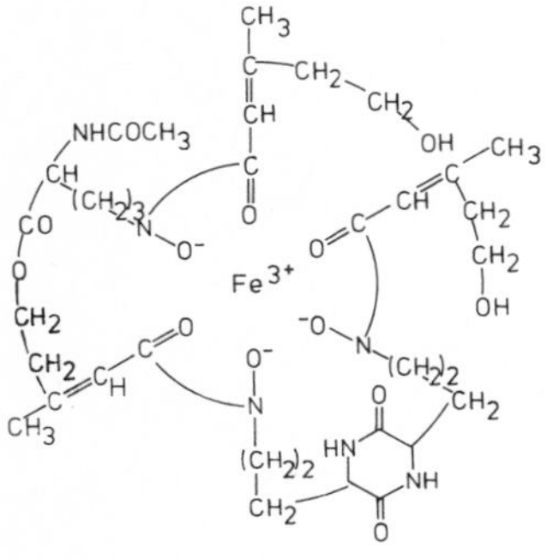

XVIII Coprogen

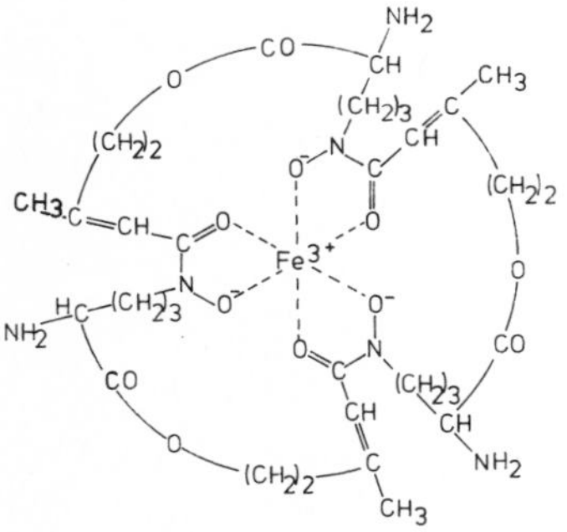

XIX Fusigen

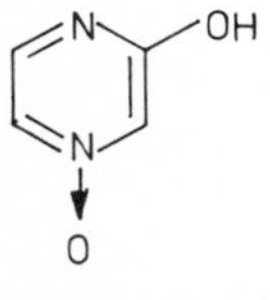

XX Emimycin

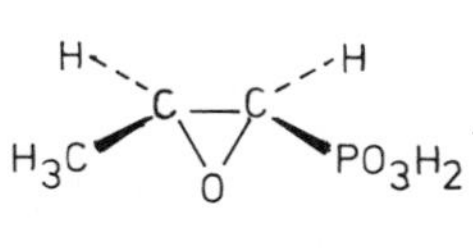

XXI Phosphonomycin

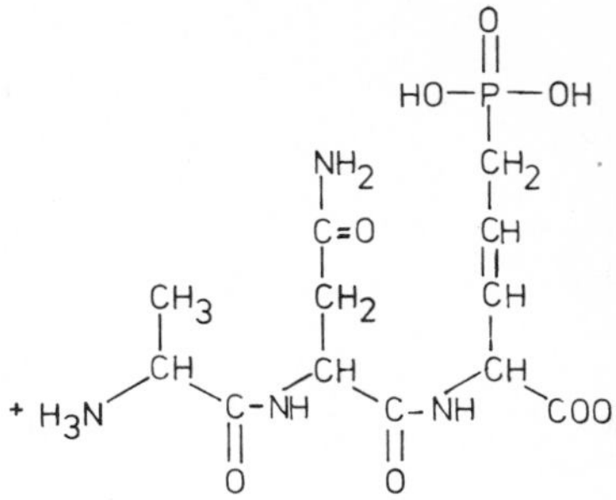

XXII Plumbemycin B

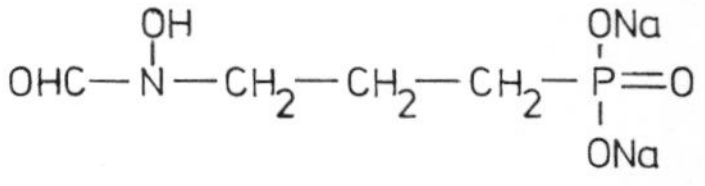

XXIII FiR 31564

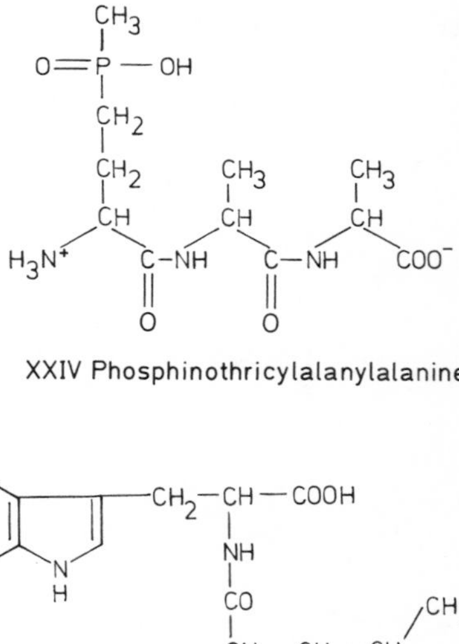

XXIV Phosphinothricylalanylalanine

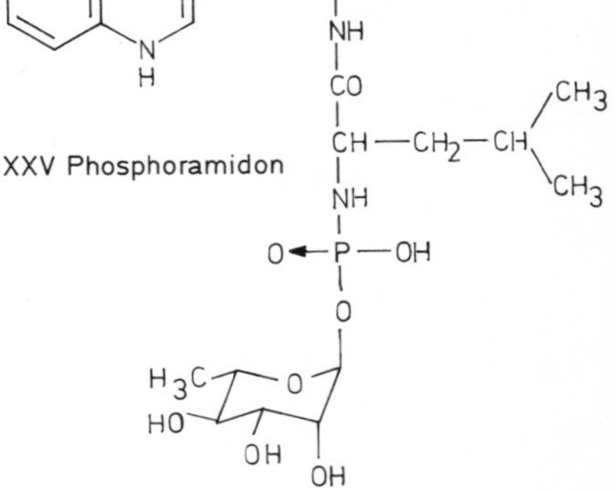

XXV Phosphoramidon

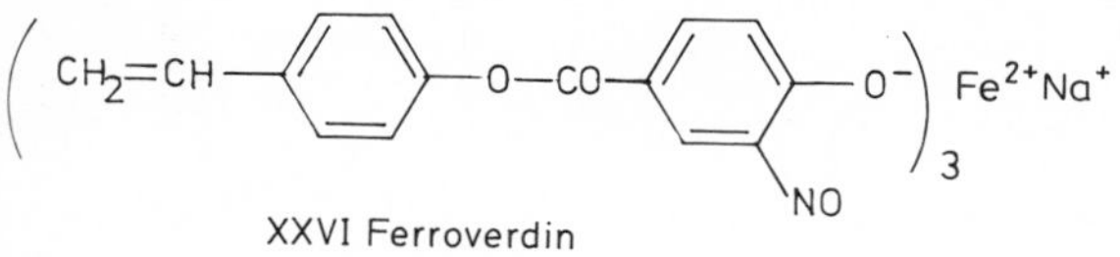

XXVI Ferroverdin

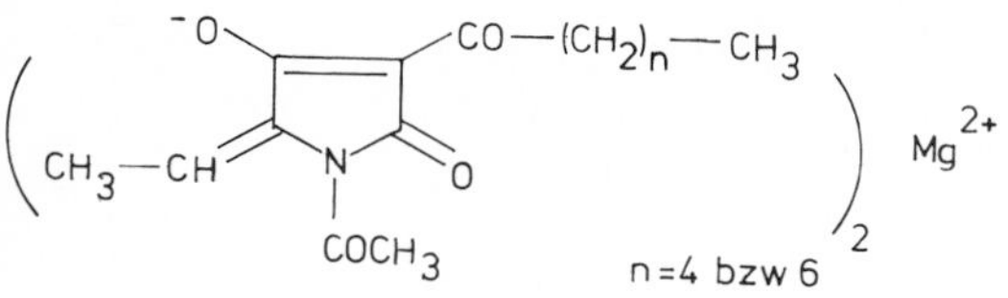

XXVII Magnesidin

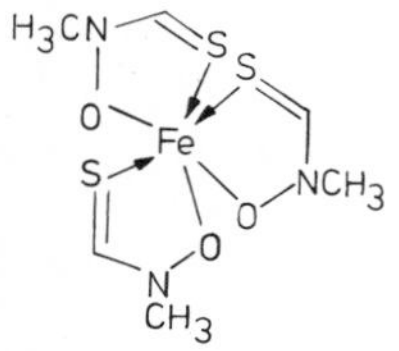

XXVIIIa Fluopsin B

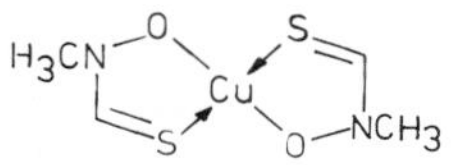

XXVIIIb Fluopsin C

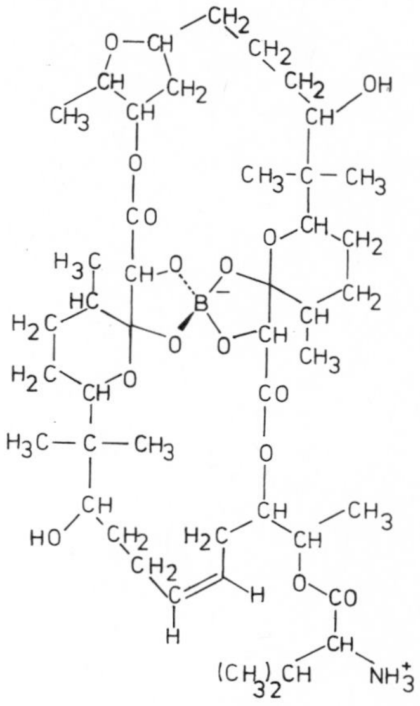

XXX Boromycin

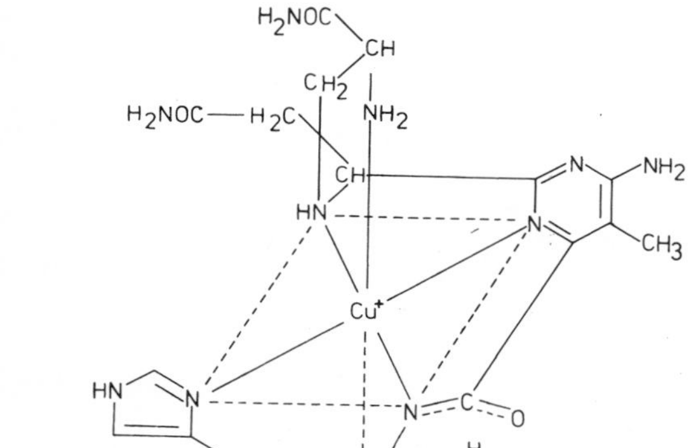

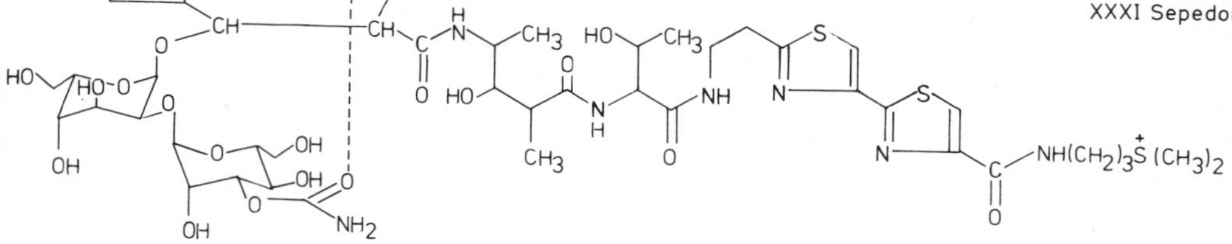

XXIX Bleomycin

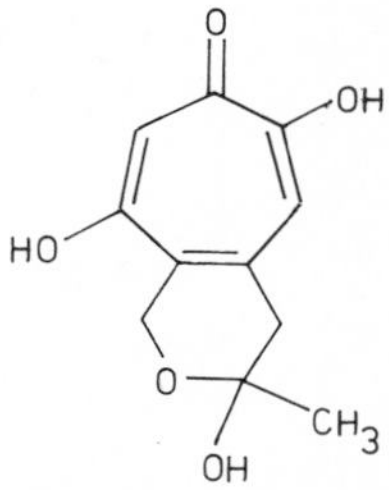

XXXI Sepedonin

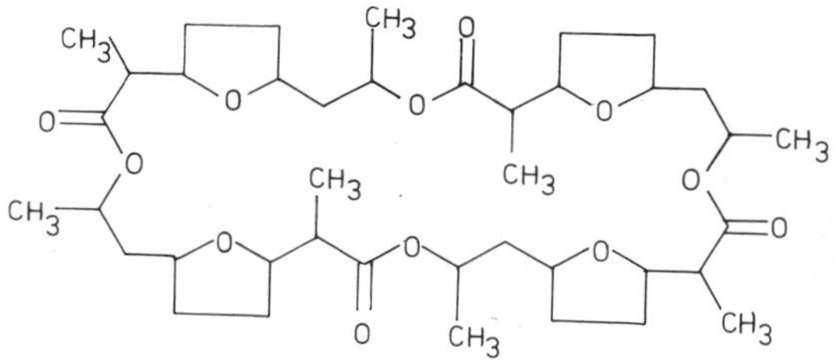

XXXII Nonactin

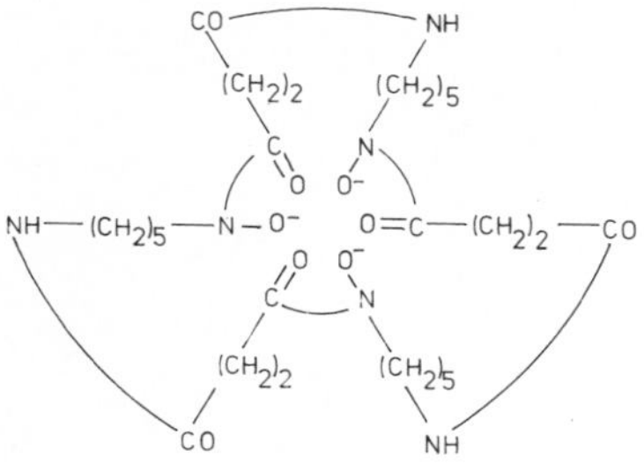

XXXIII Nocardamin

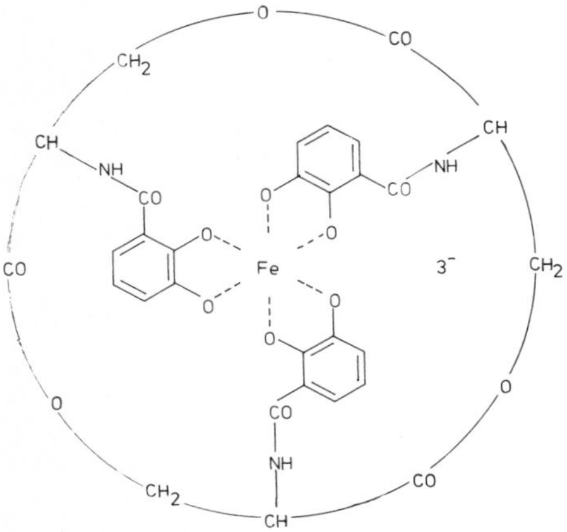

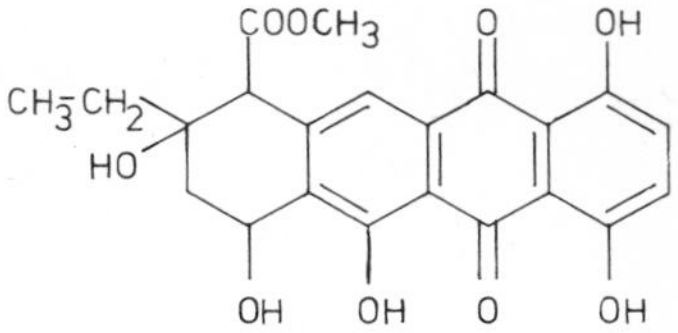

XXXVII Pyrromycinone

XXXIV Fe³⁺ Enterochelin

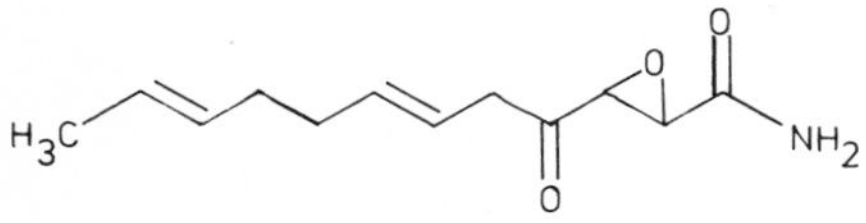

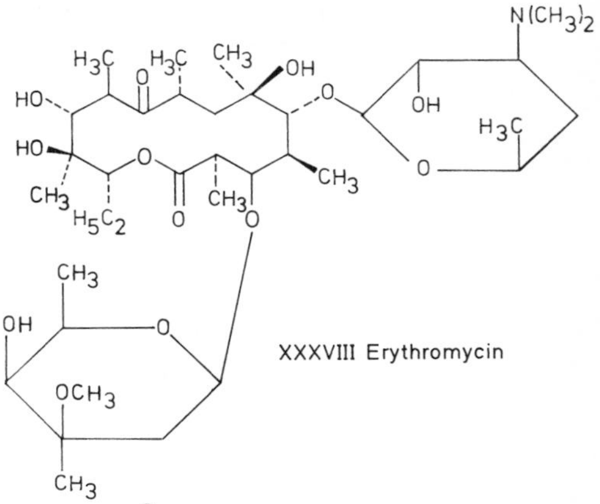

XXXVIII Erythromycin

XXXV Cerulenin

XXXIX Geldanamycin

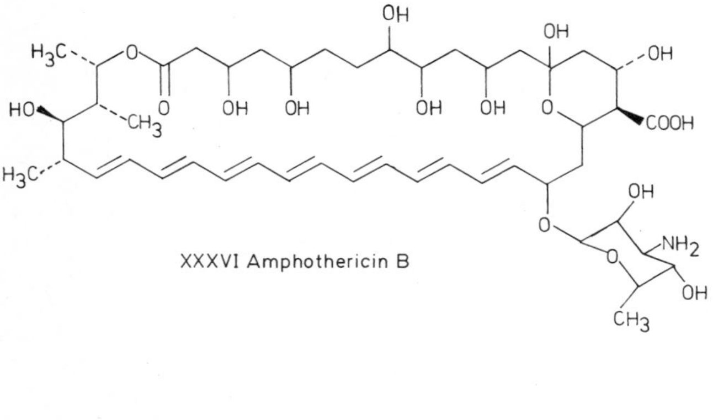

XXXVI Amphothericin B

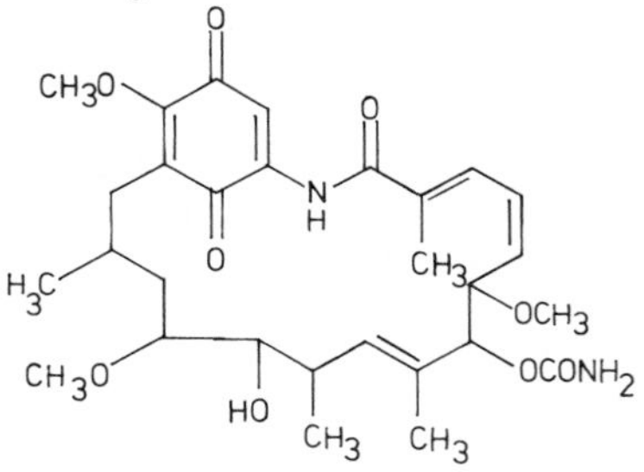

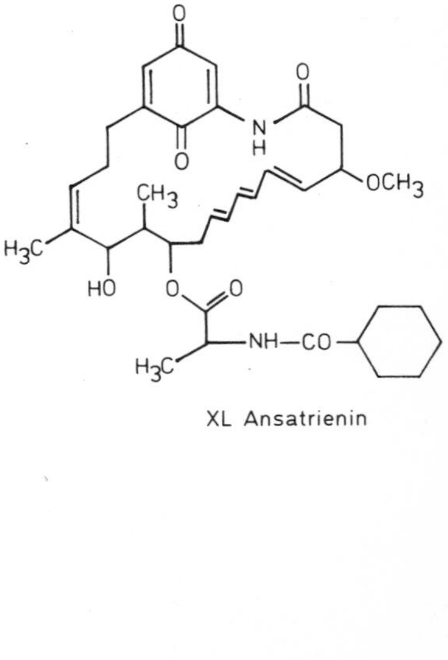

XL Ansatrienin

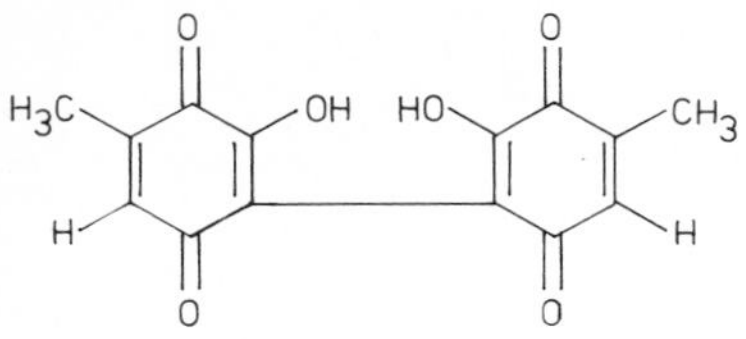

XLI Phoenicin

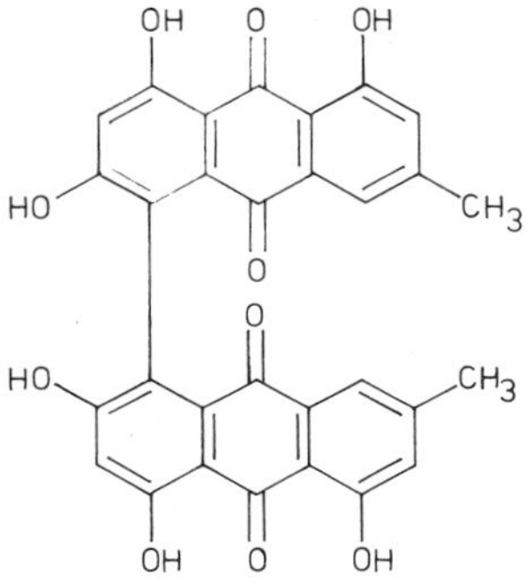

XLII Skyrin

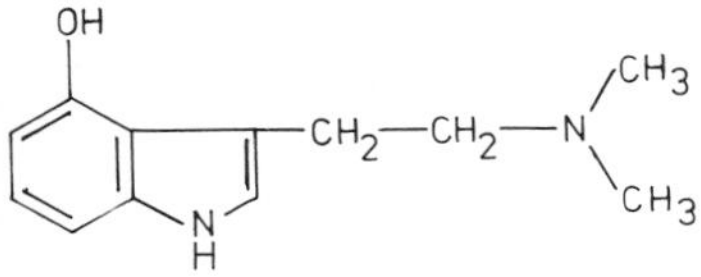

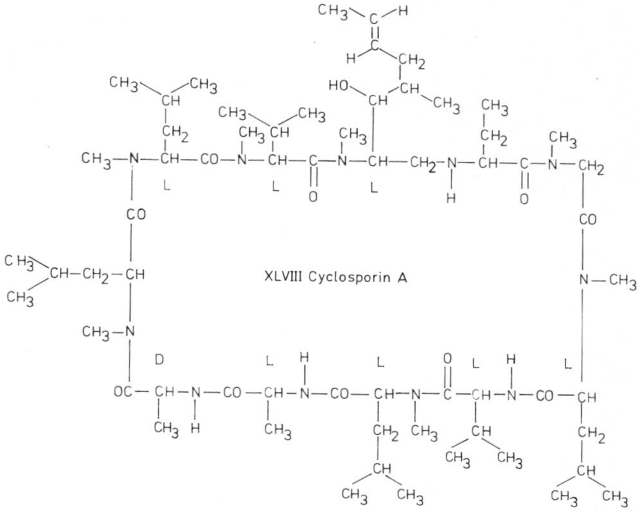

XLVIII Cyclosporin A

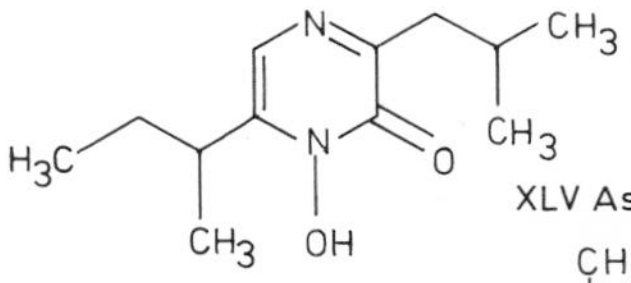

XLV Aspergillic acid

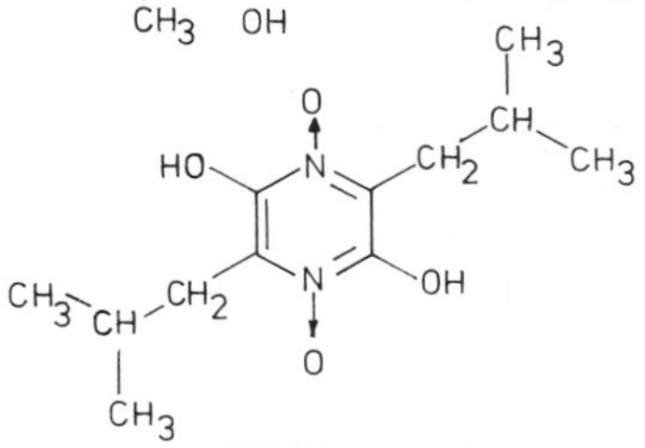

XLVI Pulcherriminic acid

XLIII Psilocine

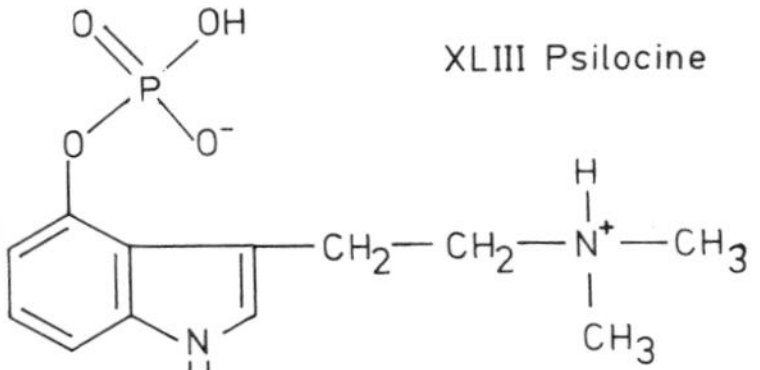

XLIV Psilocybine

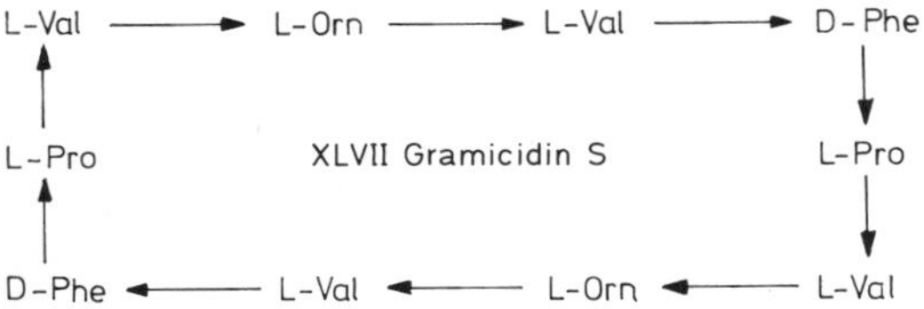

L-Val ——→ L-Orn ——→ L-Val ——→ D-Phe

↑   ↓

L-Pro   XLVII Gramicidin S   L-Pro

↑   ↓

D-Phe ←—— L-Val ←—— L-Orn ←—— L-Val

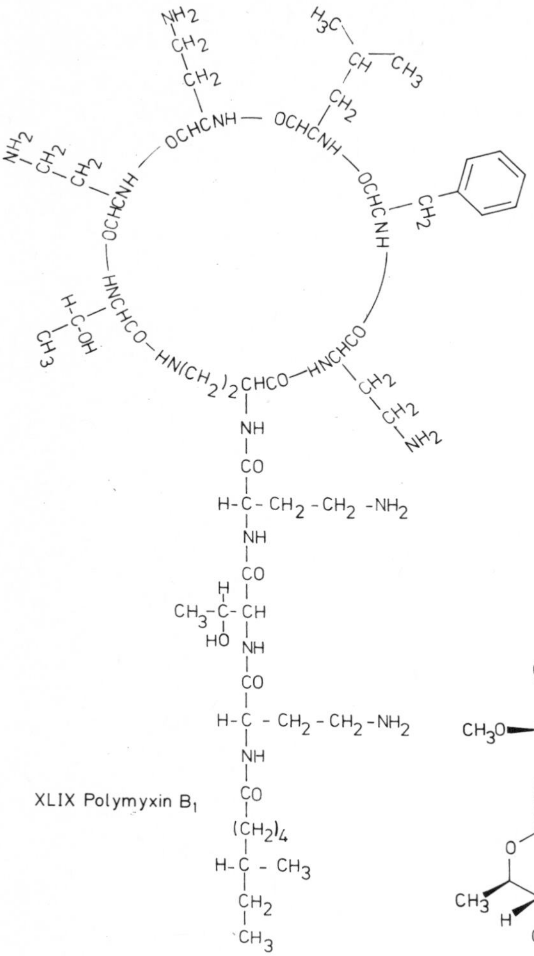

XLIX Polymyxin B₁

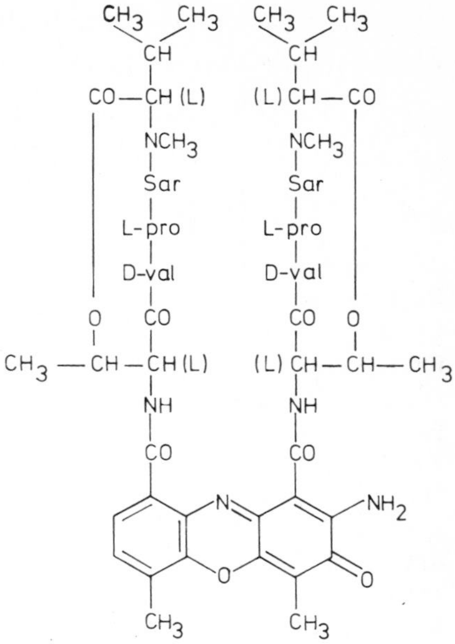

L Actinomycin D

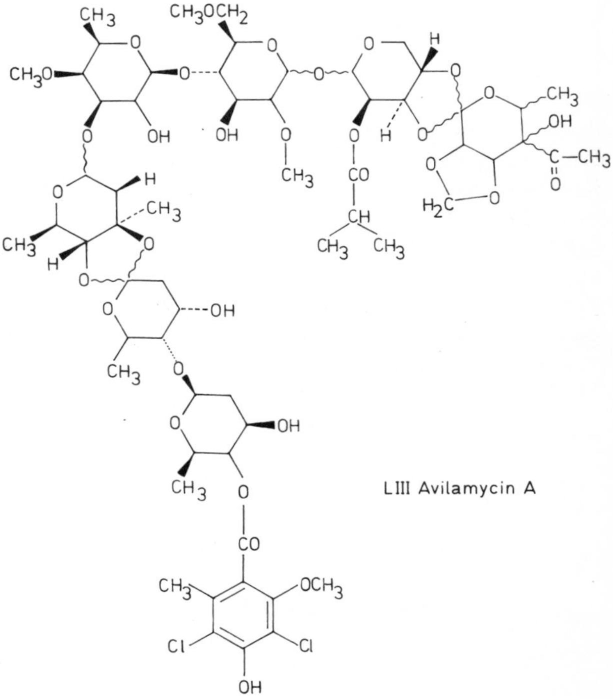

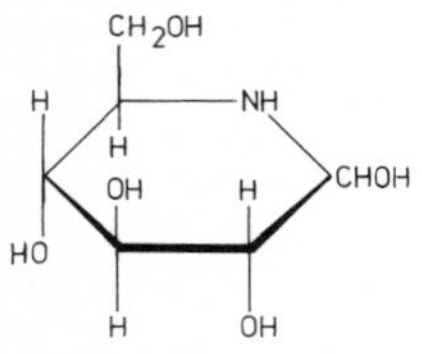

LI Nojirimycin

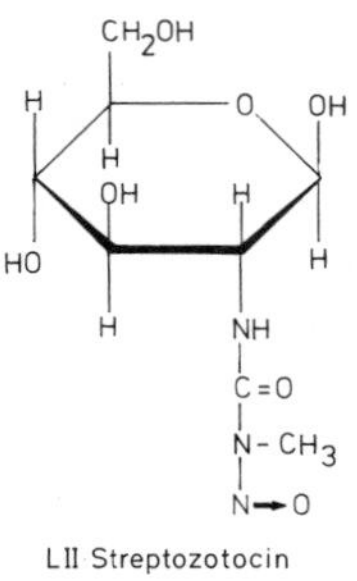

LII Streptozotocin

LIII Avilamycin A

A II.6 Technical Terms at the Fermenter

Term	Abbreviation	Unit
Bodenstein number $\left(B_{\mathrm{o}} = \dfrac{w \cdot L}{D_{\mathrm{eff}}}\right)$ (flow related to diffusion)	*Bo*	—
Bubble diameter	d_{B}	mm
Diameter of the bioreactor (tank)	D_{t}	m
Diameter of the stirrer (impeller)	D_{i}	m
Diffusion constant	D	—
Efficiency	η	%
Height of the fermenter	H_{T}	m
Henry's constant	*He*	$\mathrm{m^{3} \cdot bar \cdot kmol^{-1}}$
Level of liquid in the bioreactor	H_{L}	m
Mass exchange area (interface)	a	$\mathrm{m^{2}}$
Mass transfer number	$K_{\mathrm{L}} \cdot a$	$\mathrm{s^{-1}, h^{-1}}$
Mass transport coefficient	K_{L}	$\mathrm{m \cdot s^{-1}}$
Mixing time	t_{m}, Θ	s
Osmotic pressure	π	bar
Peripheral speed of the stirrer (tip speed)	v_{tips}	$\mathrm{m \cdot s^{-1}}$
Position of the stirrer on the shaft	S_{m}	m
Power demand with aeration	P_{g}	W
Power demand without aeration	P_{0}	W
Proportion of gas volume	ε_{G}	%
Rate of mass transport	N_{A}	$\mathrm{mol \cdot h^{-1}}$
Rate of rotation	n	$\mathrm{s^{-1}}$
Reynolds number (characterizes the flow) $(Re = v \cdot L \cdot v^{-1})$	*Re*	—
Schmidt number* $(Sc = v \cdot D^{-1})$	*Sc*	—
Sherwood number** $(Sh = K_{\mathrm{L}} \cdot d_{\mathrm{B}} \cdot D^{-1})$	*Sh*	—
Specific power input	$P \cdot V^{-1}$	$\mathrm{W \cdot L^{-1}}$
Superficial rate of flow (empty-tube velocity)	v_{s}	$\mathrm{m \cdot s^{-1}}$
Velocity gradient	$\dfrac{dv}{dx}$	$\mathrm{s^{-1}}$
Volume of the fermenter	V_{F}	$\mathrm{m^{3}}$

* Characterizing oxygen diffusion in solution.
** Characterizing oxygen transfer into the culture solution.

A II.7 Basic Physical Magnitudes (SI system) based on:

Length	(meter, m)	Temperature	(kelvin, K)
Mass	(kilogram, kg)	Luminous intensity	(candela, cd)
Time	(second, s)	Amount of substance	(mole, mol)
Current strength, electrical	(ampere, A)		

Magnitude	Symbol	Unit, Abbreviation, Relationship
Volume	V	L, m^3
Frequency	f	hertz, $Hz = s^{-1}$
Rate of rotation	n	$rpm = s^{-1}$
Velocity	v	$m \cdot s^{-1}$
Acceleration	a	$m \cdot s^{-2}$
Angular velocity	ω	$rad \cdot s^{-1}$
Angular acceleration	α	$rad \cdot s^{-2}$
Density	ρ	$kg \cdot m^{-3}$
Force	F	newton, $N = kg \cdot m \cdot s^{-2}$
Work, energy	W, E	joule, $J = N \cdot m = kg \cdot m^2 \cdot s^{-2}$
		(kilowatt hour, $kW\,h = 3.6$ MJ)
Power	P	watt, $W = J \cdot s^{-1} = kg \cdot m^2 \cdot s^{-3}$
Pressure	p	pascal, $Pa = N \cdot m^{-2} = kg \cdot s^{-2} \cdot m^{-1}$
		technical atmosphere, $at = 0.980665$ bar
		physical atmosphere, $atm = 760$ torr
		$torr = 133.3$ Pa
		$bar = 10^5$ Pa
		meter water column, $m\,H_2O = 0.1$ at
Surface tension	σ	$N \cdot m^{-1} = kg \cdot s^{-2}$
Viscosity, dynamic	η	pascal-second, $Pa \cdot s = N \cdot m^{-2} \cdot s$
kinematic	v	stokes, $St = 10^{-4}\ m^2 \cdot s^{-1}$
Amount of heat Q	Q	joule, $J = W \cdot s = N \cdot m$
		calorie, $cal = 4.1868$ J
Coefficient of heat transmission k		$cal \cdot m^{-2} \cdot h^{-1} \cdot K^{-1} = 4.868\ J \cdot m^{-2} \cdot h^{-1} \cdot K^{-1}$
		$= 1.163 \cdot 10^{-3}\ Wm^{-2}\ K^{-1}$
Thermal conductivity	λ	$W \cdot (m \cdot K)^{-1} = kg \cdot m \cdot s^{-3} \cdot K^{-1}$
Current strength, electrical	I	ampere, A
Amount of electricity, charge	Q	coulomb, $C = A \cdot s$
Tension, electrical	U	volt, $V = W \cdot A^{-1} = kg \cdot m^2 \cdot s^{-3} \cdot A^{-2}$
Resistance, electrical	R	ohm, $\Omega = V \cdot A^{-1} = kg \cdot m^2 \cdot s^{-3} \cdot A^{-2}$
Capacity	C	farad, $F = C \cdot V^{-1} = A \cdot s \cdot V^{-1}$

Appendix III
Laws, Guidelines, and
Instructions

**Arbeiten und Verkehr mit Krankheitserregern
[Handling and Trading with Disease-Producing
Agents],**
Bundesseuchengesetz §§ 19–24, Gesetzestext
pp. 12–13.

The Manufacture of Drugs and Ensuring their
Quality (publication of the revised basic rules
of the World Health Organization, 12. 1.
1977).

Richtlinien zum Schutze vor Gefahren durch
in vitro **neukombinierte Nukleinsäuren** [Guide-
lines for Protection against Risks due to **Nucleic Acids Newly Combined in vitro**],
Bundesminister für Forschung und Technologie, 2nd revised edition. Bundesanzeiger Ver-
lagsges. mbH, Cologne 1979.

Report of the Working Party on the **Practice
of Genetic Manipulation.**
Williams Committee, Her Majesty's Station-
ery Office, London 1976.

Biohazards in Biological Research,
Hellmann, A., Oxman, M. N. & Pollack, R.,
Cold Spring Harbor Laboratory, Cold Spring
Harbor 1973.

Guidelines for Testing of **Single Cell Protein**
destined as Protein Source for Animal Feed –
II,
Pure Appl. Chem. **51**, 2537–2560 (1979).

Microbiological Hazards,
Barry, R. D., Biochem. Soc. Spec. Publ. **5**, 39–
46 (1977).

Safety in Biological Laboratories,
Hartree, E., Booth, V., Biochemical Society,
London 1977.

Good Laboratory Practice Regulations of the
Food and Drug Administration,
Pharm. Ind. **41**, 259–268 (1979).

Richtlinien für die **Prüfung chemischer Desin-
fektionsmittel** [Guidelines for the **Testing of
Chemical Desinfectants**],
Deutsche Gesellschaft für Hygiene und Mikrobiologie. Gustav Fischer Verlag, Stuttgart,
2nd edition, 1969.

Vorläufige Empfehlung für den Umgang mit
pathogenen Mikroorganismen und für die
Klassifikation von Mikroorganismen und
Krankheitserregern nach den im Umgang mit
ihnen auftretenden Gefahren [Provisional
Recommendation for Handling Pathogenic
Microorganisms and for the Classification of
Microorganisms and Disease-producing
Agents in the Light of the Risks Arising in
their Handling]. Bundesgesundheitsblatt 24,
No. 22, 10. 30. 1981.

Health and Safety Aspects of Working with
Enzymes,
Flindt, M., Process Biochemistry, August
1980, S. 3–7.

General Standards for **Enzyme Regulations,**
The Association of Microbial Food Enzyme
Producers, Brussels.

Mikroorganismen für die **Lebensmitteltechnik**
[Microorganisms for **Foodstuffs Technology**],
Kommission für Ernährungsforschung. Ha-
rald Boldt-Verlag, 5407 Boppard 1974.

Sammlung von Vorschriften zur mikrobiologischen Untersuchung von **Lebensmitteln**
[Collection of Instructions for the Microbiological Investigation of **Foodstuffs**],
Schmidt-Lorenz, W. Verlag Chemie, Weinheim 1980.

Definition und Verwendung von **Pflanzenpro-
tein in Lebensmitteln** [Definition and Use of
Plant Protein in Foodstuffs],

Direction Generale de l'Administration et du Financement, German Translation of the Circular DGAF/SRF/C-1375, of 8. 27. 1975.

Bekanntmachung der Neufassung der **Richtlinien zum Schutz vor Gefahren durch in-vitro neukombinierte Nukleinsäuren** [Publication of the New Version of the **Guidelines for Protection Against Risks Due to Nucleic Acids Newly Combined in vitro**],
Bundesminister der Justiz, Bundesanzeiger, Year 33, No. 169a, of 8. 7. 1981.

Appendix IV
Basic Information for
Working in Biotechnology

A IV.1   Selection of Culture Collections

A IV.1.1   Important collections

ATCC American Type Culture Collection, 12301 Parklawn Drive, Rockville/Maryland 20852, USA.

CBS Centraalbureau voor Schimmelcultures, Oosterstraat 1, Baarn, The Netherlands.

CMI Commonwealth Mycological Institute, Ferry Lane, Kew/Surrey, England.

DSM Deutsche Sammlung von Mikroorganismen, Grisebachstr. 8, 3400 Göttingen

IAM Institute of Applied Microbiology, Tokyo, Japan, University of Tokyo, Mukogaoka I-I-I.

IFO Institute for Fermentation, Osaka, Japan, 4–54 Juso-nishinocho, Higashuyodogawaku.

NCIB National Collection of Industrial Bacteria, Aberdeen, AB9 8DG, Torry Research Station, P.O. Box 31, 135 Abbey Road, Scotland.

NRRL Northern Regional Research Laboratories, N. S. Dept. of Agriculture, Peoria, Illinois 61604, 1815 Northern University Street, USA.

UNESCO Institut für Bakteriologie, 19 Ave. Cesar Roux, CH-1004 Lausanne, Switzerland.

A IV.1.2   Literature giving further information

Martin, S. M., Quadling, C., Jones, M. L., and Skerman, V. B. D.: *World Directory of Collections of Cultures of Microorganisms*. Wiley-Interscience, New York, London, Sydney, Toronto 1972.

A IV.2   Substrates for Fermentation

A IV.2.1   Carbohydrates

A IV.2.1.1   Monosaccharides

Carbohydrates that cannot be cleaved further by hydrolysis

Classification:

Aldehyde-alcohols (aldoses) $CHO(CHOH)_nCH_2OH$ are oxidation products of polyhydric alcohols at **primary** hydroxy groups.

The most important representatives are:
L-arabinose, D-ribose, **D-glucose,** D-mannose, and D-galactose.
Specification of D-glucose (Maizena Industrieprodukte, Hamburg):

Water	max.	9.0%
DE	min.	99.9%
Spec. rotation $[\alpha]_D$ (German Pharmacopoeia 7):	$+52.2-+52.3°$	
Chlorides	max.	40.0 ppm
Ash	max.	0.02%
SO_2	max.	10 ppm

Ketone-alcohols (ketoses)
$CH_2OH-CO-(CHOH)_n-CH_2OH$ are oxidation products of polyhydric alcohols at **secondary** hydroxy groups.
The most important representative is D-fructose, obtained from potatoes, cereals, maize, and rice.
Specification of D-fructose (Merck, Darmstadt):

Spec. rotation $[\alpha]_D^{20}$:	$-91--93°$	
Water		0.5%
Heavy metals		0.001%

Maize starch (Maizena, Hamburg):

Water	max.	14%
pH	ca.	4.5
Total germ count	max.	1000
Yeasts	max.	100
Fungi	max.	100
Protein	max.	0.5%
Iron	below	1.0 ppm

Cornsteep liquor, obtained from maize.

Dry matter	48–49%
pH	3.5–4
Density	1.20
Ash	9%
Lactic acid	11–13%
Phosphorus	16–19%
Glucose	16–29 g/kg

The hydrolysis of maize starch gives:

Dextrin	enzyme system:	α-amylase
Starch		
sugars	enzyme system:	amyloglucosidase
Dextrose	enzyme system:	amyloglucosidase
Fructose	enzyme system:	glucose isomerase

A IV.2.1.1.2   Oligosaccharides

Are composed of monosaccharides or their derivatives linked to one another by glycosidic bonds. Compounds with 2 to 10 monosaccharide units.

Classification:

Disaccharides ($C_{12}H_{22}O_{11}$)
The most important representatives are **ordinary sugar** (sucrose, from beet or cane), **milk sugar** (lactose), **malt sugar** (maltose), and **cellobiose**.
Specification of cane sugar (Südzucker):

Purity	99.9%
Water	0.02%
Ash	0.0018%
Heavy metals	1 mg/kg

Trisaccharides ($C_{18}H_{32}O_{16}$)
The most important representative is **raffinose,** which occurs in sugar beet.

A IV.2.1.1.3   Polysaccharides

Constructed from monosaccharide units and their derivatives. Ten to several thousand units. D-Glucose is the most common unit; insoluble and nonreducing. The most important representatives are: **starch, glycogens, cellulose.**
Starch: mixture of amylose and amylopectin, saccharification by malt and fungal amylases.

A IV.2.1.2   Hydrocarbons

A IV.2.1.2.1   Aliphatic Hydrocarbons

Normal paraffins, C_1-C_4 compounds, are used for the production of SCP.
Longer-chain normal paraffins (from C_5) are converted via alcohols, aldehydes, and fatty acids into cell substances such as proteins, vitamins, and fats.

A IV.2.1.2.2   Aromatic Hydrocarbons

Limited technical importance. Starting materials are naphthalene, phenanthrene, and anthracene.

A IV.2.1.3   Fats and Oils

Glycerol esters of higher even-numbered fatty acids (glycerides).
Animal fats contain mixed glycerides of palmitic, stearic, and oleic acids.
The higher the amount of oleic acid, the more easily does the fat liquefy on heating (lard, whale oil). If the saturated acids predominate, the fats have higher melting points (beef fat/mutton fat).
Vegetable oils (olive oil, rapeseed oil, coconut oil, linseed oil, castor oil) are primarily glycerol esters of multiply unsaturated fatty acids.
It is mainly **soybean oil,** groundnut oil, and sunflowerseed oil that are used in fermentation.

	Percentage of		
	Oleic acid	Linoleic acid	Linolenic acid
Soybean oil	25–30	50–55	5–8
Groundnut oil	56–65	17–21	–
Sunflowerseed oil	30–35	55–65	–

They also contain about 15% of saturated fatty acids (palmitic and stearic acid).

Specification of soybean oil (Soja Mainz):

Free fatty acids	max.	0.05%
Gardner color		2–3
Flashpoint		150°C
Iodine No.		
according to Wijs		114–138
Peroxide No.	max.	1.0
Saponification No.		188–195
Viscosity	ca.	0.5 mPa·s at 20°C
Specific gravity	ca.	0.93

On a weight/weight basis, oils have about 2.5 times the calorific value of carbohydrates.

Advantages: heat-stable, meterable separately, antifoaming action, filterable.

Disadvantages: difficult to determine analytically, oils dissolve much oxygen, interfere in the recovery procedure.

A IV.2.1.4   Alcohols

Monohydric alcohols
The most important representatives are methanol, CH_3OH and ethanol, C_2H_5OH, which find use in protein fermentation.

Dihydric alcohols
Glycol = ethane-1,2-diol, $CH_2OH—CH_2OH$

Trihydric alcohols
Glycerol = $CH_2OH—CHOH—CH_2OH$. Constructional unit of the glycerides, present in animal fats and plant oils. Fermentation substrate.

Tetrahydric alcohols
Erythritol = $CH_2OH—CHOH—CHOH—CH_2OH$. The meso form occurs in algae.

Pentahydric alcohols
Pentitol = $CH_2OH—CHOH—CHOH—CHOH—CH_2OH$. Adonitol, xylitol, D-arabitol, L-arabitol: differentiating substrates (e.g., colored series).

Hexahydric alcohols
Hexitol = $CH_2OH—CHOH—CHOH—CHOH—CHOH—CH_2OH$. Sorbitol, mannitol, dulcitol: fermentation substrates.

A IV.2.1.5   Various Sources of Carbon

Molasses
Slightly purified sucrose; concentrated mother liquor from the crystallization of sucrose.

Beet sugar molasses:
48.5% sucrose
1% raffinose
1% invert sugar
20.7% organic nonsugar substances
18% H_2O
2% nitrogen

Cane sugar molasses:
33.4% sucrose
21.2% invert sugar
19.6% organic nonsugar substances
16% H_2O

Cellulose waste liquor (sulfite waste liquors)
Arise in the hydrolysis of wood with H_2SO_4. The total sugar content is

in the case of coniferous wood wastes	2–3.5%
in the case of broad-leaved wood wastes	3–4%

Main constituents: hexoses (mannose, glucose, galactose), pentoses (xylose, arabinose).

Slops
are residual liquids from fermentations in the manufacture of, for example, alcohol, acetone, and citric acid. They contain mostly residual sugars and organic acids.

A IV.2.2   Sources of Nitrogen

A IV.2.2.1   Organic Sources of Nitrogen

The most important technical N-containing raw materials for fermentation are:

Flour and glumes of:
cotton seeds
peanuts
soybeans
linseed
corn steep liquor
distillers' solubles, dry

yeast
fishmeal
meat- and bonemeal
blood meal
maizeseed meal
maize gluten meal

Protein peptones, hydrolysates of:

casein	yeast extract
lactalbumin	cotton seeds
milk protein	gelatine
soybeans	blood
fish	meat.
peanuts	

A IV.2.3.1   Microelements or trace elements (10^{-6}–10^{-8} mol)

Salts of manganese, molybdenum, zinc, copper, cobalt, nickel, vanadium, boron, chlorine, sodium, and silicon are required by many forms of life.

A IV.2.3.2   Macroelements (10^{-3}–10^{-4} mol)

Potassium, calcium, magnesium, and iron, together with nitrogen, sulfur, and phosphorus.

Important organic sources of nitrogen and their composition (figures in %)

	Dry matter	Crude protein	Crude fat	N	S	P
Soybean meal	92	45	2.5	8.2	0.4	0.7
Pharmaceutical media	95	58	4.0	9.0	0.6	1.5
Peanut meal	90	40–50	1.5–4.2		1.5	0.7
Wheat germ	92	28	1.0	4.8	0.3	1.2
Corn steep liquor	50	20–23	0.3–0.5	6.9	1.2	0.6
Skim milk powder	96	34	1.5	7.7	% Mineral matter	
Yeast extract	70	43	1.3	7	–	1.9

Peptones are cleavage products of animal or plant proteins.

Casein peptone: 85% protein content
4.5% amino nitrogen
2% phosphorus compounds

Bacterial peptone: 90% protein content
2% nucleic acids
1% fat.

A IV.2.2.2   Inorganic Sources of Nitrogen

NH_4^+ and NO_3^- salts (the most frequent assimilable compounds), urea.

A IV.2.3   Mineral Substances

A IV.2.4   Vitamins/Growth Substances

About 15 vitamins are required for the auxotrophic growth of microorganisms. They can be subdivided into fat- and water-soluble vitamins. **Biotin** and **thiamine** are the vitamins most used.
The concentration for maximum growth is 1 to 50 ppm.

Vitamin	Auxotrophic microorganisms	Occurrence
Thiamine (vitamin B$_1$)	*Lactobacillus fermenti 36* (ATCC 9338)	yeast, wheat germs
Biotin	*Lactobacillus arabinosus 17-5* (ATCC 8014)	corn steep liquor

Growth factors for microorganisms

Growth factors	Chemical groups transferred	Occurrence
Thiamine (vitamin B_1)	decarboxylation, C_1-aldehyde groups	rice husks, wheat germs, yeast
Riboflavine (vitamin B_2)	hydrogen	cereals, corn steep liquor
Pyridoxine (vitamin B_6)	amino groups, decarboxylations	residues of Penicillium mycelium, yeast, rice husks, wheat and maize, corn steep liquor
Nicotinic acid or nicotinamide	hydrogen	residues of Penicillium mycelium, wheat, liver
Pantothenic acid	acyl groups	sugar beet molasses, residues of Penicillium mycelium, corn steep liquor
Cyanocobalamine (vitamin B_{12})	carboxy groups displacement, methyl group synthesis	liver, cow dung, *Streptomyces griseus* mycelia, silage, meat
Folic acid	formyl group	residues of Penicillium mycelium, spinach, liver
Biotin	fixation of carbon dioxide	corn steep liquor, residues of Penicillium mycelium
α-Lipoic acid	hydrogen and acyl groups	liver
Purines		meat, blood meal
Pyrimidines		meat
Inositol		corn steep liquor
Choline		egg yolk, hops
Hemins	electrons	blood

A IV.2.5 Exotic Substrates

Lignin
Constituent amounting to 18 to 30% of plants. Is a mass plant product which is the slowest to undergo biological degradation.

Chitin
Is an important constituent of the cell walls of large groups of fungi and crustaceans. Consists of N-acylglucosamine residues linked with one another by β-glycosidic bonds.

Agar
Polysaccharide of complex composition from marine algae.

Cellulose
The organic compound that occurs most frequently in nature. Skeletal substance of plants. Slowly biologically degradable.

Peat

Coal
Anthracite, brown coal

A IV.3   Basic Operations of Fermentation and Recovery Technique

Basic operations in biotechnology describe working procedures that are necessary to perform fermentations or the recovery of bioproducts.

Common to basic operations both in biotechnology and in chemical production is the fact that they take place in accordance with scientific laws. These basic operations are carried out with fundamentally the same technical devices with the essential aim of ensuring the uniformity, profitability, and safety of a manufacturing process and the products resulting from it.

A IV.3.1   Fermentation Technique

The technically defined basic operations of fermentation processes are shown schematically in Table A-1, below.

Table A-1. Basic Operations in Fermentation Technique.

Process step	Performance
1. Plant cleaning	
2. Making up of the medium	batch
	continuous
3. Sterilization of the medium	batch
	continuous
4. Sterilization of vessels	empty
	filled
5. Calibration of the measuring probes and measuring devices before and after sterilization	in the vessel
	at the vessel
	externally (e.g. laboratory)
6. Preparation of the inoculum	monoculture
	mixed culture
7. Fermentation	batch
	fed batch
	repeated fed batch
	semicontinuous
	continuous
8. Aeration	feed air
	waste air
9. Stirring	mechanical
	pneumatic
	hydrodynamic
10. Process control	on line
	off line
11. Sampling	
12. Harvesting	total
	semitotal
	partial

A IV.3.1.1   Plant (Vessel) Cleaning

In addition to the external cleaning of vessels that must be carried out regularly, an internal cleaning of them must be carried out at regular intervals. A thorough internal cleaning of vessels is necessary when the product to be manufactured is changed – which usually runs in parallel with a change in the strain and in the medium – in order to remove encrusted residues of nutrient media or old growths of microbes on the walls from previous charges, particularly from the region of the spray zones.

The following methods of cleaning vessels are used:

a) mechanical/hydraulic jet cleaning
b) boiling out with dilute alkali, and
c) boiling out with formaldehyde.

A very effective method that can sometimes be applied manually consists in the insertion of **hydrojet** apparatuses which achieve a combined hydraulic-mechanical-chemical effect at low or elevated temperatures. Another method of cleaning consists in boiling out the vessel with water to which, for example, NaOH and Na_3PO_4 are added in equal parts; here total filling of the vessel is desirable.

When the solution is heated at $+95\,°C$ with moderate stirring, the encrustations present in the fermenter head or in the spray zone of the vessel are detached and washed off. After the washing process, the liquid is cooled, neutralized with dilute H_2SO_4, and fed to the clarification plant. Subsequently, the vessel is rinsed out several times with water.

If several contaminated batches are run after one another in a fermentation vessel, it is cleaned by adding formaldehyde (up to 0.1%) to the water in place of the mixture of NaOH and Na_3PO_4, with the maintenance of all the safety precautions for dealing with dangerous chemicals, and washing is then carried out with a rise in the temperature and with stirring. After this procedure, the vessel must be rinsed several times very thoroughly with pure water in order to eliminate the very last traces of formaldehyde, which otherwise have a toxic effect on the microbial growth of the following process batch.

A IV.3.1.2   The making up of the Medium

The making up of the nutrient medium can be carried out in the fermenter. For this purpose, the substrates, weighed out individually, are added to a predetermined amount of water already present and are predissolved (in the case of nondissolving substrates, slurried). After this, the solution or slurry is made up to the calculated total working volume – in the case of steam sterilization with allowance for the condensate that will arise and must be counted in. Another method of preparing the medium makes use of a preparation vessel with a stirrer provided specially for this purpose in which the total formulation is made up separately with dissolution or homogenization and is then pumped to the bioreactor. The advantage of this method is, in particular, that the transport of the substrates to the bioreactor and any external pollution by the formation of dust when filling the substrate into the bioreactor are absent. In both methods (heat-) sensitive substrates or components of the nutrient medium (glucose, vitamins, growth substances) should not be added to the main charge but must be weighed out separately and added in the sterilized state to the reactor before inoculation.

These complicated and time-consuming processes also harbor certain dangers (infection). The continuous making up of the medium has advantages, since, as a rule, this is followed by continuous sterilization which guarantees a gentle treatment of thermolabile substrates. The continuous making-up of nutrient media is used particularly in continuous fermentations, but also in the large batch production of natural microbial products (antibiotics, enzymes, amino acids, etc.). Here, a number of bioreactors run through all the basic operations of fermentation in an economically devised time plan.

A IV.3.1.3   Sterilization of the Medium

Basically, nutrient media can be made germ-free by filtration or the addition of suitable chemicals (β-propiolactone, ethylene oxide). The most common in fermentation is thermal sterilization, which can be carried out batchwise or continuously. In batchwise sterilization of the nutrient solution this can be heated and sterilized together with the vessel by blowing direct steam into the medium. The condensate formed is thereby lost to the boilerhouse, but it must be taken into account – so far as the final volume is concerned – in the making up of the medium; or the process can be carried out by indirect heating of the medium (by means of an internal or external heating steam coil. With the direct injection of steam, the time of heating up – to the predetermined final temperature (e.g., 120°C) – is relatively short, while on indirect heating this time becomes considerably longer.

While the holding time after the sterilization temperature has been reached is independent of any particular features of direct or indirect heating, the time of cooling to the operating temperature is functionally and temporally highly dependent on the cooling and heating capacity of the medium and fermenter that is available. For energy-saving reasons, continuous sterilization of the nutrient medium is always to be preferred to a batch sterilization. Not only are savings of of the order of 70 to 80% achieved in the use of steam and cooling water but by the use of a higher temperature (135°C) the sterilization time is reduced to 5 to 8 minutes, which contributes to a gentle treatment of thermolabile substrate and components in the medium.

Thermal sterilization in batch methods of preparation is carried out particularly with media having high proportions of insoluble solids, while the continuous thermal sterilization of media is used preferentially on media with completely soluble components of the substrates. Alternatively, soluble substrates can be sterile-filtered. Sterile filtration can also take place batchwise provided that the sterile-filtered nutrient medium can be fed through sterile conduits to a sterile, empty or partially water-filled, vessel.

Chemical sterilization is rarely used in production. The costs of the chemical agents and possible adverse effects of their degradation products on the growth of the highly bred production strains makes its use in large-scale fermentations appear questionable.

A IV.3.1.4   Sterilization of Vessels

In a sterilization of vessels in the filled state, the nutrient medium, the vessel, filters, connecting pieces, conduits, and sampling devices are subjected to the sterilization cycle synchronously.

Sterilization of the empty vessel is employed particularly where the nutrient medium to be used can be made germ-free rapidly either by a continuous thermal process or by filtration. In comparison to the filled (batch) fermenter sterilizations, separate sterilizations of vessel (empty) and of medium (thermal-continuous process or filtration) are more economic, take less time, have a gentler effect on material and substrate, and are more readily controllable, but they make slightly more intensive use of personnel and apparatus.

A IV.3.1.5   Calibration of the Measuring Probes and Measuring Devices before and after Sterilization (Instrument Calibration)

Fermentations require certain fixed conditions of the medium for microbial growth and the formation of the desired product. So that predetermined process magnitudes can be set, monitored, and to some extent regulated, sterilizable measuring probes must (in some cases) be post-calibrated and checked after the sterilization process, while the large number of measuring devices for fermentative parameters that do not come into contact with the sterilization process directly must be checked for their functional capacity before every new starting-up operation.

The following main criteria must be set for the measuring and control instruments to an even greater extent than for ordinary automatic measuring technique:

– reliability
– reproducibility of the measured value
– accuracy
– repeated sterilizability of the probe.

The first two points apply particularly when measuring instruments are used in continuous systems.

All the necessary calibrations, e.g., of apparatuses for measuring the speed of stirrers, the temperature, the pressure, the weights of the reactor, etc., must be checked in a daily routine at fixed times.

A IV.3.1.6   Preparation of the Inoculum

A fermentative preparation of an inoculum differs from a product fermentation primarily by the fact that it is designed for a rapid multiplication of the microorganisms. This multiplication of biomass can take place under special conditions in one, two, or more stages, using precultivation nutrient media that contain readily metabolizable N and C substrates in low concentrations and, frequently, specific inducers and precursors in order to avoid a long lag phase in the main cultivation.

Inoculation is carried out with 0.5 to 5.0 vol%, referred to the next volume stage to be inoculated, preferably from the logarithmic growth phase, where the morphological form and physiological state of the microorganism have their optimum expression. Microorganisms in the spore form, in vegetative form, as monocultures or as mixed cultures are used as the inoculation material and, in inoculation, must be transferred into the main bioreactor under contamination-free conditions.

A IV.3.1.7   Fermentation

The fermentation proper consists of an aerobic or anaerobic microbial process which is carried out to obtain natural products (antibiotics, enzymes, amino acids, etc.), usually in submerged, closed, or open processes. Depending on the nature and manner in which the system is operated – whether it is totally closed and partially periodic or continuous – a distinction is made between:

batch fermentation: closed system
fed-batch fermentation: closed system
repeated fed-batch fermentation: closed system
semicontinuous fermentation: closed/
                                           open system
continuous fermentation: open system

A IV.3.1.7.1   Batch Fermentation

Batch fermentation exists when in a closed system (fermenter) a nutrient medium is sterilized, fermentation conditions (e.g., stirrer speed, temperature, pressure, aeration, pH, pO_2) are adjusted, and the system is inoculated with a definite amount of inoculum and operated. The growth of the microorganisms in such a system will – after passing through the individual growth phases – arrive at a complete standstill, whether by the total exhaustion of the nutrient medium or because of the enrich-

ment of one or more of the products (product inhibition). In batch fermentations, with a few exceptions (e.g., adjustment of pH), no correction by the addition of any agents or substrates whatever during the whole duration of the cultivation takes place nor is there any removal of culture solution with microorganisms. They therefore frequently differ in course and result. In spite of these known uncertainties, main types of fermentations are based on batch fermentation, and these can be classified into fermentation types in the following way:

Fermentation Type I

Growth and the formation of product take place in parallel as the result of the primary energy metabolism. Biosynthesis of simple molecules.

Fermentation Type II

Growth and formation of product may – but need not – be coupled in parallel. The reaction rates are very complex in comparison with type I.

Fermentation Type III

Growth and the formation of product are strictly separated and cannot be derived directly from the energy metabolism. Biosynthesis of complex molecules.

A IV.3.1.7.2   Fed-batch Fermentation

In fed-batch fermentation, sterile nutrient solution is metered into the fermenter at intervals or continuously. The advantages of fed-batch fermentation reside particularly in the facts that an increased formation of biomass can be observed, that catabolite repression can be avoided, and that, consequently, critical partial pressures of oxygen (at constant stirrer speed and rate of aeration) can be avoided by additions of the substrate as a function of metabolic parameters.

The specific rate of growth μ in a fed-batch culture can be controlled and be raised or lowered by the rate of addition of substrate. Fed-batch fermentation with substrate-limited growth can also be used in large-scale production (e.g., in penicillin and cephalosporin fermentations), since they are technically simpler to manage than chemostat cultures (in which the volume is kept constant) and nevertheless permit quasi-equilibrium conditions to be established with high yields of products running in parallel.

A IV.3.1.7.3   Repeated Fed-batch Fermentation

A repeated fed-batch fermentation is characterized by the fact that portions of the culture solution and the microorganism are removed from the system at intervals. The closed fermentation system – fed-batch fermentation – has given rise to a partially open fermentation system in which the working volume, the rate of feed, and therefore the specific rates of growth may undergo cyclic changes. With constant time cycles, it can again be assumed that the culture passes through equilibrium conditions, so that oscillations arise which end in each case with a high secretion of product.

A IV.3.1.7.4   Semicontinuous Fermentation

Semicontinuous fermentation is also a partially open fermentation system which can be subdivided into a cyclic-continuous fermentation and a semi-continuous cell-recycling stage. The reason for the performance of a semicontinuous fermentation is the realization of the long-term and high-degree utilization of the biosynthetic potential by the periodic addition of new sterile nutrient solution and the removal for exploitation of the same amount of culture solution, whereupon the residue remaining in the tank acts as inoculum. The culture solution removed can be used for recovery of the required natural product or it may also serve as an inoculum for other fermenters with the same conditions and nutrient media. Semicontinuous fermentations are less economic than fully continuous ones but they must exhibit considerable process-engineering advantages and simplifications and an improved utilization of capacity as compared with batch fermentations.

Semicontinuous cell recycling

Semicontinuous cell recycling is used practically only with aseptically operated fermentations. The total cell mass of a fermentation charge is separated and used as an inoculum for a new batch.

A IV.3.1.7.5   Continuous Fermentation

A continuous fermentation – as an open system – is arranged in such a way that, with a constant working volume and a constant specific rate of growth of the microorganism, fresh medium containing a substrate is metered at a constant rate of flow into the system under sterile conditions and, simultaneously, the same amount of culture solution with the microorganisms is removed. Continuous fermentation processes can be systematically subdivided:

- according to the nature of their end product, e.g., biomass or metabolic products;
- according to the type of process or operation, e.g., homogeneous/heterogeneous systems, simple/multiple systems, and systems with and without the return of microorganisms; and also
- according to the principle of *control,* i.e., the chemostat or the turbidostat principle.

Whatever process principle is used in continuous fermentation, typical advantages in comparison with the classical batch fermentation lead to a better, more economic, yield which, in addition, can be controlled and calculated beforehand by mathematical derivations for the growth of the microorganisms and the formation of product.

A IV.3.1.8   Aeration

Aeration, as a fundamental operation of fermentation, for supplying the microorganisms with oxygen is basically carried out with filtration-sterilized air in strictly aerobic systems under pressure. The necessary amount of air can be determined with the aid of measuring diaphragms, suspended bodies, etc., and it can be distributed into the medium through various types of aeration distributors, which are usually installed in the bottom of the bioreactor. The oxygen demand of a fermentation depends on the substrate and the microorganism and can be calculated. The rate of aeration for an adequate economic supply of oxygen to the medium and the microorganism can be measured precisely and accurately with oxygen-analyzing probes and apparatuses in the liquid and/or gas phase and be controlled. Since the rate of respiration of most microorganisms is independent of the concentration of dissolved oxygen, in aerobic fermentation it is sufficient always to keep the partial pressure above 10% of the saturation level.

A IV.3.1.9 Stirring

As a basic operation of fermentation, stirring can be carried out mechanically, pneumatically, or hydrodynamically. An optimum circulation and mixing of all the constituents in the medium as a 3- or 4-phase mixture must be achieved, new phase-separation boundaries for the exchange of matter and energy must be formed continuously, and microturbulences must be produced, i.e., the stirring and mixing process includes the following tasks:

- the dispersion of the entering and rising bubbles of air,
- the homogeneous mixing of the nutrient medium,
- the production of sufficiently high turbulences for the transfer of heat,
- the maintenance of high relative velocities between air bubbles, substrate, and microorganism cells for the optimum exchange of matter. The many sided terminology and analysis of stirring and mixing processes is summarized in Table A-2.

It is convenient to consider aeration and stirring in aerobic fermentation technology together, since they represent mutually supplementing basic operations and, moreover, as cost- and energy-intensive methods, determine the profitability of a fermentation process.

A IV.3.1.10 Process Control

The knowledge and determination of specific parameters in a fermentation, e.g., the conditions of the medium, the growth of the microorganisms, and the formation of the product, together with the calculation of additional primary control parameters, which, for their part, have the aim of regulating and intervening in the process, today form an indispensable basic operational unit in biotechnology.

Important automatic (on-line) controls in and on the fermenter are, for example, the adjustment of the temperature, the measurement of the pH, and foam control, while parameter control outside the fermenter – waste gas analysis and all analyses of products and substrates from fermenter samples in the laboratory – represent off-line controls.

Process control makes use of a large number of physicochemical methods of determination and can be supported by the use of process computers to such an extent that fermentations can run in an automatically controlled and programmed manner.

Table A-2. Stirring and Mixing Processes.

Name	Purpose	Characterization Method of measurement
Stirring	moving the liquid	P/V; velocity profile
Mixing (stirring effect)	suspension of solid particles	homogeneity (static measurement)
	mixing of miscible liquids	mixing times (dynamic measurement)
	dispersion of gases	$K_L \cdot a$, a, OTR
	dispersion of immiscible liquids	degree of emulsification
	heat exchange	temperature

A IV.3.1.11   Sampling

Sampling is an important process in fermentation. Only with homogeneous samples taken under sterile conditions can the analyses necessary for following the process then be performed in the laboratory and the sterility be tested. Depending on the technical equipment of the fermenter, the sample may be taken through a sterilizible sample valve or through a continuous sampling device.

A IV.3.1.12   Harvesting

The harvesting of a fermentation process and the transfer of the product-containing culture solution to the recovery step can be designed according to various aspects and considerations: e.g.:

- maximum amount of product,
- lowest specific costs,
- optimum yield.

These harvesting criteria are applied particularly in the case of classical batch fermentations. For semi-continuous and fully continuous fermentations, the product $D \cdot X$ (or $D \cdot P$) is evaluated for the continuous harvesting stream from the rate of inflow and the concentration of biomass or product, i.e., the true productivity, and is used as a basis for evaluation.

A IV.3.2   Product Recovery

The recovery of the various fermentation products from the harvested culture solution is done by separating off the solids and then by various types of liquid-liquid extraction. Other basic mechanical and thermal operations such as precipitation, crystallization, drying, etc., that are customary in chemical engineering and have been taken over into recovery technique are necessary to arrive at the desired purity of the fermented product. If desired, aseptic methods can often be used.

The most important basic operations of recovery technique are listed and characterized individually in Table A-3 (exhaustive descriptions applied to special processes and products will be found parti-

Table A-3. Basic Operations of Recovery Technique (see Table A-1).

Process step	Basic operation
1. Sedimentation 2. Centrifugation 3. Filtration of solids 4. Flocculation and flotation	Separation
5. Physical disintegration of cells 6. Chemical disintegration of cells 7. Enzymatic disintegration of cells	Methods of disintegration
8. Evaporation 9. Extraction 10. Membrane filtration 11. Freeze-drying 12. Adsorption 13. Precipitations	Enrichment
14. Crystallization 15. Chromatography 16. Ultrafiltration and reverse osmosis	Purification
17. Drying	

cularly in Chapter 8, and also in Chapters 11, 12, and 15).

The first step in the isolation of a microbial product prepared by fermentation usually consists in the separation of the culture solution into a soluble fraction and a fraction that contains all insoluble constituents such as microorganisms and unconsumed ingredients of the nutrient solution. The most important basic mechanical operations of solid-body separation include:

- sedimentation
- centrifugation
- filtration
- flocculation and flotation.

A IV.3.2.1   Sedimentation

Sedimentation is the deposition of the particles suspended in a fluid medium by the action of the force of gravity. The sedimentation processes that are of technical importance almost all take place in the region of laminar flow, i.e., in the range of validity of Stokes' law. Deviations from this law that occur are due to agglomerations (combinations of small particles into larger ones) or to the formation of swarms. In concentrated suspensions, all the particles – regardless of their size – frequently sink as closed swarms, so that a sharp boundary forms between the falling suspension and the clarified liquid above it. Another deviation from Stokes' law is due to inhibition of sedimentation by neighboring particles and by friction on the walls of the vessel.

Sedimentations are used in certain fermentation processes, e.g., in the case of cell recycling. They are cheap and require little investment in material, apparatus, and energy.

A IV.3.2.2   Centrifugation

By centrifugation is understood sedimentations that are carried out in a centrifugal field. The most important element is a rotating container in which the separation of a mixture of liquid and solid is carried out by sedimentation (according to density differences) or filtration (solid from liquid).

A IV.3.2.3   Filtration of solids

By filtration is understood the separation of particles of solids from a fluid medium (liquid or gas) by means of a porous filter medium that permits the fluid phase to flow through it but retains the solid particles. In the case of liquid-solid filtrations, the Hagen-Poiseuille law can be taken as a basis for the theoretical consideration of filtration under idealized assumptions.

Depending on the purpose of filtration, a distinction is made between clarification and separation filtration. A clarification filtration is usually employed for the purification of a liquid, while a separation filtration has the aim of recovering the separated solid. Depending on the nature of the separating layer, a distinction is made between surface and depth filtration. Filtrations are less expensive with respect to apparatus, maintenance, and costs but – unless pressure filters are concerned – relatively personnel-intensive.

A IV.3.2.4   Flocculation and Flotation

By various operations, solid particles in turbid media can be caused to agglomerate into larger groups. This process increases the velocity of settling, e.g., in sedimentation, and makes the filter cake more permeable in filtration.

Flocculants that may be used include natural and synthetic substances. They are either electrolytes or organic substances with long-chain molecules having side chains that tend to form hydrogen bonds. Since the "flocs" are unstable formations, in practical use care must be taken that they do not break down. The precipitate or sludge composed of the flocs is very voluminous with a high water content.

The opposite of flocculation is flotation, by which is understood the separation of a material dispersed in a liquid by utilizing different boundary surface properties of the particles.

Three groups of flotation agents are known: collectors, foamers, and controlling flotation agents, and in addition there are flotation poisons (e.g., aluminium, iron) and also hydrophilic colloids (humins, proteins, tannic acids), which can suppress flotations.

In recovery technique, great importance is attached to flocculations, in particular, for facilitating sedimentation, filtration, or centrifugation. On the other hand, flotation processes are used mainly in the biotechnology of sewage and other effluents.

To obtain natural materials formed in cells or specific constituents of cells, a disintegration of the cells is usually necessary, which can be carried out physically, chemically, or enzymatically.

A IV.3.2.5   *Physical Disintegration of Cells*

The physicomechanical methods of digesting cells include wet milling, changing and releasing the pressure, and thermolytic processes. Shearing forces, cavitation, and thermoshock or shock-freezing are the effects that bring about the breakdown of the cell wall.

A IV.3.2.6   *Chemical Disintegration of Cells*

Alkalis or acids are mainly used to achieve the disintegration of the cells. However, the pH shock often leads to undesirable side reactions such as the denaturation of protein and precipitations.

A IV.3.2.7   *Enzymatic Disintegration of Cells*

The gentlest and most selective method is digestion with enzymes. Disadvantages of this process are the sometimes high material costs and – if fixed enzymes are not used – the loss of enzyme after only one treatment.

A IV.3.2.8   *Evaporation*

By evaporation is understood the conversion of a liquid into the gaseous state of aggregation by changing the temperature or the pressure or by varying both parameters. The aim of an evaporation process is to enrich a component of a solution or to recover the solvent.

Bioproducts are frequently thermolabile and can therefore be concentrated only by the use of relatively low temperatures.

A IV.3.2.9   *Extraction*

A frequently used method of concentrating natural materials is their extraction from solutions of solids with various solvents. The basic operation of extraction is subdivided into liquid/liquid extraction and solid/liquid extraction. If, for example, a liquid system cannot be distilled because of the risk of decomposition on heating, extractive separation may be used, because in extractions no supply of heat or cooling water is necessary. Generally, liquid/liquid extraction is of greater importance in biotechnological recovery technique than solid/liquid extraction (e.g., in the enrichment and isolation of lipophilic natural materials). Since many natural materials undergo denaturation in organic solvents, extraction is generally carried out with the shortest possible residence time in the seconds or minutes range. Also important is the fact that in the case of bioproducts only narrow pH ranges must be maintained during extraction, so that the predetermined conditions often do not permit the optimum utilization of the distribution factors.

A IV.3.2.10   *Membrane Filtration*

Methods of filtration in the area of the enrichment of bioproducts are, for example, special membrane processes which are also carried out in combination with applied electric fields (dialysis, electrophoresis). In membrane filtration – in contrast to classical filtration – dissolved particles are transported to membrane surfaces by convection and are separated there. When a hydrostatic pressure is used, some particles can pass through the membrane while particles with a larger molecular weight are retained at the membrane.

A IV.3.2.11   *Freeze-drying*

By freeze-drying or sublimation drying is understood the basic operation of recovery technique in which a material is obtained by the evaporation or volatilization (sublimation) of the frozen substance contained in the material with bypassing of the liquid state of aggregation. The conditions for a sublimation exist only below the triple point where all three states of aggregation are possible together. This type of drying has a very mild effect on the product.

A IV.3.2.12   Adsorption

Adsorption is the attachment of particles of a substance to a condensed phase as the result of the action of surface forces. This leads to an enrichment of substances at liquid boundaries or at the surfaces of solids. The amount of substance being adsorbed is functionally dependent on the phase boundary area available. Adsorption methods are used, in particular, for the enrichment of hydrophilic natural substances that cannot be extracted with organic solvents. The main agents used are ion-exchange resins, special polymer resins, and activated carbon.

The most important characteristics of adsorbents are their selective properties, which can be classified on the basis of characteristics such as pore volume, specific surface, mean pore diameter, pore distribution, and also chemical structure, activity, and physical properties.

A IV.3.2.13   Precipitations

Precipitations are, in principle, fast crystallizations which are brought about by the sudden pronounced decrease in the solubility of a substance or by its becoming almost completely insoluble in the mother liquor. Precipitation is usually preceded by a rapid chemical reaction forming the reactant that later precipitates.

Commonly used precipitants for proteins are sodium sulfate, Na_2SO_4, and ammonium sulfate, $(NH_4)_2SO_4$, which have the advantage that they can be used even at low temperatures. In the industrial area, organic precipitants such as alcohols, ketones, and polymers are also used.

Important magnitudes in precipitations are the type of mixing or the rate of inflow of the reagents, and also the temperature and the pH, which have a decisive influence on the particle size of the precipitate.

A IV.3.2.14   Crystallization

By crystallization is understood the separation of a dissolved solid in crystalline form after supersaturation by cooling or condensation. The crystallization takes place in two stages, i.e., crystallization nuclei must first be formed or be present before crystal growth can set in.

Basically, all methods of crystallization can be subdivided into two groups:

- crystallizations by the elimination of part of the solvent, and
- crystallizations without elimination of the solvent.

Continuous crystallization processes give very good homogeneous products, while in discontinuous processes less homogeneous end products may frequently occur. In comparison with other basic operations of recovery technique, the transfer from laboratory crystallization to the pilot plant and to large-scale technical crystallizations is substantially more difficult than with other processes. The theory of crystallization is not yet well developed, so that mathematical predictions are frequently impossible. For example, in crystallization processes appreciable amounts of heat arise which, when they are inadequately removed at the cooling surface, cause pronounced supersaturation and the undesirable formation of incrustations.

A IV.3.2.15   Chromatography

Under the term chromatography are included various methods for the separation of chemically and physically similar substances from a fluid medium. It is designed as a method of separation and purification in which, by the flow of a liquid through a porous adsorbent, the fractionation of mixtures is promoted by means of differential migration, i.e., the separation of the substances dissolved in a carrier liquid takes place by the use of different forces of binding to a second, usually stationary, phase, the transport of matter being determined by flow and diffusion processes and various kinetic processes.

The most important chromatographic processes used in recovery techniques are, for example: *adsorption chromatography,* in which use is made of the different affinities of substances for solid surfaces resulting from different valence forces for the separation of substances; *ion-exchange chromatography,* in which the separation of substances takes place through reversible ion formation due to different charges; *affinity chromatography,* which is based on the reversible formation of chemical complexes; *gel chromatography,* which utilizes the sieve action of carrier materials of defined pore structure for separating mixtures of substances according to molecular size; and *partition chromatography,* which uses for separation the differential distribution of a substance in two liquids as the result of their different solubilities.

The advantages of chromatographic processes in recovery technique can be seen in their high separating power with high yields under gentle conditions, the possibility of automation, and the reusability of the carrier material.

A IV.3.2.16   Ultrafiltration and Reverse Osmosis

Ultrafiltration and reverse osmosis are methods and processes in which dissolved substances are fractionated by means of membrane filters: larger molecules are retained and smaller ones can be passed through the membrane. In analogy with dynamic, i.e., filter-cake-less, filtration, a solution flows parallel to the surface of the membrane while the passage of the permeate through the membrane takes place perpendicular to it.

The true difference between ultrafiltration and reverse osmosis lies in the range of molecular sizes. Ultrafiltrations are used with molecular masses of between 500 and 300 000, where a filtration pressure of a few bar is sufficient, while in reverse osmosis processes molecular masses smaller than 250 are separated under pressures that may range between 30 and 100 bar.

Advantages in comparison with other purification processes are achieved by the avoidance of phase changes and of thermal loadings of the product, and by the simultaneous concentration and purification of the product that take place.

After the desired product from fermentative processes has been obtained in sufficient purity, in order to be converted into the final form it must usually be dried.

A IV.3.2.17   Drying

By drying is understood the separation of moisture from a substance or a mixture of substances by evaporation or vaporization for which purpose, as a rule, heat must be supplied to the product to be dried.

A large number of methods and corresponding apparatuses are available for performing drying processes. The individual processes differ mainly by the manner in which the necessary heat is supplied to the product gently or how the product to be dried is brought into contact with the drying medium, and whether it is carried out continuously or discontinuously, and under normal pressure or under vacuum.

A IV.3.3   Literature

Rehm, H. J.: Industrielle Mikrobiologie, Springer-Verlag, Berlin, Heidelberg 1980.

Zabrieskie, W.: Arminger, B., Phillip, H., Albano, A., Traders Guide to Fermentation Media Formulation, Traders Protein Division, 1980.

AFG-Handbuch, Südzucker 1979.

Schlegel, H. G.: Allgemeine Mikrobiologie, 5. Auflage, Georg-Thieme-Verlag, Stuttgart 1981.

A IV.4 Flow Sheets of Typical Biotechnological Processes

Flow Sheet: Foodstuffs, Feedstuffs

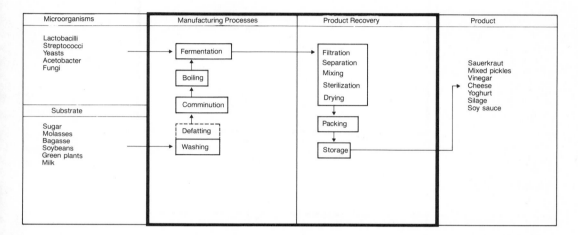

Flow Sheet: Ethanol

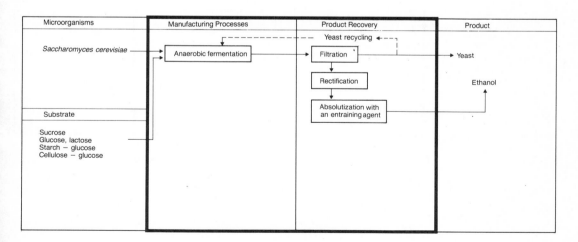

Flow Sheet: Amino Acids, L-Lysine

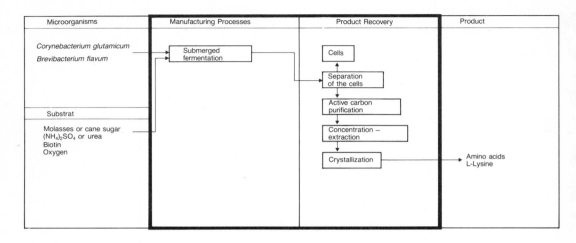

Flow Sheet: Citric Acid

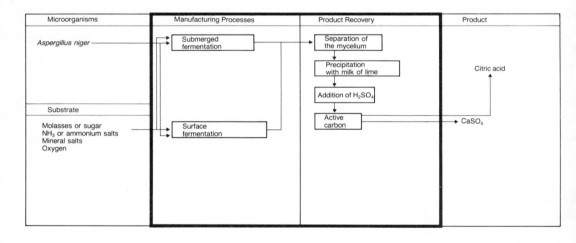

Flow Sheet: Lactic Acid

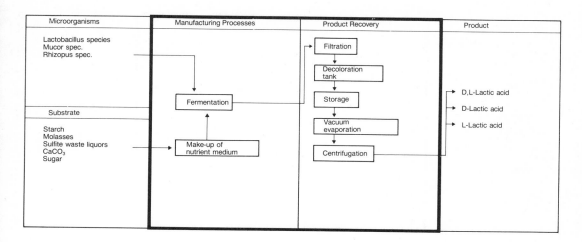

Flow Sheet: Butanol

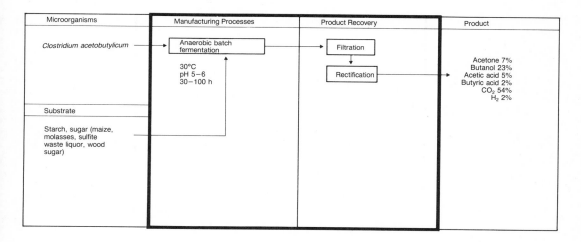

Flow Sheet: Vitamin B$_{12}$

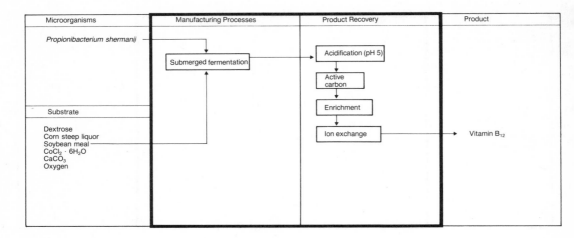

Flow Sheet: An Enzyme

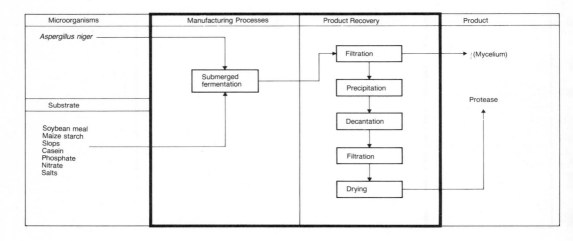

Flow Sheet: Biopolymers

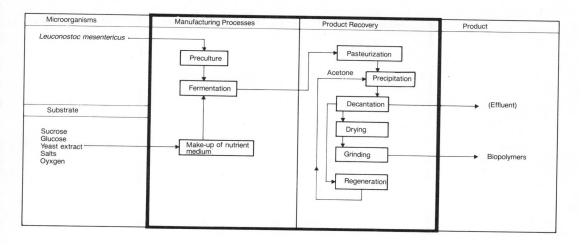

Flow Sheet: Tetracycline

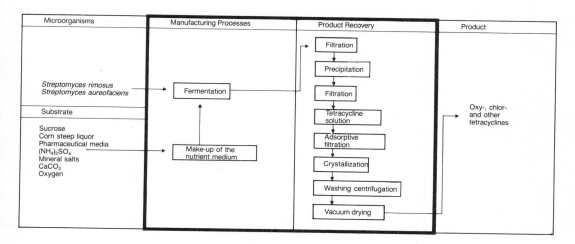

Flow Sheet: Bacitracin

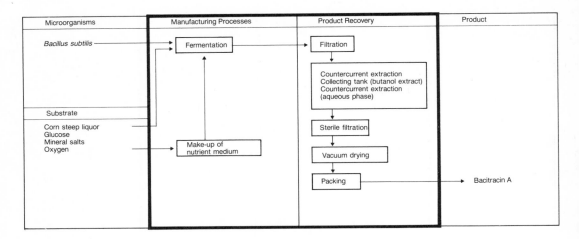

Flow Sheet: Biotransformation, Steroids

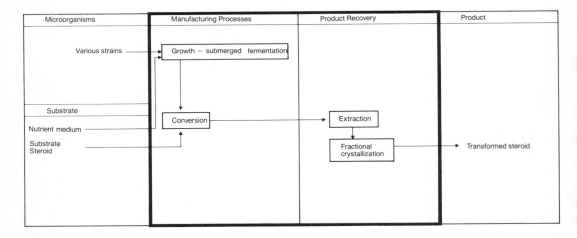

Flow Sheet: Bioprotein, Fodder Yeast

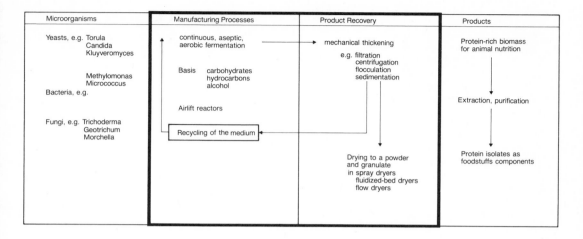

Flow Sheet: Aerobic/Anaerobic Wastewater Purification

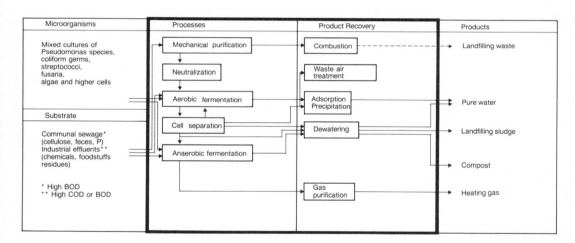

A IV.5   *Types of Reactors*

Reactor	Power	OTR	Mixing time	Gas content	v_{max}
Stirred tank	8 kW m^{-3}	4 g/L h	—	8 %	400 m^3
Stirred tank with innertube	8 kW m^{-3}	4 g/L h	—	12 %	80 m^3
High-efficiency stirred reactor	30 kW m^{-3}	15 g/L h	4 s	15 %	10 m^3
Gassing tube reactor	4 kW m^{-3}	10 g/L h	30 s	13 %	80 m^3
Stirred chamber fermenter	1.5 kW m^{-3}			20 %	120 m^3
Tube loop	3 kW m^{-3}	1 g/L h		8 %	5 m^3
Jet loop	5 kW m^{-3}	10 g/L h	60 s	30 %	500 m^3
Airlift loop	3.5 kW m^{-3}	10 g/L h	80 s	30 %	3000 m^3
Bubble column	3.5 kW m^{-3}	12 g/L h	200 s	30 %	5000 m^3
Sieve-plate column	3 kW m^{-3}	10 g/L h	300 s	50 %	1000 m^3
Plunging jet fermenter	2.5 kW m^{-3}	12 g/L h		20 %	200 m^3
Circulating nozzle reactor	0.5 kW m^{-3}	0.5 g/L h	—	85 %	100 m^3
Paddle-wheel fermenter	1.5 kW m^{-3}	3 g/L h	—	90 %	500 m^3
Immersed column fermenter	0.08 kW m^{-3}	0.12 g/L h	—	2 %	4000 m^3
Enzyme membrane reactor	10 kW m^{-3}	—	—	0 %	n · 5 L
Immersed wick fermenter	kW m^{-3}	1.6 g/L h		70 %	2000 m^3
Packed column					
Tricking film column					
Floating roller fermenter	0.1 kW m^{-3}	0.2 g/L h	—	0.01 %	1 m^3
Surface culture					

Appendix V
Manufacturing Firms

A V.1 Some Manufacturers of Important Biotechnological Apparatus

Some important groups of apparatuses are listed individually with their manufacturers.
The list makes no claim to completeness.

Literature:

ACHEMA Jahrbuch 85, Vol. 2 + 3.
Publisher: DECHEMA, Frankfurt/M. 1985.

A V.1.1 Sterilizers

Ahlborn Voss GmbH,
Voss-Str. 11–13, Postfach 1340, D-3203 Sarstedt.
Ahrens & Bode GmbH & Co., Maschinen und Apparatebau,
Alversdorfer Weg 1, D-3338 Schöningen, Federal Republic of Germany.
Aigner Medizin Apparate GmbH,
19 Avenue Dubonnet, F-92401 Courbevoie, France.
Alfa-Laval Industrietechnik GmbH,
Wilhelm-Bergner-Str., D-2056 Glinde bei Hamburg, Federal Republic of Germany.
Alliages Frittés s. a.,
54, Avenue Rhin et Danube, F-38100 Grenoble, France.

Balston Ltd.,
Springfield Mill, Maidstone, Kent, United Kingdom.
Biotronik, Wissenschaftliche Geräte GmbH,
Borsigallee 22, D-6000 Frankfurt/M. 60, Federal Republic of Germany.
Ing. F. De Lama & C. S.p.A.,
Via Piemonte 21, I-27028 San Martino Siccomario, Pavia, Italy.
Deutsch & Neumann GmbH & Co. KG,
Richard-Wagner-Str. 48/50, D-1000 Berlin 10, Federal Republic of Germany.

Fedegari Autoclavi S.p.A.,
I-27010 Albuzzano, Pavia, Italy.

Getinge Industrial Division,
Ekebergsvägen 26, S-31044 Getinge, Sweden.
Gilowy GmbH & Co.,
Bussardstr. 5, D-6078 Neu-Isenburg 2, Federal Republic of Germany.

Heinicke Instruments, Laborgerätebau GmbH,
Friedrich-Ebert-Str. 10, D-8223 Trostberg, Federal Republic of Germany.
W. C. Heraeus GmbH,
Heraeusstr. 12–14, D-6450 Hanau, Federal Republic of Germany.
Holstein und Kappert GmbH, Unternehmensbereich Unna,
Zechenstr. 49, D-4750 Unna-Königsborn, Federal Republic of Germany.
Horo Dr. Ing. A. Hofmann,
Rudolf-Diesel-Str. 8, D-7302 Ostfildern 2, Federal Republic of Germany.

KSG Klinik-Service-Gesellschaft mbH & Co., Sterilisatorenbau KG,
Bahnhofstr. 28, D-8031 Gröbenzell, Federal Republic of Germany.

Willi Memmert KG, Wärme-, medizin- und labortechnische Elektrogeräte,
Postfach 1520, D-8540 Schwabach, Federal Republic of Germany.
MMM Münchener Medizin Mechanik Ges. mbH,
Semmelweisstr. 6, D-8033 Planegg, Federal Republic of Germany.

New Brunswick Scientific Sales Co., Inc.,
44 Talmadge Road, Edison N.J. 08817, USA.

Olsa S.p.A.,
P.za Duca D'Aosta 4, I-20124 Milano, Italy.

Sterico AG, Techn. Apparate und Anlagen,
Staffelackerstr. 10, CH-8953 Dietikon 1, Switzerland.
C. Stiefenhofer KG,
Landsberger Str. 79, D-8000 München 2, Federal Republic of Germany.

Vismara Associate S.p.A.,
Via Boccaccio 27, I-20090 Trezzano s/Nav., Italy.

Tecnomara AG, Labor- und Industriebedarf,
Rieterstr. 59, CH-8059 Zürich, Switzerland.

Webecke & Co.,
Mühlenstr. 38, D-2407 Bad Schwartau, Federal Republic of Germany.

Zander Aufbereitungstechnik,
Breitscheider Weg 121, D-4030 Ratingen, Federal Republic of Germany.

A V.1.2   Incubators

Biotronik Wissenschaftliche Geräte GmbH,
Borsigallee 22, D-6000 Frankfurt/M. 60, Federal Republic of Germany.

Ehret, Emmendingen, Dipl.-Ing. W. Ehret GmbH, Fabrik für Elektro-Wärmegeräte,
Fabrikstr. 2, D-7830 Emmendingen 14, Federal Republic of Germany.

Flow, Laboratories GmbH,
Diezstr. 10, D-5300 Bonn 1, Federal Republic of Germany.

Heidolph-Elektro KG,
Starenstr. 23, D-8420 Kelheim, Federal Republic of Germany.

Heinicke Instruments, Laborgerätebau GmbH,
Friedrich-Ebert-Str. 10, D-8223 Trostberg, Federal Republic of Germany.

W. C. Heraeus GmbH,
Heraeusstr. 12–14, D-6450 Hanau, Federal Republic of Germany.

Horo Dr. Ing. A. Hofmann,
Rudolf-Diesel-Str. 8, D-7302 Ostfildern 2, Federal Republic of Germany

Infors AG,
Postfach, CH-4015 Basel, Switzerland.

Intermed-export-import,
Schicklerstr. 5/7, Postfach 17, DDR-102 Berlin, German Democratic Republic.

Jouan S. A.,
B. P. 403, F-44608 Saint-Nazaire Cedex, France.

Julabo Juchheim Labortechnik KG,
Eisenbahnstr. 43, D-7633 Seelbach, Federal Republic of Germany.

Köttermann GmbH & Co. KG, Fabrik für Laborapparate,
Industriestr. 2–10, D-3165 Hänigsen, Federal Republic of Germany.

Labora Mannheim – GmbH für Labortechnik,
Sandhofer Str. 176, D-6800 Mannheim 31, Federal Republic of Germany.

Labotect, Labortechnik, Schinkel & Schreder,
Weender Landstr. 3, D-3400 Göttingen, Federal Republic of Germany.

Willi Memmert KG, Wärme-, medizin- und labortech. Elektrogeräte,
Postfach 1520, D-8540 Schwabach, Federal Republic of Germany.

Millipore GmbH,
Siemensstr. 20, D-6078 Neu-Isenburg, Federal Republic of Germany.

New Brunswick Scientific Sales Co., Inc.,
44 Talmadge Road, Edison N. J. 08817, USA.

Rubarth & Co., Fabrik medizinischer und elektrischer Apparate,
Ikarusallee 2, D-3000 Hannover 1, Federal Republic of Germany.

Secfroid Sa,
Zone industrielle, Case postale, CH-1111 Aclens, Switzerland.

Tecnomara AG, Labor- und Industriebedarf,
Rieterstr. 59, CH-8059 Zürich, Switzerland.

Thermolyne/Sybron,
1721 Newport Circle, Santa Ana, Ca. 92705, USA.

A V.1.3   Shaking machines

Biotronik Wissenschaftliche Geräte GmbH,
Borsigallee 22, D-6000 Frankfurt/M. 60, Federal Republic of Germany.

B. Braun Melsungen AG,
Carl-Braunstr. 1, D-3508 Melsungen, Federal Republic of Germany.

Edmund Bühler, Laborgerätebau, Glastechnik, Umwelttechnik,
Im Schelmen 11, D-7400 Tübingen, Federal Republic of Germany.

C. Desaga GmbH, Nachf. Erich Fecht,
Maaßstr. 26/28, Postfach 101969, D-6900 Heidelberg 1, Federal Republic of Germany.

Guwina-Hofmann GmbH,
Lübecker Str. 46, D-1000 Berlin 21, Federal Republic of Germany.

Heinicke Instruments, Laborgerätebau GmbH,
Friedrich-Ebert-Str. 10, D-8223 Trostberg, Federal Republic of Germany.

Hellma GmbH & Co., Glastechn.-Opt. Werkstätten,
Klosterruns, Postfach 69, D-7840 Mülheim/Bd., Federal Republic of Germany.

Heto Lab Equipment A/S,
Klinthojvaenge 3, DK-3460 Birkerod, Denmark.

Infors AG,
Postfach, CH-4015 Basel, Switzerland.

Janke & Kunkel GmbH & Co. KG,
IKA-Werk Staufen,
Neumagenstr. 16, D-7813 Staufen, Federal Republic of Germany.

Köttermann GmbH & Co. KG,
Fabrik für Laborapparate,
Industriestr. 2–10, D-3165 Hänigsen, Federal Republic of Germany.

New Brunswick Scientific Sales Co., Inc.,
44 Talmadge Road, Edison N. J. 08817, USA.

Process technique, Günther Prehl KG,
P.O. Box 1095, D-3163 Sehude 1/Hannover, Federal Republic of Germany.

Raacke GmbH,
Hohenstaufenallee 27–29, D-5100 Aachen, Federal Republic of Germany.

Ernst Schütt jr., Laborgerätebau,
Güterbahnhofstr. 11, D-3400 Göttingen, Federal Republic of Germany.

Witeg Glasgeräte, Helmut Antlinger KG,
Am Bildacker 16, Postfach 1291, D-6980 Wertheim/M., Federal Republic of Germany.

A V.1.4 Bioreactors

Gebr. Becker, Apparatebau,
Zementstr. 112, D-4720 Beckum, Federal Republic of Germany.

Bender & Hobein GmbH, Fermentertechnik,
Junkerstr. 8, D-7500 Karlsruhe-Hagsfeld, Federal Republic of Germany.

Bioengineering AG,
Sagenrainstr. 7, CH-8636 Wald, Switzerland.

Biolafitte S. A.,
Boulevard Robespierre, F-78300 Poissy, France.

Biotronik Wissenschaftliche Geräte GmbH,
Borsigallee 22, D-6000 Frankfurt/M. 60, Federal Republic of Germany.

B. Braun Melsungen AG,
Carl-Braun-Str. 1, Postfach 110/120, D-3508 Melsungen, Federal Republic of Germany.

Büchi AG, Technische Glasbläserei,
CH-8610 Uster, Switzerland.

Burnett & Rolfe Ltd.,
Commissioners Road, Strood, Rochester, Kent ME2 4EJ, United Kingdom.

Chemap AG,
Alte Landstr., CH-8708 Männedorf, Switzerland.

Deutsche Metrohm GmbH & Co.,
Elektr. Meßgeräte,
In den Birken, D-7024 Filderstadt-Plattenhard, Federal Republic of Germany.

L. Eschweiler & Co., med. und techn. Apparate,
Holzkoppelweg 35, D-2300 Kiel, Federal Republic of Germany.

Heinrich Frings, Maschinen- und Apparatebau,
Jonas-Cahn-Str. 9, D-5300 Bonn 1, Federal Republic of Germany.

Giovanola Freres S. A.,
CH-1870 Monthey, Switzerland.

Infors AG,
Postfach, CH-4015 Basel, Switzerland.

Marubishi Lab. Equipment Co., Ltd.,
Koki Bldg, 14–24, 2-chome, Kanda Kaji-cho, Chiyoda-ku, Tokyo, Japan.

MBR Bio Reactor AG,
Postfach, CH-8620 Wetzikon, Switzerland.

Møller & Jochumsen a/s,
Vejlevej 3–5, DK-8700 Horsens, Denmark.

New Brunswick Scientific Sales Co., Inc.,
44 Talmadge Road, Edison N. J. 08817, USA.

OY JA-RO AB,
P.O. Box 15, SF-68601 Pietarsaari, Finland.

Ernst Schütt jr., Laborgerätebau,
Güterbahnhofstr. 11, D-3400 Göttingen, Federal Republic of Germany.

Setric,
Avenue Didier Daurat, Z. L. de Montaudran,
F-31400 Toulouse, France.

Tokyo Rikakikai Co., Ltd.,
No. 18 Toyama-cho, Kanda, Chiyoda-ku, Tokyo,
Japan.

A V.1.5   Centrifuges – Separators

Alfa-Laval AB,
Munkhättevägen, Fack, S-14700 Tumba, Sweden.

Baker Company,
Cooper St, Hanley, Stoke-on-Trent, ST1 4DW,
United Kingdom.
Braunschweigische Maschinenbauanstalt (BMA),
Am Alten Bahnhof 5, D-3300 Braunschweig,
Federal Republic of Germany.
Thomas Broadbent & Sons, Ltd.,
Huddersfield, Yorkshire, HD1 3EA, United Kingdom.

Etablissements Cellier,
Rue du Maroc, F-73104 Aix-les-Bains Cedex,
France.
Escher Wyss AG,
Postfach, CH-8023 Zürich, Switzerland.

Ferrum AG, Gießerei + Maschinenfabrik,
CH-5102 Rupperswil, Switzerland.
Flottweg-Werk, Dr. Georg Bruckmayer GmbH & Co. KG,
Industristr. 8, D-8313 Vilsbiburg/Bayern, Federal
Republic of Germany.

Guinard Centrifugation,
156, Boulevard du Général de Gaulle, F-92380
Garches, France.

Gebr. Heine GmbH & Co. KG,
Greefsallee 1, D-5060 Viersen 1, Federal Republic
of Germany.
Henkel Industriezentrifugen GmbH & Co.,
Gottlob-Grotz-Str. 1, D-7120 Bietigheim-Bissingen,
Federal Republic of Germany.
Heraeus-Christ GmbH,
Postfach 1220, D-3360 Osterode am Harz, Federal
Republic of Germany.

Klöckner-Humboldt-Deutz AG (KHD),
Wiesbergstr., D-5000 Köln 91, Federal Republic of
Germany.

Krauss-Maffei AG,
Krauss-Maffei-Str. 2, D-8000 München, Federal
Republic of Germany.
Adolf Kühner AG Maschinenbau,
CH-4052 Basel, Switzerland.

Carl Padberg Zentrifugenbau GmbH,
Rosenweg 43, D-7630 Lahr, Federal Republic of
Germany.
PEC, Process Engineering Company,
Alte Landstr. 415, CH-8708 Männedorf, Switzerland.

Siebtechnik GmbH,
Platanenallee 46, D-4330 Mülheim (Ruhr) 1,
Federal Republic of Germany.
Sharples Zentrifugentechnik,
Hans-Böckler-Str. 23, D-4220 Dinslaken, Federal
Republic of Germany.
Starcosa GmbH,
Am Alten Bahnhof 5, D-3300 Braunschweig,
Federal Republic of Germany.
Wilhelm Stock Maschinenbau KG,
Blegenstr. 4, D-3550 Marburg, Federal Republic of
Germany.

Westfalia Separator AG, Oelde,
Werner-Habig-Str., D-4740 Oelde 1, Federal Republic of Germany.

Veronesi Separatori S.A.S.,
Via Don Minzoni 1, I-40055 Villanova di Castenaso,
Italy.

A V.2   Some Manufacturers of Important Products

The list makes no claim to completeness.

Abbott Laboratories, North Chicago, Ill./USA.
ABM Chemicals, England.
Ajinomoto Co., Tokyo/Japan.
Aktiebolaget Astra, Södertalje/Sweden.
Aktiebolaget Kabi, Stockholm/Sweden.
Alembic Chemical Works Co. Ltd., Baroda/India.
American Cyanamid, Wayne, N.J./USA.
Aminova SpA, Italy.
Anheuser-Busch, Inc., St. Louis, Miss./USA.
Ankerfarm SpA, Milan/Italy.

Antibioticos SA, Madrid/Spain.
Apothekernes Laboratorium für Specialpraeparater SA, Oslo/Norway.
Archifer A.p.A., Milan/Italy.
Asahi Chemical Industry, Tokyo/Japan.

Bago SA, Argentina.
Banyu Pharmaceutical Co., Tokyo/Japan.
Bayer AG, Leverkusen/FR Germany.
Beckmann, Carlsberg, Ca./USA.
Beecham Pharmaceutical Co. Ltd., Surrey/England.
Joh. A. Benckiser GmbH, Ludwigshafen/FR Germany.
Biochemie GmbH, Kundl, Tyrol/Austria (Sandoz concern).
Biogal, Debrecen/Hungary.
Boehringer Mannheim, FR Germany.
C. H. Boehringer Sohn, Ingelheim/Rhein/FR Germany.
Bristol-Myers Co., Syracuse, N.Y./USA.

Carlo Erba SpA, Milan/Italy.
CCA, Brazil.
Chemibiotic Ltd., Inoshannon/Ireland.
China National Chemicals Import and Export Corp., Peking/PR China.
Chinese Petroleum Corp., Taipei/Taiwan.
Chinoin, Budapest/Hungary.
Chong-Kun-Domg Corp., Seoul/Rep. Korea.
Chugai Pharmaceutical Co., Tokyo/Japan.
Ciba-Geigy, Basel/Switzerland.
Citrique Belge, Tienen/Belgium.
Cellulose Attisholz AG, Attisholz/Switzerland.
Clinton Corn Processing Co., Clinton, Iowa/USA.
Sarl (CIPAN), Lisbon/Portugal.
Compania Española de la Penicillina y Antibioticos SA (CEPA), Aranjuez/Spain.
CPC International Inc., Argo, Ill./USA.
Croda Bowmans Chemical Ltd., Cheshire/England.
Cyanamid, USA.

Dainippon, Japan.
Dairyland Food Laboratories Inc., Waukesha, Wisc./USA.
Dawe's Laboratories Inc., Chicago Heights, Ill./USA.
Degussa, Frankfurt/M./FR Germany.
Deutsche Hefewerke AG, Hamburg/FR Germany.
Diamalt AG, Munich/FR Germany.

Diaspa SpA., Coronna/Italy.
Dista Products Ltd., Liverpool/England.
Dong-Myung Industrial Co Ltd., Seoul/Rep. Korea.
Dumex Ltd., Copenhagen/Denmark.

Eurolysine Co., Paris/France.

Farbenfabriken Bayer AG, Wuppertal/FR Germany.
Farmitalia SpA, Milan/Italy.
Fermentaciones Mexicanes, Mexico.
Fermentaciones y Sintesis, Mexico.
Fermentfarma SpA, Milan/Italy.
Fermic SA de SV, Ixapalapa/Mexico.
Fermion Oy, Tapiola/Finland.
Fervet SpA (division of Ciba-Geigy AG), Torre Annunziata/Italy.
Finnish State Alcohol Monopoly, Helsinki/Finland.
Fujisawa Pharmaceutical Co., Osaka/Japan.

Gist-Brocades, Delft/Holland.
Gist Brocades Fermentation Ind., USA.
Glaxo Laboratories Ltd., Greenford/England.
Grain Processing Corp., Muscatine, Iowa/USA.
Grindstedvaerket, Denmark.
Gruppo Lepetit SpA, Milan/Italy.

Hailsun Chemical Co. Ltd., Taipei/Taiwan.
Henkel International GmbH, FR Germany.
Hindustan Antibiotics Ltd., Primpri/India.
Hoechst AG, Frankfurt/Main/FR Germany.
Hoffmann-La Roche Inc., Nutley, N.J./USA.
F. Hoffmann-La Roche & Co. AG, Basel/Switzerland.
Hokko Kagaku Kogyo Co., Tokyo/Japan.

ICN-Chimica SpA, Milan/Italy.
IMC Chemicals Group Inc., Terre Haute, Ind./USA.
Imperial Chemical Industries Ltd., Manchester/England.
I.S.F. SpA, Rome/Italy.
Istituto Biochimico Italiano, Milan/Italy.

Kaken Chemical Co., Tokyo/Japan.
Kaken Kagaku, Japan.
Kanegafuchi Chemical Industries, Osaka/Japan.
Knoll GmbH, Ludwigshafen/FR Germany.
Kowa Co., Nagoya/Japan.
Kayaku Antibiotics Research Co. Ltd., Tokyo/Japan.

Krakow Pharmaceutical Works ("Polfa"), Krakow/ Poland.
KRKA Pharmaceutical and Chemical Works, Novo Mesto/Yugoslavia.
Kyowa Hakko Kogyo Co., Tokyo/Japan.

Lark SpA, Milan/Italy.
Leo Pharmaceutical Products, Ballerup/Denmark.
Eli Lilly and Co., Indianapolis, Ind./USA.
Linson Ltd., Dublin/Ireland.
Liquichimica, Italy.
Lohmann & Co. AG, Cuxhaven/FR Germany.
H. Lundbeck and Co., Valby/Denmark.

Meiji Seika Kaisha Ltd., Tokyo/Japan.
Meito Sangyo Co. Ltd., Tokyo/Japan.
E. Merck, Darmstadt/FR Germany.
Merck & Co., USA.
Mi-Won, Seoul/Rep. Korea.
Miles-Kali Chemie, FR Germany.
Miles Laboratories Inc., Elkhart, Ind./USA.
Mi-Poong Company, Korea.
Mitsubishi Chemical Industries, Tokyo/Japan.
Mitsubishi Gas, Japan.
Mitsui, Japan.

Nagase & Co. Ltd., Tokyo/Japan.
Nihon Kayaku Co., Tokyo/Japan.
Nikken Chemicals Co. Ltd., Tokyo/Japan.
NOVO Industri AS, Bagsvaerd/Denmark.

Orsan SA, Paris/France.

Pao Yeh Chemical Co., Ltd., Taipei/Taiwan.
Parke, Davis & Co., Detroit, Mich./USA.
Pechiney Ugine Kuhlmann, Paris/France.
S. B. Penick and Co., Lyndhurst, N.J./USA.
VEB Petrochem. Kombinat, DDR.
Pfizer Inc., New York, N.Y./USA.
Pharmachim Antibiotic Works, Razgrad/Bulgaria.
Pharmacosmos, Valby/Denmakr.
Philippine Fermentation Co., Union Chemical Corp., Philippines.
Pierrel SpA, Milan/Italy.
Pliva Pharmaceutical and Chemical Works, Zagreb/ Yugoslavia.
Premier Malt Products, Inc., Milwaukee, Wisc./ USA.
Proter SpA, Milan/Italy.

Quimasa SA, São Paulo/Brazil.

Rachelle Laboratories Inc., Long Beach, Ca./USA.
Reanal, Budapest/Hungary.
Recherche et Industrie Thérapeutique, Genval/ Belgium.
Rhône-Poulenc SA, Paris/France.
G. Richter, Budapest/Hungary.
Röhm GmbH, Darmstadt/FR Germany.
Rohm and Haas, Philadelphia, Penns./USA.
Roniprot, Curtea de Arges, Romania.
Roussel-Uclaf SA, Romainville/France.

Sandoz-Wander AG, Basel/Switzerland.
Sandoz Inc., Hanover, N.J./USA.
San Fu Chemical Co., Ltd., Taipei/Taiwan.
Sankyo Co. Ltd., Tokyo/Japan.
Sanraku Ocean Co. Ltd., Tokyo/Japan.
Schering AG, West-Berlin/FR Germany.
Schering Corp., Bloomfield, N.J./USA.
G. D. Searle and Co., Skokie, Ill./USA.
Shionogi and Co. Ltd., Osaka/Japan.
Smith-Kline, USA.
Snam Progetti, Italy.
Soc. Produtora de Leveduras Seleccionada, Mastosinhus/Portugal.
Soc. Prodotti Antibiotici (SPA), Milan/Italy.
Soc. de Chimie Org. & Biol., France.
Soc. Chimique Pointet Girard (Pharmuka), Villeneuve-La Garenne/France.
E. R. Squibb and Sons, Princeton, N.Y./USA.
Standard Brands, Inc., New York, N.Y./USA.
Stauffer Chemical Co., Westport, Conn./USA.
John and E. Sturge Ltd., Birmingham/England.
Surbhai Chemicals Ltd., Baroda/India.

Tai Nan Fermentation Industrial Co. Ltd., Taipei/ Taiwan.
Taiwan Sugar Corp., Taipei/Taiwan.
Taiwan Tobacco and Wine Monopoly Bureau, Taipei/Taiwan.
Takeda Chemical Industries, Osaka/Japan.
Tanabe Seiyaku Co. Ltd., Osaka/Japan.
Tarchomin Pharmaceutical Works ("Polfa"), Warsaw/Poland.
Tate and Lyle Ltd., Yorkshire/England.
Thomae, Biberach a. d. Riss/FR Germany.
Toray Industries/Japan.
Toyo Jozo Co. Ltd., Tokyo/Japan.
Tsin Tsin Foods Co., Taipei/Taiwan.
Tung Hai Industrial Fermentation Co. Ltd., Taipei/ Taiwan.

Universal Foods Corp., Milwaukee, Wisc./USA.
The Upjohn Co., Kalamazoo, Mich./USA.

Wallerstein Laboratories, Inc., Morton Grove, Ill./USA.
Wei Chuan Foods Corp., Taipei/Taiwan.
Wei Wang Industrial Fermentation Co., Ltd., Taipei/Taiwan.
The World Champion Co. Ltd., Taipei/Taiwan.
Wyeth Laboratories, Philadelphia, Penn./USA.

Yamanouchi Pharmaceutical Co., Tokyo/Japan.
Yamasa Shoyu Co. Ltd., Choshi/Japan.

Literature for A V.2

abc der Wirtschaft. Verlagsgesellschaft, Darmstadt 1978 (Foodstuffs manufacturers).

Perlman, D. (School of Pharmacy, University of Wisconsin, Madison, Wisconsin 53 706). In: *ASM News,* Vol. 43, No. 2, pp. 88/89.

Gwinner, E.: *Bioenergie, Biomasse, Biotechnologie,* Chemische Industrie, Schriftenreihe, Band 1. Verlag Handelsblatt GmbH, 1978.

Nature, *New Annual Directory of Biologicals,* London 1982.

Appendix VI
Products from
Biotechnological Processes

Reference work for products:
Laskin, A. I., and Lechevalier, H. A. (ed.):
Handbook of Microbiology, Vol. III (Micro-
bial Products). CRC Press, Cleveland 1973.

A VI.1   Antibiotics

For (some) formulas, see p. 708
Adriamycin
Amphomycin
Amphotericin B
Avoparcin
Azalomycin F
Ampicillin

Bacitracin
Bambermycins
Bicyclomycin
Blasticidin S
Bleomycin

Cactinomycin
Candicidin B
Candidin
Capreomycin
Cephalosporins
Chromomycin A_3
Coglistin
Cycloheximide
Cycloserine

Dactinomycin
Daunorubicin
Destomycin

Enduracidin
Erythromycin

Fortimicins
Flavomycin
Fumagillin
Fungimycin
Fusidic acid

Gentamicins
Gramicidin A
Gramicidin J (S)
Griseofulvin

Hygromycin B

Josamycin

Kanamycin
Kasugamycin
Kitasatamycin

Lasalocid
Lincomycin
Lividomycin

Macarbomycin
Mepartricin
Midecamycin
Mikamycin
Mithramycin
Mitomycin C
Mocimycin
Monensin
Myxin

Neomycins
Novobiocin
Nystatin

Oleandomycin
Oligomycin

Paromomycins
Penicillin G
Penicillin V

Penicillins (semisynthetic)
Pentamycin
Pimaricin
Polymyxins
Polyoxins
Pristinamycins

Ribostamycin
Rifamycins

Sagamicin
Salinomycin
Siccanin
Siomycin
Sisomicin
Streptomycins

Tetracyclines
   Chlortetracycline
   Democlocycline

Oxytetracycline
Tetracycline
Tetranactin
Thiopeptin
Thiostrepton
Tobramycin
Trichomycin
Tylosine
Tyrothricin
Tyrocidine

Uromycin

Validamycin
Vancomycin
Variotin
Viomycin
Virginiamycin

A VI.2   Vitamins

Vitamin B_2 (Riboflavin)
Vitamin B_{12} (Cyanocobalamine)
Coenzyme Q

A VI.3   Steroids
(microbial transformation)

Progesterones
   Progesterone
Corticosteroids
   Betamethasone
   Cortisone acetate

Hydrocortisone
Prednisolone
Prednisone
Triamcinolone

A VI.4   Alkaloids

Ergocornine
Ergocristine
Ergocryptine

Ergotamine
Ergometrine
Lysergic acid

A VI.5   Inocula

A VI.6   Organic Acids

Citric acid
Comenic acid
Erythorbic acid
Gluconic acid
Itaconic acid
Acetic acid

Butyric acid
2-Keto-D-gluconic acid
α-Ketoglutaric acid
Lactic acid
Malic acid
Urocanic acid

A VI.7   Organic Solvents

Acetone
Butanol

Ethanol
Butane-1,2-diol

A VI.8   Enzymes

Amylases
Amyloglucosidases
Anticyanase
L-Asparaginase

Catalase
Cellulase

Dextranase

Esterase-lipase

Glucanase
Glucose dehydrogenase
Glucose isomerase
Glucose oxidase

Hemicellulase

Invertase

Lactase
Lipase

Rennet (rennin,
chymosin)

Naringinase

Pectinase
Pentosanase
Proteases

Streptokinase-
streptodornase

Uricase

A VI.9   Amino Acids

L-Alanine
L-Arginine
L-Aspartic acid
L-Citrulline
L-Glutamic acid
L-Glutamine
L-Glutathione
L-Histidine
L-Homoserine
L-Isoleucine
L-Leucine

L-Lysine
L-Methionine
L-Ornithine
L-Phenylalanine
L-Proline
L-Serine
L-Threonine
L-Tryptophan
L-Tyrosine
L-Valine

A VI.10   Nucleotides and Nucleosides

5′-Ribonucleotides and -nucleosides
Orotic acid
9-β-D-Arabinofuranosyladenine
6-Azauridine
Nucleic acids

A VI.11   Starter Cultures

Lactic acid starter cultures
   Cheese   Sour cream
   Cottage cheese   Yoghurt
Starter cultures for meat products

A VI.12   Biomass Products (SCP)

Bakers' yeast
Brewers' yeast
Wine yeast
Diet yeast

Fodder yeast
Single-cell Protein
(bacteria, algae, fungi)

A VI.13   Insecticides

Bacillus thuringiensis

A VI.14   Growth Factors

Gibberellins

A VI.15   Polysaccharides

Alginates
Curdlan
Dextran

Scleroglucan
Xanthan

A VI.16   Miscellaneous Products

Acetoin
Acyloin

Desferrioxamine
Dihydroxyacetone

Subject Index